CHRONIC ILLNESS IN CANADA

IMPACT AND INTERVENTION

EDITED BY

MARNIE L. KRAMER-KILE, MEd, BScN, RN

Assistant Professor
School of Nursing
Mount Royal University
Calgary, Alberta

JOSEPH C. OSUJI, PhD, RN

Associate Professor
School of Nursing
Mount Royal University
Calgary, Alberta

JONES & BARTLETT
LEARNING

World Headquarters
Jones & Bartlett Learning
5 Wall Street
Burlington, MA 01803
978-443-5000
info@jblearning.com
www.jblearning.com

Jones & Bartlett Learning books and products are available through most bookstores and online booksellers. To contact Jones & Bartlett Learning directly, call 800-832-0034, fax 978-443-8000, or visit our website, www.jblearning.com.

Substantial discounts on bulk quantities of Jones & Bartlett Learning publications are available to corporations, professional associations, and other qualified organizations. For details and specific discount information, contact the special sales department at Jones & Bartlett Learning via the above contact information or send an email to specialsales@jblearning.com.

Chronic Illness in Canada: Impact and Intervention is an independent publication and has not been authorized, sponsored, or otherwise approved by the owners of the trademarks or service marks referenced in this product.

Some images in this book feature models. These models do not necessarily endorse, represent, or participate in the activities represented in the images.

The screenshots in this product are for educational and instructive purposes only. All trademarks displayed are the trademarks of the parties noted therein. Such use of trademarks is not an endorsement by said parties of Jones & Bartlett Learning, its products, or its services, nor should such use be deemed an endorsement by Jones & Bartlett Learning of said third party's products or services.

The authors, editors, and publisher have made every effort to provide accurate information. However, they are not responsible for errors, omissions, or for any outcomes related to the use of the contents of this book and take no responsibility for the use of the products and procedures described. Treatments and side effects described in this book may not be applicable to all people; likewise, some people may require a dose or experience a side effect that is not described herein. Drugs and medical devices are discussed that may have limited availability controlled by the Food and Drug Administration (FDA) for use only in a research study or clinical trial. Research, clinical practice, and government regulations often change the accepted standard in this field. When consideration is being given to use of any drug in the clinical setting, the health care provider or reader is responsible for determining FDA status of the drug, reading the package insert, and reviewing prescribing information for the most up-to-date recommendations on dose, precautions, and contraindications, and determining the appropriate usage for the product. This is especially important in the case of drugs that are new or seldom used.

Production Credits

Publisher: Kevin Sullivan
Acquisitions Editor: Amanda Harvey
Editorial Assistant: Sara Bempkins
Production Editor: Amanda Clerkin
Senior Marketing Manager: Elena McAnespie
V.P., Manufacturing and Inventory Control: Therese Connell
Composition: Paw Print Media
Cover Design: Kristin E. Parker
Cover Image: © Laurin Rinder/ShutterStock, Inc.
Printing and Binding: Edwards Brothers Malloy
Cover Printing: Edwards Brothers Malloy

To order this product, use ISBN: 978-1-4496-8744-1

Library of Congress Cataloging-in-Publication Data
Chronic illness in Canada: impact and intervention / Marnie Kramer-Kile ... [et al.].
    p. ; cm.
    Adaptation of: Chronic illness : impact and interventions / edited by Ilene Morof Lubkin, Pamala D. Larsen. 8th ed. c2013.
    Includes bibliographical references and index.
    ISBN 978-1-4496-8194-4 -- ISBN 1-4496-8194-8
    I. Kramer-Kile, Marnie. II. Chronic illness.
    [DNLM: 1. Chronic Disease--Canada. 2. Health Services for the Aged--Canada. 3. Long-Term Care--Canada. WT 500]

    616'.0478--dc23
                        2012016801

6048

Printed in the United States of America
16 15 14 13 12   10 9 8 7 6 5 4 3 2 1

To our families and children,
Chad, Ava, and Maya
and
Genevieve, Angel, Joy, Excell, Noble, and Bliss

Contents

Acknowledgments   xv

Preface   xvii

Contributors   xix

Part I   Impact of Disease   1

1   Introduction to Chronicity in Canada   3
Original chapter by Pamala D. Larsen
Canadian content added by Joyce K. Engel and Dawn Prentice
Introduction   3
Impact of Chronic Illness   7
Context for Chronic Care in Canada   8
Interventions   19
Going Forward: The Future of Chronic Care in Canada   23
Summary   24
Study Questions   25
References   25

2   Models of Care   29
Original chapter by Pamala D. Larsen
Canadian content added by Marnie L. Kramer-Kile
Introduction   29
Historical Perspectives   29
Chronic Care Model   30
Expanded Chronic Care Model   32
Guided Care   33
Self-Management Programs   36

Transitional Care   39
Online Disease Management   41
Telehealth   41
Outcomes   42
Study Questions   42
Internet Resources   42
References   42

3   The Illness Experience   45
Original chapter by Pamala D. Larsen
Canadian content added by Marnie L. Kramer-Kile
Introduction   45
Sick Role   46
Illness Perceptions   47
Influences on Illness Behavior   50
Impact and Issues Related to Illness Behaviour   52
The Illness Experience and Subsequent Behaviour   53
Legitimization of Chronic Illness   55
Interventions   58
Summary   64
Study Questions   64
References   65

4   Stigma   69
Original chapter by Diane L. Stuenkel and Vivian K. Wong
Canadian content added by Marnie L. Kramer-Kile
Introduction   69
Theoretical Frameworks: Stigma, Social Identity, and Labelling Theory   70
Unique Aspects of Stigma   72
Types of Stigma   74
Chronic Disease as Stigma   76
Impact of Stigma   77
Individual Living with Stigma   77
Interventions: Coping with Stigma or Reducing Stigma   83
Summary   92
Internet Resources   93
Study Questions   93
References   94

5 Adaptation   99
Original Chapter by Pamala D. Larsen and Faye I. Hummel
Canadian content added by Joseph C. Osuji
Introduction   99
Impact   100
The Self in Chronic Illness   102
Models   103
Overview of Coping   110
Summary   116
Study Questions   117
References   117

6 Social Isolation   121
Original chapter by Diana Luskin Biordi and Nicholas R. Nicholson
Canadian content added by Joseph C. Osuji
Introduction   121
Isolation: A Working Definition   121
Nature of Isolation   122
Feelings That Reflect Isolation   123
Description and Characteristics of Social Isolation   123
Social Isolation Versus Similar States of Human Apartness   123
Problems and Issues of Social Isolation   124
The Isolation Process   125
Social Isolation and Stigma   125
Social Isolation and Social Roles   126
Older Adults and Social Isolation   127
Social Isolation, Culture, and Gender   130
Social Components of Social Isolation   131
Demographics and Social Isolation   132
Illness Factors and Social Isolation   134
Healthcare Perspectives   135
Interventions: Counteracting Social Isolation   137
Support Groups and Other Mutual Aid   142
Spiritual Well-Being   142
Rebuilding Family Networks   143
Summary   148
Study Questions   148
References   149

7 Body Image   157

Original chapter by Diana Luskin Biordi and Patricia McCann Galon
Canadian content added by Joseph C. Osuji

Introduction   157
Definitions of Body Image   158
Historical Foundations of Body Image   160
Factors in the Definition of Body Image   161
Factors Influencing Adjustment to Body Image   162
Assessment of Body Image   168
Body Image Issues Important to Chronic Illness   170
Interventions   174
Summary   178
Study Questions   179
Internet Resources   179
References   179

8 Quality of Life   183

Original chapter by Victoria Schirm
Canadian content added by Marnie L. Kramer-Kile

Introduction   183
Defining Quality of Life   184
Conceptualizing and Measuring Quality of Life   185
Context of Quality of Life in Chronic Illness   189
Evidence-Informed Guidelines   192
Evidence-Informed Interventions to Promote Quality of Life   192
Overview of Nursing   196
Summary   202
Study Questions   203
Internet Resources   204
References   204

9 Uncertainty   207

Original chapter by Faye I. Hummel

Introduction   207
Nature of Uncertainty   207
Uncertainty in Chronic Illness Is Certain   208

Uncertainty and Social Networks   210
Sources of Uncertainty   211
Theoretical Underpinnings of Uncertainty   212
Uncertainty as Opportunity   214
Uncertainty as Harm   215
Interventions   218
Summary   223
Study Questions   224
References   224

Part II   Impact on the Client and Family   229

10 Sexuality   231
Original chapter by Margaret Chamberlain Wilmoth
Canadian content added by Joseph C. Osuji
Introduction   231
Definitions   231
Standards of Practice   232
Sexual Response Cycle and Sexual Physiology   234
Sexuality and Chronic Illness   236
Interventions   249
Summary   252
Study Questions   252
References   253

11 Powerlessness   257
Original chapter by Faye I. Hummel
Canadian content added by Joseph C. Osuji
Introduction   257
Phenomenon of Powerlessness in Chronic Illness   258
Paradox of Powerlessness in Chronic Illness   260
Theoretical Perspectives of Powerlessness and Power   261
Problems and Issues Associated with Powerlessness   264
Interventions   270
Summary   278
Study Questions   280
References   280

12 Self-Care and Self-Management   285
Original chapter by Judith E. Hertz
Canadian content added by Marnie L. Kramer-Kile
Introduction   285
Key Issues and Frameworks for Viewing Self-Care Within Chronic Illness   286
Strategies to Support Self-Management in Chronic Conditions   296
Self-Management Programmes   299
Outcomes   302
Summary   303
Study Questions   303
Internet Resources   303
References   304

13 Client and Family Education   307
Original chapter by Elaine T. Miller
Canadian content added by Joseph C. Osuji
Introduction   307
Teaching–Learning Process   308
Significance of Client and Family Teaching to Practice and
   Healthcare Costs   311
System Factors That Influence the Teaching and Learning Process   320
Educational Interventions for the Client and Family   325
Summary   330
Study Questions   331
References   332

14 Chronic Illness and the Family   335
Christina H. West and Linda L. Binding
Introduction   335
Understanding the Complex Interaction Between Chronic Illness and Family
   Life Cycle Development   336
Chronic Illness and Family Caregiving: An Experience Marked by Complexity,
   Uncertainty, and Ongoing Change   349
Intervention with the Family in the Context of Chronic Illness   358
Summary   364
Acknowledgement   365
References   365

15 Health Promotion   371
Original chapter by Alicia Huckstadt
Canadian content added by Joseph C. Osuji
Introduction   371
Defining Health Promotion in Chronic Illness   372
Online Resources   374
Challenges   374
Barriers   375
Models, Theories, and Frameworks   377
Interventions   379
Summary   386
Study Questions   387
References   388

16 Complementary and Alternative Therapies   393
Original chapter by Pamala D. Larsen
Canadian content added by Joyce M. Woods
Introduction   393
Definitions   393
Benefits of CAM   394
Users   395
Costs   397
Regulation of Complementary and Alternative Practitioners   397
Common Treatment Modalities   399
Chronic Disease and CAM   403
Issues   408
Standards for Nursing Practice and CAM   415
Cultural Considerations and CAM   416
Quackery   416
Professional Education   417
Ethical Decision Making   418
Interventions   420
Summary   422
Acknowledgement   422
Study Questions   422
References   423

17 Home Health Care   429
Original chapter by Cynthia S. Jacelon
Canadian content added by Joyce K. Engel
Introduction   429
History of Home Care   430
Organization and Funding of Home Health Care in Canada   435
Approaches to Home Health Services in Canada   437
Challenges for Home Health Care in Canada   438
Theoretical Frameworks for Management of Chronic Illness
    in Home Care   440
Home Health Nursing   446
Outcomes   453
Home Care Satisfaction Measures   457
Summary   457
Study Questions   457
Internet Resources   458
References   458

18 Long-Term Care   463
Original chapter by Susan J. Barnes and Kristen L. Mauk
Canadian content added by Dawn Prentice
Introduction   463
Historical Perspectives   465
Continuum of Care   466
LTC Recipients: A Vulnerable Population   469
Problems and Issues in LTC   470
Ethical Issues in LTC   472
Interventions   476
Palliative and Hospice Care   485
Research in LTC   486
Summary   487
Study Questions   488
Internet Resources   488
References   488

19 Hospice Palliative Care   493
Original chapter by Barbara M. Raudonis
Canadian content added by Gregg Trueman
Introduction   493
Historical Perspectives   494
Hospice Palliative Care Programming   495
Heart and Soul of Hospice Palliative Care   500
Hospice Palliative Care Symptom Management   505
Hospice Palliative Care Issues and Opportunities   509
Hospice Palliative Care Nursing   510
Allied Hospice Palliative Care Disciplines   511
Palliative Medicine   511
Research   512
Summary   513
Internet Resources   513
Study Questions   515
References   515

20 Rehabilitation   521
Original chapter by Kristen L. Mauk
Canadian content added by Marnie L. Kramer-Kile
Introduction   521
Definitions   522
Rehabilitation Models and Classification Systems   523
Rehabilitation Issues and Challenges   527
Interventions   530
Potential Strengths of the Client, Family, and Environment   532
Rehabilitation Settings   535
Rehabilitation Specialties   537
Outcome Measurement and Performance Improvement   541
Summary   542
Study Questions   543
Internet Resources   543
References   543

Index   549

Acknowledgments

We would like to begin by acknowledging Pamala Larsen and the original contributors of this textbook for their continued dedication to promoting an understanding of the impacts and issues for those individuals living with chronic conditions. We would also like to thank Jones & Bartlett Learning for providing us with an opportunity to adapt this seminal textbook to a Canadian context. Also, we would like to acknowledge our Jones & Bartlett Learning Nursing Development Team for all of their support during this process. Finally, a heartfelt thank you goes to our Canadian contributors who worked diligently despite their busy schedules to complete this project.

Preface

Recently we added a complex chronic illness course to our nursing program at Mount Royal University. Our search of textbooks for this course led us to the seventh edition of *Chronic Illness: Impact and Intervention*. What we initially admired about this textbook was its interdisciplinary focus and use of social theory alongside nursing-related concepts. Over time we realized that we needed to recognize the Canadian and global contexts that were absent from the U.S. edition. In Canada, we as healthcare professionals remain challenged, as do all healthcare professionals all over the world, with addressing chronic illness within our society. A stark fact is that in 2006 more people died of chronic illness throughout the world than our country's population at that time. Canada has always been a leader in health promotion (Barr et al., 2003); seminal documents such as the Lalonde Report and the Ottawa Charter for Health Promotion attest to this and have continued to guide the efforts of Canadian nurses and other healthcare practitioners. Nursing in particular has taken an approach to illness management that recognizes the social, cultural, and economic factors that play a role in illness experience and management. Rather than solely attempt to foster adherence to the biomedical frameworks of chronic disease management, nurses can act as a bridge between nature and culture to help promote healthy behaviours and self-care frameworks. To do this we need to understand the complex links between disease and illness management and to find ways to support clients, families, communities, and populations through this process. It is important to remember that how we interpret chronicity as healthcare professionals can have broader social impacts. This textbook attempts to identify these contexts from various perspectives and to offer some insights into the complexities of chronic illness. We look forward to continuing to grow the Canadian edition of this textbook.

Reference

Barr, V. J., Robinson, S., Marin-Link, B., Underhill, L., Dotts, A., Ravensdale, D., & Salivaras, S. (2003). The expanded chronic care model: An integration of concepts and strategies from population health promotion and chronic care model. *Hospital Quarterly, 7*(1), 73–82.

Contributors

Lead Editors

Marnie L. Kramer-Kile, MEd, BScN, RN
Assistant Professor
School of Nursing
Mount Royal University
Calgary, Alberta

Joseph C. Osuji, PhD, RN
Associate Professor
School of Nursing
Mount Royal University
Calgary, Alberta

Pamala D. Larsen, PhD, RN, CRRN, FNGNA
Associate Dean and Professor
Fay W. Whitney School of Nursing
University of Wyoming
Laramie, Wyoming

Contributors

Susan J. Barnes, PhD, RN
Chair, Graduate and Continuing Education
Kramer School of Nursing
Oklahoma City University
Oklahoma City, Oklahoma

Linda L. Binding, PhD, RN
Associate Professor
School of Nursing
Mount Royal University
Calgary, Alberta

Diana Luskin Biordi, PhD, RN, FAAN
Associate Dean for Nursing Research
    and Scholarship
College of Nursing
University of Akron
Akron, Ohio

Joyce K. Engel, PhD, RN
Associate Professor
Department of Nursing
Brock University
St. Catherines, Ontario

Patricia McCann Galon, PhD, CNS
Associate Professor
College of Nursing
The University of Akron
Akron, Ohio

Judith E. Hertz, PhD, RN
Associate Professor
School of Nursing and Health Studies
Northern Illinois University
DeKalb, Illinois

**Alicia Huckstadt, PhD, RN, ARNP, FNP-BC,
    GNP-BC**
Professor and Graduate Program Director
School of Nursing
Wichita State University
Wichita, Kansas

Faye I. Hummel, PhD, RN, CTN
Professor
School of Nursing
University of Northern Colorado
Greeley, Colorado

Cynthia S. Jacelon, PhD, RN, CRRN-A
Associate Professor
School of Nursing
University of Massachusetts, Amherst
Amherst, Massachusetts

Kristen L. Mauk, PhD, RN, CRRN-A, GCNS-BC
Professor of Nursing
Kreft Chair for the Advancement of
    Nursing Science
Valparaiso University
Valparaiso, Indiana

Elaine T. Miller, DNS, RN, FAAN
Professor of Nursing
Coordinator, Center for Aging
    with Dignity
College of Nursing
University of Cincinnati
Cincinnati, Ohio

Nicholas R. Nicholson, Jr., PhD, MPH, RN, PHCNS-BC
Postdoctoral Fellow
Geriatric Clinical Epidemiology and
    Aging-Related Research
Yale University School of Medicine
New Haven, Connecticut

Dawn Prentice, PhD, RN
Associate Professor
Department of Nursing
Brock University
St. Catharines, Ontario

Barbara M. Raudonis, PhD, RN
Associate Professor
School of Nursing
University of Texas, Arlington
Arlington, Texas

Victoria Schirm, PhD, RN
Director of Nursing Research
Department of Nursing
Penn State Milton S. Hershey
    Medical Center
Hershey, Pennsylvania

Diane L. Stuenkel, EdD, RN
Professor
The Valley Foundation School of Nursing
San Jose State University
San Jose, California

Gregg Trueman, RN, NP, BScN, MN-ACNP
Associate Professor
School of Nursing
Mount Royal University
Calgary, Alberta

Christina H. West, PhD, RN
Assistant Professor
School of Nursing
Mount Royal University
Calgary, Alberta

Margaret Chamberlain Wilmoth, PhD, RN, MSS, FAAN
Professor
School of Nursing
University of North Carolina, Charlotte
Charlotte, North Carolina

Joyce M. Woods, PhD, RN
Associate Professor
School of Nursing
Mount Royal University
Calgary, Alberta

Vivian K. Wong, PhD, RN
Associate Professor
The Valley Foundation School of Nursing
San Jose State University
San Jose, California

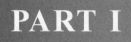
PART I

Impact of Disease

CHAPTER 1

Introduction to Chronicity in Canada

Original chapter by Pamala D. Larsen
Canadian content added by Joyce K. Engel and Dawn Prentice

INTRODUCTION

Chronic diseases are the leading cause of death in the world, accounting for 60% of all deaths worldwide (World Health Organization [WHO], 2011). Twenty percent of deaths from chronic disease occur in high-income countries, whereas the remaining 80% occur in low- and middle-income countries, where most of the world's population resides (WHO, 2011).

The statistics for chronic disease in Canada are alarming. Cardiovascular-related diseases and stroke affected 1.3 million Canadians, and, of those, 23% were aged 75 years or older (Public Health Agency of Canada [PHAC], 2009). Moreover, diabetes affected 2.4 million (6.8%) of Canadians in 2008–2009, with half of these individuals between ages 25 and 64 years (PHAC, 2011). Approximately 3.5 million Canadians have respiratory diseases (PHAC, 2008), and in 2011 there was an estimated 177,800 new cases of cancer (Canadian Cancer Society, 2011). Furthermore, 20% of Canadians will experience a mental illness in their lifetime (Canadian Mental Health Association, 2012).

These statistics are examples of the wide variety of conditions considered to be chronic, and each condition needs a diverse array of services to care for affected individuals. For example, consider clients with Alzheimer's disease, cerebral palsy, heart disease, AIDS, or spinal cord injury; each of these clients has unique physical needs and requires different services from a healthcare system that is largely attuned to delivering acute care.

The first baby boomers turned 65 in 2011, and over the next 25 years they will accelerate the aging of the Canadian population (Statistics Canada, 2010a). This has focused increased attention on the capabilities of the healthcare system. This well-educated, consumer-driven generation wants to be knowledgeable about their conditions and about all treatment options. They question their healthcare providers and do not necessarily accept healthcare advice. The baby boomer generation, in particular, has been vocal about the inability of the healthcare system to meet current needs, let alone future needs. How will the current system or a future system cope with this highly visible group of seniors and their accompanying healthcare needs?

The healthcare system also faces the challenges of a society in which there is much greater cultural diversity and where expectations of health care are more diverse than in the past. In 2006 minorities represented 16.2% of all Canadians (Statistics Canada, 2010b). By 2031 this percentage is estimated to increase to between 29% and 32% (Statistics Canada, 2010c). Data from 2001 showed that 29% of persons aged 65 to 74 were immigrants and that 28% were aged 75 to 84 years, thus further contributing to the size of the seniors' population (Turcotte & Schellenberg, 2007).

There are multiple factors for the number of individuals with chronic disease. Developments in the fields of public health, genetics, immunology, technology, and pharmacology have led to significant decreases in mortality in infancy or childhood and from acute disease. Medical success contributed, in part, to the unprecedented growth of chronic illness by extending life expectancy and by earlier detection of disease in general.

Living longer, however, leads to greater vulnerability to the occurrence of accidents and disease events that can become chronic in nature. The client who may have died from a myocardial infarction in earlier years now needs continuing health care for heart failure. The cancer survivor has healthcare needs related to the iatrogenic results of life-saving treatment. The adolescent who is a quadriplegic because of an accident may live a relatively long life with current rehabilitation efforts but needs continuous preventive and maintenance care from the healthcare system. Children with cystic fibrosis have benefited from lung transplantation but

need care for the rest of their lives. Therefore, many previously fatal conditions, injuries, and diseases have become chronic in nature.

The Canada Health Act of 1984 ensures that all Canadians have access to Medicare or publicly funded medically necessary services. Despite this guarantee, disparity in utilization of health services still exists. Quan et al. (2006) noted that some visible minorities do not use these services as frequently as Whites, possibly because of language, socioeconomic status, social supports, and other cultural factors (Newbold, 2009). Disparities also exist among Canada's aboriginal peoples in terms of health status and utilization of healthcare services. A study of the status of aboriginal patients with chronic kidney disease from Alberta suggested that these patients were twice as likely to be hospitalized than patients with chronic kidney disease in the general population (Gao et al., 2008). Although this may suggest excellent access to care by aboriginal patients, it may also suggest lack of access to primary care and to specialist services for health concerns that could be better managed in ambulatory care settings (Gao et al., 2008).

Barriers to access are complex and include both patient and environmental factors, such as rural residence and distance from care, lack of available services, and factors associated with the determinants of health, such as literacy and poverty. Lower socioeconomic status has been demonstrated to result in increased likelihood of admission to hospital for conditions that could be treated in ambulatory care settings (Gao et al., 2008). Lack of access for aboriginal patients is of particular concern in the face of the increased prevalence of chronic disorders such as obesity (74.4% of First Nations adults living on reserves were overweight or obese as compared with 51.9% of nonaboriginal adults [PHAC, 2012]), alcoholism, depression, ischemic heart disease, cerebrovascular disease, diabetes, and chronic obstructive pulmonary disease and for higher hospitalization rates for First Nations patients in Western Canada (Health Canada, 2009; MacNeil, 2008).

The effects of chronic disease are sobering. All Canadians are impacted by chronic disease, either directly or indirectly. Chronic disease threatens the individual's quality of life and accounts for one-third of potential life lost before age 65. It affects friends and family, who become caregivers, and it affects the health system, where a significant amount of expenditures is estimated to be related to chronic disorders. Chronic illness results not only in direct healthcare costs but indirectly in the loss of productivity. Productivity affects caregivers and family members who provide much of the care and support for people who have chronic conditions (Hollander, Liu, & Chappell, 2009). One in four Canadians report caring for a friend or family member with a chronic disorder. To do so, many report taking a leave of absence from work or resigning altogether, which results in lost wages, benefits, and repercussions for caregiver health. Conservative estimates show that the cost of informal caregiving in 2009 was between $25 billion and $26 billion (Hollander et al., 2009).

Disease Versus Illness

Although the terms "disease" and "illness" are often used interchangeably, there is a distinct difference between them. Disease refers to the pathophysiology of the condition, such as an alteration in structure and function. Illness, on the other hand, is the human experience of symptoms and suffering and refers to how the disease is perceived, lived with, and responded to by individuals, their families, and their healthcare providers. Although it is important to recognize the pathophysiological process of a chronic disease, understanding the illness experience is essential to providing holistic care.

> I put my elbows on my knees and let my forehead sink into my palms. I'm tired. Not just tired . . . weary. My husband's catheter went AWOL at one in the morning, and we've spent the rest of the night in the ER (How many nights does that make now? How many hours?) Noise and cold and too-bright lights and too-bright student doctors. Repeating Bruce's history, over and over. (Harleman, 2008, p. 74)

> Today is the 19th day in a row that my husband has seen a healthcare provider, and actually a few of those times, he's seen two different ones on the same day. It's either radiation therapy, receiving IV fluids and/or replacement potassium, an IV antibiotic for a resistant infection, receiving blood as an out-patient, a mishap with the jejunostomy tube . . . something every day. Will this ever stop? Will we ever have a normal life again? Right now I don't even remember what normal is.

> —*Jenny, wife of a 63-year-old cancer patient*

These patient stories chronicle part of the illness experience. The illness experience is nursing's domain. Thus, the focus here is on the illness experience of individuals and families, not specific disease processes. Although nursing cannot cure chronic disease, nursing can make a difference in the illness experience.

Acute Versus Chronic Conditions

When an individual develops an acute disease, there is typically a sudden onset, with signs and symptoms related to the disease process itself. Acute diseases end in a relatively short time, either with recovery and resumption of prior activities or with death. Chronic illness, on the other hand, continues indefinitely. Although a welcome alternative to death in most but not all cases, the illness is often seen as a mixed blessing to the individual and to society at large. In addition, the illness often becomes the person's identity. For example, an individual having any kind of cancer, even in remission, acquires the label of "that person with cancer." Chronic conditions take many forms, and there is no single onset pattern. A chronic disease can appear suddenly or through an insidious process, have episodic flare-ups or exacerbations, or remain in remission with an absence of symptoms for long periods. Maintaining wellness or keeping symptoms in remission is a juggling act of balancing treatment regimens while focusing on quality of life.

Defining Chronicity

Defining chronicity is complex. Many individuals have attempted to present an all encompassing definition of chronic illness. Initially, the characteristics of chronic diseases were identified by the Commission on Chronic Illness in the United States as all impairments or deviations from normal that included one or more of the following: permanency; residual disability; nonpathological alteration; required rehabilitation; or a long period of supervision, observation, and care (Mayo, 1956). The extent of a chronic disease further complicates attempts in defining the term. Disability may depend not only on the kind of condition and its severity but also on the implications it holds for the person. The degree of disability and altered lifestyle, part of traditional definitions, may relate more to the client's *perceptions and beliefs* about the disease than to the disease itself.

Long-term and iatrogenic effects of some treatment may constitute chronic conditions in their own right, making them eligible to be defined as a chronic illness. Take, for example, the changes in lifestyle required of clients receiving haemodialysis for end-stage renal disease. Life-saving procedures can create other problems. For instance, abdominal radiation that arrested metastatic colon cancer when an individual was 30 years old contributes to a malabsorption problem years later. Chemotherapy or radiation given to a client for an initial bout with cancer may be an influencing factor in the development of leukaemia years later.

Chronic illness, by its very nature, is never completely cured. Biologically, the human body wears out unevenly. Medical advances cause older adults to need a progressively wider variety of specialized services for increasingly complicated conditions. In the words of Emanuel (1982), "Life is the accumulation of chronic illness beneath the load of which we eventually succumb" (p. 502).

Although definitions of chronic disease are important, from a nursing perspective we are far more interested in how the illness is affecting the client and family. What is the illness experience of the client and family? Price (1996) suggested the onus of defining chronic illness, and similarly, quality of life and comfort, should be that of the client's, because only the client truly understands the illness. However, that aside, the following definition of chronic illness is offered: "Chronic illness is the irreversible presence, accumulation, or latency of disease states or impairments that involve the total human environment for supportive care and self-care, maintenance of function, and prevention of further disability" (Curtin & Lubkin, 1995, pp. 6–7).

IMPACT OF CHRONIC ILLNESS _____

This section addresses the influence of chronic illnesses and impact on society in general.

The Older Adult

Although chronic diseases and conditions exist in children, adolescents, and young and middle-aged adults, the bulk of these conditions occurs in adults age 65 years and older. Morgan, Zamora, and Hindmarsh (2007) stated as follows: "As our population ages and as medical advances continue to convert acute-life threatening diseases into chronic illnesses, our healthcare system is challenged to meet the growing burden of chronic disease" (p. 7). In 2010 approximately 4.8 million Canadians were 65 years or older. By 2036 this number is expected to reach 10.4 million (Statistics Canada, 2010a). Increased life expectancy and medical advances have contributed to these demographic changes. In 2009, 89% of Canadian seniors had at least one chronic illness, with arthritis and rheumatism reported to account for 44% (PHAC, as cited in The Chief Public Health Officer's Report, 2010). Furthermore, in 2009 one in four Canadians aged 65 to 79 experienced four chronic illnesses. The prevalence of depression in community-dwelling seniors ranged from 1% to 5% (Canadian Institute for Health Information, 2010); however, the levels are much higher for seniors living in long-term care facilities.

As people age it is clear they will have more chronic conditions and will need to access an acute care system. In Canada older adults use the emergency department significantly more than those younger than 65. Because they have multiple chronic issues their wait in the emergency department is also longer (Canadian Institute for Health Information, 2011a). How will the needs of these aging adults affect our current healthcare delivery system?

The Healthcare Delivery System

The foundation of our present day healthcare system was established when Canada became a self-governing colony. The British North American Act of 1867 (renamed the Constitution Act in 1982) essentially divided the responsibility for health care between the federal and provincial/territorial governments. The federal government was given power over marine hospitals and quarantine, and the provincial/territorial governments were given power over hospitals and asylums. Subsequently, the federal government retained primary responsibility for the direct health care of aboriginal peoples, military personnel, and prisoners; the regulation of pharmaceuticals and medical devices; and for health promotion and disease prevention.

In addition to the healthcare responsibilities for the Inuit and First Nations as laid out in the Constitution Act, the Indian Act of 1985 identified the role of the federal government in the health of Canada's First Nations, a responsibility administered through Health Canada and Indian and Northern Affairs Canada. The presence of treaties that existed before Confederation, as well as the movement towards aboriginal self-governance, has meant that the delivery of health care to aboriginal peoples is often a complex of federal, provincial, territorial, and aboriginal government decision making that challenges healthcare professionals to be responsive to the cultural, economic, and health needs of aboriginal people (Health Canada, 2011a; Kirby & LeBreton, 2001; Petrucka, 2010).

Through the division of various powers, the federal government assumed responsibility for health research first through the creation of the Medical Research Council and then through the Canadian Institute of Health Research, which replaced the Medical Research Council; both agencies have been major sources of federal funding for healthcare research in Canada. The federal government also assumes responsibility for funding support of the provincial healthcare systems, including maintenance and enforcement of the conditions of the Canada Health Act of 1984. Funds for federal support of health care come out of taxation revenues and are given to the provinces through transfer payments and taxation credits (Health Canada, 2011b; Kirby & LeBreton, 2001; Petrucka, 2010). Federal funding for health programs has been used as leverage to ensure provinces and territories abide with the criteria in the Canada Health Act, which has resulted in a delicate tension between the federal government role and interest in the delivery of health care and the responsibility of provinces and territories for delivery of healthcare services in their jurisdictions.

The division of powers for the delivery of the healthcare system has led to considerable diversity in how health care is organized and delivered in each province and territory. Each province and territory is responsible for deciding how much to budget for health care, how many healthcare personnel are required, where and how many facilities will be built, and how

health care will be organized. This has meant, for example, that home health services, which are not considered medically necessary services because they are delivered outside of hospitals, have evolved differently in the provinces and territories. Although nine provinces now have specific legislation for home health care, eligibility for home health services, the services offered, and its organization vary significantly among the provinces and territories (Health Canada, 1999; Petrucka, 2010). Similarly, although each province and territory is expected to abide by the principles of the Canada Health Act, there are differences among provinces and territories as to what drugs taken outside of hospital are covered and what ambulance services are provided, because each province and territory has its own healthcare insurance plan and is expected to plan, finance, and manage this plan (Petrucka, 2010).

CONTEXT FOR CHRONIC CARE IN CANADA

Emergence of Medicare

Before the 1940s private medicine and private insurance, with assistance from municipalities and charitable organizations, predominated in Canadian health care. The beginning of our publicly funded, comprehensive, universal health insurance (Medicare) system had its roots in Saskatchewan in 1947, when the government there introduced a province-wide, universal hospital care plan. By 1950 British Columbia and Alberta had followed the lead of Saskatchewan, and by 1957 the federal government passed the Hospital Insurance and Diagnostic Services Act, which reimbursed half of the cost of specified hospital and diagnostic services to provinces that agreed to establish universal hospital insurance. Within 4 years all provinces had agreed to provide publicly funded inpatient services.

The next step was to ensure services covered outside hospital, and again in 1962 Saskatchewan took the lead by introducing a medical insurance plan that would cover physician services. In 1964 the Royal Commission on Health Services, chaired by the Honourable Justice Emmett Hall, found that many Canadians still did not have access to medical care, or at least medical care that was adequate. The Commission recommended the establishment of a publicly funded, medical care insurance plan by the federal government that would remove economic barriers from access to physicians' services. By 1966 the federal government passed the Medical Care Act, which again reimbursed provinces and territories for half of the cost of physician services, if they adopted universal physician services plans. In 1977, under the Federal-Provincial Fiscal Arrangements and Established Programs Financing Act, cost sharing between the federal and provincial/territorial governments was replaced by a transfer of block healthcare funding to province and territories. This block funding included cash payments and a transfer of tax credits. The tax credits enabled provinces and territories to raise their tax rates by an amount equivalent to a federal reduction in taxation. The block-funding arrangement enabled provinces and territories to spend the cash transfers and tax according to their needs and priorities and preserved the autonomy of provinces and territories in the delivery of health care while committing them to the principles of a universal, publicly funded, Medicare system (Health Canada, 2011a; Kirby & LeBreton, 2001; Petrucka, 2010; Segall & Fries, 2011).

During the 1970s and 1980s, as healthcare costs began to threaten to overburden the Canadian healthcare system, the provinces and territories responded by attempting to constrain costs through physician fee schedules and hospital expenditures. In a trend that some have termed almost reprivatization, patients began to be charged a number of private fees such as extra billing by physicians in New Brunswick, Ontario, Manitoba, Saskatchewan, and Alberta and hospital user fees by New Brunswick, Quebec, Alberta, and British Columbia. A Health Services Review by Justice Emmett Hall once again warned that although health care in Canada was among the best in the world, economic circumstances were once again compromising access to services and were threatening universal health care. In response to the concerns expressed in the Health Services Review, in 1984 the Canada Health Act was unanimously passed, which replaced the previous federal hospital and medical insurance act (Health Canada, 2011b; Kirby & LeBreton, 2001; Petrucka, 2010; Segall & Fries, 2011), a structural intervention that was strongly supported by the Canadian Nurses Association.

The Canada Health Act set out five major principles or criteria that applied to all medically necessary (hospital and physician) services and to all eligible residents of a province or territory: public administration, comprehensiveness, universality, portability, and accessibility. The Canada Health Act of 1984 also prohibited extra billing and user fees (Health Canada, 2007, 2011a). The basic assumption underlying the adoption of this Act was that medical care was a human right and not a privilege for those who could afford to pay (Segall & Fries, 2011).

Despite the aspirations of the Canada Health Act, its provisions are necessarily restrictive because the principles do not apply to health promotion and health education services, extended healthcare services (nursing homes, adult residential care, home and ambulatory care), and supplementary care services (chiropractic, physiotherapy, dental services outside hospitals). With the advent of shorter stays in acute care, new technologies and pharmaceuticals, and the increased management of those with chronic disorders outside of hospitals, the Canada Health Act is applying to a shrinking number of services. The provinces and territories have responded by expanding the services that are publicly funded to specific populations, such as home care, vision care, prescription drugs, and dental care. The services that are publicly funded vary greatly from province to province and province to territory, meaning that Canada's national health care is becoming more varied and less uniform. Furthermore, there is considerable debate over what is considered medically necessary, especially as more and more of what might have been considered medically necessary in 1984 is now delivered outside hospitals (Kirby & LeBreton, 2001) and by professionals who are not physicians.

Many experts have feared and continue to fear that the current healthcare system is not sustainable, given the rate in growth of expenditures and changes in the priorities and needs of Canadians in relation to health care, including the needs of a population with increasing chronic care needs. Two influential national reports examined at length the challenges of our modern healthcare system. The federal government appointed Roy Romanow, a former premier of Saskatchewan, to head a commission to examine the healthcare system in detail and to make recommendations regarding healthcare reform. The report of the Romanow Commission, which was released in 2002, concluded that Medicare and

good health were important to Canadians and closely aligned with Canadian values. It pointed to the limitations of a system that primarily focused on episodic care and recommended sweeping changes to the healthcare system, including a focus on health promotion, illness prevention, and wellness, and the establishment of a National Health Council. Further, the report recommended a focus on specific wellness issues, such as the reduction of obesity and smoking cessation, a focus that has been criticized as too individualistic and not attuned sufficiently to the influences of the determinants of health (Oberle & Raffin Bouchal, 2009) but that has subsequently become increasingly important in our understanding of chronic disorders. The report also recommended improvement in access to health care in rural and remote areas, increases in the use of electronic technology, strengthening and expansion of home care, improvement of primary health care (PHC), catastrophic drug coverage, and appropriate funding of health care (Romanow, 2002).

The second influential report, the Kirby Report, concluded that the current healthcare system is not sustainable and also looked towards PHC as a potential solution to concerns about health care in Canada. Unlike the Romanow Report, the Kirby Report advocated stronger private sector involvement in the delivery of health care. The Report also emphasized accountability for services and funding and offered solutions to wait times, such as time limits (Kirby, 2002).

In 2003 the federal, provincial, and territorial First Ministers met and created the Health Council of Canada. The role of this Health Council, which was strengthened in the 2004 10-Year Plan to Strengthen Health Care (Health Canada, 2006), is to monitor progress on improving the effectiveness and sustainability of the healthcare system. The Health Council has reported annually and publicly on the progress of the renewal of the healthcare system in Canada since 2005. In addition to the creation of the Health Council, the 2003 First Ministers meeting affirmed the importance of PHC and agreed that the ultimate goal of PHC was access to an appropriate healthcare provider 24 hours a day, 7 days a week. In accordance with this goal an agreed-upon target was defined: that 50% of Canadian residents would have this access within 8 years.

The First Ministers' Meeting on the Future of Health Care 2004 built on the renewal agenda set out in 2003 and established the 10-Year Plan to Strengthen Health Care (Health Canada, 2006). This plan affirms the importance of both Medicare and PHC and committed $41 billion to the actions in the plan over the next 10 years. The plan set out a number of key actions (**Figure 1-1**):

- Reduction of wait times, especially in the areas of cancer, heart, diagnostic imaging, joint replacements, and sight restoration
- A Canadian Health Human Resources plan to ensure sufficient supply, type, and mix of healthcare professionals to meet the needs of the population; sufficient education; correct credentialing; and a closer collaboration among health, post-secondary education, and the labour market
- Provision of funding to cover short-term access to home care, community mental health case management, and crisis response; end-of-life care for case management nursing; palliative care medications; and personal care
- PHC reform with the objective that 50% of Canadians would have 24/7 access to a multidisciplinary healthcare team; timely implementation of the electronic health care record; and promotion of telehealth to remote and rural communities
- Increased funding to facilitate healthcare reforms to meet the needs of Northern Canadians
- Development and implementation of a national pharmaceutical strategy that would include cost options for catastrophic pharmaceutical coverage, establishment of a national drug formulary, and broaden the practice of e-prescribing
- Development of a coordinated response to infectious disease outbreaks and other public health emergencies through the new Public Health Network and a commitment to improve the health status of Canadians by addressing risk factors such as physical inactivity
- Investments in healthcare system innovation
- Recognition of the role of health promotion and disease and injury prevention in the health of Canadians through investment in resources for patients and health professionals in diabetes, HIV-AIDS, hepatitis C;

Reduction of wait times and improving access

Canadian health human resources action plans

Improving access to home care

Primary care reform

Focus on access to health care in Northern Canada

National pharmaceutical strategy

Health prevention and promotion

Health innovation

Accountability focus

FIGURE 1-1 Elements of the 10-year plan to strengthen health care.

development of a pan-Canadian public health strategy; and ensuring sufficient supplies of vaccines for immunization
- Development and implementation of health indicators to measure performance and accessible to all Canadians (Health Canada, 2006)

Evolution of Primary Health Care

Although clearly a healthcare system contributes significantly to the state of our health, it does not fully account for the many factors involved in good health, and neither does medical expertise. At one time good health was seen as merely the absence of disease, which was reflected in reliance on a biomedical model of health, in which health was a professional responsibility. Disease was considered to be a malfunctioning of body parts, and personal responsibility for health was equated with compliance with professionally prescribed treatment regimens by medical experts rather than with health promotion or health education, which offered a focus on wellness in addition to disease management. Self-care behaviour was based on the notion that medical professionals were ultimately responsible for good health because they could remove the cause, relieve symptoms, and/or replace whatever was necessary. Although medical care coexists with informal care, over-reliance on the biomedical model tended to overestimate the value of medical expertise and underemphasize other influences on health, such as personal responsibility and environment, including the social environment of families and community (Oberle & Raffin Bouchal, 2009; Segall & Fries, 2011). A key challenge to the biomedical model was the WHO statement that health was more than

simply the absence of disease and was a state of "complete physical, mental, and social well-being" (WHO, 1946, p. 100).

Lalonde (1974) is credited with introducing the concept of lifestyle into the discussion of health. The Lalonde report, *A New Perspective on the Health of Canadians*, was considered innovative at the time and moved thinking away from illness care or disease management towards a positive perspective. It suggested that health is influenced by a broad range of factors, including biology, the organization of health care, and social and physical environments. The report led to the establishment of a federal Health Promotion Directorate, the role of which was to decrease behavioural factors such as smoking, substance use and abuse, and lack of exercise, that were known to put a person at risk of disease. Although this report was highly influential in moving health towards a population-based perspective and for emphasizing the role of health education in motivating people to stay well, it was also criticized for its emphasis on personal responsibility that could lead to "blaming the victim" and for its focus on physical factors rather than on the broad spectrum of determinants of health (Oberle & Raffin Bouchal, 2009; Segall & Fries, 2011).

In 1986 Canada hosted the first International Conference on Health Promotion, which resulted in two more influential policy documents. The Ottawa Charter and *Achieving Health for All: A Framework for Health Promotion* (Epp, 1986), which envisioned health as a resource for people to manage and live their lives, established health as a social and community responsibility, and laid the groundwork for PHC. The three health challenges identified in *Achieving Health for All* are particularly relevant to chronicity in that they included reduction of inequities between those with high incomes and those with low incomes; increased effectiveness in prevention of illnesses, injuries, chronic disorders, and the resulting disabilities; and enhancement of people's ability to manage chronic illness through the provision of skills and community supports. Similarly, the framework identified three health promotion mechanisms (self-care, mutual aid, and healthy environments) that are relevant to chronicity but also to a perspective of health as a collective responsibility that includes formal and informal care and expertise. It means that "communities and regions" must work "together to create environments that are conducive to health" (Epp, 1986, p. 9). The implementation strategies included community participation in determining ways to strengthen health and strengthening community resources to provide a continuum of care and to consider all factors, including policies and health determinants, that affect health (Segall & Fries, 2011).

Within this model there is a significant shift away from professional responsibility for health and treatment to community involvement and empowerment, in which health professionals are facilitators, partners, mediators, and advocates (Oberle & Raffin Bouchal, 2009), which is a viewpoint that is more compatible with professional–patient relationships in chronic care. The population-based approach to care addresses the idea that determinants such as employment, income and social status, education, health literacy, clean water, housing, and social environments may mean that health is not a choice. The person who has chronic obstructive pulmonary disease and arthritis may have little choice as to employment or unemployment and so food security, adequate housing, and sufficient income that further impact on health may not be available as choices.

Although there is concern as to how well PHC, which is built on the concepts of community participation, empowerment, and healthy environments, is actually operationalized in Canada, PHC remains foundational to the Canadian healthcare system. "Primary health care" and "primary care" are often confused, and it is important to differentiate these two terms. Primary care refers to first point of care contact and includes treatment of diseases and injuries, basic emergency services, referrals to more specialized or higher levels of care, health promotion and education, child development care, palliative and end-of-life care, and rehabilitative care (Health Canada, 2011a). Primary care is considered a component of PHC in which interprofessional teams work together to ensure that communities have access to services at a cost the communities can afford, which includes bringing services to the client through technologies such as telehealth. Within the PHC model the community and the client are the drivers of care and are integral partners in defining the types of care and services that are needed. PHC embraces prevention, management of chronic illness, self-care, and what influences choices for health (Petrucka, 2010).

Although federal, provincial, and territorial commitments have made large commitments to provide integrated care through the *10-Year Plan to Strengthen Health Care* (Health Canada, 2006) and fuller implementation of PHC, there is still a tendency for each component of the healthcare system to view the client through its narrow window of care. Frequently, no one entity, practice, institution, or agency is managing the entire disease, and certainly none is managing the illness experience of the client and family. No one entity is responsible for the overall care of the individual, only their own independent component of care. Typically, this approach produces higher social and health costs for the client and social and economic costs for the system.

The magnitude of the interaction of chronicity, especially as the population ages, with a siloed and episodic healthcare system is captured in a cross-sectional chart audit of 2,450 patients, 65 years and older, at Sunnybrook Health Centre in Toronto (Vegda et al., 2009). This study found that older patients (80 years and older) had significantly more physician visits (an average of 4.4 visits annually), emergency department visits (0.22 visits annually), diagnostic days (5.1 test days/year), more comorbid health conditions (an average of 7.7 per patient), and more medications (an average of 8.2 per patient) than younger adults in the sample. These multiple chronic disorders, diagnostic services, and treatment plans require patients and caregivers to navigate many professional care providers and services where different foci and barriers to communication of health information may be common. Short visit times, episodic care, and lack of coordination among healthcare teams that are well versed in managing complex conditions can lead to the predominance of disease-specific guidelines over patient-centred care and care that is time consuming, impractical, and capable of producing unwarranted side effects for patients (Vegda et al., 2009). Coordination of care would be enhanced by a clinical information system that followed the patient through the healthcare system and by greater involvement of the patient and family in care planning and treatment.

Care for patients with chronic disorders needs to focus on health promotion, illness prevention, and the individual needs of the patient that takes into account optimal functioning

rather than disease-specific guidelines that may be contradictory to each other and result in increased healthcare utilization, increased need for scarce healthcare resources, and decreased quality of life for the patient (Morgan et al., 2007; Vegda et al., 2009). Most of these ideas are not new; Romanow identified the need for a nation-wide, comprehensive information technology plan in health care and for an integrated healthcare team to meet the care needs and services of the Canadian population (Romanow, 2002). The healthcare needs of the Canadian population have been clearly articulated and are highlighted in the following example; however, there is still much work to be done to ensure we move ahead to address these needs.

Think about an older adult in this system: Mr. Jones, with several comorbidities, enters an acute care institution. His admitting diagnosis is pneumonia, but now his diabetes is flaring up along with his hypertension, and his kidneys are not working as well as they should. A specialty physician is treating each of his conditions, but there is no coordinator of his care. He is taking multiple medications, and soon he becomes confused and incontinent. In addition, the focus of the acute care facility is the disease processes of this individual and not the illness experience of the patient and his elderly wife. What does our acute care system do with this older adult with multiple chronic health problems? How does our healthcare delivery system care for Mr. Jones and the multitude of others like him on the horizon?

Quality of Care

A number of initiatives have been implemented focusing on improving the quality of care in Canada. One example is the Canadian Patient

Safety Institute, a nonprofit organization with the mandate to raise awareness and facilitate best practices in regards to patient safety and quality. A second major initiative has been the establishment of the Health Council of Canada, which plays a key role in the measurement of progress towards identified health outcomes and provides evidence to support decisions made by policymakers in relation to health care. Another important initiative that is designed to improve quality of care is the Canadian Best Practices System, which enables knowledge exchange among researchers, policymakers, and healthcare practitioners; consensus building about best practices; and a centralized access point for best practices (Treasury Board of Canada Secretariat, 2007). (This system can be accessed through http://cbpp-pcpe.phac-aspc .gc.ca/system/index_e.cfm.)

The Health Council has made it clear that the burden of chronic illness is increasing in Canada and that a complete system redesign strategy, such as the chronic care model, successfully implemented in the United Kingdom, Australia, New Zealand, and the United States, needs to be broadly implemented. The Ministry of Health in British Columbia began implementation of the chronic care model in 2000, and other provinces such as Alberta, Saskatchewan, and Ontario are adapting the model as part of their quality improvement work. Collaborative techniques that bring healthcare teams together to learn how to implement tenets in the chronic care model are an important part of this process.

Appropriate reimbursement is still a major part of the quality improvement process that has to be addressed. The current fee-for-service reimbursement model was designed to support brief acute care visits and not the longer and more intense visits required with chronically ill patients. Currently, British Columbia is engaging in a demonstration project for a new reimbursement model for chronic illness care. Although these efforts are still in their infancy, they represent important steps in quality improvement in chronic illness care (The Conference, 2010).

Nursing organizations, such as the Registered Nurses Association of Ontario, provide important leadership in quality improvement for chronic illness care through the development of best practice guidelines for various chronic health concerns and care approaches, such as prompted voiding, long-term care, end-of-life, asthma, smoking cessation, and support of clients with chronic kidney disease and clients receiving methadone maintenance treatment. The Canadian Nurses Association and nursing organizations in provincial and territorial jurisdictions have provided important support to the Canada Health Council and PHC in terms of advocacy and input into practice initiatives that improve care for individuals with chronic illnesses and system design.

Culture

Illness belief systems form a cultural milieu that defines one's attitudes about illness, both acute and chronic. Conceptions or misconceptions about the source of the disease, potential treatment, and possible outcomes are all influenced by these belief systems, and one's belief system is influenced by one's culture. Providing culturally competent care may be a daunting task; however, health care is not "one size fits all," and healthcare professionals must take the extra steps to ensure culturally competent care.

Another way to view culture is to consider chronic illness as a culture. Although we often believe that each disease is different, there are multiple tasks that are similar, and illness experiences may look alike across diseases. Strauss (1975) was among the first researchers to recognize the similar issues and tasks within the culture of chronic illness. Generally, the culture of chronic illness includes preventing and managing medical crises, managing a treatment regimen, controlling symptoms, reordering time, and social isolation. In 1984 Strauss and colleagues suggested the basic strategy to cope with these issues was to normalize, not just to stay alive or keep symptoms under control but to live as normally as possible. Essentially, for a number of clients with chronic illness, a "new normal" must be created.

A number of years ago when teaching a chronic illness practicum to graduate students, this author, J. Engel, developed a mini-ethnography project of the individuals for whom the students were caring that semester. Students were caring for clients with a variety of diseases—HIV, liver disease, heart failure, rheumatoid arthritis, and breast cancer. Using grand tour questions developed as a class, students interviewed their clients over the course of the semester. During the final weeks of seminar after the practicum was completed, students compiled the data from all clients and looked at the themes that emerged. The class was able to develop a clear concept of the culture of what it is like to have a chronic illness and to understand the vast number of similarities between individuals with a variety of chronic conditions.

Social Influences

As a society we often stereotype individuals according to the colour of their skin, their culture, and their ethnicity. Unfortunately, we behave in a similar fashion with individuals with chronic conditions and disabilities. To this day some individuals will avoid others who may be in a wheelchair, have visible signs of disease (burns, paralysis, amputations, etc.), have a diagnosis of AIDS, and so forth. Although some efforts such as department store advertisements depicting individuals in wheelchairs may positively influence some behaviour, as a nation there is much progress to be made.

Publicly recognized individuals have stepped forward with stories about their own chronic conditions. The courage of these individuals to share their experiences and speak out for more comprehensive legislation to support those with chronic disease and increase re-search funding is admirable. Examples include Michael J. Fox and Muhammad Ali, with diagnoses of Parkinson's disease; Magic Johnson, with his diagnosis of HIV; and the late Christopher and Dana Reeve, as advocates for spinal cord injury research.

Financial Impact

In 2009 Canada spent 11.4% of the gross domestic product on healthcare expenditures, which equates to US$4,363 per person (Organization for Economic Cooperation and Development [OECD], 2011). This is lower than the United States (17.4%) and European countries such as the Netherlands (12%) and France (11.8%). Healthcare expenditures on average are continuing to rise faster than the economic growth (OECD, 2011). Currently, healthcare dollars spent on older adults accounts for 44% of healthcare spending for provincial and territorial budgets (Canadian Institute for Health Information, 2012). Spending on pharmaceuticals in Canada also continues to increase. In 2009 $29.7 billion was spent on pharmaceuticals and $31.1 billion in 2010, representing annual increases of 6.3% and 4.8% (Canadian Institute for Health Information, 2011b).

Chronic disorders such as cardiac diseases, cancer, respiratory conditions, and type 2 diabetes account for 60% of all deaths and 44% of all premature deaths globally (Coleman, Austin, Brach, & Wagner, 2009; Ebrahim, 2008). In 2005 it was estimated that Canada would lose $500 million from premature deaths related to these disorders, and these losses are anticipated to increase. Cumulatively, Canada could lose $9 billion between 2005 and 2015 from premature deaths (WHO, n.d.). **Table 1-1** shows information related to costs and statistics related to mortality and morbidity of selected diseases in Canada.

The Canada Health Act mandates that all Canadians have access to medically necessary hospital and physician services. Some provinces and territories provide additional coverage for benefits such as prescription drugs, dental care, and optometry services. However, the amount of financial coverage (partial or full coverage) varies across the jurisdictions. Generally, additional benefit coverage is targeted to populations such as children, seniors, or those who receive social assistance (Health Canada, 2011b). For example, an Ontario resident 65 years of age or older with a valid health care card is eligible for the Ontario Drug Benefit Program; however, the individual will still need to pay a yearly deductible and a copayment for prescription refills. Depending on income level the yearly deductible may be waived; however, it will still be necessary to pay a small copayment for prescriptions. The Ontario Drug Benefit Program does not cover equipment such as syringes or lancets for individuals with diabetes.

Preventive services, such as eye examinations, hearing tests, and preventive dental examinations, which can identify changes associated with chronic disorders not yet diagnosed (e.g., diabetes), are not generally identified as essential or medically necessary services for adults and therefore are the responsibility of private insurance providers.

For individuals without private insurance (and even for those who do have it) the limitations on funding for preventive services can lead to delayed identification of developing health problems and contribute to the long-term costs of chronic disorders. The OECD annually tracks and reports on more than 1,200 health system measures across 30 industrialized countries. Since 1998 the Commonwealth Fund has sponsored an analysis of cross-national health systems based on OECD health data. Compared with other countries, Canada has about half the average of hospital beds and fewer physicians per capita. Yet in 2007 life expectancy in Canada was 80.7 years, 1 year higher than the OECD average; however, the infant mortality rate in Canada is lower than the United States but higher than the OECD average (OECD, 2011).

In addition to services that are covered by public insurance, clients with chronic disorders, such as arthritis and diabetes, encounter additional expenses, notably for complementary and alternative medicines (CAMs). In one study of clients with osteoarthritis, approximately 43% reported using some form of CAM, such as glucosamine and chondroitin, usually after first trying conventional approaches such as nonsteroidal anti-inflammatory drugs, arthroscopy, or arthroplasty (Marsh et al., 2009). Data from the national Canadian Community Health Survey, cycles 1.1, 2.1, and 3.1, as well as related literature suggest that persons

Table 1-1   Quick Facts: Economic and Health Burden of Chronic Disease

Disease/Risk Factor	Mortality/Morbidity	Direct and Indirect Costs
Overweight/obesity	37% of Canadians are overweight and 24% are obese (Health Canada).	Estimated to cost 6 billion (based on 2006 data) or 4.1% of healthcare expenditures in Canada (Anis et al., 2010).
Chronic obstructive pulmonary disease (COPD)	Affects 4% of population aged 35 and older.	75% of persons with COPD take prescription medications; 20% report at least one visit to an emergency department within the last year, and 8% report at least one hospital stay. 21% report being referred for follow-up health education and counselling (PHAC, 2011).
Cancer	Most common cause of death in Canada. Incidence of cancer is increasing with aging and growing population. It is estimated that there will be 177, 800 new cases of cancer in 2011 and 75,000 cancer deaths. Cancer is the leading cause of death in Canada. The leading causes of cancer in women over a 10-year period are breast and colorectal and in men prostate and colorectal (Canadian Cancer Society, 2011).	Costs include direct (medical) and indirect costs. One study of occupational cancers (i.e., cancer related to exposure to carcinogens in the workplace) estimates the direct medical costs of cancer to be 15.7 million and indirect costs (e.g., lack of productivity) to be 64.1 million (based on 2,700 persons currently diagnosed) (Orenstein et al., 2010).
Cardiovascular disease	14.9% of population is diagnosed with hypertension in Canada. Nine in 10 individuals aged 20 years and older have at least one risk factor for heart disease (obesity, physical inactivity, stress, hypertension, diabetes, smoking, eating less than daily requirements for fruits and vegetables) (Dai et al., 2009).	Heart disease and strokes are the most common reasons for hospitalization in Canada, which costs the economy 20.9 billion in physician and hospital services, lost wages, and productivity (Canada Heart and Stroke, 2012).
Diabetes	Close to 2.4 million Canadians have diabetes, a number that is expected to be 56% by 2018–2019. The incidence of diabetes increases with age. Ninety to 95% of those with diabetes have type 2. Complications can occur even before diagnosis. Diabetes is the leading cause of end-stage renal disease (PHAC, 2011).	The economic burden of diabetes is estimated to be 2.5 billion annually, which does not reflect the costs of complications (eye disease, cardiovascular disease, kidney disease, nerve damage, amputation, complications in pregnancy) (PHAC, 2011).

with asthma, migraine headaches, and diabetes are the most likely to seek help from CAMs and that, overall, 12.8% of Canadians visit a CAM practitioner each year (Metcalfe, Williams, McChesney, Patten, & Jette, 2010). Although the costs of massage therapy and chiropractic treatment may be covered by private insurance plans for those patients who can afford them or are covered through employment, the costs of herbs and supplements are largely borne by individuals themselves, which adds to the economic burden of chronic disorders for individuals and families.

INTERVENTIONS

Chronic disease is an encompassing issue, such that interventions from many sources are needed to make a difference. What follows are examples of ways to decrease the impact of chronic disease.

Professional Education

One of the challenges in chronic disease care and management is educating healthcare professionals about providing care tailored to those with chronic disease. The differences are vast between caring for a person with an acute illness on a short-term basis and caring for those over the long haul with a chronic condition. WHO (2005) outlined the steps to prepare a healthcare workforce for the 21st century to appropriately care for individuals with chronic conditions. WHO (2005) called for a transformation of healthcare training to better meet the needs of those individuals with chronic conditions. The document, *Preparing a Healthcare Workforce for the 21st Century: The Challenge of Chronic Conditions* (WHO, 2005), has the support of the

World Medical Association, the International Council of Nurses, the International Pharmaceutical Federation, the European Respiratory Society, and the International Alliance of Patients' Organizations.

The competencies delineated by the WHO (2005) were identified with a process that included an extensive document/literature review and international expert agreement. All competencies were based on addressing the needs of patients with chronic conditions and their family members from a longitudinal perspective and focused on two types of "prevention" strategies: initial prevention of the chronic disease and prevention of complications from the condition. The five competencies were patient-centred care, partnering, quality improvement, information and communication technology, and public health perspective (**Table 1-2**). At first glance the competencies might not seem unique. However, in an acute care–oriented healthcare delivery system, these concepts are not as prominent. Clients are in and out of the care system quickly, and there is less need for implementation of these concepts.

Little attention is paid to educating healthcare professionals about caring for older adults. More stringent education and training standards should be available for direct-care professionals who work with persons with chronic disorders, including increasing knowledge and skills in working with patients with complex illnesses and comorbidities and working within interprofessional teams to provide direct and indirect care. Furthermore, because informal caregivers continue to play important roles in the care of older adults (with and without chronic illness), training opportunities should also be available for them.

Currently, only a small percentage of the healthcare workforce specializes in caring for

Table 1-2   WHO Core Competencies
Patient-centred care
Interviewing and communicating effectively
Assisting changes in health-related behaviors
Supporting self-management
Using a proactive approach
Partnering
Partnering with patients
Partnering with other providers
Partnering with communities
Quality improvement
Measuring care delivery and outcomes
Learning and adapting to change
Translating evidence into practice
Information and communication technology
Designing and using patient registries
Using computer technologies
Communicating with partners
Public health perspective
Providing population-based care
Systems thinking
Working across the care continuum
Working in primary healthcare–led systems
Source: World Health Organization (2005).

older adults. Data from the Canadian Nurses Association (2011) showed in 2009 only 9.6% of registered nurses were employed in geriatric or long-term care settings. The average age of the nurses was 49.5 years, which was higher than the average age of registered nurses (Canadian Nurses Association, 2011). Physicians trained in specialty care of the elderly are also low in numbers. There are less than 200 geriatricians in Canada, but estimates indicate the need for over 600 to meet the demands of the aging population (Swanson, 2007). An Institute of Medicine (2008) report recommended that financial incentives be provided to increase the number of geriatric specialists in every health profession.

Incentives would include an increase in payments for clinical services, development of awards to increase the number of faculty in geriatrics, and the establishment of programs that would provide loan forgiveness, scholarships, and direct financial incentives for individuals to become specialists in geriatrics. For the direct-care workers in long-term care facilities that typically have high levels of turnover and job dissatisfaction, the recommendation is to improve job desirability, improve supervisory relationships, and provide opportunities for career growth. Finally, models of care for older adults need to improve. The report envisioned three key principles in improving care: (1) the healthcare needs of older adults must be addressed comprehensively, (2) services need to be provided efficiently, and (3) older adults need to be encouraged to be active partners in their own care.

Chronic Disease Practitioner Competencies

The National Association of Chronic Disease Directors (NACDD) (n.d.) developed a document entitled "Competencies for Chronic Disease Practice." The organization was founded in 1988 to link the directors of chronic disease programs in each state and U.S. territory. It created these competencies to assist state and local healthcare programs with developing competent workforces and effective programs. The NACDD document is based on domains, with individual competencies within each domain. Several of the domains address the WHO competencies (i.e., partnering, evidence-informed interventions). Furthermore, the NACDD developed an assessment tool for practitioners to gauge their level of proficiency in each of the seven domains. **Table 1-3** lists the competencies for chronic disease practitioners.

Table 1-3 NACDD Competencies for Chronic Disease Practitioners	
Domain	**Competency**
Domain 1: build support	Chronic disease practitioners establish strong working relationships with stakeholders, including other programs, government agencies, and nongovernmental lay and professional groups, to build support for chronic disease prevention and control.
Domain 2: design and evaluate programs	Chronic disease practitioners develop and implement evidence-informed interventions and conduct evaluations to ensure ongoing feedback and program effectiveness.
Domain 3: influence policies and systems change	Chronic disease practitioners implement strategies to change the health-related policies of private organizations or governmental entities capable of affecting the health of targeted populations.
Domain 4: lead strategically	Chronic disease practitioners articulate health needs and strategic vision, serve as catalysts for change, and demonstrate program accomplishments to ensure continued funding and support within their scope of practice.
Domain 5: manage people	Chronic disease practitioners oversee and support the optimal performance and growth of program staff as well as themselves.
Domain 6: manage programs and resources	Chronic disease practitioners ensure the consistent administrative, financial, and staff support necessary to sustain successful implementation of planned activities and to build opportunities.
Domain 7: use public health science	Chronic disease practitioners gather, analyze, interpret, and disseminate data and research findings to define needs, identify priorities, and measure change.

World Health Organization

WHO has updated its 2000 plan for the prevention and control of noncommunicable disease. Working with partners/agencies across the world, the 2008–2013 plan focuses on cardiovascular diseases, diabetes, cancer, and chronic respiratory disease, as well as the four shared risk factors of tobacco use, physical inactivity, unhealthy diet, and the harmful use of alcohol. The action plan has six objectives (WHO, 2008):

- To raise the priority accorded to noncommunicable disease in development work at global and national levels and to integrate prevention and control of such diseases into policies across all government departments
- To establish and strengthen national policies and plans for the prevention and control of noncommunicable diseases
- To promote interventions to reduce the main shared modifiable risk factors for noncommunicable diseases—tobacco use, unhealthy diet, physical inactivity, and harmful use of alcohol
- To promote research for the prevention and control of noncommunicable diseases

- To promote partnerships for the prevention and control of noncommunicable diseases
- To monitor noncommunicable diseases and their determinants and evaluate progress at the regional, national, and global levels

Evidence-Informed Practice

The evidence-based practice movement had its beginnings in the 1970s with Dr. Archie Cochrane, a British epidemiologist. In 1971 Cochrane published a book that criticized physicians for not conducting rigorous reviews of evidence in making appropriate treatment decisions. Cochrane was a proponent of randomized clinical trials and in his exemplar case noted that thousands of low-birth-weight premature infants died needlessly (Cochrane, 1971). At the same time several randomized clinical trials had been conducted on the use of corticosteroid therapy to halt premature labour in pregnant women, but the data had never been reviewed or analyzed. After review, these studies demonstrated that this therapy was effective in halting premature labour and thus reducing infant deaths due to prematurity. Cochrane died in 1988, but as a result of his influence and call for systematic review of the literature, the Cochrane Collaboration was launched in Oxford, England, in 1993. It also hosts the Cochrane Library, which is a sophisticated collection of databases containing current, high-quality research that supports practice.

However, evidence-based practice does not rely on randomized clinical trials alone. A number of definitions have been brought forth, but Porter-O'Grady (2006) offers a clear and succinct definition: "Evidence-based practice is simply the integration of the best possible research to evidence with clinical expertise and with patient needs. Patient needs in this case refer specifically to the expectations, concerns, and requirements that patients bring to their clinical experience" (p. 1).

The term "evidence-based practice" has recently been replaced with *evidence-informed practice* within the literature. Evidence-informed practice stresses the use of research findings to build nursing knowledge, and, as appropriate, other forms of knowledge, such as quality improvement data, consensus of recognized experts, and affirmed experience to support a specific practice, are also taken into account (Wood, 2010). Nurses need to have a sound knowledge base pertaining to chronic disease management, and continued research is essential to continuing to build this knowledge (Wood, 2010).

Healthcare professionals can examine the evidence to improve the care of their clients by using a number of sources for reference. The following agencies and organizations are a sample of the resources available:

- Agency for Healthcare Research and Quality (www.ahrq.gov)
- *Clinical Evidence* (www.clinicalevidence.com)
- Cochrane Library (www.thecochranelibrary.com)
- The Joanna Briggs Institute (www.joannabriggs.edu.au)
- National Guideline Clearinghouse (www.guideline.gov)
- Task Force on Community Preventive Services (www.thecommunityguide.org)
- U.S. Preventive Services Task Force (www.ahrq.gov/clinic/uspstfab.htm)

GOING FORWARD: THE FUTURE OF CHRONIC CARE IN CANADA

Canadians value their healthcare system, as they have indicated on several occasions (Kirby & LeBreton, 2001; Romanow, 2002). As people with chronic diseases live longer and as the population ages and grows, the system needs to change from acute and episodic care models to those models that recognize the complexity of multimorbidity, such as occurs in a person who may be diagnosed with diabetes but who also has hypertension, high cholesterol levels, angina, and dementia. The complexity of multimorbidity and longer life requires the attention of health professionals and of informal caregivers and family. The trajectory of chronic conditions varies over time in response to context (including determinants of health), age, and life situations and requires approaches that include primary care, secondary care, and tertiary care.

No Canadian remains unaffected by chronic conditions. Determinants of health, such as income or genetic predisposition or lifestyle choices, may predispose individuals to later chronic disease, or they may already be living with a chronic disorder. The impact of chronicity on quality of life is greatest for the poorest in Canada, who are more likely to develop chronic disease, die younger, and suffer poverty because of disabilities resulting from chronic disorders (Fang, Kmetic, Millar, & Drasic, 2009). All Canadians are affected by the limitations of a healthcare system that is challenged by a shift towards chronicity from acute care and by the economic burdens of disease.

The Canadian Academy of Health Sciences, a nonprofit organization modelled on the U.S. Institute of Medicine and composed of membership from various disciplines, has developed a strategy for action, entitled "Transforming Care for Canadians with Chronic Health Conditions" (Canadian Academy of Health Sciences, 2010). This strategy is based on 18 months of review of research, empirical evidence, emerging practices, and consensus of an expert panel from all aspects of health care in Canada (Canadian Academy of Health Sciences, 2010). The strategy recognizes the expectations of Canadians in relation to the healthcare system and the realities facing Canadian health care, while offering recommendations to transform the system (Canadian Academy of Health Sciences, 2010).

In preparing the strategy to transform chronic care in Canada, the Canadian Academy of Health Sciences (2010, p. 9) suggested that the expectations of Canadians in relation to healthcare include the following:

- Assistance from healthcare providers to help patients and their informal caregivers to live a high-quality life
- Inclusion of family and informal caregivers as partners in care of patients with chronic disorders
- Recognition that patients and their healthcare providers know "the story"
- Encouragement from the healthcare system for health providers to spend the time they need with patients
- Multidisciplinary and interprofessional teams to care for patients with chronic disorders
- Support for health professionals to maintain their knowledge and skills
- Easy identification of and access to services that are needed
- Connection of the various services that are needed for patient care

- Guidance for the healthcare system in constant quality improvement
- Access to the best approaches to health care in every community across Canada

In relation to the healthcare system, the Canadian Academy of Health Sciences (2010) recommended that all people with chronic health conditions have access to a system with a specific team of clinicians who are responsible for their primary care and for coordinating specialty, acute, and community care throughout the lifespan as follows (pp. 1–2):

- *By aligning system funding and provider remuneration with desired outcomes.* This could be accomplished by shifting remuneration away from fee for service and enabling greater flexibility for remuneration for specialized services. Remuneration needs to be provided that recognizes the need for comprehensive care for those with chronic disorders and for health providers who are not physicians so their contribution to primary care is recognized.
- *By ensuring that quality drives system performance.* Recommendations for this strategy include the development of a pan-Canadian quality improvement strategy and development of leadership in health professionals to drive the redesign of the healthcare system.
- *By creating a culture of lifelong learning for healthcare providers.* Recommendations for this strategy focus on the development of skills and knowledge needed to effectively work with patients with chronic conditions and to shift the nature of the patient–provider relationship to one that is person focused.

- *By supporting self-management as part of everyone's care.* This could be accomplished through effective sharing of health information so that patients can manage their own health and by ensuring that services have the appropriate mix of health providers to facilitate self-management.
- *By using health information effectively and efficiently.* This refers to the effective use of technology for record keeping and information transfer and the availability of information to facilitate self-management.
- *By conducting research that supports optimal care and improved outcomes.* The recommendations for this strategy include the development of research capacity in health providers and administrators to be involved as partners in research; development of reliable, rapid evaluation of implementation of health policy initiatives; and articulation of knowledge gaps in chronic care.

SUMMARY

Although Canada boasts a healthcare system that is accessible to all citizens, this system clearly does not meet the needs of the chronically ill. Canada's Health Infoway is one initiative that offers great promise, and federal/provincial governments have renewed their commitment to PHC. However, in recognition of the impact of chronic disorders and the associated costs, it is evident that change is still required. The Canadian healthcare system must continue to evolve and move from an acute episodic system to a system that is prepared to deal with the complexities of chronic illness.

STUDY QUESTIONS

1. Summarize the state of chronic disease in Canada and globally today.
2. What factors and influences have led to the increased incidence of chronic disease in Canada?
3. What factors should be considered in defining chronicity?
4. How can we better educate healthcare professionals to care for those with chronic disease? To care for older adults with chronic disease?
5. What changes does the healthcare delivery system need to embrace to better care for those with chronic disease?
6. Compare and contrast chronic disease and chronic illness.
7. What action(s) should Canada take to decrease healthcare disparities?

For a full suite of assignments and additional learning activities, use the access code located in the front of your book and visit this exclusive website: **http://go.jblearning.com/kramer-kile**. If you do not have an access code, you can obtain one at the site.

REFERENCES

Anis, A., Zhang, W., Bansback, D., Guh, P., Amarsi, P., & Birmingham, C. (2010). Obesity and overweight in Canada: An updated cost-of-illness study. *Obesity Reviews, 11*(1), 31–40.

Canada Heart and Stroke. (2012). Statistics. Retrieved from http://www.heartandstroke.com

Canadian Academy of Health Sciences. (2010). Transforming care for Canadians with chronic health conditions. Put people first, expect the best, manage for results. Retrieved from http://www.cahs-acss.ca/wp-content/uploads/2011/09/cdm-final-English.pdf

Canadian Cancer Society. (2011). Canadian cancer statistics 2011. Retrieved from http://www.cancer.ca/canada-wide/about%20cancer/cancer%20statistics/powerpoint%20slides.aspx?sc_lang=en

Canadian Institute for Health Information. (2010). Depression among seniors in residential care. Retrieved from http://secure.cihi.ca/cihiweb/products/ccrs_depression_among_seniors_e.pdf

Canadian Institute for Health Information. (2011a). Health care in Canada 2011, a focus on seniors and aging. Retrieved from http://secure.cihi.ca/cihiweb/products/HCIC_2011_seniors_report_en.pdf

Canadian Institute for Health Information. (2011b). Drug expenditure in Canada 1985–2010. Retrieved from http://secure.cihi.ca/cihiweb/products/drug_expenditure_2010_en.pdf

Canadian Institute for Health Information. (2012). Health spending to reach $200 billion in 2011. Retrieved from http://www.cihi.ca/cihi-ext-portal/internet/en/document/spending+and+health+workforce/spending/release_03nov11

Canadian Mental Health Association. (2012). Fast facts: Mental health/mental illness. Retrieved from http://www.cmha.ca/?s=Fast+facts+mental+health+and+illness&lang=en

Canadian Nurses Association. (2011, May). RN workforce profile by area of responsibility year 2009. Retrieved from http://www2.cna-aiic.ca/CNA/documents/pdf/publications/2009_RN_Profiles_e.pdf

Chief Public Health Officer's Report. (2010). Report on the state of public health in Canada, 2010. Growing older adding life to years. Retrieved from http://publichealth.gc.ca/CPHOreport

Cochrane, A. L. (1971). *Effectiveness and efficiency: Random reflections on health services.* London, England: Nuffield Provincial Hospitals Trust.

Coleman, K., Austin, B. T., Brach, C., & Wagner, E. (2009). Evidence on the chronic care model in the new millennium. *Health Affairs: The Policy Journal of the Health Sphere, 28*(1), 75–85.

Conference. (2010). The chronic care model. Retrieved from http://theconference.ca/the-chronic-care-model.pdf

Curtin, M., & Lubkin, I. (1995). What is chronicity? In I. Lubkin (Ed.), *Chronic illness: Impact and interventions* (3rd ed., pp. 3–23). Sudbury, MA: Jones & Bartlett.

Dai, S., Bancej, C., Bienek, A., Walsh, P., Stewart, P., & Wielgosz, A. (2009). Report summary: Tracking heart disease and stroke in Canada. Retrieved from http://www.phac-aspc.gc.ca/publicat/cdic-mcbc/29-4/ar_06-eng.php

Ebrahim, S. (2008). Chronic diseases and calls to action. *International Journal of Epidemiology, 37*(2), 225–230.

Emanuel, E. (1982). We are all chronic patients. *Journal of Chronic Diseases, 35*(7), 501–502.

Epp, J. (1986). *Achieving health for all: A framework for health promotion*. Ottawa, ON: Health and Welfare Canada.

Fang, R., Kmetic, A., Millar, J., & Drasic, L. (2009). Disparities in chronic disease among Canada's low-income populations. *Preventing Chronic Disease, 6*(4), 1–9.

Gao, S., Manns, B., Culleton, B., Tonelli, M., Quan, H., Crowshoe, L., & Hemmelgarn, B. (2008). Access to health care among status Aboriginal people with chronic kidney disease. *Canadian Medical Association Journal, 179*(10), 1007–1012.

Harleman, A. (2008, January & February). My other husband. *AARP Magazine*, pp. 74–78.

Health Canada. (1999). Provincial and territorial home care programs: A synthesis for Canada. Retrieved from http://www.hc-sc.gc.ca/hcs-sss/pubs/home-domicile/1999-pt-synthes/index-eng.php

Health Canada. (2006). First Ministers' meeting on the future of health care 2004: A 10-year plan to strengthen health care. Retrieved from http://www.hc-sc.gc.ca/hcs-sss/delivery-prestation/fptcollab/2004-fmm-rpm/index-eng.php

Health Canada. (2007). Canada Health Act: Introduction. Retrieved from http://www.hc-sc.gc.ca/hcs-sss/medi-assur/cha-lcs/index-eng.php

Health Canada. (2009). A statistical profile on the health of First Nations in Canada: Health services utilization in Western Canada. Retrieved from http://www.hc-sc.gc.ca/fniah-spnia/pubs/aborig-autoch/2009-stats-profil-vol2/index-eng.php

Health Canada. (2011a). Canada's health care system. Retrieved from http://www.hc-sc.gc.ca/hcs-sss/pubs/system-regime/2011-hcs-sss/index-eng.php

Health Canada. (2011b). Canada Health Act: Frequently asked questions. Retrieved from http://www.hc-sc.gc.ca/hcs-sss/medi-assur/faq-eng.php#a3

Hollander, J., Liu, G., & Chappell, N. (2009). Who cares and how much? The imputed economic contribution to the Canadian healthcare system of middle-aged and older unpaid caregivers providing care to the elderly. *Healthcare Quarterly, 12*(2), 42–49.

Institute of Medicine. (2008). *Retooling for an aging America: Building the health care workforce*. Washington, DC: National Academies Press.

Kirby, M. J. L. (2002). *The health of Canadians: The federal role. Vol. 6: Recommendations for reform*. Ottawa, ON: Standing Senate Committee on Social Affairs, Science and Technology. Retrieved from http://www.parl.gc.ca/Content/SEN/Committee/372/SOCI/rep/repoct02vol6-e.htm

Kirby, M. J. L., & LeBreton, M. (2001). Interim report on the state of health care system in Canada: The health of Canadians: The federal role. Vol. 1: The story so far. Retrieved from http://www.parl.gc.ca/Content/SEN/Committee/371/soci/rep/repintsep01-e.htm

Lalonde, M. (1974). *A new perspective on the health of Canadians*. Ottawa, ON: Government of Canada.

MacNeil, M. S. (2008). An epidemiologic study of aboriginal adolescent health risk in Canada: The meaning of suicide. *Journal of Child and Adolescent Psychiatric Nursing, 21*(1), 3–10.

Marsh, J., Hager, C., Havey, T., Sprague, S., Bhandari, M., & Bryant, D. (2009). Use of alternative medicines by patients with OA that adversely interact with prescribed medications. *Clinical Orthopedics and Related Research, 467*(10), 2705–2722.

Mayo, L. (Ed.). (1956). *Guides to action on chronic illness*. Commission on Chronic Illness. New York, NY: National Health Council.

Metcalfe, A., Williams, J., McChesney, J., Patten, S. B., & Jette, N. (2010). Use of complementary and alternative medicine by those with a chronic disease and the general population—results of a national population based survey. *BMC Complementary and Alternative Medicine, 10*, 58.

Morgan, M. W., Zamora, N. E., & Hindmarsh, M. F. (2007). An inconvenient truth: A sustainable healthcare system requires chronic disease prevention and management transformation. *Healthcare Papers, 7*(4), 6–23.

National Association of Chronic Disease Directors. (n.d.). Competencies for chronic disease practice. Retrieved from http://www.cdph.ca.gov/programs/Documents /Competencies%20for%20Chronic%20Disease%20 Practice.pdf

Newbold, K. B. (2009). Health care use and the Canadian immigrant population. *International Journal of Health Services, 39*(3), 545–565.

Oberle, K., & Raffin Bouchal, S. (2009). *Ethics in Canadian nursing practice*. Toronto, ON: Pearson.

Orenstein, M., Dall, T., Curley, P., Chen, J., Tamburrini, A., & Peterson, J. (2010). *The economic burden of occupational cancers in Alberta*. Calgary, AB: Alberta Health Services.

Organization for Economic Cooperation and Development. (2011). Health data 2011: How does Canada compare. Retrieved from http://www.oecd.org/dataoecd /46/33/38979719.pdf

Petrucka, P. (2010). The Canadian health care system. In P. Potter, A. G. Perry, J. C. Ross-Kerr, & M. J. Wood (Eds.), *Canadian fundamentals of nursing* (pp. 14–27). Toronto, ON: Elsevier.

Porter-O'Grady, T. (2006). A new age for practice: Creating the framework for evidence. In K. Malloch & T. Porter-O'Grady (Eds.), *Introduction to evidence-based practice in nursing and health care*. Sudbury, MA: Jones & Bartlett.

Price, B. (1996). Illness careers: The chronic illness experience. *Journal of Advanced Nursing, 24*(2), 275–279.

Public Health Agency of Canada. (2008). Chronic respiratory diseases facts and figures. Retrieved from http://www.phac-aspc.gc.ca/cd-mc/crd-mrc/crd_ figures-mrc_figures-eng.php

Public Health Agency of Canada. (2009). Tracking heart disease and stroke in Canada. Retrieved from http://www.phac-aspc.gc.ca/publicat/2009/cvd-avc /report-rapport-eng.php

Public Health Agency of Canada. (2011). Diabetes in Canada: Facts and figures from a public health perspective. Retrieved from http://www.phac-aspc.gc.ca /cd-mc/publications/diabetes-diabete/facts-figures-faits-chiffres-2011/index-eng.php

Quan, H., Fong. A., De Coster, C., Wang, J., Musto, R., Noseworthy, T., & Ghali, W. A. (2006). Variations in health services utilization among ethnic populations. *Canadian Medical Association Journal, 174*(6), 787–791.

Romanow, R. J. (2002). Building on values. The future of health care in Canada (Cat. No. CP32-85/2002E-IN). Retrieved from http://publications.gc.ca/collections /Collection/CP32-85-2002E.pdf

Segall, A., & Fries, C. (2011). *Pursuing health and wellness: Healthy societies and healthy people*. Don Mills, ON: Oxford University Press.

Statistics Canada. (2010a). Population projections for Canada, provinces and territories 2009 to 2036 (Cat. No. 91-520-X). Retrieved from http://www .statcan.gc.ca/pub/91-520-x/91-520-x2010001-eng .pdf

Statistics Canada. (2010b). Ethnocultural portrait of Canada highlight tables, 2006 Census. Retrieved from http://www12.statcan.ca/census-recensement/2006 /dp-pd/hlt/97-562/pages/page.cfm?Lang=E&Geo=PR &Code=01&Table=1&Data=Dist&StartRec=1&Sort= 2&Display=Page

Statistics Canada. (2010c). Projections of the diversity of the Canadian population 2006–2031 (Cat. No. 91-551-XWE). Retrieved from http://www.statcan .gc.ca/pub/91-551-x/91-551-x2010001-eng.pdf

Strauss, A. (1975). *Chronic illness and the quality of life*. St. Louis, MO: Mosby.

Strauss, A., Corbin, J., Fagerhaugh, S., Glaser, B., Maines, D., Suczek, B., & Weiner, C. L. (1984). *Chronic illness and the quality of life* (2nd ed.). St. Louis, MO: Mosby.

Swanson, L. (2007). Geriatrics: The "sexy specialty." *Canadian Medical Association Journal, 176*(3), 310.

Treasury Board of Canada Secretariat. (2007). Analysis of program activities by strategic outcome: Health promotion and chronic disease. Retrieved from http://www.tbs-sct.gc.ca/rpp/2007-2008/PHAC-ASPC/phac-aspc02-eng.asp

Turcotte, M., & Schellenberg, G. (2007). A portrait of seniors in Canada (2006) (Cat. No. 89-519-XIE). Ottawa, ON: Statistics Canada. Retrieved from http://www.statcan.gc.ca/

Vegda, K., Nie, J., Wang, L., Tracy, C. S., Moinedden, R., & Upshur, R. (November, 2009). Trends in health services utilization, medication use, and health conditions among older adults: A 2-year retrospective chart review in a primary health practice. *BMC Health Services Research, 9*, 217.

Wood, M. J. (2010). Research as a basis for practice. In J. C. Ross-Kerr & M. J. Woods (Eds.), *Canadian fundamentals of nursing* (revised 4th ed., pp. 74–88). Toronto, ON: Elsevier Canada.

World Health Organization. (n.d.). Facing the facts: The impact of chronic disease in Canada. Retrieved from http://www.who.int/chp/chronic_disease_report/media/CANADA.pdf

World Health Organization. (1946). *Constitution of the World Health Organization: Chronicle of the World Health Organization 1.* Geneva, Switzerland: Author.

World Health Organization. (2005). *Preparing a health care workforce for the 21st century: The challenge of chronic conditions.* Geneva, Switzerland: Author.

World Health Organization (2008). *2008–2013 Action plan for the global strategy for the prevention and control of noncommunicable diseases.* Geneva, Switzerland: Author.

World Health Organization. (2011). Chronic diseases and health promotion. Retrieved from http://www.who.int/chp/en/index.html

CHAPTER 2

Models of Care

Original chapter by Pamala D. Larsen
Canadian content added by Marnie L. Kramer-Kile

INTRODUCTION

As the population age 65 and older increases and the healthcare system sees more individuals with chronic illness, healthcare providers and third-party payers are examining how to care for individuals with chronic disease long term. Increasingly, we hear about disease management models that have demonstrated better patient outcomes than "usual care." Less well publicized, however, is nursing's role in caring for individuals with chronic disease. For some of us it has always made sense that chronic care should be nursing's domain, particularly as the profession looks at care as opposed to cure. We highlight and support the role of nursing research in chronic care throughout this chapter. However, all healthcare professionals (HCPs) share the responsibility of chronic illness prevention and management. Many interdisciplinary frameworks could lend themselves to improved client outcomes. We use the term "healthcare professional" to address the following occupational titles: registered nurses, licensed practical nurses (also referred to as registered practical nurse), physicians, health behaviourists, social workers,

respiratory therapists, occupational therapists, physiotherapists, and dieticians. Chronic disease management is a collaborative effort, the client remains the central focus, and all HCPs need to be aware of how to help clients better manage their conditions. HCPs can do this by providing comprehensive and coordinated care to meet all the needs of the client.

This chapter provides an overview of models and frameworks that provide care for individuals with chronic illness and their families. Two models in particular, the chronic care model (CCM) and the expanded chronic care model (ECCM), provide a foundation for the discussion throughout this chapter. To begin this discussion it is important to first differentiate between *disease* and *illness* models of care.

HISTORICAL PERSPECTIVES

Disease Management Versus Illness Management

Most models available today for patient care are disease management models. These models monitor the physiological markers of disease, the measurement of one's glycosylated hemoglobin (HbA1c), the forced expiratory volume of a patient with chronic obstructive pulmonary disease (COPD), the number of medications prescribed to a patient, the number of visits to the healthcare provider, and so forth. However, looking at the disease, the pathophysiology, and the required medications is only one part of caring for the patient and is, quite frankly, the easier part—the measurable part. The illness experience of an individual patient, the uniqueness of the patient, and the patient's living situation, social support, and coping mechanisms— whether effective or ineffective—are the other components of the patient's life that disease management programs do not address.

Interventions

Most literature today looks at disease management models versus illness management models. However, in most studies the definition of disease management and the components of each program vary, making it hard to compare programs and health outcomes of participants. When performing a meta-analysis or systematic review, it becomes difficult to figure out inclusion criteria for studies, because each program is different. Furthermore, when looking at outcomes, the question is what specific component of the program "makes a difference" in the health outcome or is it the combination of components acting interdependently?

Mattke, Seid, and Ma (2007), in their analysis of disease management programs, suggested in broad terms that disease management refers to a system of coordinated healthcare interventions and communications to help patients address chronic disease and other health conditions. Disease management programs are "big business," with 96% of the top 150 U.S. payers

offering some form of disease management service and 83% of more than 500 major U.S. employers using programs to help individuals manage their health (as cited in Mattke et al., 2007). Revenues associated with these programs have grown significantly from $78 million in 1997 to nearly $1.2 billion in 2005 and were projected to top $1.8 billion by the end of 2008 (Mattke et al., 2007). What are the health outcomes of spending $1 to $2 billion a year? Are these programs making a difference in health outcomes, and, if so, are they reducing costs in other areas?

In their review of three evaluations of large-scale, population-based programs, 10 meta-analyses, and 16 systematic reviews covering 317 studies, Mattke and colleagues (2007) found consistent evidence of improved processes of care and disease control but no conclusive support of improved health outcomes. In addition, when the costs of the programs and/or interventions were accounted for and then cost savings subtracted, there was no evidence of a net reduction in medical costs.

Buntin, Jain, Mattke, and Lurie (2009) suggested that results from disease management programs may be skewed because of selection bias. Selection bias includes patients being recruited into programs because they are likely to attain quality and cost benefits (typically, the more engaged client interested in self-management). The conundrum is whether the disease management program itself causes the results or whether it is the selection of the appropriate patients that makes the difference (Buntin et al., 2009).

CHRONIC CARE MODEL

The best known model for providing care to those with chronic disease is the CCM. Work on this model began in the early 1990s with Dr.

Edward Wagner, an internist and director of the Seattle-based MacColl Institute for Healthcare Innovation at the Center for Health Studies, Group Health Cooperative. Wagner identified three issues in providing care to those with chronic illness through primary care (Wielawski, 2006, p. 5):

1. Primary care offices are set up to respond to acute illnesses rather than to anticipate and respond proactively to patients' needs (which is what individuals with chronic illness need).
2. Patients with chronic illness are not adequately informed about their conditions and they are not supported in the self-care of their conditions beyond the physician's office.
3. Physicians are too busy to educate and support patients with chronic illness to the degree needed for them to stay healthy.

Wagner's (1998) solution was to replace the physician-centred office with a structure that supported a team of professionals that collaborated with the patient in his or her care. Early implementation of his model took place with 15,000 diabetic patients at the Group Health Cooperative, a 590,000-member health maintenance organization in Seattle. Over 5 years the percentage of patients with up-to-date screening improved, blood sugar levels and the regularity of monitoring improved, patients reported higher satisfaction with their care, and admission to acute care facilities decreased.

During the mid- to late 1990s Wagner and associates partnered with the Robert Wood Johnson Foundation to further develop the model. The model was refined and published in its current form in 1998. Improving Chronic Illness Care (2006–2011), a national program through the Robert Wood Johnson Foundation, was launched in 1998 with the CCM as its core (**Figure 2-1**). *The CCM is not a model for individual care but for large populations of individuals.* It does not redesign patient care but redesigns clinical practices that are delivering care by implementing system and process change.

A 2009 intervention review of an earlier Cochrane Review supported the use of the CCM with clients with both type 1 and type 2 diabetes. Forty-one studies with a total of 48,000 clients were involved in the review. Renders and colleagues (2000) concluded that multifaceted professional interventions can enhance the performance of HCPs in managing clients with diabetes. Although using the model enhanced process outcomes, the effect on client health outcomes was less clear.

Studies from 2000 through 2009 were reviewed to determine the impact of the CCM in redesigning care. For this review a CCM-based intervention was defined as an intervention that integrated changes that involved most or all six areas of the model: self-management support, decision support, delivery system design, clinical information systems, healthcare organization, and community resources (Coleman, Austin, Brach, & Wagner, 2009). Eighty-two studies were retained for the final study. Published evidence suggested that practices redesigned in accord with the CCM generally improve the quality of care and outcomes for patients with various chronic illnesses (Coleman et al., 2009).

Although the CCM is a model for primary medical care, Jacelon, Furman, Rea, Macdonald, and Donaghue (2011) adapted the model for long-term care. The six constructs of the CCM were implemented to create a model for high-quality chronic disease care.

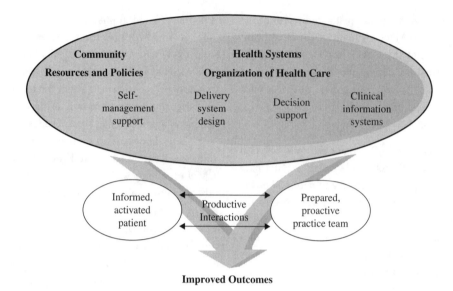

FIGURE 2-1   The chronic care model.
Source: Wagner, E. H. (1998). Chronic disease management: What will it take to improve care for chronic illness? *Effective Clinical Practice, 1,* 2–4.

EXPANDED CHRONIC CARE MODEL

A central critique of the CCM is that it places less emphasis on prevention and health promotion. The ECCM was developed in Canada by Barr et al. (2003) to address elements of population health promotion to further recognize the social determinants of health and to enhance community participation as part of the health system teams (**Figure 2-2**). This action-driven model works to broaden the focus of chronic care management towards health outcomes for individuals, communities, and populations. It expands on the CCM in two ways: (1) It includes a porous border between the formal health system and the community and (2) it re-situates four areas of focus: self-management support, decision support, delivery system design, and information systems. These four areas straddle the border between the health system and

community because they can have a significant impact on both healthcare organization and community involvement. The ECCM also modifies the previous community oval of the CCM by including significant areas for health promotion outlined by the Ottawa Charter, which includes building healthy public policy, creating supportive environments, and strengthening community action. The goals of this model are to have activated communities and clients and prepared practice teams and community partners. **Table 2-1**, created by Barr et al. (2003), compares the CCM and the ECCM.

The ECCM remains a central framework for Canadian nurses working with individuals, families, communities, and populations living with chronic conditions. Canada has been a world leader in the field of health promotion, and it has been recognized that the management of chronic illness must extend to include the community in illness support and management.

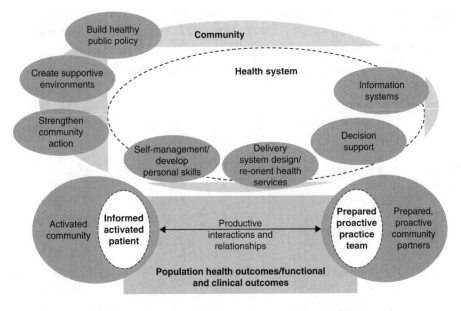

FIGURE 2-2 Expanded chronic care model: Integrating population health promotion. (*Source:* Barr, V. J., Robinson, S., Marin-Link, B., Underhill, L., Dotts, A., Ravensdale, D., & Salvaras, S. (2003). The expanded chronic care model: An integration of concepts and strategies from population health promotion and the chronic care model. *Hospital Quarterly, 7*(1), 73–82.

GUIDED CARE

Using the CCM as a basis, researchers at Johns Hopkins University developed a care model, called guided care, to improve the quality of life and efficiency of resource utilization for older adults with multiple chronic conditions. Guided care enhances the use of primary care (versus specialty care) and uses the following seven principles of chronic care: disease management, self-management, case management, lifestyle modification, transitional care, caregiver education and support, and geriatric evaluation and management (Boyd et al., 2007). The guided care model is unique in that it uses registered nurses specially trained in guided care concepts who use a computerized electronic health record in working with two to five primary care physicians to meet the needs of 50 to 60 older adults with multiple comorbidities. The guided care nurse (GCN) is based in the primary care physician's office and performs eight clinical activities, guided by scientific evidence and the patients' priorities. Pilot versions of guided care included several of the eight core activities.

The first major application of guided care occurred in a cluster-randomized controlled trial through Johns Hopkins University. The study used eight sites (49 physicians) in the Baltimore–Washington, DC area, with 904 patients in either the experimental group of guided care or the control group (usual care) (Boult et al., 2008). Patients eligible for the study were those 65 years old or older and ranking in the upper quartile of risk for using health services during the coming year.

Table 2-1   Comparison of the CCM with the ECCM

Components of the CCM		Components of the ECCM		
Component	**Definition**	**Component**	**Definition**	**Examples**
Health system—organization of health care	Program planning that includes measurable goals for better care of chronic illness			
Self-management support	Emphasis on the importance of the central role that clients have in managing their own care	Self-management/develop personal skills	Enhancing skills and capacities for personal health and wellness	Smoking prevention and cessation programs Senior walking programs
Decision support	Integration of evidence-informed guidelines into daily clinical practice	Decision support	Integration of strategies for facilitating the community's abilities to stay healthy	Development of a health promotion and prevention "best practice" guidelines
Delivery system design	Focus on teamwork and an expanded scope of practice to support chronic care	Delivery system design/re-orient health services	Expansion of mandate to support individuals and communities in a more holistic way	Advocacy on behalf of (and with) vulnerable populations Emphasis in quality improvement on health and quality of life outcomes, not just clinical outcomes
Clinical information systems	Developing information systems based on patient populations to provide relevant client data	Build healthy public policy	Development and implementation of policies designed to improve population health	Use of broad community needs assessments that take into account poverty rates, availability of public transportation, violent crime rate

Table 2-1   Comparison of the CCM with the ECCM *(continued)*

Components of the CCM		Components of the ECCM		
Component	**Definition**	**Component**	**Definition**	**Examples**
Community resources and policies	Developing partnerships with community organizations that support and meet patients' needs	Building healthy public policy	Development and implementation of policies designed to improve population health	Advocating for/ developing smoking bylaws, walking trails, reductions in the price of whole wheat flour
		Create supportive environments	Generating living and employment conditions that are safe, stimulating, satisfying, and enjoyable	Maintaining older people in their homes for as long as possible Working towards the development of well-lit streets and bicycle paths
		Strengthen community action	Working with community groups to set priorities and achieve goals that enhance the health of the community	Supporting the community in addressing the need for safe, affordable housing

Source: Reprinted with permission from Barr, V. J., Robinson, S., Marin-Link, B., Underhill, L., Dotts, A., Ravensdale, D., & Salvaras, S. (2003). The expanded chronic care model: An integration of concepts and strategies from population health promotion and chronic care model. *Hospital Quarterly, 7*(1), 73–82.

The eight clinical activities performed by the GCN were as follows:

1. *Assessment.* Initial assessments include medical, functional, cognitive, affective, psychosocial, nutritional, and environmental. Other tools used may include the Geriatric Depression Scale and the CAGE alcoholism scale. The client is also asked what his or her priorities are for improved quality of life.

2. *Planning.* The electronic health record merges the assessment data with evidence-informed practice guidelines to create a preliminary care guide that manages and monitors the patients' health conditions. The GCN and the primary care physician then personalize the care guide with input from the patient and family. The result is a patient-friendly version of the plan, called "My Action Plan," written in lay language and given to the patient.

3. *Chronic disease self-management.* The GCN encourages the patient's self-efficacy in the management of his or her chronic conditions. The patient is referred to a free, local, 15-hour chronic disease self-management course led by trained lay people and supported by the GCN. In this program—developed by Kate Lorig and associates at Stanford University—the patient learns how to operationalize the action plan.

4. *Monitoring.* The GCN monitors each patient at least monthly by telephone to address issues promptly. The electronic health record plays an important role in the monitoring by providing reminders about each patient (Boyd et al., 2007).

5. *Coaching.* Motivational interviewing is used to facilitate the patient's participation in care along with reinforcing adherence to the action plan (Boyd et al., 2007). The GCNs are trained in motivational interviewing principles and strategies to assist in this process.

6. *Coordinating transitions between sites and providers of care.* The GCN is the primary coordinator of care for patients in this program and is thus responsible for the care transitions that occur between home, the emergency department, hospitals, long-term care facilities, and other care settings.

7. *Educating and supporting caregivers.* The GCN works with family or other unpaid caregivers of the patients to educate and support them. This may include individual or group assistance, support group meetings, or ad hoc telephone consultation (Boyd et al., 2007).

8. *Accessing community resources.* Determining appropriate community resources for the patient, such as Meals on Wheels, transportation needs, and so forth, is a key function of the GCN. The idea is not to duplicate services but to utilize the services available in the community.

In April 2008, 6 months into the randomized controlled trial, data suggested that the guided care model provided improved quality of care, reduced medical care costs, and high satisfaction in both the primary care physicians and the GCNs (Boult et al., 2008). Based on these early results two of the managed care partners in the trial, Kaiser Permanente and Johns Hopkins HealthCare, agreed to continue to pay the costs of the GCNs for an additional year. However, 18-month outcomes demonstrated few results. The study examined the use of health services and included 850 older patients at high risk for using health care in the future. The only statistically significant overall effect of guided care was a reduction in episodes of home health care (Boult et al., 2011).

SELF-MANAGEMENT PROGRAMS

The term "self-management" initially appeared in a book by Thomas Creer on the rehabilitation of children with chronic illness (Lorig & Holman, 2003). Creer and colleagues used the concept to indicate that the patient was an active participant in his or her care. Creer and Holroyd (2006) stated that self-management differs from adherence in that "self-management places greater emphasis on the patient's active role in decision-making, both inside and outside the consultation room" (p. 8). Self-management is also seen as different from disease management. Creer and

Holroyd (2006) viewed disease management as being more focused on HCPs' algorithms and interventions to standardize care as opposed to self-management, which emphasizes patients' involvement in defining the problems.

Lorig and colleagues' (1999) work at Stanford University conceptualized best what we know about self-management programs. Their work is based on Corbin and Strauss' (1992) framework of medical management, role management, and emotional management. These concepts, along with how the chronic condition is perceived by the patient and family, are hallmarks of Lorig's work. Lorig's framework for self-management programs includes five core self-management skills: problem solving, decision making, resource utilization, forming of a patient–healthcare provider partnership, and taking action (Lorig & Holman, 2003).

Empirical results of self-management programs have been mixed. What follows are examples of the literature in this area. Lorig and colleagues (1999) studied 952 patients, 40 years of age and older with a diagnosis of heart disease, lung disease, stroke, or arthritis, in a 6-month-long randomized controlled trial. The chronic disease self-management program consisted of seven weekly 2.5-hour sessions on making management choices and achieving success in reaching self-selected goals as opposed to prescribing specific behaviour changes (Lorig et al., 1999).

Outcome measures included health behaviours, health status, and health service utilization. At 6 months the experimental group demonstrated improvements in weekly minutes of exercise, frequency of cognitive symptom management, communication with physicians, and self-reported health. Participants also had decreased fatigue and disability and less social/role-activity limitations with less health distress, fatigue, and disability. There were no differences between the groups in pain/physical discomfort, shortness of breath, or psychological well-being (Lorig et al., 1999).

In a more recent study of the chronic disease self-management program, researchers, using data from previous chronic disease self-management programs in English and Spanish, examined whether there were statistically significant interactions between baseline status and randomization in estimating 6-month changes in health status (Ritter, Lee, & Lorig, 2011). The researchers were looking for moderators that might affect outcome variables. Results demonstrated no moderating factors that consistently predicted improved health outcomes.

Warsi, Wang, LaValley, Avorn, and Solomon (2004) conducted a systematic review of the literature from 1964 to 1999 and reviewed 71 clinical trials. Diabetic patients had reductions in HbA1c levels and improvements in systolic blood pressure, and asthmatic patients experienced fewer attacks. Arthritis self-management education programs were not associated with statistically significant effects. Warsi and colleagues found a large number of limitations with the studies they reviewed. The methods of conducting (i.e., study design) and reporting these trials were suboptimal. There was also evidence of publication bias (Warsi et al., 2004).

Chodosh and colleagues (2005) assessed the effectiveness of self-management programs with a meta-analysis design. Of the 780 studies screened, 53 met the researchers' criteria for inclusion. Self-management interventions led to statistically and clinically significant results of decreased HbA1c (amounting to a decrease of 0.81%), a decrease of 5 mm Hg in systolic blood pressure, and a decrease of 4.3 mm Hg in diastolic blood pressure. There were no significant results for participants with osteoarthritis in either pain or function. Their conclusion was that the studies had variable quality, making it difficult to analyze, and there was possible publication bias present. In addition, it was not clear what constituted a self-management program.

One of the more recognized self-management programs is the Flinders program (formally known as the Flinders model). The Flinders program is described as an approach to help enable HCPs to empower their clients to become active partners in their care and more effective self-managers (Health Council of Canada, 2009).

According to the Flinders University website (http://www.flinders.edu.au/medicine/sites/fhbhru/self-management.cfm), the aim of the program is to provide a consistent, reproducible approach to assessing the key components of self-management that

- Improves the partnership between the client and health professional(s)
- Collaboratively identifies problems and therefore better (i.e., more successfully) targets interventions
- Is a motivational process for the client and leads to sustained behaviour change
- Allows measurement over time and tracks change
- Has a predictive ability (i.e., improvements in self-management behaviour as measured by the PIH scale) related to improved health outcomes

The Flinders care planning process is described as having five functions. The first function focuses on generic and holistic chronic condition management; this includes assessment and planning for specific disease management. This is identified as a client-centred approach that incorporates biopsychosocial aspects of care. The second function involves the use of the Partners in Health scale as a screening tool to determine which clients will benefit from full care planning and case management. It is recognized that each person living with a chronic condition will need differing levels of support. The third function of the planning process is to assess the client's self-management knowledge and to identify any behaviours or barriers that may impede self-management activities. The fourth function of the program focuses on systemic and organizational change. More specifically, the program provides a longitudinal structure to help enact specific care plans within wider institutional contexts. The fifth function of the Flinders program is to change clinicians' understanding of their practice in delivering client-centred care and to ensure that HCPs ensure clients are fully engaged in the delivery of their own care. For more information about the Flinders program please see the following link: http://www.flinders.edu.au/medicine/sites/fhbhru/self-management.cfm.

The following studies incorporated this program approach to the management of chronic conditions. Battersby and colleagues (2010) completed a pilot program for aboriginal people with diabetes in South Australia. The acceptability and impact of the Flinders model was tested by using it to guide patient self-management for community members living with diabetes. Aboriginal health workers conducted patient-centred self-management assessment and care planning (Battersby et al., 2010). Impacts were measured by patient-completed diabetes self-management assessment tools, client goal achievement, client quality of life, and clinical measures at baseline and 12 months, as well as by semistructured interviews and focus groups of the aboriginal health workers. At the end of the program self-management scores improved and the mean HbA1c was reduced from 8.74 to 8.09. It was concluded that the self-management program provided by the aboriginal health workers was accepted by the community and demonstrated appropriate client outcomes.

Lawn and Lauton (2011) reported the steps taken by HCPs to embed a chronic condition self-management program for COPD within an Australian respiratory nursing service between 2008 and 2010. This change to practice was undertaken by the respiratory nurses using the CCM and the Flinders program. These frameworks helped the nurses to recognize the importance of changing to meet clients' self-management needs and in turn also provided supportive tools for data collection, helped to assess the staff's readiness for change, mapped barriers and enablers to the program, and helped the HCP to plan short- and long-term impacts of the program. Overall, the program resulted in a coordinated service for patients with COPD across inpatient and community continuums. Both studies supported the use of the Flinders program for the development of self-management programs.

A Cochrane Review on self-management programs, led by lay leaders, was completed in 2007. The review included 17 studies with 7,442 individuals with chronic conditions such as arthritis, diabetes, hypertension, and chronic

pain. Many of the programs were similar but differed in designated conditions and the outcomes that each researcher reported. Overall, the programs led to modest, short-term improvements in patients' confidence to manage their condition and perceptions of their own health. There were increases in the amount of aerobic exercise by participants. Although there were some improvements in pain, disability, fatigue, and depression, the changes were not clinically significant. The programs did not improve quality of life for the individuals, alter the number of doctor visits for these individuals, or reduce hospitalizations (Foster, Taylor, Eldridge, Ramsay, & Griffiths, 2007).

TRANSITIONAL CARE

Naylor, Aiken, Kurtzman, Olds, and Hirschman (2011) conducted a systematic review of literature and summarized 21 randomized clinical trials of transitional care interventions targeting adults with chronic illness. Transitional care is defined as a broad range of time-limited services designed to ensure healthcare continuity, avoid preventable poor outcomes among at-risk populations, and promote the safe and timely transfer of patients from one level of care to another or from one type of setting to another (Coleman & Boult, 2003). Transitions have been associated with increased rates of potentially avoidable hospitalizations. A 2009 study reported that approximately 20% of Medicare beneficiaries discharged from hospitals were rehospitalized within 30 days and that 34% were readmitted within 90 days (as cited in Naylor et al., 2011).

The review (Naylor et al., 2011) of transitional care provided 21 studies focusing on adults with chronic illness transitioning from an acute care hospital to another setting. There was a mean sample size of 377 subjects among the studies. A variety of primary and secondary outcomes in five categories was reported: health outcomes, quality of life, patient satisfaction or perception of care, resource use, and costs. Among the 21 studies, all but 1 reported positive findings in at least one category. The 21 interventions discussed in the articles (Naylor et al., 2011) varied in terms of their nature, point of initiation, intensity, and duration. The largest group of studies could be characterized as comprehensive discharge planning and follow-up with (four studies) or without (three studies) home visits. The remainder dealt with disease or case management (four studies), education or psychoeducation (two studies), peer support (two studies), telehealth facilitation (one study), post-discharge geriatric assessment (one study), and intensive primary care (one study). Eighteen of the studies designated a nurse, most frequently an advanced practice nurse (10 studies), as the intervention's clinical manager or leader. Overall, the authors concluded a robust body of evidence supported the benefits of transitional care. Studies of nine interventions demonstrated a positive effect on at least one measure of readmissions; eight of the nine reduced all-cause readmission through at least 30 days after discharge. Three studies effectively reduced readmissions for at least 6 or 12 months after discharge. Each of these three studies included a focus on patient self-management (Naylor et al., 2011).

CASE STUDY

Mary Brown is an 80-year-old widow living alone on her farm 5 miles from town in a western rural province. Mrs. Brown's town, with a population of 10,000, has a critical access hospital. She lives in the farmhouse she moved to when she married 60 years ago. She would like to stay there as long as possible, but after her hip replacement surgery last fall her mobility is not as good as it used to be. She is mildly hypertensive and is on medication. Her type 2 diabetes is under control with diet and medication. She has lots of friends in the community, but her grown children live several provinces away. Because of her isolation and age she might be considered "at risk."

Discussion Questions

1. What are Mrs. Brown's "at-risk" variables?
2. What self-management tasks should be initiated with her?
3. What does Mrs. Brown need? What are her potential needs? This is a small community with few resources available. Be creative and develop a model of care for her.

Guided care, a model of care developed from the CCM, was evaluated in a randomized controlled trial in the Washington, DC–Baltimore, Maryland, area. Eligible patients from three healthcare systems were cluster-randomized to receive guided care or usual care for 20 months between November 1, 2006, and June 30, 2008. Eight services were provided by GCNs working in partnership with patients' primary care physicians: comprehensive assessment, evidence-informed care planning, monthly monitoring of symptoms and adherence, transitional care, coordination of HCPs, support for self-management, support for family caregivers, and enhanced access to community services. The study included 850 older patients at high risk for using health care in the future. The only statistically significant overall effect of guided care was a reduction in episodes of home health care. In a preplanned analysis, guided care also reduced skilled nursing facility admissions among Kaiser-Permanente patients.

Source: Boult et al. (2011)

ONLINE DISEASE MANAGEMENT

A retrospective, quasi-experimental cohort design evaluated program participants in an online disease management program (through Blue Cross Blue Shield) and a matched cohort of nonparticipants. The study was conducted with 413 online participants and 360 nonparticipants. The online program was a commercially available, tailored program for chronic disease self-management. Healthcare costs per person per year were $757 less than predicted for participants relative to matched nonparticipants, yielding a return on investment of $9.89 for every dollar spent on the program (Schwartz et al., 2010).

TELEHEALTH

Telehealth or home telemonitoring and telephone support provides client or caregiving support, advice, education, and follow-up by healthcare providers through telephone contact. In Canada home telehealth is most commonly used to manage diabetes, heart failure, and COPD (Canadian Agency for Drugs and Technologies in Health [CADTH], 2008). This modality of care is a useful addition to Canadian healthcare delivery, but ethical, legal, and psychological issues may arise from existing models. The research on the efficacy of telehealth has had varying results. In the case of diabetes it was found that telehealth helped clients to achieve better glycaemic control, whereas studies focusing on COPD found higher mortality rates among clients using telehealth (although the authors stated that due to a limited number of studies in this area these results should be interpreted with caution) (CADTH, 2008). Patients, particularly in rural areas, have linked increased satisfaction with this modality when used in conjunction with other models of care and access to the healthcare system. Although telehealth is often presented as a service modality that will save money for the Canadian healthcare system, further studies are needed to confirm this (CADTH, 2008).

OUTCOMES

With any model of care for individuals and families with chronic conditions, an expected outcome is that both the disease and illness experience are managed appropriately and some cost savings are realized. This chapter has demonstrated mixed results for the models currently in practice. It is still unclear how the Canadian healthcare system should be organized to best provide care for those with chronic illness. What is not "measured" in these models is how these programs or models of care affect the illness experience of the individual and family. Can we say that because an individual with a chronic illness has a lower HbA1c, or has not been hospitalized within the last 6 months, or checks his or her blood glucose level regularly, he or she has a better quality of life or experiences more life satisfaction or, in the terms of Strauss and colleagues (1984), is successful at normalizing his or her life? Perhaps in the near future managing the illness experience of the client with chronic illness will be a higher priority.

STUDY QUESTIONS

1. How do self-management components of care fit within a disease management program?
2. What role does (or should) the advanced practice nurse have in disease management?
3. What are the benefits of disease management models of care?
4. Identify the issues involved with a disease management model of care for an older adult.

STUDY QUESTIONS (Cont.)

5. How do we as nurses care for individuals and families and their *illness experience* within a disease management model?
6. After reading about different models of care in this chapter, what do you believe should be included in a model of care for an older adult with multiple comorbidities?

INTERNET RESOURCES

Chronic Disease Self-Management Program, Stanford University: patienteducation.stanford.edu/programs/cdsmp.html
Commonwealth Fund: www.commonwealthfund.org
Guided Care: www.guidedcare.org
Improving Chronic Illness Care: www.improvingchroniccare.org

For a full suite of assignments and additional learning activities, use the access code located in the front of your book and visit this exclusive website: **http://go.jblearning.com/kramer-kile**. If you do not have an access code, you can obtain one at the site.

REFERENCES

Barr, V. J., Robinson, S., Marin-Link, B., Underhill, L., Dotts, A., Ravensdale, D., & Salvaras, S. (2003). The expanded chronic care model: An integration of concepts and strategies from population health promotion and chronic care model. *Hospital Quarterly*, 7(1), 73–82.

Battersby, M. W., Kit, J. A., Prideaux, C., Collins, J. P., Harvey, P., & Mills, P. D. (2010). Implementing the Flinders model of self-management support with aboriginal people who have diabetes: Findings from a pilot study. In A. Larsen & D. Lyle (Eds.), *A bright future for rural health: Evidence based policy and practice in rural and remote Australian* (pp. 31–33). Melbourne, Australia: ARHEN.

Boult, C., Reider, L., Frey, K., Leff, B., Boyd, C. M., Wolff, J. L., . . . Scharfstein, D. O. (2008). Early effects of "guided care" on the quality of health care for multimorbid older persons: A cluster-randomized controlled trial. *Journal of Gerontology: Medical Sciences, 73A*(3), 321–327.

Boult, C., Reider, L., Leff, B., Frick, K. D., Boyd, C. M., Wolff, J. L., . . . Scharfstein, D. O. (2011). The effect of guided care teams on the use of health services: Results from a cluster-randomized controlled trial. *Archives of Internal Medicine, 171*(5), 460–466.

Boyd, C. M., Boult, C., Shadmi, E., Leff, B., Brager, R., Dunbar, L., . . . Wegener, S. (2007). Guided care for multimorbid older adults. *The Gerontologist, 47*(5), 697–704.

Buntin, M. B., Jain, A. K., Mattke, S., & Lurie, N. (2009). Who gets disease management? *Journal of General Internal Medicine, 24*(5), 649–655.

Canadian Agency for Drugs and Technologies in Health. (2008). Home telehealth for chronic disease management. Ottawa, ON: Author. Retrieved from http://www.cadth.ca/Index.php/en/hta/reports-publications/search/publication/865

Chodosh, J., Morton, S. C., Mojica, W., Maglione, M., Suttorp, M. J., Hilton, L., . . . Shekelle, P. (2005). Meta-analysis: Chronic disease self-management programs for older adults [Electronic version]. *Annals of Internal Medicine, 143*, 427–438.

Coleman, E. A., & Boult, C. (2003). Improving the quality of transitional care for persons with complex care needs. *Journal of the American Geriatrics Society, 51*(4), 556–557.

Coleman, K., Austin, B. T., Brach, C., & Wagner, E. H. (2009). Evidence on the chronic care model in the new millennium. *Health Affairs, 28*(1), 75–85.

Corbin, J., & Strauss, A. (1992). A nursing model for chronic illness management based upon the trajectory framework. In P. Woog (Ed.), *The chronic illness tra-jectory framework: The Corbin and Strauss nursing model* (pp. 9–28). New York, NY: Springer.

Creer, T., & Holroyd, K. A. (2006). Self-management of chronic conditions: The legacy of Sir William Osler. *Chronic Illness, 2*(1), 7–14.

Foster, G., Taylor, S. J. C., Eldridge, S., Ramsay, J., & Griffiths, C. J. (2007). Self-management education programmes led by lay leaders for people with chronic health conditions. *Cochrane Database of Systematic Reviews, 17*(4), CD005108.

Health Council of Canada. (2009). *Getting it right: Case studies of effective management of chronic disease using primary health care teams.* Toronto. ON: Health Council. Retrieved from www.healthcouncil canada.ca

Improving Chronic Illness Care. (2006–2011). Chronic care model. Retrieved from http://www.improvingchronic care.org/index.php?p=The_Chronic_Care_Model&s=2

Jacelon, C., Furman, E., Rea, A., Macdonald, B., & Donaghue, L. C. (2011). Creating a professional practice model for postacute care. *Journal of Gerontological Nursing, 37*(3), 53–60.

Lawn, S. J., & Lawton, K. (2011). Chronic condition self-management support within a respiratory nursing service. *Journal of Nursing and Healthcare of Chronic Illness, 3*(4), 372–380.

Lorig, K., & Holman, H. R. (2003). Self-management education: History, definition, outcomes and mechanisms. *Annals of Behavioral Medicine, 26*(1), 1–7.

Lorig, K. R., Sobel, D. S., Steward, A. L., Brown, B. W., Bandura, A., Ritter, P., . . . Holman, H. R. (1999). Evidence suggesting that a chronic disease self-management program can improve health status while reducing hospitalization: A randomized trial. *Medical Care, 37*(1), 5–14.

Mattke, S., Seid, M., & Ma, S. (2007). Evidence for the effect of disease management: Is $1 billion a year a good investment? *American Journal of Managed Care, 13*, 670–676.

Naylor, M. D., Aiken, L. H., Kurtzman, E. T., Olds, D. M., & Hirschman, K. B. (2011). The importance of transitional care in achieving health reform. *Health Affairs, 30*(4), 746–754.

Renders, C. M., Valk, G. D., Griffin, S. J., Wagner, E., vanEijk, J. T., & Assendelft, W. J. J. (2000). Interventions to improve the management of diabetes mellitus in primary care, outpatient and community settings. *Cochrane Database of Systematic Reviews,* (4), CD001481.

Ritter, P. L., Lee, J., & Lorig, K. (2011). Moderators of chronic disease self-management programs: Who benefits? *Chronic Illness, 7*(2), 162–172.

Schwartz, S. M., Day, B., Wildenhaus, K., Silberman, A., Wang, C., & Silberman, J. (2010). The impact of an online disease management program on medical costs among health plan members. *American Journal of Health Promotion, 25*(2), 126–133.

Strauss, A., Corbin, J., Fagerhaugh, S., Glaser, B., Maines, D., Suczek, B., & Wiener, C. (1984). *Chronic illness and the quality of life* (2nd ed.). St. Louis, MO: Mosby.

Wagner, E. H. (1998). Chronic disease management: What will it take to improve care for chronic illness? *Effective Clinical Practice, 1,* 2–4.

Warsi, A., Wang, P. S., LaValley, M., Avorn, J., & Solomon, D. H. (2004). Self-management education programs in chronic disease. A systematic review and methodological critique of the literature. *Archives of Internal Medicine, 164*(15), 1641–1649.

Wielawski, I. M. (2006). Improving chronic illness care. In S. L. Isaacs & J. R. Knickman (Eds.), *To improve health and health care, 10, The Robert Wood Johnson Foundation anthology* (pp. 1–17). Princeton, NJ: Robert Wood Johnson Foundation.

CHAPTER 3

The Illness Experience

Original chapter by Pamala D. Larsen
Canadian content added by Marnie L. Kramer-Kile

> *Illness is the night-side of life, a more onerous citizenship. Everyone who is born holds dual citizenship, in the kingdom of the well and in the kingdom of the sick. Although we all prefer to use only the good passport, sooner or later each of us is obligated, at least for a spell, to identify ourselves as citizens of that other place.*
> —Susan Sontag, *Illness as Metaphor*, 1988, p. 3

INTRODUCTION

Individuals living with chronic illness have to modify or adapt previous behaviours and roles to accommodate the chronicity of their condition. Societal expectations, their own expectations, and their health status all influence illness behaviour. This chapter provides an overview of the illness experience and corresponding behaviour demonstrated by those with chronic illness. It presents a sociological view of illness rather than a medical view. It is not meant to be a comprehensive review of the entire body of knowledge, which is vast.

Chronic disease involves not only the physical body, but it also affects one's relationships, self-image, and behaviour. The social aspects of disease may be related to the pathophysiological changes that are occurring but may be independent of them as well. The very act of diagnosing a condition as an illness has consequences far beyond the pathology involved (Conrad, 2005). Freidson (1970) discussed this more than 40 years ago in his writings about the meaning that is ascribed to a diagnosis by an individual.

Commonly, healthcare providers are educated in the medical model and understand its applicability and use in practice. Clients enter a healthcare system with symptoms, which are then diagnosed based on pathological findings and as such are treated and/or cured with medical treatment. For acute disease this is the pattern. One is not concerned about the client's illness behaviour associated with tonsillitis, a fractured leg, or appendicitis. An individual may be concerned the tonsillitis will return, the fractured leg may not heal normally, or there may be an adverse event associated with the appendectomy, but by and large these concerns pass quickly because of the acuteness of the event. Canada's acute care–focused healthcare system acts on the pathology that is present, with the goal that an individual will fully recover from the condition and return to prior behaviours and roles.

What happens however, when the recovery is incomplete or the illness continues or becomes chronic in nature? It is not merely pathology or a diagnosis anymore, and the individual and family develop their own meanings and perceptions of the condition, and ultimately their own, unique illness behaviours. The earliest concept of illness behaviour was described in a 1929 essay by Henry Sigerist. His essay described the "special position of the sick" (as cited in Young, 2004). Talcott Parsons developed this concept further and described the "sick role" in his 1951 work, *The Social System.* A brief examination of the sick role provides context to the illness experience, perceptions, and behaviour.

SICK ROLE

Talcott Parsons, a proponent of structural–functionalist principles, viewed health as a functional prerequisite of society. From Parsons' point of view sickness was dysfunctional and a form of social deviance (Williams, 2005). From this functionalist viewpoint social systems are linked to systems of personality and culture to form a basis for social order (Cockerham, 2001). Parsons viewed sickness as a response to social pressure that permitted the avoidance of social responsibilities. Anyone could take on the role he identified, because the role was achieved through failure to keep well. The four major components of the sick role are as follows (Williams, 2005, p. 124):

1. The person is exempt from normal social roles.
2. The person is not responsible for his or her condition.
3. The person has the obligation to want to become well.
4. The person has the obligation to seek and cooperate with technically competent help.

Although the sick role may have been previously accepted by sociologists and other disciplines that studied illness behaviour when developed by Parsons in the 1950s, it is no longer considered relevant today. Canadian culture for the most part has embraced the role of self-care and self-management of disease and participation with care providers to obtain optimal health for people living with chronic conditions. Parsons' sick role was based on assumptions about the nature of society and the nature of illness during a previous period of time that lacked these contexts (Weitz, 2007).

Using Parsons' work as a basis, Mechanic (1962) proposed the concept of illness behaviour as symptoms being perceived, evaluated, and acted (or not acted) on differently by different persons. He believed it was essential to understand the influence of norms, values, fears, and expected rewards and punishments on how an individual with illness acts. Mechanic (1995) defined illness behaviour as the "varying ways individuals respond to bodily indications, how they monitor internal states, define and interpret symptoms, make attributions, take remedial actions and utilize various sources of formal and informal care" (p. 1208).

Around the time of Mechanic's earlier work, Kasl and Cobb (1966) identified three types of health-related behaviour:

1. *Health behaviour* is any activity undertaken by a person believing him- or herself to be healthy for the purpose of preventing disease or detecting it in an asymptomatic stage.
2. *Illness behaviour* is any activity undertaken by a person who feels ill to define the state of his or her health and to discover a suitable remedy.
3. *Sick-role behaviour* is the activity undertaken for the purpose of getting well by those who consider themselves ill.

McHugh and Vallis (1986) suggested that perhaps instead of categorizing behaviour as health related, illness related, or as a sick role, it would make more sense to look at illness behaviour on a continuum. By doing this the term "illness behaviour" can be broadly defined, and this characterization may become more helpful, because the distinction between health and illness behaviours is arbitrary at times.

A more current definition of illness behaviour suggests that it "includes all of the individual's life which stems from the experience of illness, including changes in functioning and activity, and uptake of health services and other welfare benefits" (Wainwright, 2008, p. 76). Simply put, when an individual defines him- or herself as ill, different behaviours may be displayed. A behaviour could be as simple as seeking medical treatment or as complex as the individual's emotional response to the diagnosis. As more acute conditions become chronic in nature, there is more interest in how individuals behave in these circumstances. Individuals with chronic illness are living longer and are creating new norms of illness behaviour.

ILLNESS PERCEPTIONS

According to Rudell, Bhui, and Priebe (2009), two theories have dominated illness perception research: (1) the *explanatory model* (Kleinmann, 1985) and (2) *illness representations* as a part of the self-regulatory theory (Leventhal, Leventhal, & Cameron, 2001). Kleinmann, a cross-cultural psychiatrist and anthropologist, associated explanatory models with mental illness, whereas Leventhal and colleagues based their research on psychological theory. Both argue that there are cognitive and emotional representations of illness (Rudell et al., 2009). Although both models hold credence for individuals and families with chronic illness, this chapter uses the work of Leventhal and colleagues as a basis for the discussion of illness perceptions and behaviours.

Before focusing on illness behaviours, a discussion of illness perceptions is required, because they are the basis for the behaviours exhibited by individuals and families. The literature uses two terms, *illness representations* and *illness perceptions*. Both refer to how the client (and family) views the illness. Illness representations belong to clients and are interpreted by clients and may not conform to scientific beliefs (as cited in Diefenbach, Leventhal, Leventhal, & Patrick-Miller, 1996; Lee, Chaboyer, & Wallis, 2010). In most studies illness representations are measured by the Illness Perception Questionnaire, the Illness Perception Questionnaire-revised, or the Brief Illness Perception Questionnaire. Each of these questionnaires assesses the cognitive and emotional responses to illness (www.uib.no.ipq). For purposes of this chapter the terms "illness representations" and "illness perceptions" are used interchangeably, although medical sociologists might question that decision.

Why are illness perceptions of interest to healthcare providers? The primary reason is that these perceptions directly influence the emotional responses clients and families may have towards illness (Petrie & Weinman, 2006). How people behave due to their illness, the coping strategies they draw on, and how they generally responds towards their illness can be based on one's perceptions of the illness itself. Clients and their families do not simply develop their own illness beliefs and perceptions within a vacuum; instead, they are moulded by their everyday social interactions (Marks et al., 2005), their past experiences, and their culture.

The literature provides many definitions of culture. Within the nursing literature each individual with his or her model/theory of transcultural nursing has a different definition. Although there is value in those definitions, perhaps one from medical anthropology offers a broader perspective. Helman (2007) defines culture as "a set of guidelines (both explicit and implicit) that individuals use to view the world and tell them what behaviors are appropriate" (p. 2). Culture is shared, learned, dynamic, and evolutionary (Schim, Doorenbos, Benkert, & Miller, 2007). This evolution is described by Dreher and MacNaughton (2002) as follows: "People live out their lives in communities, where circumstances generate conflict, where people do not always follow the rules, and where cultural norms and institutions are massaged and modified in the exigencies of daily life" (p. 184).

Typically, one thinks of culture as associated with race and ethnicity. However, other cultures exist if a broader definition of culture is used. Examples include the culture of poverty, the culture of cancer survivors, the culture of rurality, and the culture of chronic illness, to name a few. Each of these cultures has explicit and implicit guidelines that determine how their members view the world, decide on appropriate behaviours, and perform those behaviours.

Clients and families build mental models to make sense of an event (Petrie & Weinman, 2006). Thus, when a client and family face a health threat, a model of that event is developed. The idea behind a model is that clients can then visualize the threat and become active problem solvers. Within these models are peoples' perceptions of their diagnosis as well as their illness experience of receiving treatment and potentially dealing with the consequences of the treatment not working or the illness coming to

the point where it affects their daily functioning, which in turn may forecast how they will behave and/or respond to the crisis at hand. Often, these models may not make sense to an outsider and may be built on faulty information. The model is dynamic, changing as new data from healthcare providers, their own experiences, and other sources are presented to the client and family and become incorporated into the model.

Leventhal and colleagues (2001) identified five dimensions that represent a client's view of their illness:

1. *Identity of the illness:* Connecting the symptoms with the illness and having an understanding of the illness
2. *Timeline:* Duration and progression of the illness
3. *Causes:* Perceived reason for the illness
4. *Consequences:* What will be the physical, psychosocial, and economic impact of the illness
5. *Controllability:* Can this disease be controlled or cured?

After identification of these dimensions, Leventhal and colleagues believed that coping and appraisal follow.

However, is it that simple? Leventhal and colleagues' explanation leads one to believe that everything fits into a neat little box and there is a natural, linear progression from identity to control/curability. Imagine a chronic illness has either entered your life or affected someone in your family. You may have had some sort of understanding of the disease before diagnosis, but now that the condition is "yours," that perception may change. Plus, you have the Internet to provide you with more information than you can absorb. You begin with the idea that this condition is controllable, and perhaps curable, but you find a plethora of websites and data that tell you otherwise. Thus, your beliefs and perceptions of the situation can be changed overnight, and in turn, your attitudes and behaviours do so as well.

Clients and families with chronic illness need to make sense of their illness. Their diagnosis may be complicated; at first it may not make sense or may present the person with more questions than answers. As time goes on they may change their perceptions about their disease or begin to face new challenges with their conditions. Their perceptions of illness may fluctuate over time as they reflect on the changes they have made to their daily lives; these perceptions surrounding their chronic disease conditions become an attempt to make sense of the new challenges they face. People may reconstruct their illness perceptions to help them cope through these changes.

The literature about the effects of illness perceptions and beliefs on behaviour and treatment is vast. What follows are some representative research studies that demonstrate current and continuing work in this area. Although there are studies on clients with a number of different chronic illnesses or injuries such as spinal cord injury (deRoon-Cassini, de St. Aubin, Valvano, Hastings, & Horn, 2009), most studies have focused on heart disease.

Heart Disease

Several studies have explored the relationships among quality of life, adherence to and choice of treatment, and illness beliefs/perceptions. Juergens, Seekatz, Moosdorf, Petrie, and Rief (2010) studied 56 patients undergoing coronary artery bypass grafting. Participants were assessed using the Illness Perception Questionnaire-revised before and 3 months after surgery. The

researchers concluded that patients' beliefs before surgery strongly influenced their recovery from surgery. They added that perhaps patients could benefit from presurgery cognitive interventions to change maladaptive beliefs. Similarly, Alsen, Brink, Persson, Brandstrom, and Karlson (2010) found that peoples' illness perceptions influenced health outcomes after myocardial infarction. Broadbent, Ellis, Thomas, Gamble, and Petrie (2009) indicated that a brief in-hospital illness perception intervention changed perceptions and improved rates of return to work in patients with myocardial infarction.

In a sample of clients with atrial fibrillation, clients' perceptions about their symptoms and medication at diagnosis affected their health-related quality of life (Lane, Langman, Lip, & Nouwen, 2009). Negative illness beliefs were significantly predictive of higher levels of depressive symptomology at 3 and 9 months in clients with coronary artery disease (Stafford, Berk, & Jackson, 2009). Illness beliefs were also significantly associated with depressive symptomology and health-related quality of life in clients with coronary artery disease. In a study examining adherence to secondary prevention regimens, illness beliefs contributed to adherence to those behaviours (Stafford, Jackson, & Berk, 2008).

Two representative studies in hypertension included the relationships between treatment and illness perceptions. Chen, Tsai, and Chou (2010) tested a hypothetical model of illness perception and adherence to prescribed medications. Using a sample of 355 hypertensive patients, findings suggested that adherence could be enhanced by improving the patient's perception of controllability. Other researchers argued that illness perceptions/beliefs about hypertension played a role in the choice of medication for treatment of hypertension (Figueiras et al., 2010).

Work Participation

Hoving, van der Meer, Volkova, and Frings-Dresen (2010) completed a systematic review of illness perceptions and participation in work (however, only three studies met the authors' criteria for review). They found that nonworking clients perceived more serious consequences, expected their illness to last a long period of time, and reported more symptoms and emotional responses. The working clients had a strong belief in the controllability of their condition and a better understanding of the disease (its identity).

INFLUENCES ON ILLNESS BEHAVIOUR

Illness behaviour is shaped by sociocultural and social-psychological factors (Mechanic, 1986). What follows in this section are examples of these factors. These factors may include poverty, demographic factors (such as marital status or gender), or previous experiences with illness behaviour role modelled by others (i.e., parents).

Culture of Poverty

The culture of poverty influences the development of social and psychological traits among those experiencing it. Individuals living in poverty may place health lower on their list of priorities as they attempt to live day to day without financial resources. Poverty is synonymous with a present-moment orientation, a lack of planning ahead, and a fatalistic future. The poor, who have to work to survive, often deny sickness unless it brings functional incapacity

(Helman, 2007). For example, Orpana et al. (2007) found that individuals living in households with combined incomes of less than $20,000 per year were almost three times more likely to experience a decline in self-rated health than people with the highest incomes. According to the study, job strain, financial issues, and marital problems were more common among lower income individuals. With poverty, chronic health issues such as substance abuse, smoking, obesity, and incarceration may emerge (Pearson, 2003). However, this is not to suggest that all people with lower means of financial security will face these challenges.

Demographic Status

Marital status may influence illness behaviour as well. In general, married individuals require fewer services because they are healthier but use other services because they are more attuned to preventive care (Thomas, 2003). Searle, Norman, Thompson, and Vedhara (2007) examined the influence of the illness perceptions of clients' significant others and their impact on client outcomes and illness perceptions. Differences in illness representations of significant others and clients have been shown to influence psychological adaptation in chronic fatigue syndrome and Addison's disease (cited in Searle et al., 2007). Searle and colleagues sought to understand illness representations in clients with type 2 diabetes and their partners. However, in this study, almost without exception, there was agreement between the illness representations of patients and their partners. Another aim of the study was to determine the influence of the partner or significant other on the clients' illness representation. There was some evidence to suggest that partners' representations partially mediated clients' representations on exercise and dietary behaviours (Searle et al., 2007).

Gender may influence illness behaviour and "help-seeking" behaviour in chronic conditions. The World Health Organization (n.d., para 1.) refers to gender as the "socially constructed roles, behaviours, activities, and attributes that a given society considers appropriate for men and women." The term "gender" relates to common practices among men and women, and these practices may be socially constructed and/or culturally mediated. Most importantly, not all individuals will fit into social scripts of what men and women do. However, speaking in more generalized terms surrounding gender, sociological analysis suggests that women in general are more likely than men to seek medical help for nonfatal and chronic illness (Bury, 2005). Morbidity rates demonstrate that women are more likely to be sick than men and thus seek more professional medical help (Bury, 2005). Lorber (2000) stated that women are not more fragile than men but are just more self-protective of their health status.

Some cardiac studies focused on gender revealed a different pattern in which women often do not seek help until it is too late. Pastorius Benzinger, Bernabe-Ortiz, Miranda, and Bukhman (2011) found that women in Peru were less likely to seek help for chest pain than men. Albarran, Clarke, and Crawford (2007) through their qualitative study found that symptom presentation during myocardial infarction in women may not follow "typical" patterns associated with myocardial infarction. Furthermore, these presentations along with perceptions about their cardiac symptoms may influence women's health-seeking behaviours.

Little research exists on the specific impact of gender roles for the management of health.

What is clear is that there is a greater need for the study of gender in the context of chronic disease management.

Increasing age often brings chronic conditions and disability. However, older individuals in poor health (as measured by medicine's standard measures) often do not see themselves in this way. What may influence older adults' perceptions of their illness and subsequent behaviour may not even be considered by healthcare professionals as "relevant." Kelley-Moore, Schumacher, Kahana, and Kahana (2006) identified that cessation of driving and receiving home health care influenced older adults' illness perceptions, causing them to self-identify as disabled. Therefore, the ability to maintain social roles and functioning remains a central component towards people's perceptions of their illness.

Past Experience

One's education and learning, socialization, and past experience, as defined by one's social and cultural background, mediate illness behaviour. Past experiences of observing parents being stoic, going to work when they were ill, and avoiding medical help all influence children's future responses. If children see that "hard work" and not giving in to illness pays off with rewards, they will assimilate those experiences and mirror them in their own lives. Elfant, Gall, and Perlmuter (1999) evaluated the effects of avoidant illness behaviour of parents on their adult children's adjustment to arthritis. Even after several decades children's early observations of their parents' illness behaviours appear to affect their own adjustment to arthritis. Those clients whose parents avoided work and other activities when ill with a minor condition reported greater severity of arthritis and its limitations, depression, and helplessness when compared with clients whose parents did not respond to minor illness with avoidance (Elfant et al., 1999).

What if parents and adolescents have differing views on illness perceptions? The illness perceptions of 30 adolescents and their parents were compared to see the effects on the adolescents' outcomes (Salewski, 2003). Parents' illness representations had little impact on their children's outcomes. In families with high similarity between the parents' perceptions and the adolescents' perceptions, the adolescents reported more well-being (Salewski, 2003).

In another vein, how parents respond to their children's health complaints may later influence how the children, as adults, cope with illness. Whitehead and colleagues (1994) studied the influence of childhood social learning on the adult illness behaviour of 383 women aged 20 to 40 years of age. Illness behaviour was measured by frequency of symptoms, disability days, and physician visits for menstrual, bowel, and upper respiratory symptoms. Findings included that childhood reinforcement of menstrual illness behaviour significantly predicted adult menstrual symptoms and disability days, and childhood reinforcement of cold illness behaviour predicted adult cold symptoms and disability days. The study's data supported the hypothesis that specific patterns of illness behaviour are learned during childhood through parental reinforcement and modelling, and that these behaviours continued into adulthood (Whitehead et al., 1994).

In a small study examining illness perception in clients with critical illness and their surrogates in a medical intensive care unit, it was hypothesized that perceptions would vary by demographic, personal, and clinical measures

(Ford, Zapka, Gebregziabher, Yang, & Sterba, 2010). Although client/surrogate factors, including race, faith, and precritical illness quality of life, were significant, clinical measures were not. Researchers concluded that clinicians should recognize the variability in illness perceptions and the possible implications this might have for patient/surrogate and healthcare provider communication.

One cannot minimize the impact of the past experiences of the individual and family on how they deal with their own chronic illnesses, their children's, parents', and/or siblings'. Each of those experiences affects how the individual and family perceive their current health challenge. These experiences could be positive or negative. A negative healthcare experience with a relatively minor injury/illness could have a stronger influence than that of a positive experience with serious illness. As healthcare providers it is important that we do not underestimate the client's and family's perception of their illness and its effect on outcomes.

IMPACT AND ISSUES RELATED TO ILLNESS BEHAVIOUR

As illness behaviour is described, it is important to reiterate the difference between the terms "disease" and "illness." Disease is the pathophysiology, the change in body structure or function that can be quantified, measured, and defined. Disease is the objective "measurement" of symptoms. As Wainwright (2008) stated, disease within the medical model is materialist and assumes that the mechanisms of the body can be revealed and understood in the same way that the working of the solar system can be understood through gazing at the night sky.

Illness is what the client and family experience. It is what is experienced and "lived" by the client and family and includes the "meaning" the client gives to that experience (Helman, 2007). Both the meaning given to the symptoms and the client's response, or behaviour, are influenced by the client's background and personality as well as the cultural, social, and economic contexts in which the symptoms appear.

THE ILLNESS EXPERIENCE AND SUBSEQUENT BEHAVIOUR

The diagnosis of a chronic disease and subsequent management of that disease bring unique experiences and meanings of that process to the client and family. The biomedical world, at times, disregards illness and its meaning and focuses instead on disease. Disease can be quantified and measured and can be considered a "black-and-white" concept that fits into a medical model of care.

Illness, and the unique meaning that each individual attaches to it, is complex in nature; it is not black and white but consists of many shades of grey and thus defies measurement and categorization. Illness is a subjective label that reflects both personal and social ideas about what is normal as much as the pathology behind it (Weitz, 1991). Kleinmann (1985) expressed concern that researchers have "reduced sickness to something divorced from meaning in order to avoid the hard and still unanswered technical questions concerning how to actually go about measuring meaning and objectivizing and quantifying its effect on health status and illness behavior" (p. 149). While realizing the importance of this scientific work, Kleinmann (1985) sees it as "detrimental to the understanding of illness as human experience, because they redefine the problem to

subtract that which is mostly innately human; belief [and] feelings" (p. 149).

The *common sense self-regulation model* (Leventhal et al., 2001) seeks to explain that individual illness perceptions influence coping responses to an illness. This perspective explains that clients construct their own illness representations to help them make sense of their illness experience. It is these representations that form a basis for appropriate or inappropriate coping responses (Leventhal et al., 2001). Stuifbergen Phillips, Voelmeck, and Browder (2006) used a convenience sample of 91 women with fibromyalgia to explore their illness representations. Fibromyalgia has often been a highly contested categorization of specific symptoms including chronic fatigue, generalized muscle aching, and stiffness; controversy still exists as to whether or not this diagnosis represents a unique syndrome (Ronaldson, 2010). Overall, the women had fairly negative perceptions of their illness. Emotional representations explained 41% of the variance in mental health scores. Using the model of Leventhal and colleagues (2001), less emotional distress predicted more frequent health behaviours and more positive mental health scores, whereas those women who perceived their fibromyalgia to have more serious consequences and as less controllable were more likely to have higher scores on the Fibromyalgia Impact Questionnaire.

Price (1996) described individuals with a chronic disease as developing an illness career that responds to changes in health, his or her involvement with healthcare professionals, and the psychological changes associated with pathology, grief, and stress management. This illness career is dynamic, flexible, and goes through different stages of adaptation as the disease itself may change.

Loss of Self

In the 1980s Charmaz (1983) coined the phrase "loss of self" when interviewing individuals with chronic illness through a symbolic interactionist perspective, seeking to understand how humans develop a complex set of symbols in which to give meaning to their world. The influences on the loss of self develop from the chronic condition(s) and the illness experience. Charmaz described clients' illness experience as living a restricted life, experiencing social isolation, being discredited, and burdening others. Slowly, the individual with chronic illness feels his or her self-image disappear and experiences a loss of self, without the development of an equally valued new one.

In another study of 40 men with chronic illness, Charmaz (1994) described different identity dilemmas than those seen in women. Charmaz saw these men as "preserving self." As men come to terms with illness and disability, they preserve self by limiting the effect from illness on their lives and intensifying their control over their lives. Many assume they can recapture their past self and try to do so. They may devote vast amounts of energy to keeping their illness contained and the disability invisible to maintain their masculinity. At the same time they often maintain another identity at home—thus they create a public identity and a private identity to preserve self (Charmaz, 1994).

Moral Work

Townsend, Wyke, and Hunt (2006) described the moral dimension of the chronic illness experience in their qualitative study. Their work described moral work as integral to the illness, similar to the biographical and everyday "work" of Corbin and Strauss (1988). The participants in their study spoke about the need to demonstrate their moral worth as individuals, that it was their moral obligation to manage symptoms alongside their daily life (Townsend et al., 2006).

Devalued Self

In a qualitative study of Chinese immigrant women in Canada, Anderson (1991) described how these women with type 1 diabetes have a devalued self, not only from the disease but also because of dealing with being marginalized in a foreign country where they do not speak the language. Similar to the "loss of self" described by Charmaz, Anderson discussed women who need to reconstruct a new self. Influencing this devalued self were the interactions with healthcare professionals, which were frequently negative in nature, adding to their stress.

Similarly, eight older women with a chronic disease were asked to describe the meaning of living with a long-term illness. Five themes emerged: loss and uncertainty, learning one's capacity and living accordingly, maintaining fellowship and belonging, having a source of strength, and building anew. However, clearly the guiding premise of each woman was that chronic illness brought about reassessment and formation of a new understanding of self and a sense of being revalued by the world (Lundman & Jansson, 2007).

Chronic Sorrow

The concept of chronic sorrow was first described by Olshansky in 1962 when he was working with parents of children with learning disabilities. His conclusion was that chronic sorrow was a natural response to a tragedy instead of becoming neurotic. Two more recent studies discuss the existence of chronic sorrow in individuals with chronic illness. Sixty-one clients with multiple sclerosis were interviewed about chronic sorrow and also screened for depression. Thirty-eight of the 61 clients met the criteria for chronic sorrow. The participants in the study described feeling sorrow, fear, anger, and anxiety. Frustration and sadness were constantly present or were periodically overwhelming (Isaksson, Gunnarsson, & Ahlstrom, 2007). Seven themes were identified: loss of hope, loss of control over the body, loss of integrity and dignity, loss of a healthy identity, loss of faith that life is just, loss of social relations, and loss of freedom (Isaksson et al., 2007). Implications for healthcare providers included providing psychological support for these individuals. How does one provide the appropriate help when the client perceives such significant losses? What realistic help can healthcare professionals provide?

In the other more recent study, 30 adults of working age with an average disease duration of 18 years were interviewed (Ahlstrom, 2007). Sixteen of the 30 adults experienced chronic sorrow. The losses in this study are consistent with other studies on chronic sorrow even though the group was heterogeneous regarding diagnosis.

LEGITIMIZATION OF CHRONIC ILLNESS

With some illnesses, especially when symptoms are not well defined and diagnostic tests may be ambiguous, receiving legitimization from a physician or other healthcare professionals may be difficult and frustrating. Denial of opportunity to move into the sick role leads to "doctor hopping," placing clients in problematic relationships in which they must "work out" solutions alone (Steward & Sullivan, 1982). As a result, symptomatic persons may be left to question the truth of their own illness perceptions. How do you build a mental model of your illness (as a basis for problem solving) if healthcare providers and society in general are sceptical of your symptoms?

As examples, two current chronic conditions often defy diagnosis and are slow to respond to treatment. Chronic fatigue syndrome (CFS) and fibromyalgia are typically seen as diseases of young women. In both diseases there is uncertainty with respect to aetiology, treatment, and prognosis. They are historically contested illnesses in that some question their existence (Asbring, 2001). Without legitimization from physicians or the healthcare system, these clients are labelled as hypochondriacs or malingerers. Some of these clients are referred to psychologists or psychiatrists when a physical diagnosis cannot be made and diagnostic test results are normal.

When a diagnosis is finally made the client frequently shows a somewhat joyous initial response to having a name for the recurrent and troublesome symptoms. This reaction results from the decrease in stress over the unknown. These clients have an enormous stake in how their illnesses are understood. They seek to achieve the legitimacy necessary to elicit sympathy and avoid stigma and to protect their own self-concept (Mechanic, 1995).

Asbring (2001) identified two themes from her qualitative study in which women with CFS or fibromyalgia were interviewed. She described an earlier identity partly lost and coming to terms with a new identity. Asbring used the term "identity transformation" with the women she interviewed. However, she also saw illness gains in these women. The illness and its limitations provided the women with time to think and reflect on their lives and perhaps rearrange priorities. Therefore, the illness experience of these women may be seen as a paradox with both losses and gains (Asbring, 2001).

Larun and Malterud (2007) examined 20 qualitative studies in a meta-ethnography about the illness experiences of individuals with CFS to summarize the illness experiences of the individuals as well as the physicians' perspectives. Across studies clients spoke of being "controlled and betrayed by their bodies" (Larun & Malterud, 2007, pp. 22–23). Although physical activities were mostly curtailed, individuals spoke of mental fatigue that affected memory and concentration, described difficulty with following conversations, and several believed their learning abilities had decreased. One of the themes that emerged was telling stories about *bodies that no longer held the capacity for social involvement.* For some individuals the most distressing part of the illness was the negative responses from family members, the workplace, and their physicians, who *questioned the legitimacy of their illness behaviour* because of the dynamic symptoms of CFS. Thus, their physicians' beliefs about CFS influenced the clients' perceptions of the disease and therefore their illness experience. To summarize, the researchers' analysis determined that clients' sense of identity becomes more or less invalid and that a change in identity of the individuals was experienced.

Dickson, Knussen, and Flowers (2008) described the personal loss and identity crisis in their study of 14 individuals diagnosed with CFS. Participants talked about the illness that is their life and controls every aspect of their daily lives. Self-comparison took place between the participants' former selves and their "ill selves." Scepticism from others brought further crises of self.

Finally, Nettleton (2006) described interviews with 18 neurology patients in the United Kingdom with medically unexplained symptoms. Not having a diagnosis limits legitimate access to the sick role and the ability to build a mental model of the illness. One of the biggest hurdles is that society does not grant permission to be ill in the absence of a disease with a name.

Professional Responses to Illness Behaviour and Roles

Healthcare professionals generally expect those entering the acute hospital setting to conform to sick role behaviours. Most people entering the hospital for the first time are quickly socialized and expected to cooperate with treatment, to recover, and to return to their normal roles. Provider expectations and client responses are in line with social expectations and fit with the traditional medical model of illness as acute and curable. When clients are compliant and cooperative, healthcare professionals communicate to them that they are "good patients" (Lorber, 1981). When clients are less cooperative, the staff may consider them problematic or nonadherent.

CASE STUDY

Mary Ellen is a 35-year-old woman with unexplained neurological symptoms. She is a relatively new client to the clinic where you work. However, she has been seen by your clinic several times over the last 3 months. Originally, her diagnosis was "probable multiple sclerosis." However, that diagnosis has been ruled out. Mary Ellen's clinical symptoms include double vision (at times), transient numbness and tingling down the right side of her body, and general weakness and fatigue. Although she has been employed full time as a staff associate at the county assessor's office, she has been forced to go on short-term disability. In her phone call to the office this morning she is frustrated. She states, "I feel like no one believes me—you people think that I am making this up. I'm going to lose my job if you can't figure this out. I'm not a psych case."

Discussion Questions

1. How do you make sense of this client's illness behaviour?
2. What strategies might you use to deal with this client?
3. How could you apply the frameworks for practice mentioned in this chapter to this client situation?

Self-Care

The percentage of individuals with chronic illness entering hospitals is increasing, and often these admissions are due to superimposed acute illness or exacerbations of the chronic condition. Additionally, older adults in particular may have more than one chronic condition. Many of these individuals have had their chronic illnesses for long periods and have had prior hospital experiences. Multiple contacts with the healthcare system result in loss of the "blind faith" that the individual once had in that system. Individuals with chronic illness seek a different kind of relationship with healthcare professionals in which there is "give and take" and that can empower the client. The extent to which a client with chronic

illness is included in the formulation of his or her treatment plan likely influences the assumption of responsibility for it and, ultimately, its success (Weaver & Wilson, 1994).

Thorne's (1990) study of individuals with chronic illness and their families found that their relationships with healthcare professionals evolved from what was termed "naïve trust" through "disenchantment" to a final stage of "guarded alliance." She proposed the "rules" that govern these relationships should be entirely different for acute illness and chronic illness. Although assuming sick-role dependency may be adaptive in acute illness, where medical expertise offers hope of a cure, it is not so in chronic illness. Individuals with chronic illness are the "experts" in their illnesses and should have the ultimate authority in managing those illnesses over time.

When individuals with chronic illness are hospitalized, they may view the situation quite differently from the healthcare professionals with whom they interact. Clients with multiple chronic conditions may focus on maintaining stability of their chronic conditions to prevent unnecessary symptoms, whereas their healthcare providers are more likely to focus on managing the current acute disorder. In addition, clients who have had multiple prior admissions are more likely to use their hospital savvy to gain what they want or need from the system. During hospitalization these individuals may demand certain treatments, specific times for treatment, or routines outside of hospital parameters. They may keep track of times that various routines occur or complain about or report actions of the staff as a means to an end they consider important. In a grounded theory study in the United Kingdom, Wilson, Kendall, and Brooks (2006) explored how client expertise is viewed, interpreted, defined, and experienced by both clients and healthcare professionals. With nursing playing a key role in empowering clients with chronic disease to self-manage their conditions, knowing how that client expertise is viewed (by the care provider) is extremely important. Generally, in this study of 100 healthcare professionals (physicians, nurses, physical therapists), the nurses found the expert patients to be more threatening than other healthcare professionals did. The nurses had issues with accountability, perceived threats to their professional power, and potential litigation. The data from the study demonstrated that the nurses lacked a clear role definition and distinct expertise in working with patients with chronic disease and were unable to work in a flexible partnership with self-managing patients (Wilson et al., 2006).

Lack of Role Norms for Individuals with Chronic Illness

Chronic illnesses require a variety of tasks be performed to fulfil the requirements of both the medical regimen and the individual's personal lifestyle. However, there is a lack of norms for those with chronic illness. What is expected of a client recovering from cancer surgery? An exacerbation of rheumatoid arthritis? A flare-up of inflammatory bowel disease? Assume sick-role behaviours are discouraged, or not? These individuals enter and remain in a type of impaired, "at-risk" role. Implicit behaviours for this role are not well defined by society, leading to a situation of role ambiguity. Given this lack of norms, influences on the client include the degree of disability (with different attributes of disability producing different consequences), visibility of the disability (the less the visibility, the more normal the response), self-acceptance of the disability (resulting in others' reciprocating with acceptance), and societal views of the disabled as either economically dependent or productive. Without role definition, whether disability is present or not, individuals are unable to achieve maximum levels of functioning. Individuals must adapt their definitions of themselves to their limitations and to what the anticipated future imposes on them because of the chronic condition (Watt, 2000). What is normal illness behaviour?

INTERVENTIONS

There is no "magic" list of interventions to assist and support clients and their families with the illness experience. The current healthcare system with its acute care focus, fix-and-cure model, and a prescription for each symptom does not fit with caring for individuals long term. These clients do not need their illness behaviour "fixed" or "cured"; instead, they need a healthcare professional who will listen and understand the illness experience and not the disease process. What follows are suggestions that *assist and support* clients and their families.

Frameworks and Models for Practice

A review of the literature did not yield any new frameworks for caring for those with chronic illness. With chronic illness increasing, evidence-informed frameworks need to be developed. As stated previously, not all healthcare providers have the skills to care for those with long-term illness. Meeting the psychosocial needs of clients with chronic illness is in itself an ominous task. Caring for a client with chronic illness requires a framework or model for practice that differs from that of caring for those with acute, episodic disease. The frameworks that follow are examples and are not intended to be all inclusive.

These frameworks and models should not be confused with disease management models. Disease management models address the physical symptoms of a condition. Some of those models assign an algorithm to the condition where clients receive certain "care" when their blood work is at an inappropriate level or their symptoms "measure" a certain degree of seriousness. These models manage the disease but not the illness. Illness frameworks and models address the illness experience of the individual and family that occurs as a result of changing health status.

Chronic Illness and Quality of Life

In the early 1960s Anselm Strauss, working with Barney Glaser, a social scientist, and Jeanne Quint Benoliel, a nurse, interviewed dying patients to determine what kind of "care" was needed for these clients (Corbin & Strauss, 1992). As a result of those early interviews Strauss and colleagues published a rudimentary framework that addressed the issues and concerns of individuals with chronic illness (Strauss & Glaser, 1975; Strauss et al., 1984). Although the term "trajectory" was coined at that time, it did not become fully developed until 20 years later. Strauss and colleagues' framework was simple, but it was an early attempt to examine the illness experience of the individual and family as opposed to the disease. If healthcare professionals could better understand the illness experience of clients and families, perhaps more appropriate care would be provided. Basic to this care is understanding the key problems of chronic illness (Strauss et al., 1984, p. 16):

- Prevention of medical crises and their management if they occur
- Controlling symptoms
- Carrying out of prescribed medical regimens
- Prevention of, or living with, social isolation
- Adjustment to changes in the disease
- Attempts to normalize interactions and lifestyle
- Funding—finding the necessary money
- Confronting attendant psychological, marital, and familial problems

After identifying the key problems of the individual and family with chronic illness, Strauss and colleagues (1984) suggested basic problem-solving strategies, family and organizational arrangements, and then reevaluating the consequences of those arrangements.

Trajectory Framework

From the work of Strauss and colleagues in the 1960s and 1970s the trajectory framework was further refined in the 1980s. Corbin and Strauss (1992) developed this framework so that nurses could (1) gain insight into the chronic illness experience of the client, (2) integrate existing literature about chronicity into their practice, and (3) provide direction for building nursing models that guide practice, teaching, research, and policymaking.

A trajectory is defined as the course of an illness over time, plus the actions of clients, families, and healthcare professionals to manage that course (Corbin, 1998). The illness trajectory is set in motion by pathophysiology and changes in health status, but strategies can be used by clients, families, and healthcare professionals that shape the course of dying and thus the illness trajectory (Corbin & Strauss, 1992). Even if the disease may be the same, each individual's illness trajectory is different and takes into account the uniqueness of each individual (Jablonski, 2004). Shaping does not imply that the ultimate course of the disease will be changed or the disease will be cured, merely that the illness trajectory may be shaped or altered by actions of the individual and family so that the disease course is stable, fewer exacerbations occur, and symptoms are better controlled (Corbin & Strauss, 1992).

Within the model the term "phase" indicates the different stages of the chronic illness experience for the client. There are nine phases in the trajectory model, and although it could be conceived as a continuum, it is not linear. Clients may move through these phases in a linear fashion, regress to a former phase, or plateau for an extended period. In addition, having more than one chronic disease influences movement along the trajectory. Another term used in the model is "biography." A client's biography consists of previous hospital experiences and useful ways of dealing with symptoms, illness beliefs, and other life experiences.

The initial phase of the trajectory model is the pretrajectory phase, or preventive phase, in which the course of illness has not yet begun but genetic factors or lifestyle behaviours place an individual at risk for a chronic condition. An example is the individual who is overweight, has a family history of cardiac disease and high cholesterol, and does not exercise.

During the trajectory phase signs and symptoms of the disease appear and a diagnostic workup may begin. The individual begins to cope with implications of a diagnosis. In the stable phase the illness symptoms are under control and management of the disease occurs primarily at home. A period of inability to keep symptoms under control occurs in the unstable phase. The acute phase brings severe and unrelieved symptoms or disease complications. Critical or life-threatening situations that require emergency treatment occur in the crisis phase. The comeback phase signals a gradual return to an acceptable way of life within the symptoms that the disease imposes. The downward phase is characterized by progressive deterioration and an increase in disability or symptoms. The trajectory model ends with the dying phase, characterized by gradual or rapid shutting down of body processes (Corbin, 2001).

Chronic Illness and the Life Cycle

Rolland's (1987) illness trajectory model encompasses three phases: crisis, chronic, and terminal. The crisis phase has two subphases consisting of the symptomatic period before diagnosis and the period of initial adjustment just after diagnosis. The chronic phase is the period between the beginning of treatment and the terminal phase. Rolland was one of the first authors to describe chronic illness, and in this case the chronic phase, as the "long haul," the day-to-day living with chronic illness. Finally, the terminal phase is divided into the preterminal phase, where the client and family acknowledge that death is inevitable, and the period after death (Jablonski, 2004).

Shifting Perspectives Model of Chronic Illness

This model resulted from the work of Thorne and Paterson (1998), who analyzed 292 qualitative studies of chronic physical illness published from 1980 to 1996. Of these, 158 studies became a part of a metastudy in which client roles in chronic illness were described. The work of Thorne and Paterson reflects the "insider" perspective of chronic illness as opposed to the "outsider" view, the more traditional view. This change in perspective is a shift from the traditional approach of patient-as-client to one of client-as-partner in care (Thorne & Paterson, 1998). Results from the metastudy also demonstrated a shift away from focusing on loss and burden and an attempt to view health within illness.

Analysis of these studies led to the development of the shifting perspectives model of chronic illness (Paterson, 2001). The model depicts chronic illness as an ongoing, continually shifting process where people experience a complex dialectic between the world and themselves. Paterson's model considered both the "illness" and the "wellness" of the individual (Paterson, 2003). The illness-in-the-foreground

perspective focuses on the sickness, loss, and burden of the chronic illness. This is a common reaction of those recently diagnosed with a chronic disease. The overwhelming consequences of the condition, learning about their illness, considerations of treatment, and long-term effects contribute to putting the illness in the foreground. The disease becomes the individual's identity.

Illness-in-the-foreground could also be a protective response by the individual and may be used to conserve energy for other activities. However, it could be used to maintain their identity as a "sick" person or because it is congruent with their need to have sickness as their social identity and receive secondary gains (Paterson, 2001).

With the wellness-in-the-foreground perspective the "self" is the source of identity rather than the disease (Paterson, 2001). The individual is in control and not the disease. It does not mean, though, that the individual is physically well, cured, or even in remission of the disease symptoms. The shift occurs in the individual's thinking, allowing the individual to focus away from the disease. However, any threat that cannot be controlled will transition the individual back to the illness-in-the-foreground perspective. Threats include disease progression and lack of ability to self-manage the disease, stigma, and interactions with others (Paterson, 2001).

Finally, neither the illness perspective nor the wellness perspective is right or wrong, but each merely reflects the individual's unique needs, health status, and focus at the time (Paterson, 2001). In Paterson's research published in 2003, one of her study participants was concerned that those reading about the shifting perspectives model might interpret the two perspectives as "either/or"—that one has to have either wellness or illness in the foreground. This individual stated the following:

> I think there is danger when researchers think there is a right way to have a chronic illness. There is only one way . . . the one you choose at the moment . . . generally I live in the orange. If red is illness and yellow represents wellness, then I like to be a blend of both things . . . in the orange. . . . It is not a good idea for me to be completely yellow because then I forget that I have MS and I do stupid things that I pay for later. And if I am totally in the red, I am too depressed to do anything. (Paterson, 2003, p. 990)

Dealing with Dependency

Chronic illness is fraught with unpredictable dilemmas. Even when an acute stage is past, the client's energy for recovery may be sapped by the uncertainty about the future course of the illness, the effectiveness of medical regimens, and the disruption of usual patterns of living. Awareness of behavioural responses and when they occur can help the professional avoid premature emphasis on independence until the client can collaborate in working towards a return to normal roles.

Miller (2000) recommended several strategies for decreasing clients' feelings of powerlessness as they work towards independence:

- Modifying the environment to afford clients more means of control
- Helping clients set realistic goals and expectations
- Increasing clients' knowledge about their illness and its management
- Increasing the sensitivity of health professionals and significant others to the powerlessness imposed by chronic illness
- Encouraging verbalization of feelings

Using knowledge of illness roles in planning interventions allows the healthcare professional to maximize time spent with the client. One such intervention that could be improved by integrating knowledge of illness roles is education. The client who is still in the highly dependent phase cannot benefit from education. As improvement in physical status occurs, emphasis on the desire to return to normal roles creates motivation to learn about the condition and necessary procedures for maximizing health. As the client moves into the impaired role and becomes aware of the necessity to maximize remaining potential, education provides a highly successful tool both in the hospital and at home.

Evidence-Informed Practice Box

Ten full-time nursing students, all diagnosed with at least one chronic illness, were interviewed to examine their illness experience. Participants looked for ways to be ordinary because they perceived they were different from the norm. Chronic conditions included systemic lupus erythematosus, Raynaud's syndrome, rheumatoid arthritis, psoriasis, chronic back pain, irritable bowel syndrome, fibromyalgia, relapsing-remitting multiple sclerosis, type 1 diabetes mellitus, chronic urinary tract infections, anorexia/bulimia, and adrenal hyperplasia. Using Colaizzi's (1978) phenomenological method, four major themes emerged: (1) needing to be normal, (2) dealing with the behaviours of others, (3) enduring the restrictions of illness, and (4) learning from self to care for others. Throughout the students' experiences they tried to negate their illness or their abnormal behaviour and maintain their valued social role as students. Participants believed their chronic illness created an inner strength and gave them intuitive knowledge about the body and how to better understand the needs of others.

Source: Dailey (2010)

Self-Management

The participants in the study by Kralick, Koch, Price, and Howard (2004) identified self-management as a process they initiated to bring about order in their lives. This is in sharp contrast to how most healthcare professionals describe self-management in a structured patient education program that assists clients in adhering to their medical regimen. The participants saw self-management as creating a sense of order and a process that included four themes: (1) recognizing and monitoring boundaries, (2) mobilizing resources, (3) managing the shift in self-identity, and (4) balancing, pacing, planning, and prioritizing (Kralick et al., 2004). Kralick and colleagues suggested that self-management is a combination of a process by clients and families and a structure of patient education.

The Women to Women Project has been instrumental in helping women with chronic illness in rural states manage their illnesses. Through a computer intervention model that provides education and support groups and fosters self-care, women have successfully managed their illness responses (Sullivan, Weinert, & Cudney, 2003).

Clients with chronic illness use multiple techniques to manage symptoms, maintain social roles, be the "good patient," and maintain some degree of normality. Townsend et al. (2006) described the moral obligation of individuals to self-manage their symptoms and manage their selves. Although individuals are trying to manage both symptoms and social roles, the priority is always given to behaviours that typify a "normal" life and identity management over managing the symptoms of the disease (Townsend et al., 2006).

Critical to working with clients and families in self-managing both their disease and their illness is appropriate client–healthcare provider communication. Thorne, Harris, Mahoney, Con, and McGuinness (2004) interviewed clients with end-stage renal disease, type 2 diabetes, multiple sclerosis, and fibromyalgia to determine what clients perceived as priorities. Across all diseases the concepts of courtesy, respect, and engagement were important. Certainly, courtesy and respect are fairly clear in their meaning. Engagement was described by clients as an extension of courtesy and respect. An example is a healthcare professional engaged with a client in problem solving and care management, in which they experienced a feeling of teamwork/working together. Such communication enhanced their relationships with clients.

Kaptein, Klok, Moss-Morris, and Brand (2010) reviewed 19 studies that examined how illness perceptions could impact an individual's control of asthma. Using the common sense model of self-regulation as a basis, the authors created their own model of how these perceptions affected self-management. The conclusion of the authors was that self-management was determined mainly by behavioural factors and not sociodemographic factors. One of those behavioural factors was illness perceptions.

They noted that changing a client's illness perceptions is indicated to help the client and healthcare provider achieve optimal asthma control (Kaptein et al., 2010).

Research

Do we understand and can we place in an appropriate context the meaning of illness for clients? Why do some individuals ignore symptoms and refuse to seek medical advice and others with the same condition seek immediate care and relief from their "social roles" at the slightest symptom? A relatively minor symptom in one individual causes great distress, whereas more serious health conditions in others cause little concern.

Stuifbergen and colleagues (2006) suggested that it is unclear from the literature how illness perceptions change over time and how specifically these perceptions are influenced. These researchers believed that if illness perceptions can be altered, then interactions with those in a positive manner could be encouraged. Bijsterbosch and colleagues (2009) noted that illness perceptions did change over time and were related to the progression of the disability. Illness perceptions regarding the number of symptoms attributed to osteoarthritis and the level of perceived control and perceived consequences of osteoarthritis were predictive of more disability.

Mechanic (1986, 1995) asked a question that is still pertinent today: What are the processes or factors that cause individuals exposed to similar stressors to respond differently and present unique illness behaviour? There is such variation in how individuals perceive their health status, seek or not seek medical care, and function in their social and work roles. What causes these differences?

This author poses another question. What can we do as healthcare providers to change illness perceptions of clients? A growing body of evidence shows that more negative views of illness held by clients are associated with poorer outcomes (Petrie & Weinman, 2006). What can we do to effect change in chronic sorrow? How can we give clients a sense of hope? How do we value clients so they do not believe they have devalued lives? Chronic illness is the condition as the client and family experience it. What can we do to make a difference in the lives of our clients and families?

SUMMARY

Illness behaviour is not deviant and does not need to be fixed. However, we need to support our clients and understand the lived experience of the illness. As healthcare professionals we are efficient and effective working within the disease model. However, the client lives in the illness model as well. Because nursing is an art and a science there is a strong "fit" with the illness model. The best outcome for clients with chronic illness is the healthcare professional supporting and assisting the client through the illness experience.

STUDY QUESTIONS

1. Using this chapter as a guide, how would you support and work with an individual with either CFS or fibromyalgia? How do your own past healthcare experiences influence your practice with these clients?

STUDY QUESTIONS (Cont.)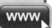

2. Dealing with "expert" patients can be difficult. Often, your own "power" as a healthcare professional is threatened. How do you deal with "expert" patients and make it a collaborative relationship?

3. There are no norms for individuals with long-term illness. What does this mean and how does it apply to the clients with chronic illness whom you have treated?

4. Differentiate between health and illness behaviours and give examples of each for someone with end-stage heart failure, endometriosis, or oesophageal cancer.

5. How do healthcare professionals influence the illness behaviour of clients and families in positive ways or negative ways?

6. Apply each of the frameworks for practice described in this chapter to clients with chronic illness whom you have treated.

7. Reflect on your own past and present health and illness experiences. What influences your own illness behaviours?

For a full suite of assignments and additional learning activities, use the access code located in the front of your book and visit this exclusive website: **http://go.jblearning.com/kramer-kile**. If you do not have an access code, you can obtain one at the site.

REFERENCES

Ahlstrom, G. (2007). Experiences of loss and chronic sorrow in persons with severe chronic illness. *Journal of Nursing and Healthcare of Chronic Illness* in association with *Journal of Clinical Nursing, 16*(3a), 76–83.

Albarran, J. W., Clarke, B. A. & Crawford, J. (2007). "It was not chest pain really, I can't explain it!" An exploratory study on the nature of symptom experienced by women during myocardial infarction. *Journal of Clinical Nursing, 16*(7), 1292–1301.

Alsen, P., Brink, E., Persson, L, Brandstrom, Y., & Karlson, B. W. (2010). Illness perceptions after myocardial infarction: Relations to fatigue, emotional distress, and health-related quality of life. *Journal of Cardiovascular Nursing, 25*(2), E1–E10.

Anderson, J. M. (1991). Immigrant women speak of chronic illness: The social construction of the devalued self. *Journal of Advanced Nursing, 16*, 710–717.

Asbring, P. (2001). Chronic illness—a disruption in life: Identity transformation among women with chronic fatigue syndrome and fibromyalgia. *Journal of Advanced Nursing, 34*(3), 312–319.

Bijsterbosch, J., Scharloo, M., Visser, A. W., Watt, I., Meulenbelt, T. W., Huzinga, T. W. J., . . . Kloppenburg, M. (2009). Illness perceptions in patients with osteoarthritis: Change over time and association with disability. *Arthritis and Rheumatism, 61*(8), 1054–1061.

Broadbent, E., Ellis, C. J., Thomas, J., Gamble, G., & Petrie, K. J. (2009). Further development of an illness perception intervention for myocardial infarction patients: A randomized controlled trial. *Journal of Psychosomatic Research, 67*, 17–23.

Bury, M. (2005). *Health and illness*. Cambridge, UK: Polity Press.

Charmaz, K. (1983). Loss of self: A fundamental form of suffering in the chronically ill. *Sociology of Health and Illness, 5*(2), 168–195.

Charmaz, K. (1994). Identity dilemma of chronically ill men. *Sociological Quarterly, 35*(2), 269–288.

Chen, S. L., Tsai, J. C., & Chou, K. R. (2010). Illness perceptions and adherence to therapeutic regimens among patients with hypertension: A structural modeling approach. *International Journal of Nursing Studies, 8*(2), 235–245.

Cockerham, W. C. (2001). The sick role. In W.C. Cockerham (Ed.), *Medical sociology* (8th ed., pp. 156–178). Upper Saddle River, NJ: Prentice Hall.

Colaizzi, P. (1978). Psychological research as the phenomenologist views it. In R. Vale & M. King (Eds.), *Existential phenomenological alternatives for psychology.* New York: NY: Oxford University Press.

Conrad, P. (2005). *The sociology of health and illness: Critical perspectives* (7th ed.). New York, NY: Worth Publishers.

Corbin, J. (1998). The Corbin & Strauss chronic illness trajectory model: An update. *Scholarly Inquiry for Nursing Practice, 12*(1), 33–41.

Corbin, J. (2001). Introduction and overview: Chronic illness and nursing. In R. Hyman & J. Corbin (Eds.), *Chronic illness: Research and theory for nursing practice* (pp. 1–15). New York, NY, Springer.

Corbin, J. M., & Strauss, A. (1988). *Unending work and care: Managing chronic illness at home.* San Francisco, CA: Jossey-Bass.

Corbin, J., & Strauss, A. (1992). A nursing model for chronic illness management based upon the trajectory framework. In P. Woog (Ed.), *The chronic illness trajectory framework: The Corbin and Strauss nursing model* (pp. 9–28). New York, NY: Springer.

Dailey, M. (2010). Need to be normal: The lived experience of chronically ill nursing students. *International Journal of Nursing Education Scholarship, 7*(1), 1–23.

deRoon-Cassini, T., de St. Aubin, E., Valvano, A., Hastings, J., & Horn, P. (2009). Psychological well-being after spinal cord injury: Perception of loss and meaning making. *Rehabilitation Psychology, 54*(3), 306–314.

Dickson, A., Knussen, C., & Flowers, P. (2008). "That was my old life; it's almost like a past-life now": Identify crisis, loss and adjustment among people living with chronic fatigue syndrome. *Psychology and Health, 23*(4), 459–476.

Diefenbach, M. A., Leventhal, E. A., Leventhal, H., & Patrick-Miller, L. (1996). Negative affect relates to cross-sectional but not longitudinal symptom reporting: Data from elderly adults. *Health Psychology, 15*(4), 282–288.

Elfant, E., Gall, E., & Perlmuter, L. C. (1999). Learned illness behavior and adjustment to arthritis. *Arthritis Care and Research, 12*(6), 411–416.

Figueiras, M., Marcelino, D., Claudino, A., Cortes, M., Maroco, J., & Weinman, J. (2010). Patients' illness schemata of hypertension: The role of beliefs for the choice of treatment. *Psychology and Health, 25*(4), 507–517.

Ford, D., Zapka, J., Gebregziabher, M., Yang, C., & Sterba, K. (2010). Factors associated with illness perception among critically ill patients and surrogates. *Chest, 138*, 59–67.

Freidson, E. (1970). *Profession of medicine.* New York, NY: Dodd, Mead.

Helman, C. G. (2007). *Culture, health and illness* (5th ed.). London, England: Arnold.

Hoving, J. L., van der Meer, M., Volkova, A. Y., & Frings-Dresen, M. H. W. (2010). Illness perceptions and work participation: A systematic review. *International Archives of Occupational & Environmental Health, 83*(6), 595–605.

Illness Perception Questionnaire. Retrieved August 2, 2011, from http://www.uib.no/ipq

Isaksson, A., Gunnarsson, L O., & Ahlstrom, G. (2007). The presence and meaning of chronic sorrow in patients with multiple sclerosis. *Journal of Nursing and Healthcare of Chronic Illness* in association with *Journal of Clinical Nursing, 16*(11c), 315–324.

Jablonski, A. (2004). The illness trajectory of end-stage renal disease dialysis patients. *Research and Theory for Nursing Practice: An International Journal, 18*(1), 51–72.

Juergens, M. C., Seekatz, B., Moosdorf, R. G., Petrie, K. J., & Rief, W. (2010). Illness beliefs before cardiac surgery predict disability, quality of life and depression 3 months later. *Journal of Psychosomatic Research, 68*(6), 553–560.

Kaptein, A. A., Klok, T., Moss-Morris, R., & Brand, P. L. P. (2010). Illness perceptions: Impact on self-management and control in asthma. *Current Opinion in Allergy and Clinical Immunology, 10*, 194–199.

Kasl, S. V., & Cobb, S. (1966). Health behavior, illness behavior, and sick-role behavior. *Archives of Environmental Health, 12*, 531–541.

Kelley-Moore, J. A., Schumacher, J. G., Kahana, E., & Kahana, B. (2006). When do older adults become "disabled"? Social and health antecedents of perceived disability in a panel study of the oldest old. *Journal of Health and Social Behavior, 47*, 126–141.

Kleinmann, A. (1985). Illness meanings and illness behavior. In S. McHugh & M. Vallis (Eds.), *Illness behavior: A multidisciplinary model* (pp. 149–160). New York, NY: Plenum.

Kralick, D., Koch, T., Price, K., & Howard, N. (2004). Chronic illness management: Taking action to create order. *Journal of Clinical Nursing, 13*, 259–267.

Lane, D. A., Langman, C. M., Lip, G. Y. H., & Nouwen, A. (2009). Illness perceptions, affective response, and health-related quality of life in patients with atrial fibrillation. *Journal of Psychosomatic Research, 66*, 203–210.

Larun, L., & Malterud, K. (2007). Identity and coping experiences in chronic fatigue syndrome: A synthesis of qualitative studies. *Patient Education and Counseling, 69*, 20–28.

Lee, B., Chaboyer, W., & Wallis, M. (2010). Illness representations in patients with traumatic injury: A longitudinal study. *Journal of Clinical Nursing, 19,* 556–563.

Leventhal, H., Leventhal, E. A., & Cameron, L. (2001). Representations, procedures, and affect in illness self-regulation: A perceptual-cognitive model. In A. Baum, T. A. Revenson, & J. E. Singer (Eds.), *Handbook of health psychology* (pp. 19–47). Mahwah, NJ: Lawrence Erlbaum Associates.

Lorber, J. (1981). Good patients and problem patients: Conformity and deviance in a general hospital. In P. Conrad & R. Kern (Eds.), *The sociology of health and illness: Critical perspectives.* New York, NY: St. Martin's Press.

Lorber, J. (2000). Gender and health. In P. Brown (Ed.), *Perspectives in medical sociology* (3rd ed., pp. 40–70). Prospect Heights, IL: Waveland Press.

Lundman, B., & Jansson, L. (2007). The meaning of living with a long-term disease: To revalue and be revalued. *Journal of Nursing and Healthcare of Chronic Illness* in association with *Journal of Clinical Nursing, 16*(7b), 109–115.

Marks, D. F., Murray, M., Evans, B., Willig, C., Woodall, C., & Sykes, C. (2005). *Health psychology: Theory, research and practice* (2nd ed.). Thousand Oaks, CA: Sage.

McHugh, S., & Vallis, M. (1986). Illness behavior: Operationalization of the biopsychosocial model. In S. McHugh & M. Vallis (Eds.), *Illness behavior: A multidisciplinary model* (pp. 1–32). New York, NY: Plenum.

Mechanic, D. (1962). The concept of illness behavior. *Journal of Chronic Diseases, 15,* 189–194.

Mechanic, D. (1986). The concept of illness behavior: Culture, situation, and personal predisposition. *Psychological Medicine, 16*, 1–7.

Mechanic, D. (1995). Sociological dimensions of illness behavior. *Social Science and Medicine, 41*(9), 1207–1216.

Miller, J. F. (2000). *Coping with chronic illness: Overcoming powerlessness* (3rd ed.). Philadelphia, PA: F. A. Davis.

Nettleton, S. (2006). "I just want permission to be ill": Towards a sociology of medically unexplained symptoms. *Social Science and Medicine, 62*, 1167–1178.

Olshansky, S. (1962). Chronic sorrow: A response to having a mentally defective child. *Social Casework, 43*, 190–193.

Orpana, H. M., Lemyre, L., & Kelly, S. (2007). Do stressors explain the association between income and declines in self-rated health? A longitudinal analysis of the National Population Health Survey. *International Journal of Behavioural Medicine, 14*(1), 40–47.

Parsons, T. (1951). *The social system.* New York, NY: The Free Press.

Pastorius Benzinger, C., Bernabe-Ortiz, A., Miranda, J. J., & Bukhman, G. (2011). Sex differences in health care-seeking behaviour for acute coronary syndrome in low income country, Peru. *Critical Pathways in Cardiology, 10*(2), 99–103.

Paterson, B. (2001). The shifting perspectives model of chronic illness. *Journal of Nursing Scholarship, 33*(1), 21–26.

Paterson, B. (2003). The koala has claws: Applications of the shifting perspectives model in research of chronic illness. *Qualitative Health Research, 13*(7), 987–994.

Pearson, L. (2003). Understanding the culture of poverty. *Nurse Practitioner, 28*, 4–6.

Petrie, K. J., & Weinman, J. (2006). Why illness perceptions matter. *Clinical Medicine, 6*(6), 536–539.

Price, B. (1996). Illness careers: The chronic illness experience. *Journal of Advanced Nursing, 24*, 275–279.

Rolland, J. S. (1987). Chronic illness and the life cycle: A conceptual framework. *Family Process, 26*, 203–221.

Ronaldson, S. (2010). Assessment and management of patients with rheumatic disorders. In R. A. Day, P. Paul, & B. Williams (Eds.), *Brunner & Suddarth's textbook of Canadian medical-surgical nursing* (2nd ed.). Philadelphia, PA: Lippincott Williams & Wilkins.

Rudell, K., Bhui, K., & Priebe, S. (2009). Concept, development and application of a new mixed method assessment of cultural variations in illness perceptions: Barts explanatory model inventory. *Journal of Health Psychology, 24*, 336–347.

Salewski, C. (2003). Illness representations in families with a chronically ill adolescent: Differences between family members and impact on patients' outcome variables. *Journal of Health Psychology, 8*(5), 587–598.

Schim, S., Doorenbos, A., Benkert, R., & Miller, J. (2007). Culturally congruent care: Putting the puzzle together [Electronic version]. *Journal of Transcultural Nursing, 18*(2), 103–110.

Searle, A., Norman, P., Thompson, R., & Vedhara, K. (2007). Illness representations among patients with type 2 diabetes and their partners: Relationships with self-management behaviors [Electronic version]. *Journal of Psychosomatic Research, 63*(2), 175–184.

Sontag, S. (1988). *Illness as metaphor*. Toronto, ON: Collins Publishers.

Stafford, L., Berk, M. & Jackson, H. L. (2009). Are illness perceptions about coronary artery disease predictive of depression and quality of life outcomes? *Journal of Psychosomatic Research, 66*, 211–220.

Stafford, L., Jackson, H. J., & Berk, M. (2008). Illness beliefs about heart disease and adherence to secondary prevention regimens. *Psychosomatic Medicine, 70*, 942–948.

Steward, D. C., & Sullivan, T. J. (1982). Illness behavior and the sick role in chronic disease: The case of multiple sclerosis. *Social Science and Medicine, 16*, 1397–1404.

Strauss, A., & Glaser, B. (1975). *Chronic illness and the quality of life*. St. Louis, MO: Mosby.

Strauss, A. L., & Strauss, A. L. (1984). *Chronic illness and the quality of life*. St. Louis: Mosby. Sullivan, T., Weinert, C., & Cudney, S. (2003). Management of chronic illness: Voices of rural women. *Journal of Advanced Nursing, 44*(6), 566–574.

Stuifbergen, A., Phillips, L., Voelmeck, W., & Browder, R. (2006). Illness perceptions and related outcomes among women with fibromyalgia syndrome. *Women's Health Issues, 16*, 353–360.

Thomas, R. (2003). *Society and health: Sociology for health professionals*. New York, NY: Kluwer.

Thorne, S. E. (1990). Constructive noncompliance in chronic illness. *Holistic Nursing Practice, 5*(1), 62–69.

Thorne, S. E., Harris, S. R., Mahoney, K., Con, A., & McGuinness, L. (2004). The context of health care communication in chronic illness [Electronic version]. *Patient Education and Counseling, 54*(3), 299–306.

Thorne, S. E., & Paterson, B. (1998). Shifting images of chronic illness. *Image, 30*(2), 173–178.

Townsend, A., Wyke, S., & Hunt, K. (2006). Self-managing and managing self: Practical and moral dilemmas in accounts of living with chronic illness. *Chronic Illness, 2*, 185–194.

Wainwright, D. (2008). Illness behavior and the discourse of health. In D. Wainwright (Ed.), *A sociology of health* (pp. 76–96). London, England: Sage.

Watt, S. (2000). Clinical decision-making in the context of chronic illness. *Health Expectations, 3*, 6–16.

Weaver, S. K., & Wilson, J .F. (1994). Moving toward patient empowerment. *Nursing and Health Care, 15*(9), 380–483.

Weitz, R. (1991). *Life with AIDS*. New Brunswick, NJ: Rutgers University Press.

Weitz, R. (2007). *The sociology of health, illness, and health care* (4th ed.). Belmont, CA: Thomson Higher Education.

Whitehead, W. E., Crowell, M. D., Heller, B. R., Robinson, J. C., Schuster, M. M., & Horn, S. (1994). Modeling and reinforcement of the sick role during childhood predicts adult illness behavior. *Psychosomatic Medicine, 56*, 541–550.

Williams, S. J. (2005). Parsons revisited: From the sick role to . . . ? *Health, 9*, 123–144.

Wilson, P. M., Kendall, S., & Brooks, F. (2006). Nurses' responses to expert patients: The rhetoric and reality of self-management in long term conditions: A grounded theory study. *International Journal of Nursing Studies, 43*, 803–818.

World Health Organization. (n.d.). *What do we mean by sex and gender?* Geneva, Switzerland: Author. Retrieved from http://www.who.int/gender/whatisgender/en/

Young, J. T. (2004). Illness behavior: A selective review and synthesis. *Sociology of Health and Illness, 26*(1), 1–31.

CHAPTER 4

Stigma

Original chapter by Diane L. Stuenkel and Vivian K. Wong
Canadian content added by Marnie L. Kramer-Kile

> *My car came to a stop at the intersection. I looked around me at all the people in the other cars, but no one there was like me. They were apart from me, distant, different. If they looked at me, they couldn't see my defect. But if they knew, they would turn away. I am separate and different from everybody that I can see in every direction as far as I can see. And it will never be the same again.*
>
> —Client with new diagnosis of cancer

INTRODUCTION

This chapter demonstrates how the concept of stigma has evolved and is a significant factor in many chronic illnesses and disabilities. It also explores the relationship of stigma to the concepts of prejudice, stereotyping, and labelling. Because stigma is socially constructed, it varies from setting to setting. In addition, individuals and groups react differently to the stigmatizing process. Those reactions must be taken into consideration when planning strategies to improve the quality of life for individuals with chronic illnesses.

Merriam Webster (2011a) defines stigma as a "mark of shame or discredit, an identifying mark or characteristic," and as a "mark of guilt or disgrace" (2011b). Although stigmatizing is common, not all individuals attach a stigma to their disease or disability. This chapter does not assume that all who come in contact with those who are disabled or chronically ill devalue them; rather, it insists that each of us examine our values, beliefs, and actions carefully. Healthcare professionals (HCPs), in particular, need to be aware of their existing values and how these beliefs affect their behaviour towards individuals with chronic illness and disabilities (Raffin Bouchal, 2009). The language that HCPs use to frame and address differing chronic disease conditions has wider social implications for the individuals living with them. For example, if health discourses surrounding type 2 diabetes only focus on its preventable nature instead of also addressing other aetiologies related to the disease, individuals may be faced with the social stigma that they brought the disease on themselves. Risk narratives may emerge that further serve to stigmatize individuals living with chronic illness. Often, it is suggested that HCPs engage in a process of *values clarification* to reflect on how their own beliefs may further perpetuate stigmas associated with chronic illness.

Sociologist Erving Goffman, known for his work on stigma (1963), traced the historical use of the word "stigma" to the Greeks, who referred to "bodily signs designed to expose something unusual and bad about the moral status of the signifier" (p. 1). He identified three classifications of stigma, discussed later in the chapter, that still have relevance for studying the role of stigma in chronic illness: (1) stigma associated with physical deformations, (2) stigma attributed to perceptions that individuals lack character or will, and (3) stigma linked to generalized perceptions according to race, culture, and religion. Stigma, then, can result from bodily appearance, behaviours associated with poor health, and assumptions made about race, culture and religion. Labelling, stereotyping, separation, status loss, and discrimination can all occur at the same time and are considered components of stigma (Link & Phelan, 2001).

THEORETICAL FRAMEWORKS: STIGMA, SOCIAL IDENTITY, AND LABELLING THEORY

Society teaches its members to categorize persons by common defining attributes and characteristics (Goffman, 1963). Daily routines establish the usual and the expected. When we meet strangers certain appearances help us anticipate what Goffman called "social identity." This identity includes personal attributes, such as competence, and structural attributes, such as occupation. For example, university students usually tolerate some eccentricities in their professors, but stuttering, physical handicaps, or diseases may bestow a social identity of incompetence. Although this identity is not based on the capacities of the individual, it may be stigmatizing.

One's social identity may include physical activities, professional roles, and the concept of self. Anything that changes one of these, such as a disability, changes the individual's identity and therefore potentially creates a stigma (Markowitz, 1998). Goffman (1963) used the idea of social identity to expand previous work done on stigma. His theory defined stigma as something that disqualifies an individual from full social acceptance. Goffman argued that social identity is a primary force in the development of stigma, because the identity a person conveys categorizes that person. Social settings and routines tell us which categories to anticipate. Therefore, when individuals fail to meet expectations because of attributes that are different and/or undesirable, they are reduced from accepted people to discounted ones—that is, they are stigmatized.

Goffman recognized that people who had stayed in a psychiatric institute or a prison were labelled. To label a person as different or deviant by powers of the society is applying a stigma (Goffman, 1963). In general, labelling theory is the way that society labels behaviours that do not conform to the norm. For instance, an individual experiencing constant drooling or the leakage of food that requires frequent wiping of the mouth exhibits behaviours different from the norm. The difficulty in swallowing may be labelled by society as deviant behaviour, despite the fact that tremor and dyskinesias associated with Parkinson's disease may be the cause (Miller, Noble, Jones, & Burn, 2006). Therefore, the concept of deviance versus normality is a social construct. That is, individuals are devalued because they display attributes that some call deviant (Kurzban & Leary, 2001).

During the two decades after Goffman's work in the 1960s, extensive criticism arose concerning the impact and long-term consequences of stigma on social identity. In the area of mental illness, critics resisted the theory that stigma could contribute to the severity and chronicity of mental illness. In a series of studies Link proposed a modified labelling theory that asserted that labelling, derived from negative social beliefs about behaviour, could lead to devaluation and discrimination. Ultimately, these feelings of devaluation and discrimination could lead to negative social consequences (Link, 1987; Link et al., 1989, 1997). Those who are labelled with mental illness often are excluded from social activities and discriminated against when they do participate.

In 1987 Link compared the expectations of discrimination and devaluation and the severity of demoralization among clients with newly diagnosed mental illness, repeat clients with mental illness, former clients with mental illness, and community residents (Link, 1987). He found that both new and repeat clients with mental illness scored higher on measures of demoralization and discrimination than community residents and former clients with mental illness. Further, he demonstrated that high scores were related to income loss and unemployment.

In 1989 Link and colleagues tested a modified labelling theory on a similar group of clients with newly diagnosed mental illness, repeat clients with mental illness, former clients, untreated clients, and community residents who were well (Link et al., 1989). They found that all groups expected clients to be devalued and discriminated against. They also found that, among current clients, the expectation of devaluation and discrimination promoted coping mechanisms of secrecy and withdrawal. Such coping mechanisms have a strong effect on social networks, reducing the size of those networks to persons considered to be safe and trustworthy.

In 1997 Link and colleagues tested modified labelling theory in a longitudinal study that compared the effects of stigma on the well-being of clients who had mental illness and a pattern of substance abuse to determine the strength of the long-term negative effects of stigma and whether the effects of treatment have counterbalancing positive effects (Link et al., 1997). They found that perceived devaluation and discrimination, as well as actual reports of discrimination, continued to have negative effects on clients even though clients were improved and had responded well to treatment. They concluded that HCPs attempting to improve quality of life for clients with mental illness must contend initially with the effects of stigma in its own right to be successful.

Fife and Wright (2000) studied stigma using modified labelling theory as a framework in individuals with HIV/AIDS and cancer. They found that stigma had a significant influence on the lives of persons with HIV/AIDS and with cancer. However, they also found that the nature of the illness had few direct effects on self-perception, whereas the effects on self appeared to relate directly to the perception of stigma. Their findings suggested that stigma has different dimensions that have varying effects on self. Rejection and social isolation lead to diminished self-esteem. Social isolation influences body image. A lack of sense of personal control stems from social isolation and financial insecurity. Social isolation appears to be the only dimension of stigma that affects each component of self.

Camp, Finlay, and Lyons (2002) questioned the inevitability of the effects of stigma on self based on the hypothesis that for stigma to exert a negative influence on self-concept, individuals must first be aware of and accept the negative self-perceptions, accept that the identity relates to them, and then apply the negative perceptions to themselves. A study of women with long-term mental health problems found that these women did not accept negative social perceptions as relevant to them. Rather, they attributed the negative perceptions to deficiencies among those who stigmatized them. These researchers found no evidence of the passive acceptance of labels and negative identities. These women appeared to avoid social interactions where they anticipated feeling different and excluded and formed new social networks with groups in which they felt accepted and understood. Whereas they acknowledged the negative consequences of mental illness, there did not appear to be an automatic link between these consequences and negative self-evaluation. Factors that contributed to a positive self-evaluation included membership in a supportive group, finding themselves in a more favourable circumstance than others with the same problems, and sharing experiences with others who had knowledge and insight about mental illness.

In summary, stigma, defined as discrediting another, arises from widely held social beliefs about personality, behaviour, and illness and is communicated to individuals through a process of socialization. When individuals display the condition that engenders the mark of discredit, they may experience social devaluation and discrimination. Stigma clearly attaches to individuals with mental illness and infectious, chronic and terminal diseases. There is increasing evidence of stigma associated with clinical obesity (Campos, 2004). Stigma may produce changes in perception of body image, social isolation, rejection, loss of status, and perceived lack of personal control. However, some evidences suggest that stigma does not attach universally to individuals with marked behaviour or conditions. Some individuals appear resistant to stigma, identifying flaws in the society conveying the negative beliefs. These individuals share experiences with others who have knowledge of and sensitivity to being stigmatized and benefit from the ability to perceive themselves as equal to or better off than others with the same condition.

UNIQUE ASPECTS OF STIGMA

There are special circumstances in which stigma can be perceived with enhanced distinction. Individuals who lack a fully developed sense of personal identity and who rely on external sources to reinforce their internal sense of worthiness may be uniquely prone to a sense of stigma. Adolescence can be used as an example. There are aspects of society that tend to be highly valued by individuals, and when that society communicates stigma, the stigmatizing beliefs are uniquely powerful. Religion and culture are examples, as well as issues concerning self-infliction and punishment.

The task of developing a stable, coherent identity is one of the most important tasks of adolescence (Erikson, 1968). To successfully complete this task the adolescent must be able to use formal operational thinking within a context of expanded social experiences to evolve a sense of self that integrates not only the similarities but also the differences observed between the self and others. Social interactions and messages from the sociocultural environment about what is desirable and what is not desirable guide and direct the adolescent towards an identity that incorporates desired similarities and rejects undesired differences. The influences and preferences of peers become important as the adolescent seeks acceptance of this newly developed sense of identity. The skill of labelling and stigmatizing individuals with intolerable differences is wielded with frightening force and sometimes terrible consequences—the 1999 Columbine High School tragedy is one example.

Intolerance often results in bullying and peer aggressiveness in the adolescent. Wang, Iannotti, Luk, and Nansel (2010) examined subtypes of bullying in a national sample of 7,475 adolescents in the United States. Bullying of all types (verbal, physical, relational, cyber, and cell phone) that occurred among students in grades 6 to 10 was related to depression, physical injuries, and increased medication use to manage nervousness and insomnia. Bullying, including cyberbullying, has also been linked to suicidal thoughts and behaviours in the adolescent (Brunstein Klomek, Sourander, & Gould, 2010; Hinduja & Patchin, 2010).

Normal adolescent maturation may include dealing with sudden growth spurts, changes in body image, and even acne associated with fluctuating hormone levels. Australian researchers explored the experience of adolescents living with very visible skin disorders (e.g., severe acne, psoriasis) (Magin, Adams, Heading, Pond, & Smith, 2006). These youth (aged 11–18 years) were stigmatized and frequently the targets of teasing and bullying behaviours by peers.

Culture may determine stigma as well. For some conditions, such as traumatic brain injury (Simpson, Mohr, & Redman, 2000), HIV/AIDS (Heckman et al., 2004), and epilepsy (Baker, Brooks, Buck, & Jacoby, 2000), stigma and social isolation cross cultural boundaries. On the other hand, in a study of attitudes about homelessness in 11 European cities, Brandon, Khoo, Maglajlie, and Abuel-Ealeh (2000) found marked differences in attitudes between countries, with high levels of stigma predominating in former Warsaw Pact countries. A determination of racial and/or cultural inferiority of a minority group by a dominant group may result in racism, discrimination, and stigma (Weston, 2003).

Religion may also play a role in stigma. In a study of five large religious groups in London that examined attitudes about depression and schizophrenia, fear of stigma among non-White groups was prevalent, particularly the fear of being misunderstood by White HCPs not of the same religious group (Cinnirella & Loewenthal, 1999).

The label and associated stigma of a disability or disease excludes individuals from social interaction or alters social relationships, whereas their intellectual or physical handicaps alone may not (Link et al., 1997). Vulnerable populations are in jeopardy of forming unhealthy relationships. Results from a South African study indicated that the stigma of disability increased participation in risky behaviours (Rohleder, 2010). Individuals with a physical or mental disability were more likely to engage in unsafe sexual practices, thereby increasing their risk of contracting HIV/AIDS. The desire to form an attachment and establish a physical relationship with another human being outweighed the need to protect oneself. The concepts of self-worth and self-esteem are interwoven with stigma.

Most stigmas are perceived as threatening by and to others. Criminals and social deviants are stigmatized because they create a sense of anxiety by threatening society's values and safety. Similarly, encounters with sick and disabled individuals also cause anxiety and apprehension, but in a different way. The encounter destroys the dream that life is fair. Sick people remind us of our mortality and vulnerability; consequently, physically healthy individuals may make negative value judgments about those who are ill or disabled (Kurzban & Leary, 2001). For example, some sighted individuals may regard those who are blind as being dependent or unwilling to take care of themselves, an assumption that is not based on what the blind person is willing or able to do. Individuals with AIDS are often subjected to moral judgment. Those with psychiatric illness have been stigmatized since medieval times (Keltner, Schwecke, & Bostrom, 2003). As a result, these individuals deal with more than their symptomatology; on a daily basis they contend with those who perceive them as less worthy or valuable, because they possess a stigma.

Some individuals are stigmatized because the behaviour or difference is considered to be self-inflicted and therefore less worthy of help. Alcoholism, drug-related problems, obesity, and mental illness are frequently included in this category (Crisp et al., 2000; Ritson, 1999). In fact, alcoholism as a disease is highly stigmatized as compared with other mental illnesses (Schomerus et al., 2010). HIV/AIDS and hepatitis B are examples of infectious diseases in which the mode of infection is considered to be self-inflicted as a result of socially unacceptable behaviour; therefore, affected individuals are stigmatized (Halevy, 2000; Heckman et al., 2004).

In the past the words "shame" and "guilt" were used to describe a concept similar to stigma—a perceived difference between a behaviour or an attribute and an ideal standard. From this perspective guilt is defined as self-criticism, and shame results from the disapproval of others. Guilt is similar to seeing oneself as discreditable. Shame is a painful feeling caused by the scorn or contempt of others. For example, a person with alcoholism may feel guilty about drinking and also feel ashamed that others perceive his or her behaviour as less than desirable.

Whenever a stigma is present the devaluing characteristic is so powerful it overshadows other traits and becomes the focus of one's personal evaluation (Kurzban & Leary, 2001). This trait, or differentness, is sufficiently powerful to break the claim of all other attributes (Goffman, 1963). As an example, the fact that a nurse has unstable type 1 diabetes may cancel her or his remaining identity as a competent health professional. The stigma attached to a professor's stutter may overshadow academic competence.

The extent of stigma resulting from any particular condition cannot be predicted. Individuals with a specific disease do not universally feel the same degree of stigma. On the other hand, very different disabilities may possess the same stigma. In writing about individuals with mental illness, Link and colleagues (1997) described variations in symptomatology among them; however, individuals without mental illness did not take those variations into account. All individuals who were disabled were seen as sharing the same stigma—mental illness—regardless of their capabilities or severity of their illness. That is, people responded to the mental illness stereotype rather than to the person's actual physical and mental capabilities.

Similarly, Herek, Capitanio, and Widaman (2003) reported on the stigmatizing effects of the label of HIV/AIDS. They found those individuals who reported a perceived reduction in the level of stigma attached to HIV/AIDS overall still generally expressed negative feelings towards people with AIDS and favoured a name-based reporting system such as that used by the public health department for other communicable diseases.

TYPES OF STIGMA

Stigma is a universal phenomenon, and every society stigmatizes. Goffman (1963) distinguished among three types of stigma. The first is the stigma of physical deformity. The actual stigma is the deficit between the expected norm of perfect physical condition and the actual physical condition. For example, many chronic conditions create changes in physical appearance or function. These changes frequently create a difference in self- or other-perception.

Stigma can arise from a normal physiological process—aging. The normal aging process creates a body far different from the television commercial "norm" of youth, physical beauty, and leanness. Younger people tend to differentiate themselves from older people based on the differences in appearances, physique, and mentality. Butler (1975) first termed "the process of systemically stereotyping and discriminating against people because they are old" as ageism (p. 894). Detrimental consequences may follow after labelling a person as elderly, senior citizen, or aged. For example, a person who is hard of hearing may refuse to use a hearing aid to avoid being labelled as "getting old." In fact, hearing loss was considered a perceived stigma in aging and the use of hearing aids was associated with being disabled in one longitudinal qualitative study (Wallhagen, 2010). Another study with 103 adults aged 60 to 70 years found them to be more sensitive to stereotyping threats affecting memory performance (Hess, Hinson, & Hodges, 2009). In other words, if the older adult is conscious of how his or her behaviour may reflect negatively on the older adult population, he or she may have increased anxiety and reduced memory capacity. Although physical decline, loneliness, and depression in the older adult have been well documented in the literature, interventions must be implemented to enhance "positive aging" (Stephens & Flick, 2010). Health promotion and positive aging attitudes can only be accomplished when the stigma of ageism is abolished.

The second type of stigma is that of character blemishes. This type may occur in individuals with HIV/AIDS, alcoholism, mental illness, or sexually transmitted diseases. For example, individuals infected with HIV face considerable stigma because many believe the infected person could have controlled the behaviours that resulted in the infection (Halevy, 2000; Heckman et al., 2004; Herek et al., 2003; Weston, 2003). Likewise, individuals with eating disorders such as anorexia nervosa fear being stigmatized (Stewart, Keel, & Schiavo, 2006). The fear of stigma can be a major barrier to seeking treatment.

The third type of stigma is tribal in origin and is known more commonly as prejudice. This type of stigma originates when one group perceives features of race, religion, or nationality of another group as deficient compared with their own socially constructed norm. Most HCPs agree that prejudice has no place in the healthcare delivery system. Although some professionals display both subtle and overt intolerance, others strive to treat persons of every age, race, and nationality with sensitivity. However, prejudice against individuals with chronic illnesses exists as surely as racial or religious prejudice.

The three types of stigma may overlap and reinforce each other (Kurzban & Leary, 2001). Individuals who are already socially isolated because of race, age, or poverty will be additionally hurt by the isolation resulting from another stigma. Heukelbach and Feldmeier (2006) stated that scabies infestations are associated with poverty in undeveloped countries, which contributes to the stigmatization of both diagnosis and treatment. Those who are financially disadvantaged or culturally distinct (that is, stigmatized by the majority of society) will suffer more stigma should they become disabled. Poor women with HIV feared the stigma associated with HIV/AIDS more than dying of the disease (Abel, 2007).

Psychologists and sociologists have built on Goffman's theory to address the concepts of felt stigma and enacted stigma (Jacoby, 1994; Scambler, 2004). Felt stigma is the internalized perception of being devalued or "not as good as" by an individual. It may be related to fears of being treated differently or of being labelled by others, even though the stigmatizing attribute is not known or outwardly apparent. The other component of felt stigma is shame (Scambler, 2004). Individuals view themselves as discreditable. The quote at the beginning of this chapter is an example of a client experiencing felt stigma.

Enacted stigma, on the other hand, refers to behaviours and perceptions by others towards the individual who is perceived as different. Enacted stigma is the situational response of others to a visible, overt stigmatizing attribute of another (Jacoby, 1994; Scambler, 2004). Hesitating or failing to shake hands with a person who has vitiligo, a dermatological condition characterized by hypopigmentation of the skin, is an example of enacted stigma.

Felt and enacted stigma may overlap. "Smoke-free" regulations are now in effect across the United States and abroad. Whereas these laws have been enacted to protect the public from the carcinogens and toxins present in second-hand smoke, the smoking behaviour may be viewed as an unfavourable attribute. By association, the individual who smokes may be seen as "less than" or as less favourable. Thus, the individuals who smoke may experience both felt stigma and enacted stigma. Indeed, some smokers and recent ex-smokers in Scotland described themselves as "lepers" (Ritchie, Amos, & Martin, 2010). The temporary segregation occurring as a result of "smoking sections" led them to stigmatize themselves as well as their behaviours and that of other smokers.

Stigma is prevalent in our society, and once it occurs it endures (Link et al., 1997). If the cause of stigma is removed, the effects are not easily overcome. An individual's social identity has already been influenced by the stigmatizing attribute. A person with a history of alcoholism or mental illness continues to carry a stigma in the same way a former prison inmate does.

CHRONIC DISEASE AS STIGMA

Individuals with chronic illness present deviations from what many people expect in daily social interchanges. In general, most people do not expect to meet someone with an electronic voice box after treatment for laryngeal cancer. Both the cancer and the assistive device may not be readily visible, but once the person begins to speak the individual is at risk of being labelled as "different" by others.

Canadian values contribute to the perception of chronic illness as a stigmatizing condition. That is, the dominant culture emphasizes qualities of youth, attractiveness, and personal accomplishment. The work ethic and heritage of the Western frontier provide heroes who are strong, conventionally productive, and physically healthy. Television and magazines demonstrate, on a daily basis, that physical perfection is the standard against which all are measured, yet these societal values collide with the reality of chronic disease. A discrepancy exists between the realities of a chronic condition, such as arthritis or HIV/AIDS, and the social expectation of physical perfection.

A disease characteristic or one having an unknown aetiology may contribute to the stigma of many chronic illnesses. In fact, any disease having an unclear cause or ineffectual treatment is suspect, including Alzheimer's disease (Jolley

& Benbow, 2000) and anxiety disorders (Davies, 2000). Clients with Alzheimer's disease also may be stigmatized because of perceptions relating to their level of decision-making competence (Werner, 2006). Diseases that are somewhat mysterious and at the same time feared, such as leprosy, are often believed to be morally contagious.

Stigma can be associated with inequitable treatment, although the relative severity of such inequitable treatment often varies with the degree of severity of the stigmatized condition. For example, public policy about HIV/AIDS has acted both to increase accessibility to treatment and potentially to limit the civil rights of the stigmatized individuals (Herek et al., 2003). In addition, the shame, guilt, and social isolation of some stigmatized individuals may lead to inequitable treatment for their families. Because of the secrecy associated with being HIV positive, affected clients and family members may not be able to access needed mental health, substance abuse rehabilitation, or infectious disease therapies (Salisbury, 2000).

Lawson et al. (2006) studied experiences of stigma, fear, and discrimination related to HIV/AIDS in individuals from African and Caribbean communities living in Toronto. Thirty individuals living with HIV/AIDS were interviewed, and 74 community members without HIV/AIDS participated in focus groups. Stigma towards people with HIV living in their community emerged as a primary finding for the study. Participants within the community focus groups often placed blame on the individual for acquiring HIV; furthermore, blame or innocence was assigned to HIV-positive people depending on how they became infected. Perceptions of social status and the notion of living at the edge of society also contributed to the amount of stigma an individual received. The thought of disclosing the

diagnosis of HIV/AIDS was thought to be a "death sentence" in itself because it would often mean exile from the community. Community members described how it was common to watch other members for signs of illness such as frequent trips to the physician's office or rapid weight loss. Stigma was also thought to intersect with racism on wider levels. Participants living with HIV/AIDS highlighted how their disease was often linked to other stereotypes associated with their culture.

This chapter has defined stigma and presented a framework for understanding stigma as a social construct. All types of stigma share a common tie: In every case an individual who might have interacted easily in a particular social situation may now be prevented from doing so by the discredited trait. The trait may become the focus of attention and potentially turn others away.

IMPACT OF STIGMA

Stigma has an impact on both the affected individual and those persons who do not share the particular trait. Responses to stigma vary and are discussed from the perspective of the person living with stigma, the layperson, and the HCP.

INDIVIDUAL LIVING WITH STIGMA

Stigmatized individuals respond to the reactions of others in a variety of ways. They are often unsure about the attitudes of others and therefore may feel a constant need to make a good impression. Individuals living with stigma each and every day may choose to accept society's or others' view of them or may choose to reject others' discrediting viewpoints. Culture may limit the coping choices available, particularly in relation to disclosing a mental illness. In a study of West Indian women coping with depression, Schreiber, Stern, and Wilson (2000) found that "being strong" was the culturally sanctioned behaviour for depression rather than disclosure.

Passing

Passing oneself off as "normal" is one strategy used by individuals living with a stigmatizing condition. Pretending to have no disability or a less stigmatic identity (Dudley, 1983; Goffman, 1963; Joachim & Acorn, 2000) may be an option if the stigmatizing attribute is not readily visible.

Passing is a viable option for those with felt stigma associated with conditions such as type 2 diabetes or a positive AIDS antibody test but no symptoms. The process of passing may include the concealment of any signs of the stigma.

Some individuals refuse to use adaptive devices, such as hearing aids, because this tells others of their disability. Another example is the abused client who provides reasonable explanations for bruises, swelling, and injuries. The practice of "passing" may significantly impair the health-seeking behaviour of the abused individual, particularly where sociocultural barriers to disclosure exist (Bauer, Rodriguez, Quiroga, & Flores-Ortiz, 2000).

CASE STUDY 1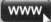

Richard Wilson is a 43-year-old, married, high school science teacher. He is 100 pounds overweight and smokes cigarettes (1 pack per day for the past 20 years). He is thankful that he is in reasonably good health, although he does state that "my doctor started making me take a blood pressure pill every day when I saw her 2 months ago." Mr. Wilson lives in a province that has recently enacted smoke-free legislation. He rarely travels because he is concerned that he "will not fit in those tiny airplane seats."

Discussion Questions

1. For what type of stigma is Mr. Wilson at risk? How would you assess this client's self-perception of stigma?
2. What strategies can the healthcare provider offer this client to reduce the effects of stigma?
3. At Mr. Wilson's next blood pressure check appointment, how can the nurse evaluate whether the client has made progress in reducing felt and/or enacted stigma?
4. What strategies can the HCP use to help break through the barriers of enacted stigma by members of the healthcare team towards individuals with negatively perceived lifestyle behaviours?
5. How can the HCP assess nutritional status and make recommendations for behavioural change without stigmatizing the individual?

CASE STUDY 2

Dr. Min Pak is a 78-year-old retired nursing professor from Korea. While visiting her son in Canada she developed nausea, vomiting, diarrhoea, and abdominal pain. She went to a nearby urgent care centre. The nurse at the urgent care centre just finished checking her vital signs.

Dr. Pak: What are my blood pressure and temperature?

Nurse: Blood pressure is a little low and you have a low-grade temperature.

Dr. Pak: Could you please tell me the numbers?

Nurse: Blood pressure is in the 90s and you have a slight fever. Trust me, you don't need to know the exact numbers. By the way, when was the last time you had something to eat or drink, sweetie?

Dr. Pak: [thinking]

Nurse: When did you last have something to eat or drink? [*speaking louder and gesturing eating and drinking with mouth and hand*]

Dr. Pak: I heard you. That was 3 hours ago.

Nurse: You marked on the health form that you have chronic pancreatitis. How often and how much do you drink? And, of what kind?

Discussion Questions

1. What type of stigma is Dr. Pak experiencing?
2. Describe the nurse's attitudes and perceptions of stigma.
3. What interventions to reduce stigma would you suggest the client and the healthcare provider implement?
4. What are the implications for professional nursing practice?

Covering

Because of the potential threat and anxiety-provoking nature of disclosing a stigmatizing difference, most people deemphasize their differentness. This response, called covering, is an attempt to make the difference seem smaller or less significant than it really is (Goffman, 1963). Covering involves understanding the difference between visibility and obtrusiveness; that is, the condition is openly acknowledged but its consequences are minimized.

Persons with special dietary requirements may deny the importance of maintaining the restriction in a social situation, even though they follow it. The goal is to divert attention from the defect, create a more comfortable situation for all, and minimize the risk of experiencing enacted stigma.

Humour, used in a skilful and light-hearted manner by the stigmatized individual, may decrease the anxiety of others and avoid an awkward encounter. This form of covering neutralizes the anxiety-producing subject; therefore, it is no longer taboo and can more easily be managed.

Disregard

A person's first response to enacted stigma may be disregard. In other words they may choose not to reflect on or discuss the painful incidents. Well-adjusted individuals who are comfortable with their identity, have dealt with stigma for a long time, and choose not to respond to the reaction of others may disregard it (Dudley, 1983).

Other examples are wheelchair athletes. These athletes disregard perceptions that their disabilities prohibit them from participating in strenuous, athletic endeavours. Any person who has observed these well-conditioned athletes racing their wheelchairs up hills in competitive meets may find it difficult to consider them discredited.

Going public with a serious medical diagnosis is another example of disregard by acting in the face of negative consequences. One positive aspect of going public is the potential for assertive political action and social change. Celebrities such as Muhammed Ali, Earvin (Magic) Johnson, Michael J. Fox, and the late Christopher and Dana Reeve, among others, have captured public attention and acted positively to reduce enacted stigma by disclosing their personal struggles with a variety of conditions.

Resistance and Rejection

Similar to disregard, resistance and rejection are additional strategies used in response to stigma (Dudley, 1983). Individuals may speak out and challenge rules and protocol if their needs are not met. More recently, Franks, Henwood, and Bowden (2007) noted that resisting and rejecting were strategies used by maternal mental health clients. These disadvantaged mothers outright rejected or actively resisted the judgments of professionals who held negative opinions. Broader societal misconceptions, such as the belief all teen mothers are on welfare, also were rejected. The use of resistance or rejection can be used to preserve or bolster a more positive self-identity and effect larger societal changes.

Isolation

Humans have a proclivity for separating themselves into small subgroups because staying with one's own group is easier, requires less effort, and, for some individuals, is more congenial. However, this separation into groups tends to emphasize differences rather than similarities (Link et al., 1989). Closed interaction from within may enhance one's feelings of normality because the individual is surrounded by others who are similar (Camp et al., 2002). The process of isolation can occur any time outsiders are seen as threatening or are reminders that the world is different from the in-group.

Staying with like others may be a source of support, but some individuals with a disability or chronic illness may feel more comfortable when they are surrounded by nondisabled individuals. A young woman, disabled since birth, feels better around nondisabled people because she has always considered herself normal. Her attitude reminds us to use caution when making assumptions about the perceptions of others.

Information Management

In addition to the stigmatized individual, family members often acquire a secondary stigma as a result of association (Goffman, 1963) and must deal with their own responses to situations of enacted stigma. Mothers who are HIV positive expend significant effort to protect their children from the negative effects of disclosure of their HIV status (Sandelowski & Barroso, 2003). Likewise, family members who care for persons with HIV/AIDS share the stigma and are discredited, resulting in rejection, loss of friends, and harassment (Gewirtz & Gossart-Walker, 2000; Salisbury, 2000).

Information management is used by both the individual and loved ones in dealing with felt and enacted stigma. The world may be divided into a large group of people to whom they tell nothing and a small group of insiders who are aware of the stigmatizing condition. HCPs may use information management in an attempt to lessen the likelihood of stigma for a client. For example, listing a diagnosis of Hansen's disease or mycobacterial neurodermatitis gives the client the option of revealing the alternate name of leprosy, with its accompanying historical stigma.

Layperson: Responses to and Effects of Stigma

Responses of an individual to a stigmatized person vary with the particular stigma and the individual's past conditioning. Because society specifies the characteristics that are stigmatized, it also teaches its members how to react to that stigma. Differences between groups based on nationality and culture have been found in attitudes towards those with disabilities (Brandon et al., 2000; Cinnirella & Loewenthal, 1999). Just as children learn to interact with others who are culturally different by watching and listening to those around them, they also learn how to treat individuals with chronic illness or disabilities by incorporating societal judgments. Sadly, these reactions are often negative.

With the advances in telecommunication and electronic communication the general public is more aware of chronic physical and mental illnesses. Yet an online survey by the American Psychiatric Association (2010) on the perception of mental illness found the stigma still persisted. Adults ($n = 2,285$) who responded to the survey revealed an increased acceptance to mental disorders, especially when they had a personal experience of the disease with family and friends. Other responders kept a more open mind after obtaining accurate information on mental illnesses from the mass media, celebrity figures, and Internet sources.

Devaluing

People may believe the person with the stigma is less valuable, less human, or less desired. Unfortunately, many of us practice more than one kind of discrimination and, by so doing, effectively reduce the life chances of the stigmatized individual (Goffman, 1963). Devaluing results in enacted stigma as demonstrated by those who categorize individuals as inferior or even dangerous. Use of words such as "cripple" or "moron" also represent a devaluing of individuals.

Stereotyping

Categories simplify our lives. Instead of needing to decide what to do in every situation, we can respond to categories of situations. Stereotypes are a negative type of category. They are a social reaction to ambiguous situations and allow us to react to group expectations rather than to individuals. When individuals meet those with physical impairments, expectations are not clear (Katz, 1981). People often are at a loss as to how to react, so placing the individual with chronic illness in a stereotyped category reduces the ambiguousness towards him or her and makes the situation more comfortable for those doing the stereotyping. Much less effort is required to sustain a bias than is required to reconsider or alter it.

Using stereotypes to understand individuals decreases our attention to other positive characteristics (Hynd, 1958). Categorizing tends to make one see the world as a dichotomy. For example, people are categorized as either mentally delayed or not, even though mental capabilities exist on a continuum, with all of us falling somewhere along the line.

Responses such as scapegoating and ostracizing people with HIV/AIDS have increased the impact of this disease and delayed treatment (Distabile, Dubler, Solomon, & Klein, 1999; Rehm & Franck, 2000; Salisbury, 2000). These responses also impede appropriate health education aimed at prevention.

Labelling

The label attached to an individual's condition is crucial and influences the way we think about that individual. The diagnosis of HIV/AIDS is a powerful label, possibly resulting in the loss of relationships and jobs. People with learning disabilities may not mind being called slow learners but may be startled by being called mentally retarded (Dudley, 1983). Their response indicates that they see this latter term as a negative label.

Professional Responses: Attitudes and Perceptions of Stigma

In the United States most HCPs share the American dream of achievement, attractiveness, and a cohesive, healthy family. These values influence our perceptions of individuals who are disabled, chronically ill, or otherwise considered "less than normal." Although the factors that contribute to these individual differences vary, the consequences of stigma associated with chronic illnesses are similar in different health conditions and cultures (Van Brakel, 2006).

Attitudes

It is not surprising that society's values and definitions of stigma affect the attitudes of HCPs. Attitudes can be changed by interactions with clients and acquaintances with chronic illness (Sandelowski & Barroso, 2003). Students' confidence in clients' ability to cope with a disease increased with professional experience. In a similar manner, knowing someone with a chronic disease increased positive attitudes. When HCPs (general practitioners, nurses, and counsellors) were asked about their perceptions of depression among older adults, they agreed the older adults displayed embarrassment and shame when disclosing feelings of depression. Older adults were perceived as reluctant to seek mental health services because depression was identified as a stigma. Whether these perceptions of the HCPs are consistent with those of the older adults requires further examination (Murray et al., 2006).

Perceptions

HCPs' perceptions of stigma affect care outcomes. Liggins and Hatcher (2005) studied the stigma of mental illness in the hospital setting. Labelling a client as mentally ill had a negative impact on both the client and the HCP. Clients believed they were ignored or treated differently because they had mental illness. They feared how the HCP would respond to them. The HCP showed disbelief towards physical ailments because the client had "mental disease." Healthcare providers also assumed mental illness was associated with an unpredictable behaviour that might affect the HCP–client relationship (Liggins & Hatcher, 2005). Clearly, interventions to reduce perceptions of stigma and episodes of enacted stigma in the hospital setting are needed.

The attitude of the healthcare provider is vital in reducing the stigma associated with chronic illness. HCPs who are nonjudgmental, empathic, and knowledgeable were observed to reduce the perception of stigma in a specialized HIV/AIDS unit. Stigma was minimized when nurses and other interdisciplinary team members identified themselves with the behaviours of the clients, held a positive view of the disease, and reached consensus in the delivery of appropriate care (Hodgson, 2006).

Another study of medical students' perspectives of illness disclosed a surprising aspect of stigma. Medical students revealed a high level of concern over the perception of social stigma attached to their own personal health problems and the resulting professional jeopardy they might encounter upon disclosure (Roberts, Warner, & Trumpower, 2000).

HCPs potentially display all the reactions and responses towards discredited individuals that laypersons do. Therefore, caregivers need a thorough understanding of these responses if we are to overcome the effects of stigmatizing behaviour or to eliminate it outright. Understanding the concept of stigma increases one's ability to plan interventions for clients with chronic illnesses (Joachim & Acorn, 2000).

INTERVENTIONS: COPING WITH STIGMA OR REDUCING STIGMA

A chronic illness or disability imposes various constraints on an individual's life. The stigma of a specific disorder adds additional burdens, often far greater than those caused by the disorder itself

(Joachim & Acorn, 2000). Individuals with chronic conditions usually receive medical treatment, but few interventions may be directed at reducing the effects of the associated stigma.

Helping others to manage the effects of stigma is not simple and should be approached with care. At best, change will be slow and uneven. However, consistent and knowledgeable interventions aimed specifically at reducing the impact of stigma are as crucial as those that reduce blood pressure or chronic pain. The following section discusses appropriate strategies healthcare providers can use in their practice to address the issue of stigma.

HCP and Client Interactions

The HCP who is aware of his or her own biases, beliefs, and behaviours has already begun to mitigate the effects of stigma for the client and family members. Being aware of the societal context and implications that a diagnosis of chronic illness carries enables the HCP to work with the client to develop strategies to prevent, reduce, or cope with potentially stigmatizing conditions. Part of this is contingent upon the HCP's ability to provide *culturally competent care*. According to Leninger and McFarland (2002), culturally competent care is

> "the use of culturally based care and health knowledge in sensitive, creative and meaningful ways to fit the general lifeways and needs of individuals or groups for beneficial and meaningful health and well-being or to help them face illness, disabilities, or death" (p. 84).

To do so HCPs must be aware of their personal attitudes towards others of different cultures. Although awareness and sensitivity are part of cultural competence, competency implies that awareness and sensitivity have been operationalized (Schim, Doorenbos, Benkert, & Miller, 2007).

Professional Attitudes: Cure Versus Care

Traditionally, the goal of health care has been to cure the client. Because chronic illness is now more prevalent than infectious disease or acute illness, this criterion of success may be inappropriate. Cure is neither essential nor necessary in order that the client benefit. Instead, caring, demonstrated by valuing and assisting, should be the criterion. With the increasing number of people with chronic illnesses, professionals must learn to accept those characteristics accompanying chronic illness: an indeterminate course of disease, relapses, and multiple treatment modalities. Cost containment is a central focus in healthcare delivery. Providers must not lose sight, however, of health policy considerations that include ideas of personhood and equitable health care sensitive to the reality of stigmatizing chronic illness (Gewirtz & Gossart-Walker, 2000; Roskes, Feldman, Arrington, & Leisher, 1999; Salisbury, 2000).

Mutual Participation Model

The manner in which health care is delivered may increase or decrease the effects of stigma. Encouraging a client's participation in health-care decision making is an outward demonstration of respect and regard for that person. Establishing the client as a partner in setting goals demonstrates one's acceptance and valuing of the individual. On the other hand, when HCPs make decisions regarding treatment or goals without consulting a client, they reinforce the person's feeling of being discredited or discreditable. Therefore, any mode of care delivery that increases client participation enhances that person's perception of self-worth and reduces the effects of stigma. The mutual participation model is the model of choice in managing chronic diseases because it enhances the client's feelings of self-worth. The client is responsible for long-term disease management, and the HCP is responsible for helping the client help him- or herself.

Mutual participation divides power evenly between professional and client and leads to a relationship that can be mutually satisfying. In other words, the client should be as satisfied with the recommendations and decisions as the provider is. In addition, each party depends on the other for information culminating in a satisfactory solution. The client needs the provider's experience and expertise; the provider does not only need the client's history and symptoms but his or her priorities, expectations, and goals as well. Sometimes a choice between treatments with relatively equal mortality rates is necessary—for example, surgery or radiation for cancer treatment. The professional can offer expert knowledge regarding long-term effects of radiation and changes in body image due to surgery. The client must decide the relative value of side effects of the alternative proposed treatments. Because the "right" decision depends on the individual, input from both client and healthcare provider is necessary to produce a course of action that is mutually acceptable.

When HCPs become more comfortable with allowing clients a greater range of participation and decision making, the relationship decreases some of the stigmatizing effects of the disability. HCPs must create an atmosphere in which individuals with chronic conditions not only are expected to cooperate but are encouraged to express their concerns, observations, expectations, and limitations. Together, they explore alternative strategies and decide on one that is agreeable to both. When a client's priorities and goals are valued and incorporated into the regimen, an increased sense of acceptance emerges. Therefore, the respect and regard for clients demonstrated by this model provide effective tools to counteract some stigmatizing effects of illness.

HCPs who establish a therapeutic relationship with their client are ideally situated to assess their client's perceptions of felt or enacted stigma. Asking open-ended questions to ascertain how the client perceives himself or herself, the meaning of the disease to the client, and types of interactions with others may elicit valuable information. Family members and significant others may be included in the assessment as well.

It is particularly important to distinguish between nonparticipation and nonacceptance when caring for stigmatized individuals. Nonparticipation is an abstinence from social activities that is based on limitations caused by a disability or illness. Nonacceptance, on the other hand, is a negative attitude—a resistance or reluctance on the part of the nondisabled person to admit the disabled person to various kinds and degrees of social relationships (Ladieu-Leviton, Adler, & Dembo, 1977). A person with a disability who chooses not to join a camping trip is a nonparticipant; the physical disability serves as the basis for that person's decision not to participate. Deciding not to invite that person to join the group, whether or not participation is possible, is nonacceptance; it pre-empts the person's choice and is a form of enacted stigma.

Commonly, individuals without a disability cannot accurately estimate the limits of potential participation for those with a disease or disability—a key point for HCPs to remember. Typically, the physical limitations imposed by a disability are overestimated by others. If nondisabled individuals incorrectly assume a disabled individual is not able to participate, that is a form of nonacceptance. Such nonacceptance is created by the difference between the degree of participation that is actually possible and the degree assumed possible by those who are not disabled. If the difference can be resolved, nonacceptance ceases to be a problem.

The remedy for this dilemma is simple. Nondisabled individuals can simply indicate that they want the disabled individual to participate, leaving to him or her the decision of whether to become involved. Perhaps the individual with the disability would like to participate, but in a different way. For example, the young adult who has juvenile arthritis may not regret being unable to actually fish if he or she can go along on the trip and spend time socializing with friends. HCPs can encourage their clients to look for these opportunities to participate as they are able.

Family members or significant others who are involved in the client's care must not be forgotten. An ethnographic study of immediate family members of burn survivors explored the perceptions of stigma (Rossi, Vila Vda, Zago, & Ferreira, 2005). The stigma associated with the burn and the accompanying feelings of loss of control affected both the client and the family. The family had fears of facing the reactions from society, which encompassed feelings of sadness, anger, denial, resignation, and/or anxiety. Some family members expressed feelings of shame when living with someone whose role and appearance changed due to the burn injuries. Thus, it is imperative that the perceptions of both the stigmatized person and the family are assessed.

Client-Centred Interventions

Strategies to Increase Self-Worth

Societal norms and values are a major determinant of an individual's sense of self-esteem and self-worth. The person who does not possess the expected attribute is quite aware of this discredit as an equal and desired individual in society. In addition, individuals with chronic conditions may find their own deformities or failings decrease their self-respect. That is, not only do stigmatized individuals have to deal with the responses of others (enacted stigma), but some experience strong negative feelings about their own self-worth (felt stigma). These internalized perceptions may be more difficult to deal with than the illness or disability itself. Examples of negative feelings were described by 60 study participants with epilepsy. More than half of the participants experienced feelings of shame, fear, worry, and low self-esteem, and one-fourth had the perception of stigma (de Souza & Salgado, 2006).

In another study obese individuals and their family members noted both stigmatization and discrimination on the basis of weight. They reported being constantly reminded by family members, peers, healthcare providers, and strangers that they were inferior as compared with those who were not obese (Rogge, Greenwald, & Golden, 2004).

In an attempt to change self-perception of stigma, Abel (2007) used an intervention of emotional writing disclosure for women with HIV. Women who participated in the intervention had more positive scores on the stigma scale tool at the end of the 12-week pilot study than women in the control group. The stigma scale is a 28-item self-report questionnaire developed to measure the stigma felt by clients with psychiatric illness (King et al., 2007). This journaling strategy may be one way the healthcare provider can help individuals change their internal perception of stigma.

With these internalized negative perceptions, some people with chronic illness choose to conceal the disease. When 14 people with a diagnosis of multiple sclerosis and their families were interviewed, it was found that the disease was purposefully concealed or selectively disclosed to shield from social judgment or to enhance social belonging at work (Grytten & Maseide, 2005). In describing studies of clients with cerebral palsy, cancer, facial deformity, arthritis, and multiple sclerosis, Shontz (1977) noted that the personal meaning of the disability to each client was uniformly regarded as crucial. For example, individuals who feel valuable because they are healthy and physically fit usually experience feelings of worthlessness if they contract a chronic condition. But people with diabetes will never be without a regimen and the necessary paraphernalia; visually impaired individuals will never see normally again. Therefore, the individuals' reactions and ability to accommodate these discrepancies determine their attitudes of worth and value.

In contrast, some individuals with chronic conditions can accept deviations from expected norms and feel relatively untouched. They have reordered life's priorities; no longer is the absence of disease or disability their major criterion for self-worth. Rather, an alternative ideology evolves to counter the "standard" ideologies. A strong sense of identity protects them, and they are able to feel acceptable in the face of the stigma (Goffman, 1963).

This identity belief system, also called cognitive belief patterns, refers to a person's perspective. It includes one's perceptions, mental attitudes, beliefs, and interpretations of experiences (Link et al., 1997). Individuals who are stigmatized by the major society may believe and perceive that their groups are actually superior or at least preferable. These belief patterns offer protection from the stigmatized reactions of others. Yet, being in a specific cultural or ethnic group does not always provide protection against stigma in certain diseases. In fact, the stigma of having a mental illness is even more prominent among some ethnic groups. A literature review by Gary (2005) found that African Americans, Asian Americans, Hispanic Americans, and Indian Americans all perceived stigma related to mental illness in addition to the prejudice and discrimination already experienced due to the affiliation with their particular ethnic group.

Cognitive belief patterns help individuals with chronic illnesses achieve identity acceptance and protection in the face of stigmatizing conditions. For example, after extensive cancer surgery, clients may consciously tell themselves they are full human beings because the missing part was diseased or useless. The body, although disfigured, is now healthy and totally acceptable. Similarly, wheelchair athletes take pride in their superb physical condition and competitiveness. That is, one's perception of self-worth influences one's reactions to disease or disability. An individual's question "Am I worthwhile?" is answered by determining his or her own values and perspective. Therefore, clients' definitions of themselves are crucial factors in self-satisfaction.

Support Groups

Goffman (1963) used the term "the own" for those who share a stigma. Those who share the same stigma can offer the "tricks of the trade," acceptance, and moral support to a person living with stigma. Self-help or support groups are examples of persons who are the own. Alcoholics Anonymous, for instance, provides a community of the own as well as a way of life for its members. Members speak publicly, demonstrating that people with alcoholism are treatable, not terrible, people.

Groups composed of people with similar conditions can be formal or informal and are enormously helpful. First, peer groups can be used to explore all the potential response options discussed previously, such as resisting and passing. Second, problem-solving sessions in these groups explore possible solutions to common situations (Dudley, 1983). Finally, others who share the stigma provide a source of acceptance and support for both the individuals with the chronic condition and their families. Maternal mental health clients developed and implemented an ongoing support group in consultation with an HCP (Franks et al., 2007). These women were able to promote and sustain their group for a 12-month period.

O'Sullivan (2006) reported on a unique twist to the self-help group. A Barcelona, Spain radio program was planned and implemented by persons with mental illness. The program sought to inform, educate, and break down the stigma and stereotypes associated with mental illness. Benefits to the participants included an increase in self-esteem and more positive self-perception.

A word of caution is needed. Sometimes stigmatized individuals feel more comfortable with nonstigmatized individuals than with like others as a result of a closer identity with the former. For example, not all women with cancer respond positively to the American Cancer Society's Reach to Recovery support groups; some may feel more discomfort than support.

Reputable online support groups present another option for people with the technological equipment and skills to access these resources. The ability to control the encounter with like others in a safe haven may be appealing to many clients. The advent of social media sites such as Facebook© may alter the way individuals access and develop support networks as well. Social sites may offer another means of establishing both social and supportive relationships with the amount of disclosure controlled by the person. One must be aware of the potential for misuse, misrepresentation, and violations of privacy that could occur. Research in this area is sorely needed. Ultimately, the "best" solution varies from individual to individual.

Other Considerations

Other points for the HCPs to consider are issues of "inclusion" and "exclusion" and how they impact stigma. Technology and assistive devices are significant factors because they underline the fact that "quality of life" is not a static entity. Until relatively recently, electric wheelchairs were not readily available. Now such wheelchairs exist, in paediatric to bariatric sizes, as well as electric scooters that allow mobility for clients with a variety of conditions. Formerly, a person with paralyzed arms could only type slowly with a stick fastened to a headband; now there are increasingly accurate voice-activated home computers that type as the person speaks. In the same vein a person whose speech is unintelligible to most others can press symbols on a display board that produces full sentences spoken in a nonrobotic, smooth human voice. The savvy HCP will attend to technological advances and assist clients in obtaining necessary aids to promote full functioning of the individual.

To that end, the opportunity to hire personal assistants is also important. Having such assistance allows individuals with severe disabilities to have a far richer life than those without such help. Many disability advocates are pressing for public money that is currently spent on nursing homes and other institutions to be redirected to enable individuals who are disabled or chronically ill to live in their own homes. Maintaining function and independence may lessen the impact of both felt and enacted stigma.

Developing Supportive Others

Supportive others are persons (professional and nonprofessional) who do not carry the stigmatizing trait but are knowledgeable and offer sensitive understanding to individuals who do carry it. These people are called "the wise" by Goffman (1963) and are accorded acceptance within the group of stigmatized individuals. Desired behaviours are simply the ones friends or acquaintances would use. The stigmatized person must be seen and treated as a full human being—viewed as more than body changes or orthopaedic equipment, seen as a person who is more than a stigmatized condition.

The AIDS epidemic has added to the impetus for the development of groups of supportive others. In many cities the model of care for those with HIV/AIDS depends on volunteer, community-based groups that supply food, transportation, in-home care, acceptance, and support. This community network is an adjunct to hospital care and provides a vivid example of wise others who are essential to the care of these clients.

Implications for Professional Practice

One way an individual can become wise is by asking straightforward, sensitive questions, such as inquiring about the disabled person's condition. Many individuals with disabilities would welcome the opportunity to disclose as much or as little as they wish, because that would mean the disability was no longer taboo. For example, the disabled person may prefer that others ask about a cane or a walker rather than ignore it. This opportunity allows the disabled individual to reply with whatever explanation he or she wishes. Therefore, the disability is acknowledged, not ignored. It goes without saying that these questions should be asked after a beginning relationship is established, as opposed to being asked out of idle curiosity.

The process of becoming wise is not simple; it may mean offering oneself and waiting for validation of acceptance. HCPs who encounter individuals with chronic illness cannot prove themselves as wise immediately. Validation requires consistent behaviour by the professional that is sensitive, knowledgeable, and accepting. Being wise is not a new role for nurses or other caring HCPs. Nurses have traditionally worked in medically underserved areas with discredited persons and are accustomed to treating clients as individuals, not as conditions. Nurses often assume the predominant role of gatekeepers to the healthcare delivery system for many devalued individuals. Often, clients with chronic illnesses receive effective and efficient care from these nurses and other HCPs, who have great opportunities to perform the role of the wise.

Evidence-Informed Practice Box

A study by Dickson and colleagues (2006) offers some insight into the impact of stigma on people living with chronic fatigue syndrome (CFS).

Purpose: To explore the impact of stigma (external and internal) on treatment-seeking behaviours of older adults with depression by race (African American, White).

Sample: Purposeful sample of 14 adults between the ages of 21 and 68 years living in the United Kingdom diagnosed with CFS.

Method: In-depth inductive interviews were completed and transcribed verbatim. Transcripts were analyzed for recurrent themes using interpretive phenomenological analysis. An interpretive phenomenological approach to analysis seeks to explore the links between what the participants say within the interviews and the way they believe about their own experiences.

Select Findings: Participants described a delay or difficulty in achieving a diagnosis of CFS from their physician. This led to heated negotiations with their physician over whether they had CFS or depression. These views purported by physicians were often perceived by participants as a personal attack on their sense of morality as if they were using

(continues)

their diagnosis to escape from their social roles. The delegitimation of their condition often prompted participants to find new physicians who would treat them. Participants also identified other forms of stigma outside of their relationships with physicians. Some described a loss of relationships due to frustration and cynicism related to their CFS. Partnered relationships also suffered because many participants did not believe they had support from their partner and had to learn to struggle with their illness alone.

Conclusions: Further research exploring the delegitimising experiences of people with CFS (particularly in the context of friends and partners) is suggested due to the small study size and lack of generalizability to larger populations of people living with CFS.

Source: Dickson, A., Knussen, C., & Flowers, P. (2007). Stigma and the delegitimation experience: An interpretive phenomenological analysis of people living with chronic fatigue syndrome. *Psychology and Health, 22*(7), 851–867.

Another strategy HCPs can use to acquire real-life knowledge about individuals with a particular illness is to increase their interaction with people who have the disorder (Heijnders & Van Der Meij, 2006). In addition to increasing exposure to and interaction with people who have a particular stigmatizing condition, Corrigan and Penn (1999) suggested it is important for HCPs to be exposed to people who are successfully coping with a condition;

those who have recovered from mental illness, who are in remission, or who have been successfully rehabilitated. This knowledge can enable them to offer not only sensitive understanding and practical suggestions to individuals with chronic illness but also hope. Nurses who work with HIV/AIDS clients, for instance, have the opportunity to find out which behaviour is really effective and can learn about outcomes and clients' reactions. This information is extremely valuable as providers advocate for similar clients and their families.

Implications for Professional Education

HCPs' attitudes are representative of general societal views and so can be expected to include prejudices. Because HCPs have prolonged relationships with chronically ill individuals, the impact of these prejudices can be great. Programs to teach professional staff to identify and correct preconceived and often subconscious notions of categories and stereotypes deserve high priority (Dudley, 1983).

Providing intensive staff education for the purpose of reducing stigma perception by all employees in any particular agency is beneficial. In addition, professional staff are then in a position to role model desired behaviours and to share information to help nonprofessional staff treat clients in an accepting manner.

One study of stigma-promoting behaviours provides ideas for HCPs who wish to change their attitudes (Dudley, 1983). In Dudley's study the most frequent stigma-promoting behaviours included staring, denial of opportunities for clients to present views, inappropriate language in referring to clients, inappropriate restrictions of activities, violation of confidentiality, physical abuse, and ignoring clients. In-service days that focus on both didactic presentation of communication strategies and role-playing–specific scenarios would be a first step to eliminating situations of enacted stigma in the workplace.

One way to increase visibility and heighten awareness about the impact of stigma is to encourage structured contact between HCPs and affected individuals (Joachim & Acorn, 2000). This approach should be preceded by group work with a knowledgeable leader who can help identify and work through attitudes and reactions. For example, many nursing students do not like skilled nursing facilities because older adults are seen as unappealing. A gerontology nurse specialist spent time with such a group of students before they began working in the skilled nursing facility. She showed slides of faces etched with character and told stories of interesting experiences these individuals had that helped the students see the elderly as human beings. A group discussion between the specialist and students confronted myths and stereotypical thinking regarding the stigma of aging. As a result these students had a more positive experience at the skilled nursing facility.

Knowledgeable preparation for contact with stigmatized individuals does not solve all problems; it is, however, one way to expose stigmatized reactions such as stereotyping, to examine them, and to provide information to caregivers. The group sessions described here may be appropriate for both nonprofessional and professional caregivers in the community or in agencies.

Implications for Community Education Programs

Educational programs that reduce the effects of stigma can be shared with the community at large. Many organizations, such as the American Cancer Society and the American Diabetes Association, provide speakers or literature for the community. Schools, scout troops, and church groups are ideal settings for sensitive introductions of individuals who have many positive values and characteristics but do not meet normal health expectations. For instance, individuals with HIV/AIDS have been the focus of group discussions in which children learn to see these people simply as other human beings. Educational programs, such as those that dispel the fears about mental illness, reduce the stigmatizing effects of that disease (Link et al., 1989).

Much of the stigma attached to chronic conditions still pervades society's attitudes and policies (Herek et al., 2003), yet situations have changed. In the 1970s an unprecedented and multilayered surge of activism grew among individuals with disabilities and their advocates and resulted in significant social and structural change. In the United States individuals with disabilities began to speak out by publishing magazines, creating films, and organizing political action on both the local and national levels. Their actions greatly influenced a landmark change, namely, the Americans with Disabilities Act, which was signed into law in 1990. This legislation requires the government and the private sector to provide disabled individuals with opportunities for jobs and education, access to transportation, and access to public buildings.

Currently, a disabilities act does not exist in Canada. According to the Council of Canadians with Disabilities there has been debate within the Canadian disability community about whether a federal act would be useful or if existing mechanisms such as the Canadian Charter of Rights and Freedoms, federal statues, and strong antidiscrimination laws are useful enough to remove barriers for individuals living with disabilities. The research has been mixed on the efficacy of federal acts within this area. The conservative government in 2005 made a promise to introduce a national disability act to promote reasonable access to medical care, medical equipment, education, employment, transportation, and housing for Canadians with disabilities (Gordon, 2006, para. 7). This promise has yet to be fulfilled.

The media can also be influenced to present a more positive portrayal of people with chronic conditions. Providers and others can write to television networks that show individuals with disabilities functioning well and commend them for these portrayals. Likewise, people can be encouraged to voice their displeasure and to point out inaccuracies surrounding chronic conditions. In late fall 2010 the National Alliance on Mental Illness called for individuals to write and email a major television network and a popular television show's producer over a disparaging, stereotypical portrayal of an historical figure's mental illness.

Mass media campaigns designed to increase awareness of certain conditions or risk factors for disease can backfire in terms of preventing or reducing stigma. Clients with lung cancer not only perceived stigma of cancer in general (such as fear of disclosure, financial impact, body image changes, and effects on family and social relationships) but also the stigma that is associated with smoking and the shame of a self-inflicted disease, regardless of whether they stopped smoking or had never smoked. They experienced fear related to death as depicted by the mass media, families and friends avoiding contact, and being looked upon as being "dirty" in relation to smoking (Chapple, Ziebland, & McPherson, 2004).

Another study identified methods of health communication that were designed to increase public awareness but actually had the opposite effect of increasing public stigma (Wang, 1998).

The health communication approaches conveyed individuals with obvious disabling characteristics with the accompanying message, "Don't be like this." Awareness was heightened at the expense of furthering the stigma of the disabled individual. HCPs who volunteer to serve on executive boards of healthcare agencies or support agencies can offer guidance to those developing marketing campaigns, public service announcements, and community education materials.

Recent social changes have suggested that internalization of stigma based on prevailing social norms may be changing for some health problems. Rehabilitation programs for substance abuse are now commonly covered by health insurance, in part as a result of active consumer demand, evidencing a change of social attitude (Garfinkel & Dorian, 2000). The impact of stigmatizing conditions in women's health, such as abortion and breast cancer with mastectomy, has been reduced (Bennett, 1997). These changes are, perhaps, evidence that visibility and disclosure may have a positive impact on the process of negative stereotyping.

SUMMARY

Determining client outcomes, like many of the psychosocial concepts associated with chronic illnesses, is difficult. Some clients may be stigmatized on a regular basis but may have overcome the personal feelings associated with it. Therefore, client outcomes of stigma might be the *lack* of other common psychosocial effects of chronic illness, such as follows:

- The client is *not* socially isolated but is continuing his or her daily and normal activities without difficulty.

- The client's self-esteem remains high despite the chronic illness and accompanying physical symptoms.
- Healthy relationships continue with family, friends, and supportive others.
- The client is *not* depressed and interacts appropriately with others.

This chapter dealt primarily with adults' perceptions of stigma and interventional strategies that healthcare providers can use to both raise awareness of and to decrease the incidence of stigma.

INTERNET RESOURCES

Mental Health Issues

Achieve Solutions website: https://www.achieve solutions.net/achievesolutions/en/tlc/Content .do?contentId=21466

U.S. Department of Health and Human Services, Substance Abuse and Mental Health Services Administration stigma homepage: http://www .whatadifference.samhsa.gov/

Stigma.org links to mental health websites: www .stigma.org

Active Minds: Changing the Conversation on Mental Health (working to reduce the stigma of mental illness on college campuses): www .activeminds.org

National Alliance on Mental Illness Stigma Busters (click on Fight Stigma to sign up for StigmaBusters alerts and to access resources): www.nami.org

HIV/AIDS Issues

HRSA Care Action—Providing HIV/AIDS Care in a Changing Environment: hab.hrsa.gov. Resources include a literature review on HIV and stigma, clinical guidelines.

HIV & AIDS: Stigma and Discrimination: www.avert.org/hiv-aids-stigma.htm (Note: Avert.org is also available on Facebook.)

STUDY QUESTIONS

1. Compare and contrast the concepts of felt stigma and enacted stigma. Are these two concepts mutually exclusive?
2. How does the process of labelling by others influence the perception of felt stigma and the incidence of enacted stigma?
3. Advanced practice nurses can implement strategies to decrease the incidence of enacted stigma in society. What might the advanced practice nurse do in each of the following roles to decrease stigma: nurse administrator, nurse educator, clinician?
4. As a change agent in your practice setting, what strategies can you readily implement to increase awareness of stigma among administrators, HCPs, and support staff?
5. What strategies can you readily implement to decrease the perceptions of stigma by your clients?
6. Discuss the similarities and differences among prejudice, stereotyping, and labelling. What is the relationship to stigma?

For a full suite of assignments and additional learning activities, use the access code located in the front of your book and visit this exclusive website: **http://go.jblearning.com/kramer-kile**. If you do not have an access code, you can obtain one at the site.

REFERENCES

Abel, E. (2007). Women with HIV and stigma. *Family and Community Health, 30*(Suppl. 1), 104–106.

American Psychiatric Association. (2010, May 3). Openness by friends, family, celebrities reduces stigma of mental illness survey (press@psych.org Release No. 10-33). Retrieved from https://www.achievesolutions.net/achievesolutions/en/tlc/Content.do?contentId=21466

Baker, G. A., Brooks, J., Buck, D., & Jacoby, A. (2000). The stigma of epilepsy: A European perspective. *Epilepsia, 41*(1), 98–104.

Bauer, H., Rodriguez, M., Quiroga, S., & Flores-Ortiz, Y. (2000). Barriers to health care for abused Latina and Asian immigrant women. *Journal of Health Care for the Poor and Underserved, 11*(1), 33–44.

Bennett, T. (1997). Women's health in maternal and child health: Time for a new tradition? *Maternal and Child Health Journal, 1*(3), 253–265.

Brandon, D., Khoo, R., Maglajlie, R., & Abuel-Ealeh, M. (2000). European snapshot homeless survey: Result of questions asked of passers-by in 11 European cities. *International Journal of Nursing Practice, 6*(1), 39–45.

Brunstein Klomek, A., Sourander, A., & Gould, M. (2010). The association of suicide and bullying in childhood to young adulthood: A review of cross-sectional and longitudinal research findings. *Canadian Journal of Psychiatry, 55*(5), 282–288.

Butler, R. N. (1975). Psychiatry and the elderly: An overview. *American Journal of Psychiatry, 132*, 893–900.

Camp, D. L., Finlay, W. M. L., & Lyons, E. (2002). Is low self-esteem an inevitable consequence of stigma? An example from women with chronic mental health problems. *Social Science and Medicine, 55*(5), 823–834.

Campos, P. (2004). *The obesity myth: Why America's obsession with weight is hazardous to your health.* New York, NY: Gotham Books.

Chapple, A., Ziebland, S., & McPherson, A. (2004). Stigma, shame, and blame experienced by patients with lung cancer: Qualitative study. *British Medical Journal, 328*(7454), 1470.

Cinnirella, M., & Loewenthal, K. M. (1999). Religion and ethnic group influences on beliefs about mental illness: A qualitative interview study. *British Journal of Medical Psychology, 72*(4), 505–524.

Corrigan, P., & Penn, D. (1999). Lessons from social psychology on discrediting psychiatric stigma. *American Psychology, 54*(9), 765–776.

Crisp, A., Gelder, M., Rix, S., Meltzer, H., & Rowland, O. J. (2000). Stigmatization of people with mental illness. *British Journal of Psychiatry, 177*, 4–7.

Davies, M. R. (2000). The stigma of anxiety disorders. *International Journal of Clinical Practice, 54*(1), 44–47.

de Souza, E. A., & Salgado, P. C. (2006). A psychosocial view of anxiety and depression in epilepsy. *Epilepsy and Behavior, 8*(1), 232–238.

Distabile, P., Dubler, N., Solomon, L., & Klein, R. (1999). Self-reported legal needs of women with or at risk for HIV infection. The HER Study Group. *Journal of Urban Health, 76*(4), 435–447.

Dudley, J. (1983). *Living with stigma: The plight of the people who we label mentally retarded.* Springfield, IL: Charles C. Thomas.

Erikson, E. (1968). *Identity: Youth in crisis.* New York, NY: W. W. Norton.

Fife, B., & Wright, E. (2000). The dimensionality of stigma: A comparison of its impact on the self of persons with HIV/AIDS and cancer. *Journal of Health and Social Behavior, 41*(1), 50–67.

Franks, W., Henwood, K., & Bowden, G. (2007). Promoting maternal mental health: Women's strategies for presenting a positive identity and the implications for mental health promotion. *Journal of Public Mental Health, 6*(2), 40–51.

Garfinkel, P. E., & Dorian, B. J. (2000). Psychiatry in the new millennium. *Canadian Journal of Psychiatry, 45*(1), 40–47.

Gary, F. A. (2005). Stigma: Barrier to mental health care among ethnic minorities. *Issues in Mental Health Nursing, 26*(10), 979–999.

Gewirtz, A., & Gossart-Walker, S. (2000). Home-based treatment for children and families affected by HIV and AIDS. Dealing with stigma, secrecy, disclosure, and loss. *Child and Adolescent Psychiatry Clinics of North America, 9*(2), 313–330.

Glasman, L. R., Weinhardt, L. S., DiFrancesico, W., & Hackl, K. L. (2010). Intentions to seek and accept an HIV test among men of Mexican descent in the midwestern USA. *AIDS Care, 22*(6), 718–728.

Goffman, E. (1963). *Stigma: Notes on management of spoiled identity.* Englewood Cliffs, NJ: Prentice Hall.

Gordon, P. (2006). *A federal disability act: Opportunities and challenges contributing to the dialogue.* Ottawa, ON: Council of Canadians with Disabilities. Retrieved from http://www.ccdonline.ca/en/socialpolicy/fda/1006#I

Grytten, N., & Maseide, P. (2005). What is expressed is not always what is felt: Coping with stigma and the embodiment of perceived illegitimacy of multiple sclerosis. *Chronic Illness, 1*(3), 231–243.

Halevy, A. (2000). AIDS, surgery, and the Americans with Disabilities Act. *Archives of Surgery, 135*(1), 51–54.

Heckman, T. G., Anderson, E. S., Sikkema, K. J., Kochman, A., Kalichman, S. C., & Anderson, T. (2004). Emotional distress in nonmetropolitan persons living with HIV disease enrolled in a telephone-delivered, coping improvement group intervention. *Health Psychology, 23*(1), 94–100.

Heijnders, M., & Van Der Meij, S. (2006). The fight against stigma: An overview of stigma-reduction strategies and interventions. *Psychology, Health & Medicine, 11*(3), 353–363.

Herek, G. M., Capitanio, J. P., & Widaman, K. F. (2003). Stigma, social risk, and health policy: Public attitudes toward HIV surveillance policies and the social construct of illness. *Health Psychology, 22*(5), 533–540.

Hess, T. M., Hinson, J. T., & Hodges, E. A. (2009). Moderators of and mechanisms underlying stereotype threat effects on older adults' memory performance. *Experimental Aging Research, 35*(2), 153–177.

Heukelbach, J., & Feldmeier, H. (2006). Scabies. *The Lancet, 367,* 1767–1774.

Hinduja, S., & Patchin, J. W. (2010). Bullying, cyberbullying, and suicide. *Archives of Suicide Research, 14*(3), 206–221.

Hodgson, I. (2006). Empathy, inclusion and enclaves: The culture of care of people with HIV/AIDS and nursing implications. *Journal of Advanced Nursing, 55*(3), 283–290.

Hynd, H. M. (1958). *On shame and the search for identity* (3rd ed.). New York, NY: Harcourt Brace Jovanovich.

Jacoby, A. (1994). Felt versus enacted stigma: A concept revisited. *Social Science and Medicine, 8*(2), 269–274.

Joachim, G., & Acorn, S. (2000). Stigma of visible and invisible chronic conditions. *Journal of Advanced Nursing, 32*(1), 243–248.

Jolley, D. J., & Benbow, S. M. (2000). Stigma and Alzheimer's disease: Causes, consequences, and a constructive approach. *International Journal of Clinical Practice, 54*(2), 117–119.

Katz, I. (1981). *Stigma: A social psychological analysis.* Hillsdale, NJ: Lawrence Erlbaum Associates.

Keltner, K., Schwecke, L., & Bostrom, C. (2003). *Psychiatric nursing* (4th ed.). St. Louis, MO: Mosby.

King, M., Dinos, S., Shaw, J., Watson, R., Stevens, S., Passetti, F., . . . Serfaty, M. (2007). The stigma scale: Development of a standardized measure of the stigma of mental illness. *British Journal of Psychiatry, 190,* 248–254.

Kurzban, R., & Leary, M. R. (2001). Evolutionary origins of stigmatization: The functions of social exclusion. *Psychological Bulletin, 127*(2), 187–208.

Ladieu-Leviton, G., Adler, D., & Dembo, T. (1977). Studies in adjustment to visible injuries: Social acceptance of the injured. In R. Marinelli & A. Dell Orto (Eds.), *The psychological and social impact of the physical disability.* New York, NY: Springer.

Lawson, E., Gardezi, F., Calzavara, L., Husbands, W., Myers, T., & Tharao, W. E. (2006). *HIV/AIDS, stigma, denial, fear and discrimination: Experiences and responses of people from African and Caribbean communities in Toronto.* Toronto, ON: The African and Caribbean Council on HIV/AIDS in Ontario (ACCHO) and the HIV Social Behavioural and Epidemiological Studies Unit, University of Toronto.

Leninger, M. M., & McFarland, M. R. (2002). *Transcultural nursing: Concepts, theories, research and practice* (2nd ed.). New York, NY: McGraw-Hill.

Liggins, J., & Hatcher, S. (2005). Stigma toward the mentally ill in the general hospital: A qualitative study. *General Hospital Psychiatry, 27*(5), 359–364.

Link, B. G. (1987). Understanding labeling effects in the area of mental disorders: An assessment of the effects of expectations of rejection. *American Sociological Review, 52*(1), 96–112.

Link, B. G., Cullen, F. T., Struening, E., Shrout, P. E., & Dohrenwend, B. P. (1989). A modified labeling theory approach to mental disorders: An empirical assessment. *American Sociological Review, 54*(3), 400–423.

Link, B. G., & Phelan, J. C. (2001). Conceptualizing stigma. *Annual Review of Sociology, 27,* 363–385.

Link, B. G., Struening, E. L., Rahav, M., Phelan, J. C., & Nuttbrock, L. (1997). On stigma and its consequences: Evidence from a longitudinal study of men with dual diagnoses of mental illness and substance abuse. *Journal of Health and Social Behavior, 38*(2), 177–190.

Magin, P., Adams, J., Heading, G., Pond, D., & Smith, W. (2007). Psychological sequelae of acne vulgaris: Results of a qualitative study. *Australian Family Physician, 52,* 978–979.

Markowitz, F. E. (1998). The effects of stigma on the psychological well-being and life satisfaction of persons with mental illness. *Journal of Health and Social Behavior, 39,* 335–347.

Merriam Webster. (2011a). Stigma. Retrieved from http ://www.merriam-webster.com/dictionary/stigma

Merriam Webster. (2011b). Stigma. Retrieved from http ://www.merriam-webster.com/thesaurus/stigma

Miller, N., Noble, E., Jones, D., & Burn, D. (2006). Hard to swallow: Dysphagia in Parkinson's disease. *Age and Ageing, 35*(6), 614–618.

Murray, J., Banerjee, S., Byng, R., Tylee, A., Bhugra, D., & Macdonald, A. (2006). Primary care professionals' perceptions of depression in older people: A qualitative study. *Social Science and Medicine, 63*(5), 1363–1373.

O'Sullivan, M. (2006). Making radio waves. *A Life in the Day, 10*(2), 6–8.

Raffin Bouchal, S. (2009). Nursing values and ethics. In J. C. Ross-Kerr & M. J. Woods (Eds.), *Potter & Perry's Canadian fundamentals of nursing* (Revised 4th ed.). Toronto, ON: Elsevier Canada.

Rehm, R. S., & Franck, L. S. (2000). Long-term goals and normalization strategies of children and families affected by HIV/AIDS. *Advances in Nursing Science, 23*(1), 69–82.

Ritchie, D., Amos, A., & Martin, C. (2010). Original investigation: "But it just has that sort of feel about it, a leper." Stigma, smoke-free legislation and public health. *Nicotine and Tobacco Research, 12*(6), 622–629.

Ritson, E. B. (1999). Alcohol, drugs, and stigma. *International Journal of Clinical Practice, 53*(7), 549–551.

Roberts, L. W., Warner, T. D., & Trumpower, D. (2000). Medical students' evolving perspectives on their personal health care: Clinical and educational implications of a longitudinal study. *Comprehensive Psychiatry, 41*(4), 303–314.

Rohleder, P. (2010). Rehabilitation in practice: "They don't know how to defend themselves": Talk about disability and HIV risk in South Africa. *Disability and Rehabilitation, 32*(10), 855–863.

Rogge, M. M., Greenwald, M., & Golden, A. (2004). Obesity, stigma, and civilized oppression. *Advances in Nursing Science, 27*(4), 301–315.

Roskes, E., Feldman, R., Arrington, S., & Leisher, M. (1999). A model program for the treatment of mentally ill offenders in the community. *Community Mental Health Journal, 35*(5), 461–472.

Rossi, L. A., Vila Vda, S., Zago, M. M., & Ferreira, E. (2005). The stigma of burns perceptions of burned patients' relatives when facing discharge from hospital. *Burns, 31*(1), 37–44.

Salisbury, K. M. (2000). National and state policies influencing the care of children affected by AIDS. *Child and Adolescent Psychiatry Clinics of North America, 9*(2), 425–449.

Sandelowski, M., & Barroso, J. (2003). Motherhood in the context of maternal HIV infection. *Research in Nursing and Health, 26,* 470–482.

Scambler, G. (2004). Reframing stigma: Felt and enacted stigma and challenges to the sociology of chronic and disabling conditions. *Social Theory and Health, 2,* 29–46.

Schim, S., Doorenbos, A., Benkert, R., & Miller, J. (2007). Culturally congruent care: Putting the puzzle together [Electronic version]. *Journal of Transcultural Nursing, 18*(2), 103–110.

Schomerus, G., Lucht, M., Holzinger, A., Matschinger, H., Carta, M. G., & Angermeyer, M. C. (2010, December 18 epub). The stigma of alcohol dependence compared with other mental disorders: A review of population studies. *Alcohol Alcohol, 46*(2), 105–112.

Schreiber, R., Stern, P. N., & Wilson, C. (2000). Being strong: How black West-Indian Canadian women manage depression and its stigma. *Journal of Nursing Scholarship, 32*(1), 39–45.

Shontz, E. (1977). Physical disability and personality: Theory and recent research. In R. Marinelli & A. Dell Orto (Eds.), *The psychological and social impact of physical disability*. New York, NY: Springer.

Simpson, G., Mohr, R., & Redman, A. (2000). Cultural variations in the understanding of traumatic brain injury and brain injury rehabilitation. *Brain Injury, 14*(2), 125–140.

Stephens, C., & Flick, U. (2010). Health and ageing—challenges for health psychology research. *Journal of Health Psychology, 15*(5), 643–648.

Stewart, M., Keel, P., & Schiavo, R. S. (2006). Stigmatization of anorexia nervosa. *International Journal of Eating Disorders, 39*(4), 320–325.

Van Brakel, W. H. (2006). Measuring health-related stigma: A literature review. *Psychology of Health and Medicine, 11*(3), 307–334.

Wallhagen, M. I. (2010). The stigma of hearing loss. *The Gerontologist, 50*(1), 66–75.

Wang, C. (1998). Portraying stigmatized conditions: Disabling images in public health. *Journal of Health Communication, 3*(2), 149–159.

Wang, J., Iannotti, R. J., Luk, J. W., & Nansel, T. R. (2010). Co-occurrence of victimization from five subtypes of bullying: Physical, verbal, social exclusion, spreading rumors, and cyber. *Journal of Pediatric Psychology, 35*(10), 1103–1112.

Werner, P. (2006). Lay perceptions regarding the competence of persons with Alzheimer's disease. *International Journal of Geriatric Psychiatry, 21*, 674–680.

Weston, H. J. (2003). Public honor, private shame, and HIV: Issues affecting sexual health service delivery in London's South Asian communities. *Health and Place, 9*(2), 109–117.

CHAPTER 5

Adaptation

Original chapter by Pamala D. Larsen and Faye I. Hummel
Canadian content added by Joseph C. Osuji

INTRODUCTION

Persons with chronic illness chart a life course to successfully navigate the challenges that are inherent within themselves and their families, their relationships, or the setting in which they find themselves. Throughout the course of their illness individuals must rely on a healthcare system in which pharmaceuticals, machines, and a wide array of technology have become the hallmarks of "quality health care." Although the disease focus may be appropriate intermittently during the trajectory of a chronic illness to meet acute physical needs of the individual, this perspective does not meet the social, psychological, and emotional needs of clients with chronic conditions. In other words, the disease or biomedical focus of the healthcare system does not address the holistic needs of the individual and therefore is not enough to manage the illness experience of the client and family.

Early work by Visotsky, Hamburg, Goss, and Lebovits (1961) in studying clients with polio posed some initial questions regarding adaptation. They asked their clients how they dealt with this stressor, polio, and what coping behaviour(s) could predict favourable outcomes. Fifty years later the same questions are being asked. Although we have made progress in understanding certain components of adaptation, many questions remain unanswered.

The lens for viewing chronic illness is determined by numerous variables within the individual affected as well as how healthcare professionals, the system, and the setting providing care view the chronic condition. The elderly woman with arthritis who has been socialized to the primacy of medicine in the healthcare system may rely solely on her physician-prescribed pharmaceutical treatment of her joint pain and fatigue. On the other hand, a young man with hepatitis C gathers information from a wide variety of sources regarding the treatment and management of his chronic condition and maintains control of his treatment plan. The adaptation mechanisms of the elderly woman and the young man are very different as well. Each individual brings to the illness his or her own uniqueness—personality traits, past experiences, culture, values—to influence the adaptation process in his or her own way.

Defining Adaptation

The terms "adjustment" and "adaptation" are used interchangeably in the literature (Stanton & Revenson, 2007) and in this chapter as well. Sharpe and Curran (2006) define adjustment as a response to a change in the environment that allows an organism to become more suitably adapted to that change. Most definitions of adjustment or adaptation, however, allude to the lack of a psychological disorder being present. An early description of adjustment (and a continuing one) is the absence of a diagnosed psychological disorder, psychological symptoms, or negative mood (Stanton, Revenson, & Tennen, 2007). Even in Visotsky et al.'s study in 1961 in clients with polio, there was a movement to discount that definition. Although the presence or absence of a psychological disorder may be a part of adjustment, it is only one indicator of it.

Adjustment to illness has been operationalized as good quality of life, well-being, vitality, positive affect, life satisfaction, and global self-esteem (Sharpe & Curran, 2006). Conversely, "adjustment disorder" is defined as the development of clinically significant emotional or behavioural symptoms in response to an identifiable stress or stressor (American Psychiatric Association, 2000).

There is little consistency in the literature in defining adaptation or adjustment. Each author/researcher defines adaptation or adjustment differently based on their own theoretical framework or outcome measurement. As one example, Kiebles, Doerfler, and Keefer (2010) in their study of adjustment to inflammatory bowel disease defined adjustment as a composite of perceived disability, psychological functioning, and disease-specific and health-related quality of life.

This chapter provides an overview of adaptation in individuals with chronic illness. With entire books devoted to coping and adaptation, the depth of this chapter is limited. However, classic sources from different parts of the globe and models are included, along with interventions appropriate for individuals and families with chronic illness.

IMPACT

Conceptualization of Adjustment

The psychological and social consequences of chronic diseases demand significant adjustments from individuals. Stanton and Revenson (2007) identified five attributes of adjustment: (1) chronic illness necessitates adjustment in multiple life domains, (2) there are positive and negative outcomes of adjustment, (3) adjustment is dynamic, (4) adjustment can be described only within the context of each unique individual, and (5) heterogeneity is the rule rather than the exception in adjustment. Each of these concepts is further described below.

Chronic Illness Necessitates Adjustment in Multiple Life Domains

Adjustment in chronic illness is multifaceted and is more than just physical; it crosses interpersonal, cognitive, emotional, and behavioural domains. Adjustment is a holistic event in the client, with all domains being interrelated. Therefore, a change in one domain may affect adjustment in another domain (Stanton, Collins, & Sworowski, 2001; Stanton & Revenson, 2007; Stewart, Ross, & Hartley, 2004). According to Stanton and colleagues (2007), related conceptualizations of adjustment to chronic illnesses include "mastery of disease related adaptive tasks, preservation of functional status, perceived quality of life in several other domains, absence of psychological disorder and low negative affect" (p. 567). Cognitive adaptation might involve personal self-evaluation or self-reflection. Adaptation in the behavioural domain includes returning to work or resuming the role of the "breadwinner" of the family. Anxiety, in the emotional domain, may affect the ability to socialize in the interpersonal domain or influence blood pressure in the physical domain. Emotional adaptation could be the absence of depression, and interpersonal adaptation may be the willingness to be "social" again. Again, each domain may affect the other.

Adjustment Involves Both Positive and Negative Outcome Dimensions

Typically, we think of outcomes of chronic illness as being negative, as evidenced by distress, psychological dysfunction, relationships in disarray, and so forth. As stated previously, one definition of positive adjustment is the absence of a diagnosed psychological disorder, psychological symptoms, or negative mood (Stanton et al., 2007). However, there may be a positive side of chronic illness as well.

It is not unusual to hear individuals with chronic illness say things like "having this disease has been the best thing that ever happened to me—it made me wake up to see what was important." There may be positive aspects of chronic disease, but how clients come to view it in this way is not known. Folkman, Moskowitz, Ozer, and Park (1997), in their study of HIV-positive and HIV caregiving partners of men with AIDS, found that although study participants reported high levels of depressive symptoms, they also demonstrated positive morale and positive states of mind when compared with the general population norms.

One way to describe these paradoxical findings is a concept called *response shift*. Sprangers and Schwartz (2000) coined this phrase to describe a change in the meaning of one's self-evaluation of a target construct as a result of (1) change in an individual's internal standards of measurement, (2) change in the individual's values, or (3) reconceptualization of the target construct.

Although anecdotally we consider negative outcomes of chronic illness more common, research demonstrates that positive adjustment may more accurately represent the adjustment experience of most individuals with chronic disease (Stanton & Revenson, 2007). This is because it is understood that a disease that disrupts life should not only preclude the experience of joy but sometimes create avenues for positive coping and growth.

Adjustment Is a Dynamic Process

Adjustment to chronic illness is neither linear nor lockstep (Stanton & Revenson, 2007). As exacerbations occur—as in rheumatoid arthritis or multiple sclerosis—the cancer recurs, or the physical limitations of heart failure increase, each change requires readjustment or readaptation. In addition, changes may not be limited to changes in one's physical condition that affect adaptation but changes in the rest of the individual's life. A spouse losing his or her job, a child getting seriously injured, and a parent no longer able to care for him- or herself are examples of factors that affect the adaptation of the client with chronic illness.

Adjustment Can Be Viewed Only from Within the Context of the Individual

There is variability in adaptation, and that is to be expected. From the context of the individual, the physical symptoms, the functional changes, and the uncertainty may or may not be pertinent to the individual. Each stressor of the illness has a different relevance for each individual and as a result elicits a different reaction from each individual. The context of each individual is different, whether it is age, gender, ethnicity, or socioeconomic status. Other influencing contextual variables to adaptation to chronic illness include "interpersonal processes, personality attributes, cognitive appraisals, and coping processes" (Stanton et al., 2007, p. 570). The 35-year-old married woman newly diagnosed with breast cancer with three grade school–aged children has a different context than the 80-year-old woman with the same diagnosis. Although that is an extreme example, the variation that exists among individuals cannot be underestimated.

Heterogeneity Is the Rule, Not the Exception

Anecdotally, we know that if we put 20 women of the same age with the same stage of breast cancer and same prognosis in a room, each of those individuals will adapt to their chronic condition differently. Some will be considered by most as "well adjusted," whereas others might be considered maladjusted. The remaining individuals may fall somewhere in the middle. The person's individual determinants and uniqueness affect the ability of the individual to adapt to the illness. Although commonalities exist among individuals with chronic illness, there is significant variability as well.

Differences in individual adjustment abound in the literature. Helgeson, Snyder, and Seltman (2004) in a study of women with breast cancer from 4 to 55 months after diagnosis found that 43% of the sample evidenced high and stable psychological quality of life, 18%

had a somewhat lower quality of life, 26% evidenced low psychological functioning, and 12% had an immediate and substantial decline in psychological function.

Dew and colleagues (2005) identified five groups of distinct distress profiles in heart transplantation patients over several years: (1) consistently low distress, (2) consistent, significant levels of distress, (3) high distress for the initial 3 months, (4) high distress at 3 years, and (5) fluctuating distress.

THE SELF IN CHRONIC ILLNESS

Chronic illness changes the body and forces identity changes (Brink, 2009). Before illness, most individuals take their health for granted. Any disruption of normality may cause a threat to the self (Charmaz, 1995). Bury (1982) conceptualized this as a biographical disruption. The meaning of the illness and biographical disruption vary in significance for the individual and family. One's self-concept and self-confidence may change due to chronic illness. Morea, Friend, and Bennett (2008) refer to the illness self-concept. According to the authors, the illness self-concept is the integration of illness into the self that in turn affects the adjustment to chronic illness.

Brink (2009), in her study with patients post-myocardial infarction, identified two different behaviours in her model: self-modifying and self-protecting behaviours. For example, self-protecting behaviours may block lifestyle changes. Individuals with self-modifying behaviour reoriented themselves to the situation and accepted the consequences of the illness. Identifying a client's behaviour can better help the healthcare professional in planning appropriate interventions.

MODELS

As researchers we have a broad goal to understand the process of adaptation, predict outcomes, and modify interventions to meet the needs of our clients. A model that is able to perform all those activities is preferable for practice; however, a perfect model does not exist at this time. What follows are sample models from the literature.

Biomedical Model

The medical model provides a framework for assumptions about the nature of health and illness. The client is a complex set of anatomical parts and interrelated systems. Anatomical, physiological, and/or biochemical failures translate into aetiologies of ill health, thus promoting a disease-oriented approach to care. This theoretical perspective of chronic illness is reflected in the language and actions of healthcare professionals who refer to "the diabetic in room 328" rather than to Mrs. Sanchez, who has diabetes.

Pathophysiology, pharmacotherapy, and technology are emphasized and become prominent in the diagnosis and intervention of all illness and disease, albeit acute or chronic. Antonovsky (1979) considered the medical model a dichotomous model. If pathology is present, then there is illness, and wellness or health is not possible. Explanatory assumptions and theories are used for determining the cause of symptoms, and uniformity of causality and treatment of disease are inferred.

The biomedical paradigm tends to medicalise all human conditions in which symptoms can be controlled and cured with biomedical strategies. This model reduces the individual to a disease and fails to recognize the human aspects and experiences of the individual who happens to have a chronic illness (Sakalys, 2000) and diminishes social and cultural explanation of disease (Mirowsky & Ross, 2002). Physical complaints and signs or symptoms of disease become the hallmarks of interaction and discourse within the healthcare arena.

The relationship between the healthcare professional and the client with chronic illness is one of objectivity, biological pathology, diagnosis, and signs and symptoms, all of which require medical interventions. Healthcare professionals tend to shield themselves from the human aspects of chronic illness, whereas their skill sets, techniques, and procedures become the focus of interaction with the client (Freeth, 2007). Power and expertise are held exclusively by the healthcare system, and the interactions between the healthcare professional and the client are directive and unbalanced. The individual with chronic illness becomes disempowered to engage in his or her own healthcare decisions and relies solely on the healthcare professional.

The biomedical model is insufficient in providing health care to individuals with chronic illness (Waisbond, 2007), because it fails to acknowledge the breadth and depth of the illness experience. This model reduces chronic illness to just biological processes, conceptualises a separation of a mechanistic body from other aspects of the individual, and emphasises finding a cure or a fix. The medical model does not acknowledge the person with the chronic condition, who holds knowledge and expertise about the factors that influence his or her physical symptoms of chronic disease; in other words, the expert patient. For example, at the end of the month Mrs. Jones, who is retired and surviving on old age security payments, becomes anxious that she will not have enough money to purchase her prescriptions for her hypertension. Although she is able to financially manage otherwise, Mrs. Jones' stress and worry exacerbate her hypertension. Mrs. Jones' physician does not anticipate that the probable cause of her elevated blood pressure is related to her stress. The physician responds to Mrs. Jones' hypertension with a change of medication to manage her symptoms. The quantification of all signs and symptoms of disease fails to address the total illness experience of the individual. With increased attention to genetic research and gene technologies, the biomedical theories of disease continue to be reinforced, with less emphasis on the individual's social context and experiences (Dixon-Woods, 2001).

Despite the limitations of the biomedical model in adaptation, its usefulness is apparent during the acute phase of chronic illness. Although the focus of the biomedical model is limited to disease and organic dysfunction, this model is central for adaptation to chronic illness, particularly at the time of diagnosis when individuals and families are overwhelmed with a new diagnosis and sorting out the facts about the illness. In addition, during periods of illness exacerbations the biomedical model helps explain signs and symptoms and may provide a source of retreat and relief, depending on the stage of the chronic illness. There are times when individuals and families need current information about the chronic illness, signs and symptoms, the anticipated trajectory of the illness course, the array of treatment modalities, and traditional as well as alternative strategies. The biomedical model is the foundation for evidence-informed healthcare practice and provides the gold standard for treatment and intervention. Consequently, this model provides measurable goals for treatment and client outcomes relative to morbidity and mortality.

Lazarus and Folkman Model

Although there are other stress and coping models, none is better known than the one developed by Richard Lazarus and Susan Folkman (1984). Their model, a cognitive-phenomenological theory of stress, views adaptation to chronic illness through the lens of adapting to stressors. It is a transactional model of stress and coping, meaning that antecedent variables, such as personality traits, past experiences, and disease and treatment variables, act via mediating variables, such as coping strategies, to facilitate outcomes and, in this case, adaptation. Stressors are mediated by primary appraisal, which is the individual's gauge of the significance and importance of the stressor. Primary appraisal is influenced by the background, experiences, culture, ethnicity, and personality of the individual and is therefore characterized by stability across situations (Folkman, Lazarus, Gruen, & DeLongis, 1986).

The second step of the model is secondary appraisal of the situation. The individual asks the question, "What can I do about this situation?", and this leads to the coping strategies used to manage the stressor. Secondary appraisal is influenced by the physical and social environment and may be context specific (Stewart et al., 2004). To adapt involves applying the coping strategies that are most appropriate to the situation. Individuals use both problem-focused coping and emotion-focused coping. Originally, Lazarus and Folkman presumed the goal for all individuals was to use problem-focused coping and that emotion-focused coping yielded poor adaptation to the stressor, in this case the illness. However, work since 1986 has supported a place for emotion-focused coping as well as problem-focused coping (Stewart et al., 2004).

Engel's Biopsychosocial Model

Clearly, a model that could address both the biological and psychosocial aspects of chronic disease is a preferred one for health care. Engel (1977) was perhaps one of the earliest authors of such a model that offered a welcome alternative to the narrow biomedical model of understanding illnesses. Engel's model suggests "that to understand and respond adequately to patients suffering and to give them a sense of being understood, clinicians must attend simultaneously to the biological, psychological, and social dimensions of illness" (Borrell-Carrio, Suchman, & Epstein, 2004, p. 576).

Engel's model outlined three ways in which a psychosocial factor could influence a health outcome: direct, indirect, and moderating. A direct effect is a belief or value of the client that would preclude him or her from a specific medical intervention. An indirect effect is defined through a mediational process (Stewart et al., 2004). An example is an individual's current symptoms, for instance, nausea and vomiting, decreasing the client's motivation to participate in a prescribed exercise regimen and thereby decreasing physical functioning. A moderating effect alters the causal relationship between a psychosocial factor and a health outcome.

Livneh and Antonak Model

Livneh and Antonak (1997), working from previous models, proposed that variables associated with chronic illness and disability could be organized into four main categories/steps: (1) disability related (e.g., type of condition, such as terminal vs. nonterminal), (2) sociodemographic factors of the individual (e.g., gender, age, ethnicity), (3) individual differences or personality (e.g., coping strategies, locus of control, personal meaning of the condition), and (4) physical and social environmental factors (e.g., social support, stigma). The interactions of these classes of variables significantly affected adaptation.

Livneh and Antonak (1997) also saw the adaptation process as different from adaptation itself. They theorized that the process of adaptation was fluid and dynamic, whereas adaptation status was the result or outcome of the process (Stewart et al., 2004).

Common Sense Model of Self-Regulation

The common sense model of self-regulation posits that the client's illness beliefs and representations of that illness influence adaptation to the illness and health outcomes (Leventhal, Leventhal, & Cameron, 2001). According to the model patients develop cognitive and emotional representations of their condition to "make sense" or find meaning in the illness. Leventhal and colleagues (2001) identified five dimensions that represent a client's view of their illness:

1. *Identity of the illness:* connecting the symptoms with the illness and having an understanding of the illness
2. *Timeline:* duration and progression of the illness
3. *Causes:* perceived reason for the illness
4. *Consequences:* the physical, psychosocial, and economic impact of the illness
5. *Controllability:* whether the disease could be controlled or cured

After identification of these dimensions, Leventhal and colleagues believed that coping and appraisals follow. Significant evidence showed that an individual's representation and perception of the illness will determine what common sense health behaviours and coping mechanisms were used to deal or cope with it. As such, "coping decisions will differ as a function of the meaning individuals assign to their symptoms (i.e., their illness representations), and this interpretive process will reflect their past illness experiences, social expectations, information from friends, media and medical practitioners" (McAndrew et al., 2008, p. 196).

Moos and Holahan Model

Stewart and colleagues (2004) suggested that an ideal model for adaptation should address four criteria: (1) the reciprocal influences of biological, psychological, social, and behavioural variables of the client and the disease process; (2) the broad application to clients with a wide range of chronic illnesses and conditions; (3) the ability to address the influences

of culture, gender, ethnicity, and life stage of the client; and (4) the ability to predict the level of client adaptation, which will then lead to appropriate interventions for the client.

Currently, a search of the literature does not identify any "ideal" models that can meet the preceding criteria. Moos and Holahan (2007), however, developed a simple model that provides a framework to view adaptation. Because of its ease of use and understanding, more detail is provided on this model. Moos and Holahan's framework (**Figure 5-1**) is a way of conceptualizing coping and integrating it into a broader model.

The common sense model has been used extensively as a framework in research in chronic illness. Several examples follow:

• Curable/controllable illness is related to better health and functioning (Hagger & Orbell, 2003)

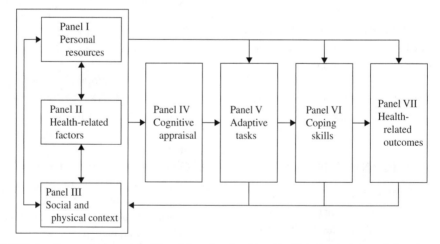

FIGURE 5-1 Conceptual model of the determinants of health-related outcomes of chronic illness and disability.
Source: Moos, R. H., & Holahan, C. J. (2007). Adaptive tasks and methods of coping with illness and disability. In E. Martz & H. Livneh (Eds.), *Coping with chronic illness and disability* (pp. 107–128). New York, NY: Springer

- Prediction of disability by illness beliefs in clients with rheumatoid arthritis (Graves, Scott, Lempp, & Weinman, 2009)
- Use of common sense model to improve adherence with cardiac rehabilitation programs among women with heart disease (Shifren, 2003)
- Application of the model to understand diabetes-related distress (Paddison, Alpass, & Stephens, 2010)
- Using common sense model to analyze patient descriptions of cancer-related fatigue (Barsevick, Whitmer, & Walker, 2001)

According to the model, five sets of factors are associated with the selection of appropriate coping skills and the resulting health-related outcomes, in this case, adaptation. The model includes three factors that influence cognitive appraisal: (1) personal resources (panel I), (2) health-related factors (panel II), and (3) the social and physical context (panel III). Cognitive appraisal (panel IV) then dictates what adaptive tasks (panel V) need to be accomplished. Panels I through V mediate the choice of coping skills (panel VI), leading to Panel pII, the outcome.

Personal Resources and Culture

This broad category includes intellectual ability, ego and self-confidence, religion, and prior health-related and coping experiences. Demographic characteristics, such as age, gender, ethnicity, culture, and education, are included in this category as well. Personal resources include personality—which may be viewed as either a risk factor or protective factor (Stanton et al., 2007)—locus of control, optimism, and autonomy. Individuals who have a more internal locus of control, higher self-confidence

and self-efficacy, and a stronger sense of coherence are more likely to rely on problem solving than other aspects of coping (Moos & Holahan, 2007).

In Canada a discussion on coping and adaptation must encompass the sociopolitical realities of the country. Canada as a country presents itself as a model for multiculturalism, described by Leong and Wong (2003) as a "socio-political policy that endorses diversity, inclusiveness and equality, while recognizing the legitimacy and values of ethnic differences and cultural heritage" (p. 4). Ethnic group membership is associated with many psychological processes such as identity, group pride, and discrimination (Stanton et al., 2007). Each ethnic group or culture may have different values and beliefs that affect illness perceptions that, in turn, may affect adaptation (Cohen & Welch, 2000). For some cultures chronic disease and disability may produce stigma such that adaptation is not possible. Degazon (1995), while exploring ethnic identification and coping strategies, found a significant relationship between the ethnic groups with which the individual is identified and the coping strategy used.

Social and cultural factors are known to influence individuals' appraisal of stress and shape their coping responses. Iwasaki and Bartlett (2006) emphasized that "culture plays a central role in explaining leisure stress-coping mechanisms" of people with First Nations origin who have diabetes "whether these are tied to collective strengths, cultural identity, spiritual renewal, or physical/behavioural benefits" (p. 321). Aboriginal people's seemingly positive adaptation and coping with diabetes mellitus could be explained by "their recognition of the importance of spirituality, culture, values and traditions," which reinforces their "hopes for healing" (Sunday et al., 2001, p. 80). In a similar study Demers, Robichaud, Gelinas, Noread, and Desroisiers (2009) explored the association of behavioural strategies and social participation among older adults and suggested that behavioural coping strategies were important as a mechanism for reducing the effects of stressful events or difficulties associated with aging. These studies examined coping specifically; however, the relationship of coping with adaptation is uncertain. In addition, it is clear that little is known about the implications of culture and ethnicity in disease-related adaptation (Stanton et al., 2007).

The uniqueness of each individual influences how the chronic condition is appraised, what coping strategies are used, and how and if adaptation can be achieved. For instance, pessimists report higher levels of hostility and depression on the day before coronary artery bypass graft surgery than do optimists (Maes, Leventhal, & deRidder, 1996). Clients who are optimists tend to cope in a more active, problem-oriented way as opposed to pessimists, who tend to use more avoidant or passive ways of coping. It is not clear how specifically these personality traits influence and affect coping. Carver, Scheier, and Weintraub (1989) noted that the impact of personality characteristics on coping is modest and that coping preferences exist independently of personality factors. Although coping preferences could be viewed as personality attributes, they may influence coping indirectly through their impact on appraisal (Maes et al., 1996).

Socioeconomic class affects health outcomes directly and through environmental mechanisms, including access to care and risky and protective health behaviours (Stanton et al., 2007). Although it can be conceptualized as a determinant of adaptation, the pattern is not unidirectional (Stanton et al., 2007). Chronic conditions often influence work patterns and work disability. Work-related disability and loss of a job can decrease an individual's socioeconomic status.

Health-Related Factors

These factors include the type of onset and progression of the chronic condition, the location of symptoms, the prognosis, and the type of disability. Disease and treatment-related factors are often considered exogenous variables in adaptation (Stanton et al., 2001). A disease factor could be the stigma that the individual (and/or family) associates with the condition. Other disease factors could include a change in body image, declining mobility, extreme fatigue, and so forth. However, the existence and impact of disease factors may actually be influenced significantly by other determinants, such as ethnicity, socioeconomic status, and social support. For example, aboriginal individuals with diabetes suggested their stress was compounded by broader structural systems and dynamics at different levels: "socio-economic, cultural, historical and political levels" (Iwasaki & Bartlett, 2006, p. 321). Many studies do not reveal significant relationships of disease-related factors with adjustment (Stanton et al., 2001). The disease stage of a chronic condition is related inconsistently to adjustment (van't Spijker, Trijsburg, & Duivenvorrden, 1997).

The characteristics of the disease and of treatment contribute to the appraisal of the disease-related event. Surgery, monitoring of physical symptoms (e.g., blood glucose), diet, radiation, chemotherapy, and all the side effects of treatment are important components in how the client appraises the situation.

Social and Physical Context

This context includes the relationships between the individuals with the chronic disease, their family members, caregivers, and social network. House (1981) described social support as supportive behaviours and resources of individuals' social ties that include emotional support, intimacy, positive interaction, and tangible support. A supportive social context can enhance self-efficacy, transforming appraisal of a health condition as a challenge rather than a threat, and enhance reliance on approach coping. When family members or friends do not convey interest, individuals with serious chronic conditions may avoid talking about their problem and be less likely to cope with the illness-related demands (Norton et al., 2005).

In general, social support is related to positive adaptation in several chronic diseases (Stanton et al., 2001). However, studies differ in how social support is conceptualized. Social support has been used as a coping strategy, a coping resource in the environment, and considered dependent on personality attributes and coping of the individual (Schreurs & deRidder, 1997). Interpersonal relationships can both aid and hinder adaptation to chronic illness, especially in cultures such as the aboriginal people of Canada. For such cultures, "the potential for social support to negatively influence health becomes increasingly apparent" (Richmond & Ross, 2008, p. 1425). For women in particular, interpersonal relationships are vital components of their adjustment to major stressors (Cummins, Ireland, Resnick, & Blum, 1999; Revenson, 1994).

Cognitive Appraisal

Appraising the illness is the first step in deciding the adaptive tasks that need to be accomplished. This is also the step in the adaptation process where the illness is appraised as either a challenge or a threat. How the illness is appraised, whether it is controllable or threatening, determines appropriate adaptive tasks and subsequent coping strategies. Using Lazarus and Folkman's model, primary appraisal of the "threat" or "event" includes the appraisal of harm or loss that has already occurred, or threatened harm or loss (Folkman & Greer, 2000), and includes an evaluation of its personal significance (Walker, Jackson, & Littlejohn, 2004). Secondary appraisal occurs when one assesses the situation's controllability and compares it with one's available coping resources.

The individual who appraises a diagnosis of multiple sclerosis as a death sentence will make very different decisions regarding treatment than another individual who sees hope. With such different appraisals, coping and adjustment will be very different in these two individuals.

Adaptive Tasks

Moos and Holahan (2007) identified seven adaptive tasks. Three of the seven tasks are related to the health condition and its treatment and the other four are more general and could apply to all life crises and transitions, not just chronic illness. The tasks are (1) managing symptoms, (2) managing treatment, (3) forming relationships with healthcare providers, (4) managing emotions, (5) maintaining a positive self-image, (6) relating to family members and friends, and (7) preparing for an uncertain future (Moos & Holahan, 2007).

CASE STUDY

It was 5 months after Dan was reunited with his wife and two daughters that he began to experience sleep disorders, night sweats, nightmares, and "flashbacks" of the horrors of war he had experienced while he was deployed to Afghanistan. There he had seen many of his buddies killed and injured. He, too, was injured by enemy fire but had healed and recovered. Dan found himself withdrawing from his family, and he no longer wanted to participate in his children's sporting events. He was experiencing conflict and difficulty at work. At a recent visit with his healthcare provider Dan was diagnosed with posttraumatic stress disorder. Dan was devastated. He believed he had left his fears and memories of violence in Afghanistan. Dan had assumed he would return to his previous happy life with his family. Doubts and questions about his future rushed over him. What would he and his family need to do to return to and maintain secure and safe relationships? Would he be able to return to work? Would he be able to enjoy his children's activities and events? Would his life ever return to "normal"? Where would all of this end?

Discussion Questions

1. What personal resources, health-related factors, and social and physical factors are contributing to Dan's cognitive appraisal of the situation?
2. Compare and contrast the biomedical model and the Moos and Holahan model for adaptation for Dan and his chronic condition.
3. Discuss the role of the nurse for Dan and his family.

OVERVIEW OF COPING

Richard Lazarus's 1966 book, *Psychological Stress and the Coping Process*, was an initial scholarly work that expanded how coping was conceptualized. Since that time the coping literature has increased significantly, with researchers undertaking studies to understand why some individuals fare better than others when encountering stress in their lives (Folkman & Moskowitz, 2004). Coping is described by Folkman and Moskowitz as "the thoughts and behaviours used to manage the internal and external elements of situations that are appraised as stressful" (p. 745). It is a process that unfolds in the context of a situation or condition that is appraised as personally significant and as taxing or exceeding the individual's resources (Lazarus & Folkman, 1984). The coping process is initiated in response to the individual's appraisal that important goals have been harmed, lost, or threatened (Folkman & Moskowitz, 2004). What we have learned in the last 45 years is that coping is a complex, multidimensional process that is sensitive both to the environment and its demands and resources and to personality traits that influence the appraisal of stress, in this case chronic illness, and the resources for coping (Folkman & Moskowitz, 2004). Coping is not a stand-alone concept or phenomenon but embedded in a complex, dynamic process that involves the person, the environment, and the relationship between them.

Lazarus and Folkman (1984) described problem-focused and emotion-focused coping strategies. Problem-focused strategies alter person–environment relationships, and the purpose of emotion-focused strategies is to regulate internal states. Initially, problem-focused strategies were seen as "better" or as able to influence health outcomes in a more positive manner. However, since Lazarus and Folkman posited their original work, that view has changed. Emotion-focused coping strategies may specifically assist in developing and sustaining a sense of psychological well-being, despite unfavourable circumstances (Folkman & Greer, 2000).

Other theorists have used different terms to describe coping. In addition to problem-focused and emotion-focused coping, meaning-focused coping has been identified as a type of coping in which cognitive strategies are used to manage the meaning of the situation (Folkman & Moskowitz, 2004). *Passive* coping, which includes avoidance, and *active* coping, which is nonavoidance coping, were described by Shaw (1999). This two-factor structure of coping is incorporated into the coping framework as an antecedent to the behavioural intention to cope as well as to carry out the coping behaviour. It is likely that individuals may have a number of coping responses at their disposal, although each individual may have their own preferred styles based on their personality attributes (Shaw, 1999).

An issue in studying coping is that the coping strategy needs to be evaluated in the specific context in which it is used (Folkman & Moskowitz, 2004). Coping strategies are not inherently good or bad, but instead their effectiveness depends on the context in which they are used. Evaluation of the effectiveness of coping requires, first, selecting the appropriate outcomes and, second, paying attention to the fit between the coping and the situation (Folkman & Moskowitz, 2004).

Adaptation/Adjustment

What do we know about adaptation? It is a complex construct (like coping), it is multidimensional, and it is holistic. However, it is rarely measured holistically in studies. Consensus does exist regarding the centrality of an individual's appraisal of their adjustment. It is the client's adjustment and perception, not the healthcare professional's (Stanton et al., 2001).

We also understand that emotionally supportive relationships set the stage for positive adjustment, whereas criticism, social constraints, and social isolation induce risk (Stanton et al., 2007). Active approach-oriented coping strategies manage disease-related challenges and may bolster adjustment, whereas concerted efforts to avoid disease-related thoughts and feelings are predictors of distress. Two basic conclusions come from the descriptive research literature: Most individuals appear to "adjust" well to chronic illness, and there is considerable variability in adjustment both across studies and across individuals within single studies (Stanton et al., 2001).

In a review article on psychological adjustment to chronic disease, deRidder, Geenen, Kuijer, and van Middendorp (2008) identified five elements of successful adjustment: (1) successful performance of adaptive tasks, (2) absence of psychological disorders, (3) presence of low negative affect and high positive affect, (4) adequate function status (e.g., going to work), and (5) satisfaction and well-being in various life domains. Some of these are easily "measured." For example, absence or presence of a psychological disorder could be ascertained with a degree of certainty. However, other conceptualizations cannot.

Maes and colleagues (1996) believed that definitions of adjustment are too simplistic, as many studies operationalise adjustment in terms of psychological outcomes and neglect the medical, cognitive, or social outcomes. Positive adjustment is not merely the absence of pathology. Typical indicators of adjustment in research are positive and negative effects and represent two very different dimensions. Therefore, using only lack of depressive symptoms to indicate adjustment will yield a partial picture of adjustment (Stanton et al., 2001). Maes and colleagues posit that although anxiety and depression are important markers of adjustment, assessment of everyday life behaviours and activities may be much more relevant.

deRidder and colleagues' 2008 article appears to typify Maes and colleagues' concern. The primary emphasis is on psychological effects, as noted by the title of the article, "Psychological Adjustment to Chronic Disease." The more appropriate term, from this author's point of view, is *psychosocial adaptation*, because it more clearly defines and describes the whole person than does *psychological adaptation*, which is too narrow.

The concept of hardiness was studied in the 1970s (Kobasa, 1979) and into the late 1980s (Pollock, 1989). Brooks (2003) analyzed 125 articles published from 1966 to 2002 to determine the significance of hardiness in adaptation. This "personal resource," within Moos and Holahan's (2007) framework, demonstrated a significant relationship to psychological, psychosocial, and physiological adaptation. Higher levels of hardiness had positive outcomes in clients with chronic illness (Brooks, 2003).

The current literature on hardiness is scarce; however, Brooks (2008) used a cross-sectional survey design involving 60 participants to look at the effect of health-related hardiness. Individuals who had higher health-related hardiness had better psychosocial adjustment to their illness. Additionally, individuals with higher health-related hardiness had a higher self-perception of their health status (Brooks, 2008).

How coping is related specifically to adjustment has not been clearly described (Sharpe & Curran, 2006). Intellectually, we believe coping strategies do contribute to adaptation and may be a mediator, but they probably interact with other factors in contributing to adaptation (Stanton & Revenson, 2007).

Berg and Upchurch (2007) advanced a model that speaks to dyadic coping and adjustment. Their development–contextual model of couples coping with chronic illness views chronic illness as affecting the adjustment of both the client and the spouse such that coping strategies enacted by the patient are related to those enacted by the spouse and vice versa. In a sample of 190 couples in which the women had rheumatoid arthritis, Sterba and colleagues (2008) demonstrated that couple congruence concerning women's personal control over rheumatoid arthritis and its cyclic nature predicted better psychological adjustment in women longitudinally.

In the chronic pain literature acceptance is a more common concept than coping variables used to described how clients adapt to chronic pain. Acceptance includes responding to pain-related experiences without attempts at control or avoidance (Esteve, Ramirez-Maestre, & Lopez-Martinez, 2007).

Resilience

Resilience represents the "ability to survive and even thrive in the face of adversity" (Smith, Boutte, Zigler, & Finn-Stevenson, 2004, p. 214). It is linked to the constructs of coping and adaptation (Maluccio, 2002). Although resilience captures a wide range of experiences, it is most notably understood as the ability to adapt in the face of adversity. Resilience helps people cope (Black & Ford-Giboe, 2004). Kralik, vanLoon, and Visentin (2006) used interactional processes inherent in participatory action research to explore the concept of resilience. In this collaborative inquiry, data were gathered through email discussion groups. Data analysis revealed resilience meant having a strong sense of self-worth, the ability to benefit from experiences, and the capacity to adapt. Resiliency is a process of reflection, learning, and action directed at overcoming adversity.

Interventions

The literature provides an abundance of descriptive studies measuring coping and/or adaptation, but few interventional studies exist. It appears that we can measure coping or adaptation but are unable to conceptualize those results into interventions or ways we can help clients better cope with or adapt to chronic illness.

Stanton and Revenson (2007) suggested that we improve the interpersonal context of our clients by teaching them to develop and maintain social ties, recognize and accept others' help and emotional encouragement, or change their appraisals of the support they are receiving. Psychosocial interventions are directed toward individual-level change and may include cognitive-behavioural, educational, and interpersonal support components. Support groups may provide emotional support as well as an educational focus. The education is expected to strengthen one's sense of control over the disease, reduce feelings of confusion, and enhance decision making (Stanton & Revenson, 2007). The peer support provides emotional support and thus enhances self-esteem, minimizes aloneness, and may reinforce coping strategies.

An earlier study that is still referred to frequently in the literature is that of Folkman and colleagues' (1997) coping effectiveness training with HIV-positive men. This interventional study, based on Lazarus and Folkman's (1984) stress and coping theory, was effective in increasing the quality of life in these men. The training included (1) appraisal training to disaggregate global stressors into specific coping tasks, (2) coping training to tailor application of strategies, and (3) social support training.

Nurses may be wise to capitalize on a client's religious beliefs and partner with clergy to effect adaptation (Loeb, 2006). Programs related to health education and screening, support groups, and physical activity that are based in a church may be helpful. Barg and Gullatte (2001) explained that church-based health programming can frame health information in a way that may better fit with a client's view of life, that is, their relationship with God. It is also important for health practitioners to recognize and encourage culturally appropriate coping methods for diverse cultures. Cultural resilience, according to Walters and Simoni (2002), represents culturally relevant coping strategies that in the case of aboriginal women may include enculturation, spiritual coping, and traditional healing practices. These Walters and Simoni described as "indigenist" stress coping models.

From another perspective, Pakenham (2007) highlighted the need for practitioners to facilitate clients' cognitive processing of the implications and meaning of their illness. A blend of cognitive-restructuring strategies, client-centred approaches, and existential approaches may be helpful to the client and family.

Cognitive-Behavioural Strategies

Cognitive-behavioural strategies can be used to teach coping skills to clients with chronic illness (Folkman & Moskowitz, 2004). Sharpe and Curran (2006) also encouraged the use of cognitive-behavioural treatments, as the research literature is clear that cognitive-behavioural treatment is effective in managing psychological distress associated with illness. Such programs include strategies with the aim of facilitating a realistic, but optimistic, attitude toward illness and/or facilitating more adaptive coping strategies. Programs typically include education about the illness, goal setting and pacing, relaxation strategies and attention diversion skills, cognitive therapy, communication skills, and management of high-risk situations (such as exacerbations of the illness).

McAndrew and colleagues (2008) developed two interventions based on the common sense model of self-regulation. The first intervention is a bottom-up concrete/behavioural approach that was used with clients with diabetes. The approach begins with a focus on behaviour to create an overarching view of diabetes as a chronic condition that requires constant self-regulation. The second intervention is conceived as a top-down or abstract/cognitive strategy that provides clients who have asthma with a conceptual framework that focuses on asthma being present even when it is asymptomatic (McAndrew et al., 2008). The authors suggest that clients may benefit from starting with one strategy or the other. However, it is expected that successful interventions will combine both approaches.

Emotional Intelligence

Emotional intelligence describes the ability to understand, perceive, use, and manage the emotions of self and others (McKenna, 2007). Emotional intelligence training includes six spheres of emotional competence: emotional openness/adaptation, the impact on and of others, self-esteem/identity, management of stress, communication skills/social functioning, and goal management and motivation. It is suggested that emotional self-management can affect the adjustment of individuals with chronic illness, and this can be enabled by the use of emotional intelligence techniques by healthcare professionals (McKenna, 2007).

Psychosocial Rehabilitation

Breast cancer survivors attended a 1-week psychosocial rehabilitation course consisting of moderate physical activity, lectures, group work, and addressing concerns about returning to work. The workshop was led by a multidisciplinary team. The researchers used the common sense model of self-regulation as a framework for the study. Results demonstrated that illness perceptions of breast cancer survivors were not changed by a short psychosocial rehabilitation program (Jorgensen, Frederiksen, Boesen, Elsass, & Johansen, 2009).

Self-Management Programs

Based on the literature on chronic illness self-management, Swendeman, Ingram, and Rotheram-Borus (2009) identified three broad categories in chronic disease self-management: physical health, psychological functioning, and social relationships. Elements related to physical health were knowledge and behaviour to maintain health status, whereas elements related to psychological functioning included self-efficacy and empowerment as well as emotional status and identity shifts. Social relationship elements related to collaborative partnerships with healthcare professionals and family members and social support. Self-management programs based on enhancing self-efficacy are highly successful in reducing symptoms and encouraging behaviour change in many chronic illnesses (Newman, 2006). Self-efficacy could be considered a personal context variable and thus may be a determinant in the appraisal of the illness, the coping strategies used by the individual, and the outcome (the physical, emotional, and social adaptation). Although self-efficacy is task and situation specific, programs that encourage that concept could influence adaptation. Significant improvements in health dimensions were recorded for clients with chronic illness who attended a self-management course in Australia (Bell & Orpin 2006).

Self-Help Groups

As common as self-help and self-support groups are for those with chronic illness, one would expect the research literature to be clear as to their value. Unfortunately, that is not the case. Anecdotal articles exist, but there are few research-based articles. In addition, research commonly examines such support groups for a short period—6, 10, 12, and 15 weeks—whereas a chronic illness can be present for 30, 40, or 50 years. Therefore, the outcome that we might see in such studies is greatly diminished as the studies demonstrate outcomes at one point in time.

Dibb and Yardley (2006) investigated the role that social comparison might play in adaptation using a self-help group as the context. Social comparison proposes that individuals with similar problems compare each other's health status. Often, this comparison occurs within self-help groups, which consist of individuals with similar circumstances. It has been suggested that downward comparison, where comparison is made with a person who is doing less well, will initiate positive affect as it increases self-esteem. Conversely, upward comparison with a person doing less well may result in hope (Dibb & Yardley, 2006). Results of the study with 301 clients with Ménière's disease demonstrated that positive social comparison was associated with better adjustment after controlling for other baseline variables, whereas negative social comparison was associated with worse adjustment over time.

Positive Life Skills

In a sample of 187 HIV-infected women, a positive life skills workshop was effective in increasing antiretroviral adherence, improving mental well-being, and reducing stress (Bova, Burwick, & Quinones, 2008). The workshop consisted of 10 weekly sessions with 6 to 15 women in each group. Workshop facilitators shared a vision of a safe, positive, and respectful environment for women to learn and experience. Part of the workshop involved reframing negative meanings.

SUMMARY

The literature on adjustment has been mostly spearheaded by the discipline of psychology. Thus, the theme of that literature is psychological adaptation versus psychosocial adaptation. Unfortunately, this narrow focus only addresses one component of adaptation. Psychosocial adaptation or adjustment better encompasses the totality of caring for the client and family. Examining the literature also demonstrates the lack of studies that focus on clients from different ethnicities, cultures, and socioeconomic groups. Most studies have been done with White, middle-class populations (deRidder et al., 2008). Thus, the generalisability of these studies is limited. What is clear is that we have a long way to go in understanding, effecting, measuring, and influencing adaptation. With the increasing number of individuals with chronic disease, continuing research and study need to be pursued in this area.

Evidence-Informed Practice Box

Adaptation in chronic illness is a multidimensional construct. Adjustment to chronic illness requires attention to medical management of the disease as well as cognitive, emotional, behavioural, and psychological factors of daily life. Multiple sclerosis (MS) is a chronic illness noted for unpredictability of symptoms and progression of illness as well as variability in day-to-day symptoms. The chronic and uncertain nature of MS requires coping and adjustment not only for persons with MS but for their families as well. Little research has been conducted to identify successful or unsuccessful adaptation to MS. Previous research focused on the experience of caregivers rather than how couples work in concert to navigate alterations in their roles and responsibilities.

Starks, Morris, Yorkston, Gray, and Johnson (2010) conducted a mixed methods study with couples in which one partner had MS. The purpose of the research was to identify strengths and adaptive coping behaviours as well as risk factors for relational stress. Data were collected through semistructured interviews with eight couples to explore how these couples defined and identified their relationships, how they navigated role changes, and how they received external support. Data analysis was guided by a conceptual framework of family adaptation to chronic illness. Results included two patterns of adaptation to MS: "in sync" or "out of sync." Couples in sync were able to transition to managing MS as a chronic illness and to continue to do things of importance to them, including work and leisure activities with family and friends. These couples were able to adjust their goals and expectations to the realities of their lives and maintain a collaborative problem-solving style. Couples out of sync had experienced loss of roles, identity, and self-worth as a result of the rapid progression of functional losses. Differences in personal styles in these couples shifted from being complementary to oppositional in the face of increased demands and struggles.

This research identified mechanisms for adaptation that can assist healthcare professionals in caring for persons with MS and their families. This study provides a guide for healthcare professionals to assess the possible risk factors for relational strain in couples with MS and identify families who might benefit from referrals to family therapy or other relational support. Further, results from this research have applicability for persons with other chronic illnesses and their families and provide a resource for healthcare professionals for interventions to facilitate adaptation to chronic conditions.

Source: Starks et al. (2010)

STUDY QUESTIONS

1. Why is adaptation to chronic illness important to the client and family with chronic illness?

2. Describe how different personal resources could affect adaptation.

3. Compare and contrast the key concepts of the models discussed in this chapter. What are the overlaps in these models? What are the missing elements in these models that would facilitate adaptation?

4. Apply the adaptation framework of Moos and Holahan to one of your clients with chronic illness. What fits? What does not fit?

5. From your perspective, what is social support's relationship to adaptation? What is your experience with the role of social support in the adaptation of your clients?

6. Develop a generic teaching plan that addresses adaptation to chronic illness. What are key points that could then be individualized to clients?

For a full suite of assignments and additional learning activities, use the access code located in the front of your book and visit this exclusive website: **http://go.jblearning.com/kramer-kile**. If you do not have an access code, you can obtain one at the site.

REFERENCES

American Psychiatric Association. (2000). *Diagnostic and statistical manual of mental disorders* (4th ed., revised). Washington, DC: Author.

Antonovsky, A. (1979). *Health, stress, and coping.* San Francisco, CA: Jossey-Bass.

Barg, F. K., & Gullatte, M. M. (2001). Cancer support groups: Meeting the needs of African Americans with cancer. *Seminars in Oncology Nursing, 17,* 171–178.

Barsevick, A. M., Whitmer, K., & Walker, L. (2001). In their own words: Using the common sense model to analyze patient descriptions of cancer related fatigue. *Oncology Nursing Forum, 28*(9), 1363–1369.

Bell, E., & Orpin, P. (2006). Self management of chronic conditions: Implications for rural physicians of a demonstration project down under. *Canadian Journal of Rural Medicine, 11*(1), 33–42.

Berg, C. A., & Upchurch, R. (2007). A developmental-contextual model of couples coping with chronic illness across the adult life span [Electronic version]. *Psychological Bulletin, 133*(6), 920–954.

Black, C., & Ford-Giboe, M. (2004). Adolescent mothers: Resilience, family health work and health-promoting practices. *Journal of Advanced Nursing, 48*(4), 351–360.

Borrell-Carrio, F., Suchman, L. A., & Epstein, R. M. (2004). The biopsychosocial model 25 yrs later: Principles, practice and scientific inquiry. *Annals of Family Medicine, 2*(6), 576–582.

Bova, C., Burwick, T. N., & Quinones, M. (2008). Improving women's adjustment to HIV infection: Results of the positive life skills workshop project [Electronic version]. *Journal of the Association of Nurses in AIDS Care, 19*(1), 58–65.

Brink, E. (2009). Adaptation positions and behavior among post-myocardial infarction patients. *Clinical Nursing Research, 18*(2), 119–135.

Brooks, M. (2003). Health-related hardiness and chronic illness: A synthesis of current research [Electronic version]. *Nursing Forum, 38*(3), 11–20.

Brooks, M. (2008). Health-related hardiness in individuals with chronic illnesses. *Clinical Nursing Research, 17*(2), 98–117.

Bury, M. (1982). Chronic illness as biographical disruption. *Sociology of Health and Illness, 4,* 167–182.

Carver, C. S., Scheier, M. F., & Weintraub, J. K. (1989). Assessing coping strategies: A theoretically based approach. *Journal of Personality and Social Psychology, 56,* 267–283.

Charmaz, K. (1995). The body, identity, and self: Adapting to impairment. *Sociological Quarterly, 36,* 657–680.

Cohen, J. A., & Welch, L. M. (2000). Attitudes, beliefs, values and culture as mediators of stress. In V. Rice (Ed.), *Handbook of stress, coping and health: Implications for nursing research, theory and practice* (pp. 335–366). Thousand Oaks, CA: Sage.

Cummins, J. R., Ireland, M., Resnick, M. D., & Blum, R. W. (1999). Correlates of physical and emotional health among Native American adolescents. *Journal of Adolescent Health, 24,* 338–344.

Degazon, C. E. (1995). Coping, diabetes, and the older African American. *Nursing Outlook, 43*(6), 254–259.

Demers, L., Robichaud, L., Gelinas, I., Noread, L., & Desroisiers, J. (2009). Coping strategies and social participation in older adults. *Gerontology, 55,* 233-239.

deRidder, D., Geenen, R., Kuijer, R., & van Middendorp, H. (2008). Psychological adjustment to chronic disease. *Lancet, 372,* 246–254.

Dew, M. A., Myaskovsky, L., Switzer, G. E., DiMartini, A. F., Schulberg, H. C., & Kormos, R. L. (2005). Profiles and predictors of the course of psychological distress across four years after heart transplantation [Electronic version]. *Psychological Medicine, 35,* 1215–1227.

Dibb, B., & Yardley, L. (2006). How does social comparison within a self-help group influence adjustment to chronic illness? A longitudinal study. *Social Science and Medicine, 63,* 1602–1613.

Dixon-Woods, A. (2001). Writing wrongs? An analysis of published discourses about the use of patient information leaflets. *Social Science & Medicine, 52,* 1432–1437.

Engel, G. L. (1977). Need for a new medical model. *Science, 196,* 129–136.

Esteve, R., Ramirez-Maestre, C., & Lopez-Martinez, A. E. (2007). Adjustment to chronic pain: The role of pain acceptance, coping strategies, and pain-related cognitions. *Annals of Behavioral Medicine, 33*(2), 179–188.

Folkman, S., & Greer, S. (2000). Promoting psychological well-being in the face of serious illness: When theory, research, and practice inform each other. *Psycho-Oncology, 9,* 11–19.

Folkman, S., Lazarus, R. S., Gruen, R. J., & DeLongis, A. (1986). Appraisal, coping, health status, and psychological symptoms. *Journal of Personality and Social Psychology, 50*(3), 571–579.

Folkman, S., & Moskowitz, J. T. (2004). Coping: Pitfalls and promise. *Annual Review of Psychology, 55,* 745–774.

Folkman, S., Moskowitz, J. T., Ozer, E. M., & Park, C. L. (1997). Positive meaningful events and coping in the context of HIV/AIDS. In B. H. Gottlieb (Ed.), *Coping with chronic stress* (pp. 293–314). New York, NY: Plenum.

Freeth, R. (2007). Working within the medical model. *Healthcare Counseling & Psychotherapy Journal, 7*(4), 3–7.

Graves, H., Scott, D. L., Lempp, H., & Weinman, J. (2009). Illness beliefs predict disability in rheumatoid arthritis. *Journal of Psychosomatic Research, 67,* 417–423.

Hagger, M. S., & Orbell, S. (2003). A meta-analytic review of the common-sense model of illness representations. *Psychology and Health, 18,* 141–184.

Helgeson, V. S., Snyder, P., & Seltman, H. (2004). Psychological and physical adjustment to breast cancer over 4 years: Identifying distinct trajectories of change [Electronic version]. *Health Psychology, 23,* 3–15.

House, J. C. (1981). *Work, stress and social support.* Reading, MA: Addison-Wesley.

Iwasaki, Y., & Bartlett, J. (2006). Culturally meaningful leisure as a way of coping with stress among aboriginal individuals with diabetes. *Journal of Leisure research, 38*(3), 321–338.

Jorgensen, I. L., Frederiksen, K., Boesen, E., Elsass, P., & Johansen, C. (2009). An exploratory study of associations between illness perceptions and adjustment and changes after psychosocial rehabilitation in survivors of breast cancer. *Acta Oncologica, 48,* 1119–1127.

Kiebles, J. L., Doerfler, B., & Keefer, L. (2010). Preliminary evidence supporting a framework of psychological adjustment to inflammatory bowel disease. *Inflammatory Bowel Disease, 16*(10), 1685–1695.

Kobasa, S. C. (1979). Stressful life events, personality and health: An inquiry into hardiness. *Journal of Personal and Social Psychology, 37*(1), 1–11.

Kralik, D., vanLoon, A., & Visentin, K. (2006). Resilience in the chronic illness experience. *Educational Action Research, 14*(2), 187–201.

Leong, F. T., & Wong, P. T (2003). Optimal functioning from cross-cultural perspectives. In W. B. Walsh (Ed.), *Counselling psychology and optimal human functioning* (pp. 123–150). Mahwah, NJ: Lawrence Erlbaum Associates.

Lazarus, R. S. (1966). *Psychological stress and the coping process*. New York, NY: McGraw-Hill.

Lazarus, R. S., & Folkman, S. (1984). *Stress appraisal and coping*. New York, NY: Springer.

Leventhal, H., Leventhal, E. A., & Cameron, L. (2001). Representations, procedures, and affect in illness self-regulation: A perceptual-cognitive model. In A. Baum, T. A. Revenson, & J. E. Singer (Eds.), *Handbook of health psychology* (pp. 19–47). Mahwah, NJ: Lawrence Erlbaum Associates.

Livneh, H., & Antonak, R. F. (1997). *Psychosocial adaptation to chronic illness and disability*. Gaithersburg, MD: Aspen.

Loeb, S. (2006). African American older adults coping with chronic health conditions [Electronic version]. *Journal of Transcultural Nursing, 17*(2), 139–147.

Maes, S., Leventhal, H., & deRidder, D. (1996). Coping with chronic diseases. In M. Zeidner & N. S. Endler (Eds.), *Handbook of coping: Theory, research, applications* (pp. 221–251). New York, NY: Wiley.

Maluccio, A. (2002). Resilience: A many-splendored construct? *American Journal of Orthopsychiatry, 72*(4), 596–599.

McAndrew, L. M., Musumeci-Szabo, T. J., Mora, P. A., Vileikyte, L., Burns, E., Halm, E., Leventhal, E., & Leventhal, H. (2008). Using the common sense model to design interventions for the prevention and management of chronic illness threats: From description to process. *British Journal of Health Psychology, 13*, 195–204.

McKenna, J. (2007). Emotional intelligence training in adjustment to physical disability and illness [Electronic version]. *International Journal of Therapy and Rehabilitation, 14*(12), 551–556.

Mirowsky, J., & Ross, C. (2002). Measurement for a human science [Electronic version]. *Journal of Health and Social Behavior, 43*, 152–170.

Moos, R. H., & Holahan, C. J. (2007). Adaptive tasks and methods of coping with illness and disability. In E. Martz & H. Livneh (Eds.), *Coping with chronic illness and disability* (pp. 107–128). New York, NY: Springer.

Morea, J. M., Friend, R., & Bennett, R. M. (2008). Conceptualizing and measuring illness self-concept: A comparison with self-esteem and optimism in predicting fibromyalgia adjustment. *Research in Nursing and Health, 31*, 563–575.

Newman, A. (2006). Self-efficacy. In I. Lubkin & P. Larsen (Eds.), *Chronic illness: Impact and interventions* (6th ed., pp. 105–120). Sudbury, MA: Jones & Bartlett.

Norton, T. R., Manne, S. L., Rubin, S., Hernandez, E., Carlson, J., Bergman, C., . . . Rosenblum, N. (2005). Ovarian cancer patients' psychological distress: The role of physical impairment, perceived unsupportive family and friend behavior, perceived control, and self-esteem [Electronic version]. *Health Psychology, 24*, 143–152.

Paddison, C. A. M., Alpass, F. M., & Stephens, C. V. (2010). Using the common-sense model of illness self regulation to understand diabetes-related distress: The importance of being able to "make sense" of diabetes. *New Zealand Journal of Psychiatry, 39*(1), 45–50.

Pakenham, K. I. (2007). Making sense of multiple sclerosis [Electronic version]. *Rehabilitation Psychology, 52*(4), 380–389.

Pollock, S. E. (1989). The hardiness characteristic: A motivating factor in adaptation. *Advances in Nursing Science, 11*(2), 53–62.

Revenson, T. (1994). Social support and marital coping with chronic illness. *Annals of Behavioral Medicine, 16*, 122–130.

Richmond, C. A. M., & Ross, N. A. (2008). Social support, material circumstance and health behaviour: Influences on health in First Nation and Inuit communities of Canada. *Social Science and Medicine, 67*, 1423–1433.

Sakalys, J. A. (2000). The political role of illness narratives. *Journal of Advanced Nursing, 31*(6), 1469–1475.

Schreurs, K. M. G., & deRidder, D. T. D. (1997). Integration of coping and social support perspectives: Implications for the study of adaptation to chronic diseases [Electronic version]. *Clinical Psychology Review, 17*, 89–112.

Sharpe, L., & Curran, L. (2006). Understanding the process of adjustment to illness [Electronic version]. *Social Science & Medicine, 62*, 1153–1166.

Shaw, C. (1999). A framework for the study of coping illness behavior and outcomes. *Journal of Advanced Nursing, 29*(5), 1246–1255.

Shifren, K. (2003). Women with heart disease: Can the common-sense model of illness help? *Health Care for Women International, 24*(4), 355–368.

Smith, E. P., Boutte, G. S., Zigler, E., & Finn-Stevenson, M. (2004). Opportunities for schools to promote resilience in children and youth. In K. Maton, C. J., Schellenback, B. J. Leadbeater, & A. L. Solarz (Eds.), *Investing in children, youth, families and communities: Strengths based research and policy* (pp. 213–232). Washington, DC: American Psychological Association.

Sprangers, M. A. G., & Schwartz, C. E. (2000). Integrating response shift into health-related quality-of-life research: A theoretical model. In C. E. Schwartz & M. A. G. Sprangers (Eds.), *Adaptation to changing health: Response shift in quality-of-life research* (pp. 11–23). Washington, DC: American Psychological Association.

Stanton, A. L., Collins, C. A., & Sworowski, L. A. (2001). Adjustment to chronic illness: Theory and research. In A. Baum, T. A. Revenson, & J. E. Singer (Eds.), *Handbook of health psychology* (pp. 387–403). Mahwah, NJ: Lawrence Erlbaum Associates.

Stanton, A. L., & Revenson, T. A. (2007). Adjustment to chronic disease: Progress and promise in research. In H. S. Friedman & R. C. Silver (Eds.), *Foundations of health psychology* (pp. 203–233). New York, NY: Oxford University Press.

Stanton, A. L., Revenson, T. A., & Tennen, H. (2007). Health psychology: Psychological adjustment to chronic disease [Electronic version]. *Annual Review of Psychology, 58*, 565–592.

Starks, H., Morris, M. A., Yorkston, K. M., Gray, R. F., & Johnson, K. L. (2010). Being in- or out-of-sync: Couples' adaptation to change in multiple sclerosis. *Disability and Rehabilitation, 32*(3), 196–206.

Sterba, K. R., DeBellis, R. F., Lewis, M. A., DeVeillis, B. M., Jordan, J. M., & Baucom, D. H. (2008). Effects of couple illness perception congruence on psychological adjustment in women with rheumatoid arthritis. *Health Psychology, 27*(2), 221–229.

Stewart, K. E., Ross, D., & Hartley, S. (2004). Patient adaptation to chronic illness. In T. J. Boll, J. M. Raczynski, & L. C. Leviton (Eds.), *Handbook of clinical health psychology*. Vol. 2, *Disorders of behavior and health* (pp. 405–421). Washington, DC: American Psychological Association.

Sunday, J., Eyles, J., & Upshur, R. (2006). Applying Aristotle's doctrine of causation to aboriginal and biomedical understandings of diabetes. *Culture, Medicine and Psychiatry, 25*, 63–85.

Swendeman, D., Ingram, B. L., & Rotheram-Borus, M. J. (2009). Common elements in self-management of HIV and other chronic illnesses: An integrative framework. *AIDS Care, 21*(10), 1321–1334.

van't Spijker, A., Trijsburg, R. W., & Duivenvorrden, H. J. (1997). Psychological sequelae of cancer diagnosis: A meta-analytical review of 58 studies after 1980 [Electronic version]. *Psychosomatic Medicine, 59*, 280–293.

Visotsky, H. M., Hamburg, D. A., Goss, M. E., & Lebovits, B. Z. (1961). Coping behavior under extreme stress: Observations of patients with severe poliomyelitis. *Archives of General Psychiatry, 5*, 27–52.

Waisbond, S. (2007). Beyond the medical-informational model: Recasting the role of communication in tuberculosis control [Electronic version]. *Social Science & Medicine, 65*(10), 2130–2134.

Walker, J. G., Jackson, J. J., & Littlejohn, G. O. (2004). Models of adjustment to chronic illness: Using the example of rheumatoid arthritis [Electronic version]. *Clinical Psychology Review, 24*, 461–488.

Walters, K. L., & Simoni, J. M. (2002). Reconceptualizing native women's health: An indigenist stress-coping model. *American Journal of Public Health, 92*, 520–524

CHAPTER 6

Social Isolation

Original chapter by Diana Luskin Biordi and Nicholas R. Nicholson
Canadian content added by Joseph C. Osuji

INTRODUCTION

Humans are social animals who are supposed to actively seek human companionship or relationships. The lives of hermits or cloistered, solitary existences are extraordinary because they so vividly remind us that, usually, life is richer for the human contact we share. As valuable as life may be when we engage in a variety of relationships, time reserved for solitude is also necessary as we seek rest or contemplative opportunity in "our own space." The weaving together of individual possibilities for social engagement or solitude develops a certain uniqueness and texture in personal and community relationships. These distinctive personal configurations of engagement and disengagement have consequences for our health, work, and social lives. It is critical, therefore, that healthcare professionals understand the value of social engagement and of solitude.

ISOLATION: A WORKING DEFINITION

"Belonging" is a multidimensional social construct of relatedness to persons, places, or things and is fundamental to personality and social well-being (Hill, 2006). If belonging is connectedness, then social isolation is the distancing of an individual, psychologically, physically, or both, from his or her network of desired or needed relationships with other persons. Social isolation is described as an "objective measure of contacts with other people" (Havens, Hall, Sylvestre, & Jivan, 2004, p. 130) that results in a loss of place within one's group(s). The isolation may be voluntary or involuntary. In cognitively intact persons social isolation can be identified as such by the isolate. Although some may consider isolation as purely subjective, the various dimensions of isolation argue against this singular position, as discussed in this chapter.

The literature portrays social isolation as typically accompanied by feelings related to loss or marginality. Apartness or aloneness, often described as solitude, may also be a part of the concept of social isolation in that it is a distancing from one's network, but this state may be accompanied by more positive feelings and is often voluntarily initiated by the isolate. Some researchers debate whether apartness should be included in or distinguished as a separate concept from social isolation. As seen in the literature that follows, social isolation has several definitions and distinctions, dependent on empirical research and the stance of the observer.

When Is Isolation a Problem?

Social isolation ranges from the voluntary isolate who seeks disengagement from social intercourse for a variety of reasons to those whose isolation is involuntary or imposed by others. Privacy or being alone, if actively chosen, has the potential for enhancing the human psyche. On the other hand, involuntary social isolation occurs when an individual's demand for social contacts or communications exceeds the human or situational capability of others. Involuntary isolation is negatively viewed because the outcomes are the dissolution of social exchanges and the support they provide for the individual or his or her support system(s). Some persons, such as those with cognitive deficits, may not understand their involuntary isolation, but their parent, spouse, or significant other may indeed understand that involuntary social isolation can have a negative and profound impact on the caregiver and care recipient.

Social isolation experienced negatively by an individual or his or her significant other becomes a problem that requires management. In fact, according to much of the literature, only physical functional disability ranks with social isolation in its impact on the client and the client's social support network (family, friends, fellow workers, and so forth). Therefore, social isolation is one of the two most important aspects of chronic illness to be managed in the plan of care.

Distinctions of Social Isolation

Social isolation is viewed from the perspective of the number, frequency, and quality of contacts; the longevity or durability of these contacts; and the negativism attributed to the isolation felt by the individual involved. Social isolation has been the subject of the humanities for hundreds of years. Who has not heard of John Donne's exclamation, "No man is an island," or, conversely, the philosophy of existentialism—that humans are ultimately alone? Yet the concept of social isolation has been systematically researched during only the last 50 years. Unlike some existentialists and social scientists, healthcare professionals, with their problem-oriented, clinical approach, tend to regard social isolation as negative rather than positive.

NATURE OF ISOLATION

Isolation can occur at four layers of the social concept. The outermost social layer is community, where one feels integrated or isolated from the larger social structure. Next is the layer of organization (work, schools, churches), followed by a layer closer to the person, that is, confidantes (friends, family, significant others). Finally, the innermost layer is that of the person, who has the personality, the intellectual ability, or the senses with which to apprehend and interpret relationships (Lin, 1986).

In the healthcare literature the primary focus is on the clinical dyad, so the examination of social isolation tends to be confined to the levels of confidante and person and extended only to the organization and community for single clients, one at a time. For the healthcare professional the most likely relationships are bound to expectations of individually centred reciprocity, mutuality, caring, and responsibility. On the other hand, health policy literature tends to focus on the reciprocity of community and organizations to populations of individuals, and so it deals with collective social isolation.

Four patterns of social isolation or interaction have been identified at the level of the clinical dyad. Although these were originally formulated with older adults in mind, they can be analogized easily to younger persons by making them age-relative:

- Persons who have been integrated into social groups throughout their lifetime
- The "early isolate," who was isolated as an adult but is relatively active in old age
- The "recent isolate," who was active in early adulthood but is not in old age
- The "lifelong isolate," whose life is one of isolation

FEELINGS THAT REFLECT ISOLATION

Social isolation can be characterized by feelings of boredom and marginality or exclusion (Weiss, 1973). Boredom occurs because of the lack of validation of one's work or daily routines; therefore, these tasks become only busy work. Marginality is the sense of being excluded from desired networks or groups. Other feelings ascribed to social isolation include loneliness, anger, despair, sadness, frustration, or, in some cases, relief.

DESCRIPTION AND CHARACTERISTICS OF SOCIAL ISOLATION

The existence of social isolation increases our awareness of the need for humans to associate with each other in an authentic intimate relationship, whether characterized by caring or some other emotion, such as anger. When we speak of social isolation we think first of the affected person; then we almost immediately consider that individual's relationships. This chapter demonstrates that, as a process, social isolation may be a feature in a variety of illnesses and disabilities across the life cycle.

As an ill person becomes more aware of the constricting social network and declining participation, he or she may feel sadness, anger, despair, or reduced self-esteem. These emotions factor into a changed social and personal identity but are also separate issues for the person who is chronically ill. Moreover, depending on their own emotional and physical needs, friends and acquaintances may drop out of a person's social support system until only the most loyal remain (Tilden & Weinert, 1987). Families, however, are likely to remain in the social network. As the social network reaches its limitations it may itself become needful of interventions, such as respite care for the parents of a child who is chronically ill or support groups for the siblings of children with cancer (Heiney, Goon-Johnson, Ettinger, & Ettinger, 1990).

SOCIAL ISOLATION VERSUS SIMILAR STATES OF HUMAN APARTNESS

Social isolation has been treated either as a distinct phenomenon or has been combined or equated with other states relating to human apartness. The literature is replete with a variety of definitions of social isolation, many of which are interrelated, synonymous, or confused with other distinct but related phenomena.

Social Isolation and Alienation

Social isolation and alienation have been linked together or treated as synonymous in much of the healthcare literature, although these two concepts differ from one another. Alienation encompasses powerlessness, normlessness, isolation, self-estrangement, and meaninglessness (Holocomb-McCoy, 2004). Powerlessness refers to the belief held by an individual that one's own behaviours cannot elicit the results one desires or seeks. In normlessness the individual has a strong belief that socially unapproved behaviours are necessary to achieve goals. Isolation means the inability to value highly held goals or beliefs that others usually value. Self-estrangement has come to mean the divorce of one's self from one's work or creative possibilities. Finally, meaninglessness is the sense that few significant predictions about the outcomes of behaviour can be made. Thus, one can see that isolation is only one psychological state of alienation. However, authors frequently merge the finer points of one or more of the five dimensions of alienation and call the result isolation.

Social Isolation and Loneliness

Although social isolation is typically viewed today as a deprivation in social contacts, Peplau and Perlman (1986) suggested it is loneliness, not social isolation, that occurs when an individual perceives her or his social relationships as not containing the desired quantity or quality of social contacts. In an even more subtle distinction, loneliness has been referred to as an alienation of the self and "the painful and agonizing longing to be related to, to connect to others, and to be accepted and valued" (Ami, 2004, p. 29). Loneliness has been linked to anxiety, interpersonal hostility, and depression (Lau & Kong, 1999) but differs from depression in that in loneliness one attempts to integrate oneself into new relationships, whereas in depression there is a surrendering of oneself to the distress (Weiss, 1973).

Although loneliness does relate to social isolation, to use social isolation and loneliness as interchangeable terms can be confusing. To maintain clarity, loneliness should be considered the subjective emotional state of the individual, whereas social isolation is the objective state of deprivation of social contact and content (Bennet, 1980). Therefore, loneliness refers to the psychological state of the individual, whereas social isolation relates to the sociological status. Although it is true that social isolation might lead to loneliness, loneliness is not, in itself, a necessary condition of social isolation. Both conditions can exist apart from each other.

Social Isolation and Aloneness

Tightly linked with social isolation is the need for social support, which is the social context or environment that facilitates the survival of human beings (Lin, 1986) by offering social, emotional, and material support needed and received by an individual, especially one who is chronically ill. Although social support literature has focused on the instrumental and material benefits of support, recent literature on social isolation relates isolation more to the negative feeling state of aloneness (Lasgaard et al., 2010; Nelson, 2009). This feeling is associated with deficits in social support networks, diminished participation in these networks or in social relationships, or feelings of rejection or withdrawal.

PROBLEMS AND ISSUES OF SOCIAL ISOLATION

Regardless of how social isolation occurs, the result is that basic needs for authentic intimacy remain unmet. Typically, this is perceived as alienating or unpleasant, and the social isolation that occurs can lead to depression, loneliness, or other social and cognitive impairments that then exacerbate the isolation.

Several predisposing reasons for social isolation have been proposed: status-altering physical disabilities or illnesses, frailties associated with advanced age or developmental delays, personality or neurological disorders, and environmental constraints, which often refer to physical surroundings but are also interpreted by some to include diminished personal or material resources (Tilden & Weinert, 1987).

THE ISOLATION PROCESS

A typical course of isolation that evolves as an illness or disability becomes more apparent in the change in social network relationships. Friends or families begin to withdraw from the isolated individual or the individual from them. This process may be slow or subtle, as with individuals with arthritis, or it may be rapid, as with the person with AIDS. Unfortunately, the process of isolation may not be based on accurate or rational information.

On the other hand, self-perception in chronic illness can also influence disease progression and management. Self-perception "is a set of features, which one identifies with . . . , it consists of convictions about one's general appearance, physical and intellectual condition, abilities, activity, social position etc" (Korwin-Piotrowska, Korwin-Piotrowska, & Samochowiec, 2010, p. 63). Individuals with serious chronic illnesses come to perceive themselves as different from others and outside the mainstream of ordinary life (Williams & Bury, 1989). This perception of being different may be shared by others, who may then reject them, their disability, and their differentness. Part of this sense of being different can stem from the ongoing demands of the illness. For example, social relationships are

interrupted because families and friends cannot adjust the erratic treatment to acceptable social activities. From such real events or from social perceptions, social isolation can occur either as a process or as an outcome.

Individuals with chronic illness often face their own mortality more explicitly than do others. According to Jim and Anderson (2007), meaning is conceptualized in four dimensions: feelings of inner peace and thoughts of satisfaction with one's life, the benefits accruing from spirituality and the absence or loss of meaning-negative emotions, confusion, and loss of life's value. Cancer patients lose meaning in their lives as a result of negative social and physical consequences associated with heightened distress (Jim & Anderson, 2007).

Even if death does not frighten those with chronic illness, it frequently frightens those in their social networks, which leads to guilt, uncertainty, and perhaps strained silences and withdrawal. In the case of individuals with cancer (Bachner, O'Rourke, & Camel, 2011; Turner-Cobb, Bloor, Whittemore, West, & Spiegel, 2006; Yasemin & Seher, 2010), heart disease (Bennett et al., 2001; Bobsworth et al., 2000), fibromyalgia (Franks, Cronan, & Oliver, 2004), or systemic lupus erythematosus (Mazzoni & Cicognani, 2011), social support is significant to their survival. For those who lack this social support, social isolation is not merely a metaphor for death but can hasten it.

SOCIAL ISOLATION AND STIGMA

Social isolation may occur as a result of stigma. Many persons will risk anonymity rather than expose themselves to a judgmental audience. Because chronic illnesses can be stigmatizing, the concern about the possibility of revealing a discredited or discreditable self can slow or paralyze social interaction. In studies investigating stigma and HIV, it was observed that stigma resulted in feelings of rejection among HIV-positive South Asians in Toronto (Vlassoff & Ali, 2010), it adversely affected uptake of facility-based labour and delivery services and quality of care in Kenya (Turan, Miller, Bukusi, Sande, & Cohen, 2007), and it resulted in discrimination against HIV-positive individuals in Russia (Balabanova, Cooker, Atun, & Drobniewski, 2006).

For fear of negative consequences, individuals with chronic illness such as HIV and their families grapple with how much information about the diagnosis they should share, with whom, and when. This eventually results in "negative psychological and physical outcomes and continued spread of the disease" (Sowell & Philips, 2010, p. 394). If an illness is manageable or reasonably invisible, its presence may be hidden from all but a select few, often for years. Parents of children with chronic illnesses were reported to manage stressful encounters and uncertainty by disguising, withholding, or limiting information to others (Cohen, 1993), an action that may add to limiting their social network.

As siblings of children with cancer deal with the isolation of their brother or sister, they become vulnerable to social isolation themselves (Bendor, 1990). Social isolation not only burdens those with chronic illness, it also extends into family dynamics and requires the healthcare professional to consider how the family manages. Thus, with social isolation being a burden for the family, it requires the healthcare professional to consider how the family manages the illness and the isolation.

Where the stigmatized disability is quite obvious, as in the visibility of burn scars or the odour of colitis, the person who is chronically ill might venture only within small circles of understanding individuals (Gallo, Breitmayer, Knafl, & Zoeller, 1991). Where employment is possible, it will often be work that does not require many social interactions, such as night work or jobs within protected environments (sheltered workshops, home offices). Regardless of what serves as reminders of the disability, the disability is incorporated into the isolate's sense of self; that is, it becomes part of his or her social and personal identity.

SOCIAL ISOLATION AND SOCIAL ROLES

Any weakening or diminishment of relationships or social roles might produce social isolation for individuals or their significant others. Clients who lose family, friends, and associated position and power are inclined to feelings of rejection, worthlessness, and loss of self-esteem (Ravish, 1985). These feelings become magnified by the client's culture if that culture values community (Litwin & Zoabi, 2003; Siplic & Kadis, 2002). An example of social isolation of both caregiver and care recipient occurred in a situation of a woman whose husband had Alzheimer's disease. The couple had been confined for more than 2 years in an apartment in a large city, from which her confused husband frequently wandered. Her comment, "I'm not like a wife and not like a single person either," reflected their dwindling social network and her loss of wifely privileges but not obligations. This ambiguity is common to many whose spouses are incapacitated. Moreover, after a spouse dies the widow or widower often grieves as much for the loss of the role of a married person as for the loss of the spouse.

The loss of social roles can occur as a result of illness or disability, social changes throughout the lifespan (e.g., in school groups, with career moves, or in unaccepting communities), marital dissolution (through death or divorce), or secondary to ostracism incurred by membership in a "wrong" group. The loss of social roles and the resultant isolation of the individual have been useful analytic devices in the examination of issues of the aged, the widowed, the physically impaired, or in psychopathology.

OLDER ADULTS AND SOCIAL ISOLATION

Older age, with its many losses of physical and psychological health, social roles, mobility, bereavement, economic status, and physical living arrangements, can contribute to decreasing social networks and increasing isolation (Cloutier-Fisher, Kobayashi, & Smith, 2011; Havens et al., 2004; Howat, Iredell, Grenade, Nedwetzky, & Collins, 2004; Kobayashi, Cloutier-Fisher, & Roth, 2009; Victor et al., 2002). In 2003 the Canadian Federal/Provincial and Territorial Taskforce on Seniors identified social isolation as an important determinant of vulnerability and poor health outcomes among seniors (Cloutier-Fisher & Kobayashi, 2009). This will become even more of an issue as the number of older adults in Canada and across the globe increases proportionately in the next two decades. The United Nations reported that 11% of the world population was aged 60 and above, and this number is estimated to rise to 22% by 2050 (United Nations, 2007). According to Statistics Canada, seniors represent one of the fastest growing population sections in Canada, and currently make up 13.1% of the overall Canadian population. This number has been projected to grow from 4.2 million in 2005 to 9.8 million in 2039 (Statistics Canada, 2011). According to Kobayashi et al. (2009), a Canadian body of research in this area has paid limited attention to the increasing prevalence of social isolation among older adults or its relationships with health status.

Social isolation has been linked with functional disability. One definition of functional disability is "the degree of difficulty or inability to independently perform basic activities of daily living (ADLs) or other tasks essential for independent living" (Mendes de Leon, Gold, Glass, Kaplan, & George, 2001, p. S179). Social networks may influence the functional disability process by preventing decline or facilitating recovery (Mendes de Leon et al., 1999). Consequently, functional disability may impact social networks by preventing older adults from seeking engagement with other members. Network size and social interaction are significantly associated with functional disability risk (Mendes de Leon et al., 2001). Older adults who are more socially engaged report less functional disability (Mendes de Leon, Glass, & Berkman, 2003), and those who are a strong part of a social network have been found to have reduced risk of functional disability (Mendes de Leon et al., 1999).

Social isolation has been shown to be a serious health risk for older adults (Findlay, 2003), with studies indicating a relationship between all-cause mortality (Ceria et al., 2001), coronary disease (Eng, Rimm, Fitzmaurice, & Kawachi, 2002), and cognitive impairments (Barnes, Mendes de Leon, Wilson, Bienias, & Evans, 2004; Beland, Zunzunegui, Alvarado, Otero, & Del Ser, 2005; Holtzman et al., 2004; Zunzunegui, Alvarado, Del Ser, & Otero, 2003). In a converse finding, older adults with extensive social networks were protected against dementia

(Fratiglioni, Paillard-Borg, & Winblad, 2004; Fratiglioni, Wang, Ericsson, Maytan, & Winblad, 2000; Seidler, Bernhardt, Nienhaus, & Frolich, 2003; Wang, Karp, Winblad, & Fratiglioni, 2002). And, as described earlier, although low social engagement may not be a form of social isolation per se, it is a psychological isolator and thus a risk factor in social isolation (Howat et al., 2004). For example, depressive symptoms in older adults were shown to be decreased by social integration (Ramos & Wilmoth, 2003). Isolated older adults were shown to have increased risk for coronary heart disease (Brummett et al., 2001; Eng et al., 2002), and death related to congestive heart failure was predicted by social isolation (Murberg, 2004). Similarly, poststroke outcomes, for example, additional strokes, myocardial infarction, or death, were predicted by prestroke isolation (Boden-Albala, Litwak, Elkind, Rundek, & Sacco, 2005). Isolated women before a diagnosis of breast cancer, when compared with socially integrated women, were found to have a 66% increase in all-cause mortality (Kroenke, Kubzansky, Schernhammer, Holmes, & Kawachi, 2006). Quality of life among breast cancer survivorship is impacted negatively by social isolation (Michael, Berkman, Colditz, Holmes, & Kawachi, 2002). Finally, and perhaps most relevant to health and cost outcomes, socially isolated older adults were found to be four to five times more likely to be rehospitalized within a year from their previous hospitalization (Mistry et al., 2001).

The extent (from local to community and integrated to contained) and nature (positive or negative social relationships) of a social network (Litwin, 1997; Wenger, Davies, Shahtahmasebi, & Scott, 1996) affected health as well as social isolation (Seeman, 2000; Wenger, 1997). In fact, the quality of the social relationship may have more impact than the number of ties (Pinquart & Sorensen, 2001), which suggests that a few solid relationships may be more beneficial than many ties of poor quality.

CASE STUDY

Thomas is an 85-year-old man with severe chronic obstructive pulmonary disease, depression, and type 2 diabetes. He currently smokes cigarettes and has smoked for the last 45 years. Thomas is a widower, but he has a common law partner for the past 8 years named Gretchen. Gretchen has high care demands due to a recent cerebrovascular accident, which left her with expressive aphasia and incontinence. Thomas is a member of the local Legion chapter and was in charge of fundraising until recently. He had to give up his position because he needed to be at home more to watch over Gretchen. When talking about his home situation Thomas states, "I hate to give up all the time with my buddies. I've been a member for 50 years, but since she can't tell me she's wet, I have to check all the time. If I'm not at home, who's going to check?" Despite the fact that she is a lot of work physically and sometimes her inability to speak is discouraging, Thomas says he loves her company. He states that it is wonderful to have a constant companion even though direct conversations are extremely difficult, but you are unsure if this is really how he feels.

Before retirement Thomas was a certified general accountant who worked for a local accounting office. He enjoyed the interaction with his clients and was described as a very social

CASE STUDY   (Continued)   **www**

person with numerous friends. He made lots of new friends through his skills in bringing in high returns on taxes for his clients. In fact, the best man at his wedding, Frank, initially was his tax client. Frank had bought Thomas a steak dinner to thank him for saving him and his wife lots of money, after which the two became best friends. The two men and their wives had shared many social occasions, but when Frank died years ago Thomas became depressed and stopped wanting to go out socially. At that time Thomas' wife of 50 years, Frances, had encouraged him to continue to go out and meet new people. He began to get out more and started to feel like his old self, when Frances died suddenly of a myocardial infarction. After her death Thomas refused to be social. He said, "What's the point of going out and meeting people, if they are just going to die on you? I'd rather stay in." He also attended church services every week but now doesn't go anymore; instead, he watches the services on TV. Thomas says, "God knows I'm still dedicated, so I don't need to go out and chat about how great things are with a bunch of busybody church types—especially when things aren't that great at all." About a year after his wife Frances died, he met Gretchen in the supermarket, and they have been partners ever since—both are happy to stay in most of the time.

Thomas was functioning at a moderate to high level but recently had a fall secondary to shortness of breath related to emphysema and an acute syncopal episode. He was hospitalized for the shortness of breath, the mild abrasions from the fall, and to have a neurological workup. His respiratory status returned to baseline with the addition of a new inhaler, his neurological status checked out well, and, thankfully, there were no broken bones. Because he is Gretchen's primary caretaker, her granddaughter flew in from out of town to take care of her until Thomas was released. He was released after 3 days in the hospital with home care follow-up at their home.

You are the home care nurse on your first visit to his home. Having completed your reading of Thomas' chart you wonder how this man turned from a social accountant to someone who has been hospitalized for an injurious fall. Additionally, you wonder about how the many psychosocial factors play into his well-being and the well-being of Gretchen. Thomas has stopped seeing his friends, has stopped attending church, has had a decline in his overall health, has implied he doesn't really belong anywhere, and, aside from Gretchen, has a lack of fulfilling relationships—all leading to a possible diagnosis of social isolation. As you walk to the front door with your chart and admissions paperwork you see Thomas through the window silently crying by himself in the kitchen.

Discussion Questions

1. Given Thomas' history, identify the factors that put him most at risk for social isolation.
2. When considering nursing interventions for Thomas, what would be the number one health issue to address? In your opinion is Thomas a social isolate? Why or why not?
3. Do you consider Gretchen, Thomas' common law partner, a positive or negative influence on his life? Explain your answer.

Although much of the current research in social isolation with older adults has focused on community-dwelling adults, one growing segment of study is on assisted-living arrangements, which is one of the fastest growing segments of senior housing (Hawes, Phillips, Rose, Holan, & Sherman, 2003). In assisted-living settings where there are many internal (to the setting) social networks, life satisfaction, quality of life, and perception of home were positively reported (Street, Burge, Quadagno, & Barrett, 2007). Assisted living has the potential to focus on health promotion and function maintenance, such as the identification of social isolation and appropriate interventions (Resnick, 2007).

Strictly speaking, social isolation is not confined to a place. The socially isolated are not necessarily homebound or place-bound, although that is typically the case. That being said, however, environments that are removed (such as rural locations) or those not conducive to safety (such as high-crime areas) can contribute to social isolation (Klinenberg, 2001). Social isolation as a function of location has been demonstrated, particularly for the older adult in urbanized settings, in a number of countries other than Canada (Klinenberg, 2001; Lillyman & Und, 2007; Russell & Schofield, 1999). In these cases elderly individuals cannot leave their homes because of lack of transportation or for fear of assault, so they increasingly isolate themselves from others. This situation is intensified by distrust, socioeconomic status, or locale, and it is worse if the older adult has a chronic illness compounding those constraints. The inability to drive a car may be an eventual reality as one ages. Limited or no driving confines activities outside the home (Marottoli et al., 2000) and thus limits interactions with others for the older adult.

One objective of planned senior housing is to provide individuals with a readymade social network within a community (Mahmood, Chaudhury, Kobayashi, & Valente, 2008; Mashburn, 2006), although this objective is not always met. The frail elderly are found to be less interactive with more mobile, healthier older adults, possibly because healthier older adults have few extra resources to expend on others who may have even fewer resources, or they may have better health and networks that are incongruent with, and less likely to cross, those of the frail elderly (Heumann, 1988).

Nursing home residents with chronic illness or sensory impairments tend to be more isolated than other elderly persons. In England, for instance, those in residential care who are ill or disabled are considered socially dead, impoverished by the inactive nature of institutionalization and unable to occupy any positive, valued role in the community (Watson, 1988). Stephens and Bernstein (1984) found that older, sicker residents were more socially isolated than healthier residents. The investigators found that family and longer standing friendships served as better buffers to social isolation than did other residents.

SOCIAL ISOLATION, CULTURE, AND GENDER

Andresen and Brownson (2000) noted that the experience, prevalence, and meanings of chronic illness are determined by factors such as age, culture, gender, sexual orientation, socioeconomic and geographical factors. In the Canadian context Cloutier-Fisher and Kobayashi (2009) explored the differences among socially isolated older adults by gender and geography and concluded that social isolation is a "multidimensional social construct, and when individual characteristics such as gender are considered together with contextual variables like place of residence, a more comprehensive and layered portrait of vulnerability among the socially isolated persons begins to emerge" (p. 181).

As globalization and sensitivity to Canadian multiculturalism increases, with its concurrent absorption of multiethnic, multilingual, and multireligious individuals into yet other cultures, there is an overlap into mainstream healthcare systems. This is especially true of cultural groups that have not assimilated into the dominant culture. Language differences and traditional living arrangements may impede social adaptation. In addition, many immigrants, especially those who are chronically ill, are less able to engage in support networks, given their long working hours, low-paying jobs, socioeconomic difficulties, and changes in family lifestyles and living arrangements.

An extensive literature review on health care and its relationship with culture demonstrated two overarching issues: (1) the definitions of culture are conceptually broad and/or indistinct, and (2) mainstream health care struggles to integrate these multicultural groups with varying degrees of success. When one speaks of "culture," many concepts are mixed or even confused (Habayeb, 1995). According to Jong-Gieveld and Havens (2004), there is a wide variation among lonely and not lonely older Canadian adults and adults from European countries, demonstrating that diverse cultures determine social isolation and its perception among older adults. Van-Tilburg, Havens, and De Jong Grieveld (2004) compared older adults from Canada (Manitoba), the Netherlands, and Italy (Tuscany) and concluded that loneliness is culture bound, because location and culture did

matter in the intensity of loneliness suffered. The dominant White society in Canada and its healthcare system is secular, individualistic, technology and science oriented, and tends to be male dominated (Borman & Biordi, 1992; Smith, 1996). Other European-based cultures have similar situations. Social isolation must be viewed from the client's cultural definition of the number, frequency, and quality of contacts; the longevity or durability of these contacts; and the negativism attributed to the isolation felt by the individual involved.

Studies in the United States and Canada indicate how women, aboriginals, minority groups, the poor, and others have not received the same care as the dominant male White middle or upper classes (Fiscella, Franks, Gold, & Clancy, 2000; Prasad, 2007; Webster, 2005). Many ethnic and religious groups in Canada value community closeness, family kinship, geographical proximity, and social communication. These values must be integrated into the mainstream healthcare industry if we are to target and improve access by minority and multicultural groups. The task of attempting to deliver "tailored," culturally competent care to so many groups is overwhelming and lacks an integrating strategy that appeals to all groups. One can now find a large number of articles targeting mainstream healthcare providers that provide hints, tips, or insights into cultural groups.

SOCIAL COMPONENTS OF SOCIAL ISOLATION

Mere numbers of people surrounding someone do not cure negative social isolation; an individual can be socially isolated even in a crowd if one's significant social network is lost. This situation is true for such groups as those living or working in sheltered-care workshops, residents in long-term care facilities, or people in prisons. What is critical to social isolation is that, because of situations imposed on them, individuals perceive themselves as disconnected from meaningful discourse with people important to them.

Associated with social isolation is reciprocity or mutuality, that is, the amount of give and take that can occur between isolated individuals and their social networks. Throughout the years much evidence has accumulated to indicate that informal networks of social support offer significant emotional assistance, information, and material resources for a number of different populations. These support systems appear to foster good health, help maintain appropriate behaviours, and alleviate stress (DiMatteo & Hays, 1981; Stephens & Bernstein, 1984).

Examining reciprocity in the relationships of social networks focuses not only on social roles and the content of the exchange but also on the level of agreement between the isolated person and his or her "others" in the network (Randers, Mattiasson, & Olson, 2003). The incongruence between respondents in a social network regarding their exchanges can help alert the healthcare professional to the level of emotional or material need or exhaustion that exists in either respondent. For example, the senior author observed, during a home visit by a nurse, that a homebound older woman complained that her children had done very little for her. However, it was discovered the children visited every day, brought meals, shopped for their mother, and managed her financial affairs. In this case the elderly mother felt isolated despite her children's visits and assistance.

DEMOGRAPHICS AND SOCIAL ISOLATION

Few studies focus directly on demographic variables and social isolation; typically, this topic is embedded in other research questions across a variety of illnesses. Nevertheless, when these disparate studies are taken together, the impact of demographics on social isolation in the individual with chronic illness is evident. Issues of gender, marital status, family position and context, and socioeconomic standing (such as education or employment) have been shown to affect social isolation.

Socioeconomic Factors

Changes in socioeconomic status, such as employment status, have been correlated with social isolation. The lack of employment of both caregiver and care recipient, cited in much of the caregiver literature, can have an adverse effect. A study of caregivers of frail elderly veterans noted that these caregivers are more at risk for physical, emotional, and financial strain than are other populations, because disabled elderly veterans receive fewer long-term care services than do other elderly populations (Dorfman, Homes, & Berlin, 1996).

Unemployment of the older adult is just one component of the maturational continuum; parents worry about the potential for employment and insurance for their children with chronic illnesses (Wang & Barnard, 2004). Lower income status, especially when coupled with less education, negatively influences health status and is associated with both a limiting social network and greater loneliness, which, in turn, impacts health status and social isolation (Cox, Spiro, & Sullivan, 1988; Williams & Bury, 1989). For instance, almost half of the head-injured clients in one study could not work, which then affected their families' economic status and increased their social isolation (Kinsella, Ford, & Moran, 1989). Financial concerns were found to be a reason older adults did not participate socially, thus leading to increased risk of social isolation. The study by Howat and colleagues (2004) used focus groups and interviews with adults aged 65 and older to help explain factors that contribute to social isolation, in addition to identifying barriers and facilitators to social participation.

In addition to problems of employment potential, there are economic and social concerns over the costs incurred by health care, employment discrimination, subsequent inability to secure insurance, and loss of potential friendship networks at work—all of which are factors in increasing social isolation or reducing social interactions. In fact, economics exaggerates the costs of chronic illness. People with disabilities suffer disproportionately in the labour market, which then affects their connections with family and community social networks (Christ, 1987). This is particularly evident in the examination of those with mental illness and their social isolation (Chinman, Weingarten, Stayner, & Davidson, 2001; Melle, Friis, Hauff, & Vaglum, 2000).

General Family Factors

As chronic illness persists and tasks must be managed, relationships are drained, leaving individuals with chronic illness at high risk for social isolation (Berkman, 1983; Tilden & Weinert, 1987). When isolation does occur, it can be a long-term reality for the individual and family. However, people with chronic illnesses tend toward psychological well-being when there is social support and involvement. Particularly

important is the adequacy, more than the availability, of social relationships (Wright, 1995; Zimmer, 1995).

There is evidence that social isolation does not necessarily occur in every situation. In fact, the negative impact of social isolation on families with children who are chronically ill has been questioned. One study, which used a large community-based, random sample, found that families with children who are chronically ill did not experience a greater degree of social isolation than those with healthy children, nor did they function differently, except for modest increases in maternal dysfunction (Cadman, Rosenbaum, Boyle, & Offord, 1991). Cadman and his associates argued that prior studies were subject to biases because the families in those studies were in the clinic populations of the hospital or agency. By definition, such populations were receiving care for illnesses or responses to illnesses and hence were experiencing an unusual aggregate of problems, which is why they were at the clinic or hospital. Therefore, such families were not representative of families throughout the community.

In another study, classroom teachers evaluated children with cancer or sickle cell disease with a matched sample of control subjects. The authors found the children who were chronically ill were remarkably resilient in the classroom setting, although those who survived their brain tumours and could attend regular classes were perceived as more sensitive and isolated (Noll et al., 1992). On the other hand, adolescents with chronic illnesses have been marginalized, which predisposes them to feelings of isolation and low self-worth (DiNapoli & Murphy, 2002).

Similarly, some studies of older adults found that isolation does not always occur with increasing age (Victor et al., 2002). Childless older individuals tend to be more socially isolated than those with children, and when adult children live nearby older people frequently interact with at least one of them (Mullins & Dugan, 1990). It is also interesting to note that older people tend to be less influenced by their children than by contacts with other relatives, friends, and associates (Berkman, 1983; Ryan & Patterson, 1987).

Findings indicate that in every group from age 30 to older than 70 years, primarily those with the fewest social and community ties were nearly three times as likely to die as those with more ties (Berkman, 1983). In other words, maintaining social contacts enhanced longevity. These individuals tended to be widowers or widows and lacked membership in formal groups (Berkman, 1983), thereby limiting their social contacts. In another study older adults who lived in senior housing complexes showed little difference in friendship patterns and life satisfaction (Poulin, 1984). Both studies found that living alone, being single, or not having family does not necessarily imply social isolation. Rather, if older people have social networks, many developed throughout a lifetime, and if these networks remain available to them, they are provided with support when needed (Berkman, 1983).

Gender and Marital Status

Typically, women have more extensive and varied social networks than do men (Antonucci, 1985). However, if one spouse has a chronic illness, married couples spend more time together and less time with networks and activities outside the home (DesRosier, Catanzaro, & Piller, 1992; Foxall, Eckberg, & Griffith, 1986). Although gender differences in caregiving occur (Miller, 1990; Tilden & Weinert, 1987), women

caregivers indicate greater isolation, increased loneliness, and decreased life satisfaction than do men. Yet both genders show psychological improvement if social contacts, by telephone or in person, increase (Foxall et al., 1986). After the death of a spouse it has been suggested that men have higher psychological distress (Umberson, Wortman, & Kessler, 1992) and increased mortality rates (Stroebe & Stroebe, 1983) when compared with women.

Although women caregivers may have professional, community, and social networks to aid them in coping with their disabled spouses, over time they reduce their links to these potential supports. Physical work, social costs and barriers, preparation time for care and outings, and other demands of caregiving become so extreme that women curtail access to and use of support networks external to home. As these caregivers narrow their use of social networks, they unwittingly isolate their spouse with chronic illness as well. Although women reported needing personal or psychological time alone for relief, the subject of their isolation, the person with chronic illness, also became their greatest confidante as the pair struggled in their joint isolation (DesRosier et al., 1992).

ILLNESS FACTORS AND SOCIAL ISOLATION

Chronic illness is multidimensional, and persons with chronic illness and their networks must assume a variety of tasks: managing treatment regimens, controlling symptoms, preventing and managing crises, reordering time, managing the illness trajectory, dealing with healthcare professionals, normalizing life, preserving a reasonable self-image, keeping emotional balance, managing social isolation, funding the costs of health care, and preparing for an uncertain future (Strauss et al., 1984). As people with chronic illnesses struggle to understand their body failure and maintain personal and social identities they may become fatigued, sicker, or lose hope more readily. Should this happen, they may more easily withdraw from their social networks. Individuals who have four or more chronic illnesses were shown to be at risk for social isolation (Havens & Hall, 2001).

It has been suggested that isolation not only influences the individual's social network (Newman, Fitzpatrick, Lamb, & Shipley, 1989) but also can lead to depression and even suicide (Lyons, 1982; Trout, 1980), particularly in the elderly (Frierson, 1991). Women whose illnesses required more physical demands on themselves and greater symptom management reported greater depression but no effect on their relationship with their partner. Women who had concerns about the meaning of their illness reported greater marital distress and lower satisfaction with their family network (Woods, Haberman, & Packard, 1993).

Persons with HIV or AIDS had psychological effects that depended not only on the diagnosis but also on the age of the person. Older individuals showed significant differences in a number of variables, including social isolation (Catalan, 1998). In addition, HIV-negative men who cared for their partners or friends often lived in social isolation with their care recipients (Mallinson, 1999).

In severely head-injured individuals it was not the chronic physical disability that disrupted family cohesion as much as the resulting social impairment (Kinsella et al., 1989). The greatest burden identified was social isolation brought on by the impaired self-control of the head-injured person and their inability to learn from social experience. However, the social isolation was particularly burdensome for the families, because the head injury reduced the client's capacity for recognition of and reflection on the deficiencies in social relationships and precluded formation of new close relationships. Consequently, although friendships and employment possibilities were reduced for the client, the real impact was felt by the constrained family (Kinsella et al., 1989).

HEALTHCARE PERSPECTIVES

People with chronic illnesses struggle to understand their body failure and its effect on their activities and lives (Corbin & Strauss, 1987). In doing so they also struggle to maintain their sense of personal and social identity, often in the face of altered self-image and enormous financial, psychological, and social obstacles. If individuals with chronic illness lose hope or become otherwise incapacitated, they may withdraw from their social networks, isolating themselves and others important to them. Frequently, the daily management of illness means working with healthcare professionals who often do not recognize the inconspicuous but daily struggles of the person's realities of a "new" body, the issues of care, and the development of a new self-identity (Corbin & Strauss, 1987; Dropkin, 1989; Hopper, 1981).

With increased technology, the aging of the population, and changes in economics, chronic illness has begun to assume major proportions in Canada and across the globe. Concomitantly, the literature contains more articles describing various chronic illnesses, the strategies used to manage them, and issues of social and psychological well-being, including social isolation (Russell et al., 2008).

The impact of prevailing paradigms of care interventions held by various constituencies is evident. For example, most healthcare professionals still see clients only episodically, using the medical model of "cure" and remaining within the model of the dominant healthcare system. In the case of children with cancer, however, the child focuses on the meaning of his or her impairment (which varies by age); the parents focus first on the immediate concern with their child's longevity and cure and later on the impairment and long-term effects; the healthcare professional focuses on client survival; the mental health professional focuses on identifying and minimizing impact, impairments, and social barriers; and the public (third-party payers, employers, schoolmates, partners) focuses on contributions and cost. All of these views centre on the interaction and exchange, as well as the specific responsibilities and obligations, incurred by the various networks that touch them. Interactions are intensified by the potential withdrawal of any party from the network (Christ, 1987).

Given the variety of care-versus-cure paradigms, the real, daily micro-impositions of chronic illness on social identity and social networks are often lost. The compassion felt by many healthcare professionals is evident in the increasing number of articles available and the attempts to present evidence of the isolation felt by clients and their networks. Nevertheless, these articles may not be explicit; therefore, the proposed interventions for the isolate are unclear, irrelevant, or even discouraging. For example, when discussing facial disfigurement one article noted the healthcare professional expected evidence of the client's image integration as early as 1 week after surgery (Dropkin, 1989). That same article suggested and reiterated that although the surgery was necessary for removal of the cancer,

the resulting defect was confined to a relatively small aspect of the anatomy and that the alteration in appearance or function did not change the person (Dropkin, 1989). The terminology and the interventions in this article focused on the acute postoperative period and did not take into account what disfigured clients were likely to feel later than 1 week after surgery or that the word "defect" gives a strong clue to the understanding that the disfiguring surgery is obviously and emotionally charged toward the negative.

For a clearer view of the impact of such surgery as seen by the client, Gamba and colleagues (1992) asked postsurgical patients, grouped by the extent of their facial disfigurement, questions about their self-image, relationship with their partner and social network, and overall impact of the therapy. Those with extensive disfigurement reported that it was "like putting up with something undesirable" (p. 221), and many patients were unable to touch or look at themselves. Those with extensive disfigurement also reported more social isolation, poor self-image, and/or a worsened sexual relationship with their partner, even though they maintained satisfactory relationships with their children. In another study reported in the Gamba article, half of the individuals who underwent hemi-mandibulectomy for head and neck cancers became social recluses, compared with 11% of patients who had laryngectomies. As can be seen, in more than one study respondents attached a negative meaning to their disfiguring surgery and its results.

Such findings take into account the client's personal meaning of illness and treatment and their effects on social isolation, demonstrating the isolating treatment or illness (e.g., disfigurement) often is not associated with objective disability. In fact, others have found the degree of isolation is not directly proportional to the extent of disability (Creed, 1990; Maddox, 1985; Newman et al., 1989). It is important that healthcare professionals not ignore or discount the meaning of illness to the client, regardless of any professional opinion about objective disability or the desirability of treatment.

INTERVENTIONS: COUNTERACTING SOCIAL ISOLATION _____

In social isolation the interventions of choice need to remain at the discretion of the client or caregiver. As can be seen from this chapter, writers focus largely on definitions and correlates of social isolation and relatively less on interventions. When interventions are reported they often relate to the aggregate, such as the policy-related interventions of community housing. The results of many of these larger-scale interventions have been noted in this chapter. Other interventions are mentioned herein, although the list is not all inclusive.

Because the situation of each person with chronic illness is unique, interventions can be expected to vary (for examples, see Dickens, Richards, Greaves, & Campbell, 2011; Holley, 2007). Nonetheless, certain useful techniques and strategies can be generalized (Dela Cruz, 1986). Basically, these strategies require that a balance of responsibilities be developed between the healthcare professional and the client, with the following aims:

- Increasing the moral autonomy or freedom of choice of the isolate
- Increasing social interaction at a level acceptable to the client
- Using repetitive and recognizable strategies that are validated with the client, which correlate to reducing particular isolating behaviours

The approach to interventions can also be matched, layer by layer, to the social layering model presented earlier in this chapter, that is, from community, to organization, to network, to person. Therefore, interventions might be cast as ranging from community-based empowerment (transportation-system improvements, for example), work-related enhancements (computer telecare), network and family support group enhancements (nursing), case management, neighbourhood watches, or client–professional clinical treatments or care. Examples of these are discussed in this chapter.

Another point to remember is that evaluation is a key principle in any problem-solving system, such as the evaluation found in the nursing process. Throughout the assessment and intervention phases the healthcare professional should explicitly consider how effective the intervention is or was. The effect of cultural and social differences should be taken into account. The willingness and flexibility to change an ineffective strategy is the mark of the competent professional.

Assessment of Social Isolation

When social isolation occurs a systematic assessment can help determine proposed interventions, which the professional must validate with the client before taking action. Guiding people, rather than forcing them to go along with interventions, requires the healthcare professional to offer a rationale for the proposed interventions. One must ask if one is giving reasonable rationales, assurances, or support. At the same time the professional should remember that some cultures value the authority and the expertise of other family members over that of the individual. Consequently, the healthcare professional may have to provide a rationale for suggested interventions to the ranking authority within the support group. Frequently, this is a male figure, often older, who is considered most deserving of any explanation. Other cultures may be matriarchal, so a woman is the ranking authority.

The key to assessing social isolation is to observe for three distinct features: negativity, involuntary or other imposed solitude, and declining quality and numbers within the isolate's social networks. Social isolation must be distinguished from other conditions such as loneliness or depression, both of which are often accompanied by anxiety, desperation, self-pity, boredom, and signs of attempts to fill a void, such as overeating, substance abuse, excessive shopping, or kleptomania. In addition, loneliness is often associated with losses, whereas depression is frequently regarded as anger turned inward. Because social isolation, loneliness, and depression can all be destructive, the healthcare professional must be resourceful in assessing which issue predominates at any particular point in time.

Properly conducted, an assessment yields its own suggestions for responsive intervention. For instance, the assessment may indicate the client is a lifelong isolate and that future isolation is a desired and comfortable lifestyle. In this case the professional's best intervention is to remain available and observant but noninterfering.

If, on the other hand, the client has become isolated and wants or needs relief, then the intervention should be constructed along lines consistent with his or her current needs and history. If the healthcare professional discovers that a support network is lax in calling or contacting a client, the provider can help the client and support network rebuild bridges to each other. There are usually support groups to which those in a social network can be referred for aid. As an illustration, if the network is overwhelmed, information can be provided about respite programs. Interventions such as these will help members of the social network maintain energy levels necessary to help their chronically ill relative or friend.

Assessment typically involves the clinical dyad of caregiver and client. It is at this level that assessment is critical to the development of appropriate and effective interventions. Without an adequate and sensitive assessment, interventions are likely to be ineffective or incomplete.

Measurement of Social Isolation

The major issue in measuring social isolation is that the instrumentation does not fully capture the conceptual definition of social isolation. For example, social isolation, as described in this chapter, has no specific instrument of measurement. Despite Sabir et al.'s (2009) recommendation for a social isolation measure that has a specific capacity to identify isolated older adults, some researchers have used instruments that define social isolation as an extreme lack of social networks or support, whereas others use a group of questions that purport to measure social isolation. The closely related concept of social networks has two frequently used research measures that may be useful when assessing social isolation. Because there is some conceptual overlap of both constructs, specifically the number of social contacts, measures used to assess social networks may serve as a useful initial assessment for social isolation.

A literature review revealed the two most commonly used and reported research measures of social networks are the Lubben social network scale (LSNS) (Lubben, 1988) and the Berkman-Syme social network index (SNI) (Berkman & Syme, 1979). Both tools measure, essentially, the amount of contact one has with others.

The SNI was cited in 209 articles and the LSNS was cited in 38 articles found in MEDLINE, CINAHL, EMBASE, and PsycINFO. The SNI is a nontheoretical summed aggregation of several items that examined a range of social ties and networks and how they directly affected people. Both the relative importance and the number of social contacts are aggregated into four weighted sources. The LSNS was developed to measure social networks among older adults (Lubben, 1988) and is based on the SNI and its original questionnaire. The LSNS has 10 equally weighted items, which place individuals into four quartiles with a cut-off score for social isolation. Reliability and validity have been examined (Lubben, 1988; Lubben & Gironda, 1996; Rubenstein, Josephson, & Robbins, 1994). The LSNS is typically administered prospectively during data collection and is difficult to use in secondary data analysis, although this has been attempted (Lubben, Weiler, & Chi, 1989).

Given the state of the science, when measuring social isolation the SNI or LSNS should be chosen based on one's research purpose and question, and also semistructured interviews or questionnaires should be used to confirm a diagnosis of social isolation. The SNI or LSNS score will give some indication as to whether the individual may be at risk for social isolation, warranting further assessment through interview. Once social isolation is identified in an older adult, it is important to use evidence-informed recommendations as interventions to decrease negative health-related consequences.

Management of Self: Identity Development

The need for an ongoing identity leads an individual to seek a level where he or she can overcome, avoid, or internalize stigma and, concomitantly, manage resulting social isolation. Social networks can be affected by stigma. Managing various concerns requires people who are chronically ill to develop a new sense of self consistent with their disabilities. This "new" life is intertwined with the lives of members of their social networks, which may now include both healthcare professionals and other persons with chronic illnesses. Lessons must be learned to deal with new body demands and associated behaviours. Consequently, the individual with chronic illness must redevelop an identity with norms different from previous ones.

The willingness to change to different and unknown norms is just a first step, one that often takes great courage and time. For instance, one study indicated that clients with pronounced physical, financial, and medical care problems after head and neck surgery exhibited prolonged social isolation 1 year after surgery (Krouse, Krouse, & Fabian, 1989). Although no single study has indicated the time necessary for such identity transformations, anecdotal information suggests it can last several years; indeed, for some it is a lifelong experience.

Identity Transformation

Clarifying how networks form and function is a significant contribution to the management of the struggles of the client who is chronically ill and isolated. The perceptive healthcare worker should know that much of the management done by the chronically ill and their networks is not seen or well understood by healthcare professionals today (Corbin & Strauss, 1987). However, we can use Charmaz's (1987) findings as guides for assessing the likely identity level of the individual as we try to understand potential withdrawal or actual isolation.

Charmaz (1987), using mostly middle-aged women, developed a framework of hierarchical identity transformations useful in diagnosing a chronically ill individual's proclivity to social networking and in discovering which social network might be most appropriate. This hierarchy of identity takes into account a reconstruction toward a desired future self, based on past and present selves, and reflects the individual's relative difficulty in achieving specific aspirations. Charmaz's analysis progresses toward a "salvaged self" that retains a past identity based on important values or attributes while still acknowledging dependency.

Initially, the individual takes on a supernormal identity, which assumes an ability to retain all previous success values, social acclamation, struggles, and competition. At this identity level the individual who is chronically ill attempts to participate more intensely than those in a nonimpaired world despite the limitations of illness. The next identity level is the restored self, with the expectation of eventually returning to the previous self despite the chronic illness or its severity. Healthcare workers might identify this self with the psychological state of denial, but in terms of identity the individual has simply assumed there is no discontinuation with a former self. At the third level, the contingent personal identity, one defines oneself in terms of potential risk and failure, indicating the individual still has not come to terms with a future self but has begun to realize the supernormal identity will no longer be viable. Finally, the level of the salvaged self is reached, whereby the individual attempts to define the self as worthwhile, despite recognizing that present circumstances invalidate any previous identity (Charmaz, 1987).

Not only does social isolation relate to stigma; it can develop as an individual loses hope of sustaining aspirations for a normal or supernormal self, which are now unrealistic. As persons with chronic illness act out regret, disappointment, and anger, their significant others and healthcare professionals may react in kind, perpetuating a downward spiral of loss, anger, and subsequent greater social isolation. The idea of identity hierarchies thus alerts the caregiver to a process in which shifts in identity are expected.

The reactions, health advice, and the experiences of individuals with chronic illness must be taken into account in managing that particular identity, as must the various factors that help shape that identity. Both the social network and adapted norms now available play a role at each stage in identity transformation. At the supernormal identity level, individuals who are chronically ill were in only limited contact with healthcare professionals but presumably in greater contact with healthier individuals who acted as their referents; at the level of the salvaged self, home care was used (Charmaz, 1987).

Integrating Culture into Health Care

Isolation, by its very definition, must include a cultural screening through which desired social contacts are defined. When one speaks of social isolation among unique ethnic groups, the number, type, and quality of contact must be sifted through a particularistic screen of that person's culture. Not only the clients' but the provider's communication patterns, roles, relationships, and traditions are important elements to consider for both assessment and intervention (Barker, 1994; Cheng, 1997; Groce & Zola, 1993; Hill, 2006; Kim, 1998; Margolin, 2006; Treolar, 1999; Welch, 1998).

Some believe that matching culturally similar providers to clients would be a way to meet needs with effective interventions (Welch, 1998). However, healthcare educators and service providers recognize the issues of a smaller supply of providers and the greater numbers of clients in a struggling dominant healthcare system coping with multiculturalism. To meet supply and demand issues, as well as cultural needs, the idea of cultural competence is promoted. Cultural education is advanced as the key to effective interventions that intersect the values of two disparate groups of individuals (Davidhizar, Bechtel, & Giger, 1998; Jones, Bond, & Cason, 1998; Mc–Namara, Martin, Waddel, & Yuen, 1997; Smith, 1996). Cultural education not only results in outcomes of culturally relevant compliance (Davidhizar et al., 1998) but also helps alleviate the isolation of individuals with chronic illness (Barker, 1994; Hildebrandt, 1997; Treolar, 1999).

For those who find that such culturally based education is unavailable, and assuming there are more groups and more traditions than can possibly be understood by a single healthcare provider, a fail-safe strategy remains. This approach requires the provider to approach each person, regardless of his or her cultural milieu, with respect and dignity in an explicit good-faith effort to inquire, understand, and be responsive to the client's culture, needs, and person. The provider must set aside prejudices and stereotypes and instead use an authentic, sensitive inquiry into the client's beliefs and well-being (Browne, 1997; Treolar, 1999).

By seeking to understand differences, one can find pleasure in the differences and move beyond them to enjoy the similarities of us all. This approach is undergirded by a culture of "caring" and moves toward a model of actively participating groups exchanging concerns of identity, egalitarianism, and needed care (Browne, 1997; Catlin, 1998; Keller & Stevens, 1997; Treolar,

1999). In so doing, social isolation can be managed within the context most comfortable to the client, who is the raison d'être of the healthcare professional.

Respite

The need for respite has been cited as one of the greatest necessities for isolated older adults with illness and their caregivers, many of whom are themselves elderly (Dickens et al., 2011; Miller, 1990). Its purpose is to relieve caregivers for a period of time so they may engage in activities that help sustain them or their loved ones, the care recipients. Respite involves four elements: purpose, time, activities, and place. The time may be in short blocks or for longer (but still relatively short-term) periods, both of which temporarily relieve the caregiver of responsibility. Activities may be practical, such as grocery shopping; psychological, such as providing time for self-replenishment or recreation; or physical, such as providing time for rest or medical/nursing attention.

Respite may occur in the home or elsewhere, such as senior centres, day-care centres, or long-term care facilities. Senior centres usually accommodate persons who are more independent and flexible, often offering social gathering places and events, meals, and health assessment, exercise, and/or maintenance activities. Day-care centres typically host individuals with more diminished functioning. Other places, such as long-term care facilities, manage clients with an even greater inability to function.

Finally, respite may be delivered by paid or unpaid persons who may be friends, professionals, family, employees, or neighbours. Although many care recipients welcome relief for their caregiver, some may fear abandonment. The family caregiver and professional must work together to assure the care recipient that he or she will not be abandoned (D. Biordi, 1993, unpublished data). Therefore, the professional has a great deal of latitude in using the four elements to devise interventions tailored to the flexible needs of an isolated caregiver and care recipient.

SUPPORT GROUPS AND OTHER MUTUAL AID

Support groups, or even peer counsellors (Holley, 2007), have been identified for a wide variety of chronic illnesses and conditions, such as breast cancer (Reach to Recovery), bereavement (Widow to Widow), and alcoholism (Alcoholics Anonymous), or for other conditions such as multiple sclerosis or blindness. These groups or individuals assist those with chronic illness or disabilities to cope with their illness and the associated changes in identities and social roles of their chronic illness or disability. Such counselling can help enhance one's self-esteem, provide alternative meanings of the illness, suggest ways to cope, assist in specific interventions that have helped others, or offer services or care for either the isolate or caregiver (Holley, 2007). Almost every large city or county has lists of resources that can be accessed: health departments, social work agencies, schools, and libraries. Even the telephone book's yellow pages can assist in finding support groups or other resources. The Internet is also a source of information about support groups and resource listings. Some resources list group entry requirements or qualifications.

Because of their variety and number, support groups are not always available in every community, so healthcare professionals may find themselves in the position of developing a group. Therefore, as part of a community assessment the healthcare professional should not only note the groups currently available but also identify someone who might be willing to develop a needed group. The healthcare professional also may have to help find a meeting place, refer clients to the group, assist clients in discussing barriers to their care, and, if necessary, develop structured activities (such as exercise regimens for arthritic individuals). In addition, the use of motivational devices, such as pictures, videos, audio recordings, reminiscence therapy, or games, may be helpful in developing discussion. Demonstrations of specific illness-related regimens, such as exercises, clothing aids, or body mechanics, are also useful to support groups. Professionals should be alert to problems the isolate may have in integrating into groups, such as resistance to meeting new people, low self-esteem, apprehension over participation in new activities, or the problems of transportation, building access, and inconvenient meeting times (Matteson, McConnell, & Linton, 1997).

Social activity groups are one way of integrating isolated institutionalized individuals or of reversing hospital-induced confusion; such groups could be recreational therapy groups or those developed particularly to address a special interest (e.g., parents facing the imminent death of a child). Given the limited financial resources typical of most persons who are chronically ill, support groups that are not costly to the chronically ill or their families are more likely to be welcomed.

SPIRITUAL WELL-BEING

For many, religious or spiritual beliefs offer an important social connection and give great meaning to life. Spiritual well-being typically affirms the unity of the person with his or her environment, often expressed in oneness with his or her god(s) (Matteson et al., 1997). Consequently, ensuring isolates some means of connection to their religious support may help them find newer meaning in life or illness and provide them with other people with whom to share that meaning. The healthcare professional should assess the meaning of spirituality or religion to the individual, the kind of spiritual meeting place he or she finds most comforting, and the types of religious support available in the community. Religious groups range from formal gatherings to religiously aided social groups.

Frequently, the official gathering places of religious or spiritual groups, for example, churches, temples, or mosques, have outreach or social groups that make visits, arrange for social outings, or develop pen pals or other means of human connectedness. The nurse or other healthcare professional may have to initiate contact with these groups to assist in developing the necessary outreach between them and the isolate.

REBUILDING FAMILY NETWORKS

Keeping, or rebuilding, family networks has much to offer. However, families that have disintegrated may have a history of fragile relationships. The healthcare professional must assess these networks carefully to develop truly effective interventions. The professional must also take into account the client's type of isolation (lifelong vs. recent) and the wishes of the isolate: With whom (if anyone) in the family does the isolate wish contact? How often? What members of the family exist, and which care about the isolate? What is their relationship to the isolate— parent, sibling, child, friend-as-family, other

relative? The professional can then make contact with the individuals indicated to be most accommodating to the isolate, explain the situation, make future plans to bring them and the isolate together, and afterward assess the outcome. However, it may not be possible to bring uninterested family members back into the isolate's social network.

For family members who are interested and willing, rebuilding networks means the professional must take into account the location or proximity of family members to the isolate. If they live near each other, and because a "space of one's own" is a critical human need, a balance of territorial and personal needs must be managed if the isolate is to be reintegrated. If the isolate and family agree to live together, the family's physical environment will require assessment for safety, access, and territorial space. Not only are factors such as sleeping space and heat and ventilation important, but personal space and having one's own possessions are as important to the family members as they are to the ill person. Teaching the family and isolate how to respect each other's privacy (such as by getting permission to enter a room or look through personal belongings, speaking directly to one another, and so forth) is a way to help them bridge their differences.

Understanding Family Relationships

The nature of the relationship between family and isolate must be understood. The family's meanings and actions attached to love, power, and conflict and observations of the frequency of controlling strategies by various individuals inform the professional of potential interventions. For example, some clients who live alone were found to be more likely to be satisfied with support when they were feeling depressed, whereas clients living with others were more satisfied with supporters who cared about them (Foxall et al., 1994).

In some families love is thought to indicate close togetherness, whereas in other families love is thought to provide members with independence. Love and power can be developed and thought of either as a pyramidal (top-down) set of relationships or as an egalitarian circle. Conflict may be a means of connection or of distancing and can be expressed by shouting and insults or by quiet assertion.

Community Resources to Keep Families Together

Using community resources, such as support groups, is a way to help keep a family together. Families draw on each other's experiences as models for coping. For example, families in which there is a child with cancer find ways to help their child cope with the isolation induced by chemotherapy. When necessary, the health-care professional may wish to refer the isolate and family to psychiatric or specialty nurses, counsellors, psychiatrists, or social workers to help them overcome their disintegration. Successful implementation of the wide range of family-related interventions requires sensitive perceptions of the needs not only of the isolate but also of the various family members with whom that individual must interact.

Two interesting community resources that could help alert families to potential problem situations for isolates are the post office and newspaper delivery services. If these delivery persons observe a build-up of uncollected mail or newspapers, they can call or check the house to see if there is an older adult isolate in distress. Families who are concerned about their isolated family member can provide their post office,

regular mail carrier, or news delivery service with information about the isolate that can be used in the event of a problem. Nurses and social workers can also contact mail and news services or help families make these contacts. This intervention can be expanded to include any regular visitor, such as a rental manager, janitor, or neighbour, who might be willing to check on the welfare of the isolate.

In some communities employees at banks and stores also react to older individuals who may be isolated. If unusual financial activities or changes in shopping patterns are noticed, the individual can be contacted to make sure everything is satisfactory. Although in some communities mail and newspaper services and banks and stores are not involved with people in their areas, these resources are valuable and should be expanded throughout the country.

Communication Technologies

Telephone

The telephone is a method used to counteract the effects of place-boundedness. Although findings of its effectiveness are equivocal (Kivett, 1979; Praderas & MacDonald, 1986), the telephone is considered almost a necessity in reducing the isolation of a place-bound individual. In literature other than that of the socially isolated, nurses using telephone contact reduced health problems and costs of readmission for patients (Norbeck, DeJoseph, & Smith, 1996).

Computers

For many persons, including homebound older adults or people with disabilities, computers have helped offset social isolation and loneliness through features such as access to the Internet and social network platforms like

Facebook©, which allows the person to reach family and friends or to find new friends, activities, and other common interests (Gatto & Tak, 2008). Computers can also be used to provide fun activities, such as games. In Canada computers are more widely available than elsewhere, more so among those within higher socioeconomic status and the more highly educated.

Increasingly, online groups offer support, such as that described for breast cancer patients (Hoybye, Johansen, & Tjornhoj-Thomsen, 2005), parents with children diagnosed with cancer (Helga, 2007), and support for health issues of aboriginal women (Hoffman-Goetz & Donelle, 2007). Advances in computer technology have created special attachments, such as cameras, breath tubes, or special keyboards and font sizes, that customize computers to the needs of the isolated or disabled, including those with visual impairment (Imel, 1999; Salem, 1998).

The use of information and other communication technologies has been helpful in alleviating barriers to the return to work for those with spinal cord injuries and the resulting disabilities (Bricout, 2004). Telecommuting enables home-based work and has proven effective for those with mobility or transportation limitations or whose illnesses or disabilities necessitate rest periods incompatible with typical work environments. Computers have also been used to relieve isolation or loneliness and assist in the management of chronic illness and support groups located in rural environments (Clark, 2002; Hill & Weinert, 2004; Johnson & Ashton, 2003; Weinert, Cudney, & Winters, 2005).

Whether connecting via the Internet, using word processing, corresponding via email, taking classes, or joining social networking sites, computers also allow isolates to actively fill many hours of otherwise empty time, bringing a measure of relief to tedium while expanding their intellectual and social lives. The caveat, of course, is that the use of the computer, and especially the Internet, could itself be an isolating factor for many individuals. This creates a danger of virtual reality overrunning actual reality, in which case isolates compound their isolation. That having been said, however, the computer offers many more advantages than disadvantages in the possibilities for overcoming some elements of isolation.

Evidence-Informed Practice Box

Methodologically rigorous, evidence-informed practice research about social isolation is difficult to find. One such study, however, was undertaken by Fyrand (2003). This study examined the effect of a social network intervention on 264 women participants with rheumatoid arthritis (RA). Participants were randomized into three groups, that is, one intervention and two control groups, labelled as the Intervention Group, the Attention Control Group, and the No-Treatment Control Group, respectively.

The *research questions* guiding this study were as follows: "To what extent, if any, will network intervention influence (1) the total size of the patients' social network, (2) the amount of the patients' daily emotional support, and (3) the patients' social functioning" (Fyrand, 2003, p. 72). The *intervention* in this study consisted of two separate but related sessions: (1) a preparatory assessment session and (2) the network meeting. Participants randomized into the attention control group were given the opportunity to attend a single 2-hour meeting in which they were presented information about RA from a panel of experts who also responded to their questions about RA. The third control group had no intervention or meeting.

Three *findings* indicated that (1) the intervention group experienced a statistically significant increase in their social network size; (2) at time 2 in the study, emotional social support was higher for the intervention group; and (3) less social dysfunction occurred in the intervention group.

The *intervention* basically assessed a patient participant's social network and then helped the patient and the social network to assist the patient in socially functional problem solving about the illness. Through the meeting process in the intervention group, a change in attitude was observed when the patient developed an increased awareness of the need for social network members. In addition, the network members often shared problems about their own lives, which normalized any feelings of stigma experienced by the patient. The author called this a "response shift" (p. 83), where both parties change their self-evaluation and make a concerted effort to support each other.

During the preparatory assessment session three important areas were covered: (1) information about the research project, (2) the relationship between health and social networks, and (3) how the patient experienced chronic illness. During this 2-hour preparatory assessment the researchers mapped the participant's present social network. The social network map helped the participants to obtain a deeper analysis of the makeup of their social networks and allowed the researcher and participant to make decisions about which member of the network should be invited to the network meeting (the second element of this intervention). In this initial preparatory session participant patients also discussed, in depth, how their chronic disease (RA) impacted their lives. As feelings were explored researchers took great care to ensure the participants had adequate time and attention regarding these important topics.

The network meeting consisted of network members, typically the friends and family who were listed in the preparatory assessment, getting together to problem solve. An average of seven network members, in addition to a network research therapist, attended for an average of 2 hours. The research network therapist acted as a leader and catalyst of the group, mobilizing the participant and the group of network members to dialogue about the participant patient's problem-solving process. The group leader opened the meeting with the expectations of the meeting and a presentation of the topics that were deemed important, as derived from the preparatory meeting. The general goal for the group was to share how they viewed the participant's life with RA and to describe their hopes and expectations of the meetings. The goal for the participant was to elicit free discussion of those topics that were of highest importance. A consensus was formed within the group about how to best solve the problems raised, with the further intention to develop trust and involvement between members of the network. In addition to the participant learning how to best present problems to social network members, the aim of the network meeting was to help the participant and members change dysfunctional network behaviours. The researchers suggested that by clustering the network members and the participant together in a single room, the network and participant would better sense their collective power and the participant could re-bond with any hitherto damaged social network relationships.

This article lays out a sensible intervention that targets social network members. Through a pair of relatively short meetings, the researchers created an exportable, effective intervention that reduced social isolation and rehabilitated, to some extent, dysfunctional social networks. Furthermore, not only is this intervention brief, but it also does not require technology that requires extra training. It does require the network therapist to be a professional, such as a nurse, social worker, or psychologist, who is skilled in group therapy and mapping social networks. Therefore, this cost-effective intervention can be easily conducted in a variety of settings with a variety of patients who have social networks willing to meet together for a minimum of only 4 hours.

Source: Fyrand (2003).

Touch

In cultures where touch is important, families and professionals must learn the use and comfort of touch. Pets may be useful alternatives to human touch and human interaction; pet therapy is increasingly used as an intervention in families, communities, and group settings such as nursing homes (Banks, 1998; Collins et al., 2006). Feeling loved and having it demonstrated through touch can do much to reduce isolation and its often concomitant lowered self-esteem. Because some individuals find touch uncomfortable, professionals must assess (by simply asking or observing flinching, grimacing, or resignation) the family's or isolate's responsiveness to touch.

Behaviour Modification

Behaviour modification is a technique best used by skilled professionals. It involves the systematic analysis of responses and their antecedent cues and consequences; the use of cognitive therapy to change awareness, perceptions, and behaviours; and the specification of realistic, measurable goals or actual behaviours. In addition, reward structures and understanding support persons are necessary in the definition of the problem and its solution. Consistency is needed to develop stable patterns of responses. The timeframe of such modification can vary with the problem.

Behaviour modification is particularly useful for addressing specific problems, for example, the isolate who is fearful of going outside the house. It is also an important intervention when the environment can be held stable, such as in an institutional setting. Matteson and colleagues (1997) noted that where groups are small or the motivation intense, successful behavioural interventions have been instituted for the socially isolated in institutions as well as in the home.

SUMMARY

Ideally, the reduction of social isolation and the maintenance of the integrity of the person who is chronically ill and his or her caregiver(s) are preferred outcomes of interventions. However, so many factors can affect social isolation, its assessment, and intervention that it is difficult to draw simple linear relationships between structure, process, and outcomes. As shown throughout this chapter, a professional must be sensitive to, and prioritize, interventions within the cultural milieu in which the client and support network reside. Handling the emotionally charged issues surrounding every social isolate requires that professionals recognize in their clients, as well as in themselves, those values that most drive their relationships and build solutions that best deliver culturally and personally competent care toward a better life for their clients.

STUDY QUESTIONS www

1. Is loneliness the same thing as social isolation? Why or why not?
2. How might the distance that a manually powered or an electrically powered wheelchair can go relate to social isolation?
3. List six characteristics that identify a client who may be at risk for social isolation. What criteria did you use to develop these characteristics?
4. Suppose another healthcare professional said about a very new client, "Oh, we must make certain Mrs.

STUDY QUESTIONS (Cont.) www

Jones has company. She's a widow, you know." With regard to social isolation, what arguments could you make, pro or con, about this statement?

5. Develop at least five questions you could use to assess and validate social isolation in a client. Consider how you might approach identity levels, actual isolation, network assessment, and feelings of the isolate. Add other priorities as you wish, but offer rationales for each of them.

6. Name three community resources you could use to reduce the social isolation of clients.

7. What two principles should guide a healthcare professional when developing any intervention with an isolated client? Why are these important?

8. Suppose a client said to you, "I have had arthritis in my fingers and hands for a long time now. I simply can't do what I used to do. I now have new handles for my kitchen cabinets because the knobs hurt my hands, and new clothes especially made for people like me who can't work buttons. My daughter was shopping and she saw them and told me about them. Now I feel better when I get together with them to see my grandchildren." At what stage of identity might you expect this client to be? Why? Is this person an isolate? Explain your answer.

STUDY QUESTIONS (Cont.)
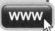

9. A gay teenager is your client. He has recently "come out" and is now depressed because his schoolmates shun him, his parents are going through a grief reaction to his announcement, and he has few other friends who share his interests or sexual orientation. Is he at risk for social isolation? Loneliness? How would you assess his social network? What interventions, if any, would you recommend? Explain your answers.

For a full suite of assignments and additional learning activities, use the access code located in the front of your book and visit this exclusive website: **http://go.jblearning.com/kramer-kile**. If you do not have an access code, you can obtain one at the site.

REFERENCES

Ami, R. (2004). Loneliness then and now: Reflections on social and emotional alienation in everyday life. *Current Psychology, 23*(1), 24–40.

Andresen, E., & Brownson, R. (2000). Disability and health status: Ethnic differences among women in the United States. *Journal of Epidemiology and Community Health, 54,* 200–206.

Antonucci, T. (1985). Social support: Theoretical advances, recent findings, and pressing issues. In I. G. Sarason & B. R. Sarason (Eds.), *Social support: Theory, research, and application* (pp. 21–37). Boston, MA: Martinus Nyhoff.

Bachner, Y., O'Rourke, N., & Camel, S. (2011). Fear of death, mortality communication and psychological distress among secular and religiously observant family caregivers of terminal cancer patients. *Death Studies, 35*(2), 163–187.

Balabanova, Y., Cooker, R., Atun, R. A., & Drobniewski, F. (2006). Stigma and HIV infection in Russia. *AIDS Care, 18*(7), 846–852.

Banks, M. R. (1998). *The effects of animal-assisted therapy on loneliness in an elderly population in long-term care facilities.* Louisiana State University Health Sciences Center School of Nursing.

Barker, J. C. (1994). Recognizing cultural differences: Health care providers and elderly patients. *Gerontology & Geriatric Education, 15*(1), 9–21.

Barnes, L. L., Mendes de Leon, C. F., Wilson, R. S., Bienias, J. L., & Evans, D. A. (2004). Social resources and cognitive decline in a population of older African Americans and whites. *Neurology, 63*(12), 2322–2326.

Beland, F., Zunzunegui, M. V., Alvarado, B., Otero, A., & Del Ser, T. (2005). Trajectories of cognitive decline and social relations. *Journals of Gerontology. Series B, Psychological Sciences and Social Sciences, 60*(6), P320–P330.

Bendor, S. (1990). Anxiety and isolation in siblings of pediatric cancer patients: The need for prevention. *Social Work in Health Care, 14*(3), 17–35.

Bennet, R. (1980). *Aging, isolation, and resocialization.* New York, NY: VanNostrand Reinhold.

Bennett, S, J., Perkins, S. M., Lane, K. A., Deer, M., Brater, D. C., & Murray, M. D. (2001). Social support and health-related quality of life in chronic heart failure patients. *Quality of Life Research, 10*(8), 671–681.

Berkman, L. (1983). The assessment of social networks and social support in the elderly. *Journal of the American Geriatrics Society, 31*(12), 743–749.

Berkman, L. F., & Syme, S. L. (1979). Social networks, host resistance, and mortality: A nine-year follow-up study of Alameda County residents. *American Journal of Epidemiology, 109*(2), 186–204.

Bobsworth, H. B., Siegler, I. C., Olsen, M. K., Brummett, B. H., Barefoot, J. C., Williams, R. B., Clapp-Channing, N. E., & Mark, D. B. (2000). Social support and quality of life in patients with coronary artery disease. *Quality of Life Research, 9*(7), 829–839.

Boden-Albala, B., Litwak, E., Elkind, M. S., Rundek, T., & Sacco, R. L. (2005). Social isolation and outcomes post stroke. *Neurology, 64*(11), 1888–1892.

Borman, J., & Biordi, D. (1992). Female nurse executives: Finally, at an advantage. *Journal of Nursing Administration, 22*(9), 37–41.

Bricout, J. C. (2004). Using telework to enhance return to work outcomes for individuals with spinal cord injuries. *Neurorehabilitation, 19*(2), 147–159.

Browne, A. J. (1997). The concept analysis of respect applying the hybrid model in cross-cultural settings. *Western Journal of Nursing Research, 19*(6), 762–780.

Brummett, B. H., Barefoot, J. C., Siegler, I. C., Clapp-Channing, N. E., Lytle, B. L., Bosworth, H. B., Williams, R. B., & Mark, D. B. (2001). Characteristics of socially isolated patients with coronary artery disease who are at elevated risk for mortality. *Psychosomatic Medicine, 63*(2), 267–272.

Cadman, D., Rosenbaum, P., Boyle, M., & Offord, D. (1991). Children with chronic illness: Family and parent demographic characteristics and psychosocial adjustment. *Pediatrics, 87*(6), 884–889.

Catalan, J. (1998). Mental health problems in older adults with HIV referred to a psychological-medicine unit. *AIDS Care: Psychological and Socio-medical Aspects of AIDS/HIV, 10*(2), 105–112.

Catlin, A. J. (1998). Editor's choice. When cultures clash, comments on a brilliant new book. *The spirit catches you and you fall down*. New York, NY: Farrar, Straus, and Giroux.

Ceria, C. D., Masaki, K. H., Rodriguez, B. L., Chen, R., Yano, K., & Curb, J. D. (2001). The relationship of psychosocial factors to total mortality among older Japanese-American men: The Honolulu heart program. *Journal of the American Geriatrics Society, 49*(6), 725–731.

Cheng, B. K. (1997). Cultural clash between providers of majority culture and patients of Chinese culture. *Journal of Long Term Home Health Care, 16*(2), 39–43.

Chinman, M. J., Weingarten, R., Stayner, D., & Davidson, L. (2001). Chronicity reconsidered: Improving person-environment fit through a consumer-run service. *Community Mental Health Journal, 37*(3), 215–229.

Christ, G. (1987). Social consequences of the cancer experience. *American Journal of Pediatric Hematology/ Oncology, 9*(1), 84–88.

Clark, D. J. (2002). Older adults living through and with their computers. *Computers, Informatics, Nursing, 20*(3), 117–124.

Cloutier-Fisher, D., & Kobayashi, K. (2009). Examining social isolation by gender and geography: A conceptual and operational challenge using population health data in Canada. *Gender, Place and Culture, 16*(2), 181–199.

Cloutier-Fisher, D., Kobayashi, K., & Smith, A. (2011). The subjective dimension of social isolation: A qualitative investigation of older adults in small social networks. *Journal of Aging Studies, 25*(4), 407–414.

Cohen, M. (1993). The unknown and the unknowable—managing sustained uncertainty. *Western Journal of Nursing Research, 15*(1), 77–96.

Collins, D., Fitzgerald, S., Sachs-Ericsson, N., Scherer, M., Cooper, R., & Boninger, M. (2006). Psychosocial well-being and community participation of service dog partners. *Disability and Rehabilitation, 1*(1), 41–48.

Corbin, J., & Strauss, A. (1987). Accompaniments of chronic illness: Changes in body, self, biography, and biographical time. In J. Roth & P. Conrad (Eds.), *Research in the sociology of health care*. Greenwich, CT: JAI Press.

Cox, C., Spiro, M., & Sullivan, J. (1988). Social risk factors: Impact on elders' perceived health status. *Journal of Community Health Nursing, 5*(1), 59–73.

Creed, F. (1990). Psychological disorders in rheumatoid arthritis: A growing consensus? *Annual Rheumatic Disorders, 49*, 808–812.

Davidhizar, R., Bechtel, G. L., & Giger, J. N. (1998). Model helps CMs deliver multicultural care: Addressing cultural issues boosts compliance. *Case Management Advisor, 9*(6), 97–100.

Dela Cruz, L. (1986). On loneliness and the elderly. *Journal of Gerontological Nursing, 12*(11), 22–27.

DesRosier, M., Catanzaro, M., & Piller, J. (1992). Living with chronic illness: Social support and the well spouse perspective. *Rehabilitation Nursing, 17*(2), 87–91.

Dickens, A. P., Richards, S. H., Greaves, C. J., & Campbell, J. L (2011). Interventions targeting social isolation in older people: A systematic review. *BMC Public Health, 11*(1), 647–668.

DiMatteo, M. R., & Hays, R. (1981). Social support and serious illness. In B. H. Gottlieb (Ed.), *Social networks and social support*. Beverly Hills, CA: Sage.

DiNapoli, P., & Murphy, D. (2002). The marginalization of chronically ill adolescents. *Nursing Clinics of North America, 37*(3), 565–572.

Dorfman, L., Homes, C., & Berlin, K. (1996). Wife caregivers of frail elderly veterans: Correlates of caregiver satisfaction and caregiver strain. *Family Relations, 45*, 46–55.

Dropkin, M. (1989). Coping with disfigurement and dysfunction. *Seminars in Oncology Nursing, 5*(3), 213–219.

Eng, P. M., Rimm, E. B., Fitzmaurice, G., & Kawachi, I. (2002). Social ties and change in social ties in relation to subsequent total and cause-specific mortality and coronary heart disease incidence in men. *American Journal of Epidemiology, 155*(8), 700–709.

Findlay, R. (2003). Interventions to reduce social isolation amongst older people: Where is the evidence? *Aging & Society, 23*, 647–658.

Fiscella, K., Franks, M., Gold, M., & Clancy, D. (2000). Social support, disability, and depression: A longitudinal study of rheumatoid arthritis. *Journal of the American Medical Association, 283*, 2579–2584.

Foxall, M., Barron, C., Dollen, K., Shull, K., et al. (1994). Low vision elders: Living arrangements, loneliness, and social support. *Journal of Gerontological Nursing, 20*, 6–14.

Foxall, M., Eckberg, J., & Griffith, N. (1986). Spousal adjustment to chronic illness. *Rehabilitation Nursing, 11*, 13–16.

Franks, H. M., Cronan, T. A., & Oliver, K. (2004). Social support in women with fibromyalgia: Is quality more important than quantity? *Journal of Community Psychology, 32*(4), 425–438.

Fratiglioni, L., Paillard-Borg, S., & Winblad, B. (2004). An active and socially integrated lifestyle in late life might protect against dementia. *Lancet Neurology, 3*(6), 343–353.

Fratiglioni, L., Wang, H. X., Ericsson, K., Maytan, M., & Winblad, B. (2000). Influence of social network on occurrence of dementia: A community-based longitudinal study. *Lancet, 355*(9212), 1315–1319.

Frierson, R. L. (1991). Suicide attempts by the old and the very old. *Archives of Internal Medicine, 151*(1), 141–144.

Fyrand, L. (2003). The effect of social network intervention for women with rheumatoid arthritis. *Family Process, 42*(1), 71.

Gallo, A. M., Breitmayer, B. J., Knafl, K. A., & Zoeller, L. H. (1991). Stigma in childhood chronic illness: A well sibling perspective. *Pediatric Nursing, 17*(1), 21–25.

Gatto, S. L., & Tak. S. H. (2008). Computer, Internet and e-mail use among older adults: Benefits and barriers. *Educational Gerontology, 34*(9), 800–811.

Gamba, A., Romano, M., Grosso, I., Tamburini, M., Cantu, G., Molinari, R., & Ventafridda, V. (1992). Psychosocial adjustment of patients surgically treated for head and neck cancer. *Head and Neck, 14*(3), 218–223.

Groce, N. E., & Zola, I. (1993). Multiculturalism, chronic illness, and disability. *Pediatrics, 91*(5), 32–39.

Habayeb, G. L. (1995). Cultural diversity: A nursing concept not yet reliably defined. *Nursing Outlook, 43*(5), 224–227.

Havens, B., & Hall, M. (2001). Social isolation, loneliness, and the health of older adults in Manitoba, Canada. *Indian Journal of Gerontology, 1*(15), 126–144.

Havens, B., Hall, M., Sylvestre, G., & Jivan, T. (2004). Social isolation and loneliness: Differences between older rural and urban Manitobans. *Canadian Journal of Aging, 23*(2), 129–140.

Hawes, C., Phillips, C. D., Rose, M., Holan, S., & Sherman, M. (2003). A national survey of assisted living facilities. *The Gerontologist, 43*(6), 875–882.

Helga, B. (2007). Computer-mediated support group intervention for parents. *Journal of Nursing Scholarship, 40*(1), 32–38.

Heiney, S., Goon-Johnson, K., Ettinger, R., & Ettinger, S. (1990). The effects of group therapy on siblings of pediatric oncology patients. *Journal of Pediatric Oncology Nursing, 7*(3), 95–100.

Heumann, L. (1988). Assisting the frail elderly living in subsidized housing for the independent elderly: A profile of the management and its support priorities. *The Gerontologist, 28*, 625–631.

Hildebrandt, E. (1997). Have I angered my ancestors? Influences of culture on health care with elderly black South Africans as an example. *Journal of Multicultural Nursing and Health, 3*(1), 40–49.

Hill, D. L. (2006). Sense of belonging as connectedness, American Indian worldview and mental health. *Archives of Psychiatric Nursing, 20*(5), 210–216.

Hill, W. G., & Weinert, C. (2004). An evaluation of an online intervention to provide social support and health education. *Computers, Informatics, Nursing, 22*(5), 282–288.

Hoffman-Goetz, L., & Donelle, L. (2007). Chatroom computer-mediated support on health issues for aboriginal women. *Health Care for Women International, 28*(4), 397–418.

Holley, U. A. (2007). Social isolation: A practical guide for nurses assisting clients with chronic illness. *Rehabilitation Nursing, 32*(2), 51–56.

Holocomb-McCoy, C. (2004). Alienation: A concept for understanding low-income, urban clients. *Journal of Humanistic Counselling, Education and Development, 43*(2), 188–196.

Holtzman, R. E., Rebok, G. W., Saczynski, J. S., Kouzis, A. C., Wilcox Doyle, K., & Eaton, W. W. (2004). Social network characteristics and cognition in middle-aged and older adults. *Journals of Gerontology, Series B, Psychological Sciences and Social Sciences, 59*(6), P278–P284.

Hopper, S. (1981). Diabetes as a stigmatized condition: The case of low income clinic patients in the United States. *Social Science and Medicine, 15*, 11–19.

Howat, P., Iredell, H., Grenade, L., Nedwetzky, A., & Collins, J. (2004). Reducing social isolation amongst older people implications for health professionals. *Geriaction, 22*(1), 13–20.

Hoybye, M. T., Johansen, C., & Tjornboj-Thomsen, T. (2005). Online interaction: Effects of storytelling in an internet breast cancer support group. *Psychooncology, 14*(3), 211–220.

Imel, S. (1999) *Seniors in cyberspace. Trends and issues alerts*. Washington, DC: Office of Educational Research and Improvement.

Jim, S. H., & Anderson, B. L. (2007). Meaning of life mediates the relationship between social and physical functioning and distress in cancer survivors. *British Journal of Health Psychology, 12*, 363–381.

Johnson, D., & Ashton, C. (2003). Effects of computer-mediated communication on social support and loneliness for isolated persons with disabilities. *American Journal of Recreational Therapy, 2*(3), 23–32.

Jones, M. D., Bond, M. L., & Cason, C. L. (1998). Where does culture fit in outcomes management? *Journal of Nursing Care Quality, 13*(1), 41–51.

Jong-Gieveld, J., & Havens, B. (2004). Cross-national comparison of social isolation and loneliness: Introduction and overview. *Canadian Journal on Aging, 23*(2), 109–113.

Keller, C. S., & Stevens, K. R. (1997). Cultural considerations in promoting wellness. *Journal of Cardiovascular Nursing, 11*(3), 15–25.

Kim, L. S. (1998). Long term care for the Korean American elderly: An exploration for a better way of services. *Journal of Long Term Home Health Care, 16*(2), 35–38.

Kinsella, G., Ford, B., & Moran, C. (1989). Survival of social relationships following head injury. *International Disability Studies, 11*(1), 9–14.

Kivett, V. (1979). Discriminators of loneliness among the rural elderly: Implications for interventions. *The Gerontologist, 19*(1), 108–115.

Klinenberg, E. (2001). Dying alone: The social production of urban isolation. *Ethnography, 2*(4), 501–531.

Kobayashi, K., Cloutier-Fisher, D., & Roth, M. (2009). Making meaningful connections: A profile of social isolation and health among older adults in small town and small city, British Columbia. *Journal of Aging and Health, 21*(2), 374–397.

Korwin-Piotrowska, K., Korwin-Piotrowska, T., & Samochowiec, J. (2010). Self perception among patients with multiple sclerosis. *Archives of Psychiatry and Psychotherapy, 3*, 63–68.

Kroenke, C. H., Kubzansky, L. D., Schernhammer, E. S., Holmes, M. D., & Kawachi, I. (2006). Social networks, social support, and survival after breast cancer diagnosis. *Journal of Clinical Oncology, 24*(7), 1105–1111.

Krouse, J., Krouse, H., & Fabian, R. (1989). Adaptation to surgery for head and neck cancer. *Laryngoscope, 99*, 789–794.

Lasgaard, M., Nielsen, A., Eriksen, M. E., & Goossens, L. (2010). Loneliness and social support in adolescent boys with autism spectrum disorders. *Journal of Autism Development Disorder, 40*, 218–226.

Lau, S., & Kong, C. K. (1999). The acceptance of lonely others: Effects of loneliness and gender of the target person and loneliness of the perceiver. *Journal of Social Psychology, 139*(2), 229–241.

Lillyman, S., & Und, L. (2007). Fear of social isolation: Results of a survey of older adults in Gloucestershire. *Nursing Older People, 19*(10), 26–28.

Lin, N. (1986). Conceptualizing social support. In N. Lin, A. Dean, & W. Ensel (Eds.), *Social support, life events, and depression*. New York, NY: Academic Press.

Litwin, H. (1997). Support network type and health service utilization. *Research on Aging, 19*(3), 274–299.

Litwin, H., & Zoabi, S. (2003). Modernization and elder abuse in an Arab-Israeli context. *Research on Aging, 25*(3), 224–246.

Lubben, J. (1988). Assessing social networks among elderly populations. *Family Community Health, 11*(3), 42–52.

Lubben, J., & Gironda, M. (1996). Assessing social support networks among older people in the United States. In H. Litwin (Ed.), *The social networks of older people: A cross-national analysis* (p. 144). Westport, CT: Praeger.

Lubben, J., Weiler, P., & Chi, I. (1989). Gender and ethnic differences in the health practices of the elderly poor. *Journal of Clinical Epidemiology, 42*(8), 725–733.

Lyons, M. J. (1982). Psychological concomitants of the environment influencing suicidal behavior in middle and later life. *Dissertation Abstracts International, 43*, 1620B.

Maddox, G. L. (1985). Intervention strategies to enhance well-being in later life: The status and prospect of guided change. *Health Services Research, 19*, 1007–1032.

Mahmood, A., Chaudhury, H., Kobayashi, K., & Valente, M. (2008). The housing and community characteristics of South Asian immigrant older adults in greater Vancouver, British Columbia: A comparison between older adults in ethno-specific seniors housing and community dwelling older adults. *Journal of Architectural and Planning Research, 25*(1), 54–75.

Mallinson, R. K. (1999). The lived experiences of AIDS-related multiple losses by HIV-negative gay men. *Journal of the Association of Nurses in AIDS Care, 10*(5), 22–31.

Margolin, S. (2006). African American youths with internalizing difficulties: Relation to social support and activity involvement. *Children and Schools, 28*(3), 135–144.

Marottoli, R. A., deLeon, C. F. M., Glass, T. A., Williams, C. S., Cooney, L. M., & Berkman, L. F. (2000). Consequences of driving cessation: Decreased out-of-home activity levels. *Journal of Gerontology Series B: Psychological Sciences and Social Sciences, 55*(6), S334–S340.

Mashburn, S. (2006). A place called home: Not for profit organizations provide innovative housing and services for older adults. *Generations, 29*(4), 58–60.

Matteson, M. A., McConnell, E. S., & Linton, A. (1997). *Gerontological nursing: Concepts and practice* (2nd ed.). Philadelphia, PA: Saunders.

Mazzoni, D., & Cicognani, E. (2011). Social support and health in patients with systemis lupus erythematosus: A literature review. *Lupus, 20*(11), 1117–1125.

McNamara, B., Martin, K., Waddel, C., & Yuen, K. (1997). Palliative care in a multicultural society: Perceptions of health care professionals. *Palliative Medicine, 11*(5), 359–367.

Melle, I., Friis, S., Hauff, E., & Vaglum, P. (2000). Social functioning of patients with schizophrenia in high income welfare societies. *Psychiatric Services, 51*(2), 223–228.

Mendes de Leon, C. F., Glass, T. A., Beckett, L. A., Seeman, T. E., Evans, D. A., & Berkman, L. F. (1999). Social networks and disability transitions across eight intervals of yearly data in the new haven EPESE. *Journals of Gerontology. Series B, Psychological Sciences and Social Sciences, 54*(3), S162–S172.

Mendes de Leon, C. F., Glass, T. A., & Berkman, L. F. (2003). Social engagement and disability in a community population of older adults: The New Haven EPESE. *American Journal of Epidemiology, 157*(7), 633–642.

Mendes de Leon, C. F., Gold, D., Glass, T., Kaplan, L., & George, L. (2001). Disability as a function of social networks and support in elderly African Americans and whites: The Duke EPESE 1986–1992. *Journals of Gerontology. Series B, Psychological Sciences and Social Sciences, 56B*(3), S179–S190.

Michael, Y. L., Berkman, L. F., Colditz, G. A., Holmes, M. D., & Kawachi, I. (2002). Social networks and health-related quality of life in breast cancer survivors: A prospective study. *Journal of Psychosomatic Research, 52*(5), 285–293.

Miller, B. (1990). Gender differences in spouse caregiver strain: Socialization and role explanations. *Journal of Marriage and the Family, 52*, 311–322.

Mistry, R., Rosansky, J., McGuire, J., McDermott, C., Jarvik, L., & UPBEAT Collaborative Group. (2001). Social isolation predicts rehospitalization in a group of older American veterans enrolled in the UPBEAT program. *International Journal of Geriatric Psychiatry, 16*(10), 950–959.

Mullins, L., & Dugan, E. (1990). The influence of depression, and family and friendship relations, on residents' loneliness in congregate housing. *The Gerontologist, 30*(3), 377–384.

Murberg, T. A. (2004). Long-term effect of social relationships on mortality in patients with congestive heart failure. *International Journal of Psychiatry in Medicine, 34*(3), 207–217.

Newman, S. P., Fitzpatrick, R., Lamb, R., & Shipley, M. (1989). The origins of depressed mood in rheumatoid arthritis. *Journal of Rheumatology, 16*(6), 740–744.

Nicholson, N. R. (2009). Social isolation in older adults: An evolutionary concept analysis. *Journal of Advanced Nursing, 65*(6), 1342–1352.

Noll, R., Ris, M. D., Davies, W. H., Burkowski, W., & Koontz, K. (1992). Social interactions between children with cancer or sickle cell disease and their peers: Teacher ratings. *Developmental and Behavioral Pediatrics, 13*(3), 187–193.

Norbeck, J., DeJoseph, J., & Smith, R. (1996). A randomized trial of an empirically derived social support intervention to prevent low birthweight among African-American women. *Social Science and Medicine, 43*, 947–954.

Peplau, L. A., & Perlman, D. (Eds.). (1986). *Loneliness: A sourcebook of current theory, research, and therapy*. New York, NY: John Wiley & Sons.

Pinquart, M., & Sorensen, J. (2001). Influences on loneliness in older adults: A meta-analysis. *Basic and Applied Social Psychology, 23*(4), 245–266.

Poulin, J. (1984). Age segregation and the interpersonal involvement and morale of the aged. *The Gerontologist, 24*(3), 266–269.

Praderas, K., & MacDonald, M. (1986). Telephone conversational skills training with socially isolated, impaired nursing home residents. *Journal of Applied Behavior Analysis, 19*(4), 337–348.

Prasad, G. V. R (2007). Remnal transplantation for ethnic minorities in Canada: Inequity in access and outcomes? *Kidney International, 72*(4), 390–392.

Ramos, M., & Wilmoth, J. (2003). Social relationships and depressive symptoms among older adults in southern Brazil. *Journal of Gerontology, Series B, Psychological Sciences and Social Sciences, 58*(4), S253–S261.

Randers, I., Mattiasson A., & Olson T. H. (2003). The "social self": The 11th category of integrity—implications for enhancing geriatric nursing care. *Journal of Applied Gerontology, 22*(2), 289–309.

Ravish, T. (1985). Prevent isolation before it starts. *Journal of Gerontological Nursing, 11*(10), 10–13.

Resnick, B. (2007). Assisted living: The perfect place for nursing. *Geriatric Nursing, 28*(1), 7–8.

Rubenstein, L. Z., Josephson, K. R., & Robbins, A. S. (1994). Falls in the nursing home. *Annals of Internal Medicine, 121*(6), 442–451.

Russell, C., & Schofield, T. (1999). Social isolation in old age: A qualitative exploration of service providers' perceptions. *Ageing and Society, 19*(1), 69–91.

Russell, G., Thille, P., Hogg, W., & Lemelin, J. (2008). Beyond fighting fires and chasing tails? Chronic illness care plans in Ontario, Canada. *Annals of Family Medicine, 6*(2), 146–153.

Ryan, M., & Patterson, J. (1987). Loneliness in the elderly. *Journal of Gerontological Nursing, 13*(5), 6–12.

Sabir, M., Wethington, E., Breckman, R., Meador, R., Reid, M. C., & Pillemer, K. (2009). A community-based participatory critique of social isolation intervention research for community dwelling older adults. *Journal of Applied Gerontology, 28*(2), 218–234.

Salem, P. (1998). *Paradoxical impacts of electronic communication technologies*. Paper presented at the International Communication Association/National Communication Association Conference, Rome, Italy, July 15–17.

Seeman, T. E. (2000). Health promoting effects of friends and family on health outcomes in older adults. *American Journal of Health Promotion, 14*(6), 362–370.

Seidler, A., Bernhardt, T., Nienhaus, A., & Frolich, L. (2003). Association between the psychosocial network and dementia—a case-control study. *Journal of Psychiatric Research, 37*(2), 89–98.

Siplic, F., & Kadis, D. (2002). The psychosocial aspect of aging. *Socialno Delo, 41*(5), 295–300.

Smith, J. W. (1996). Cultural and spiritual issues in palliative care. *Journal of Cancer Care, 5*(4), 173–178.

Sowell, R. L., & Philips, K. D. (2010). Understanding and responding to HIV/AIDS stigma and disclosure: An international challenge for mental health nurses. *Issues in Mental Health Nursing, 31*, 394–402.

Stephens, M., & Bernstein, M. (1984). Social support and well-being among residents of planned housing. *The Gerontologist, 24*, 144–148.

Strauss, A., Corbin, J., Fagerhaugh, S., Glaser, B., Maines, D., Suczek, B., & Wiener, C. L. (1984). *Chronic illness and the quality of life* (2nd ed.). St. Louis, MO: Mosby.

Street, D., Burge, S., Quadagno, J., & Barrett, A. (2007). The salience of social relationships for resident well-being in assisted living. *Journals of Gerontology, Series B, Psychological Sciences and Social Sciences, 62*(2), S129–S134.

Stroebe, M., & Stroebe, W. (1983). Who suffers more? Sex differences in health risks of the widowed. *Psychological Bulletin, 93*(2), 279.

Tilden, V., & Weinert, C. (1987). Social support and the chronically ill individual. *Nursing Clinics of North America, 22*(3), 613–620.

Treolar, L. L. (1999). People with disabilities—the same, but different: Implications for health care practice. *Journal of Transcultural Nursing, 10*(4), 358–364.

Trout, D. (1980). The role of social isolation in suicide. *Suicide and Life Threatening Behavior, 10*, 10–22.

Turan, J. M., Miller, S., Bukusi, E. A., Sande, J., & Cohen, C. R. (2007). HIV/AIDS and maternity care in Kenya: How fears of stigma and discrimination affect uptake and provision of labour and delivery services. *AIDS Care, 20*(8), 938–945.

Turner-Cobb, J. M., Bloor, L. E., Whittemore, A. S., West, D., & Spiegel, D. (2006). Disengagement and social support moderate distress among women with family history of breast cancer. *The Breast Journal, 12*(1), 7–15.

Umberson, D., Wortman, C., & Kessler, R. (1992). Widowhood and depression: Explaining long-term gender differences in vulnerability. *Journal of Health and Social Behavior, 33*(1), 10.

United Nations. (2007). *Magnitude and speed of population ageing. World population aging 2007.* New York, NY: United Nations.

Van Tilburg, L., Havens, B., & De Jong Grieveld, J. (2004). Loneliness among older adults in the Netherlands, Italy and Canada: A multi-faceted comparison. *Canadian Journal on Aging, 23,* 169–179.

Victor, C., Scambler, S. J., Shah, S., Cook D. G., Harris, T., Rink, E., & De Wilde, D. (2002). Has loneliness amongst older people increased? An investigation into variations among cohorts. *Ageing and Society, 22*(5), 585–597.

Vlassoff, C., & Ali, F. (2010). HIV related stigma among South-Asians in Toronto. *Ethnicity and Health, 16*(1), 25–42.

Wang, H. X., Karp, A., Winblad, B., & Fratiglioni, L. (2002). Late-life engagement in social and leisure activities is associated with a decreased risk of dementia: A longitudinal study from the Kungsholmen Project. *American Journal of Epidemiology, 155*(12), 1081–1087.

Wang, K. W., & Barnard, A. (2004). Technology-dependent children and their families: A review. *Journal of Advanced Nursing, 45*(1), 34–46.

Watson, E. (1988). Dead to the world. *Nursing Times, 84*(21), 52–54.

Webster, P. (2005). Minority health care remains a problem for Canada leaders. *Lancet, 365*(9470), 1531–1533.

Weinert, C., Cudney, S., & Winters, C. (2005). Social support in cyberspace: The next generation. *Computers, Informatics, Nursing, 23*(1), 7–15.

Weiss, R. S. (1973). *Loneliness: The experience of emotional and social isolation.* Cambridge, MA: Massachusetts Institute of Technology Press.

Welch, C. M. (1998). The adult health and development program: Bridging the racial gap. *International Electronic Journal of Health Education, 1*(3), 178–181.

Wenger, G. C. (1997). Social networks and the prediction of elderly people at risk. *Aging and Mental Health, 1*(4), 311.

Wenger, G. C., Davies, R., Shahtahmasebi, S., & Scott, A. (1996). Social isolation and loneliness in old age: Review and model refinement. *Aging & Society, 16,* 333–358.

Williams, S., & Bury, M. (1989). Impairment, disability, and handicap in chronic respiratory illness. *Social Science and Medicine, 29*(5), 609–616.

Woods, N., Haberman, M., & Packard, N. (1993). Demands of illness and individual, dyadic, and family adaptation in chronic illness. *Western Journal of Nursing Research, 15*(1), 10–30.

Wright, L. (1995). Human development in the context of aging and chronic illness: The role of attachment in Alzheimer's disease and stroke. *International Journal of Aging and Human Development, 44,* 133–150.

Yasemin, Y., & Seher, K. (2010). The relationship between social support and loneliness in Turkish patients with cancer. *Journal of Clinical Nursing, 19*(5/6), 832–839.

Zimmer, M. (1995). Activity participation and well being among older people with arthritis. *The Gerontologist, 351,* 463–471.

Zunzunegui, M. V., Alvarado, B. E., Del Ser, T., & Otero, A. (2003). Social networks, social integration, and social engagement determine cognitive decline in community-dwelling Spanish older adults. *Journals of Gerontology, Series B, Psychological Sciences and Social Sciences, 58*(2), S93–S100.

CHAPTER 7

Body Image

Original chapter by Diana Luskin Biordi and Patricia McCann Galon
Canadian content added by Joseph C. Osuji

INTRODUCTION

Of all the prisms through which culture can be viewed, body image is one of the most prevalent and profound. From the abstract concepts of beauty, sexuality, and community to the tangibles of health, mobility, and communication, the ideal of the perfect body prevails. Against that culturally normed model of the perfect body, one forms an image of one's own body that is reflective of the culture and social environments.

Contemporary preoccupation with body image issues has permeated our culture and ways of life. Nearly 50% of North American women experience some degree of body image dissatisfaction, and millions of Canadian women spend unnecessary time and energy in the pursuit of thinness (Olmsted & McFarlane, 2004).

The perfect body changes from culture to culture and across time. Models of ancient Greeks, for example, show muscular young men and women with broad shoulders, small waists, and narrow pelvises, whereas today's prevalent North American model is waif-like thin with body tone for women and defined muscularity for men.

Body image is contingent upon social and cultural perceptions of how a body should look and perform. Therefore, individuals use a frame of reference for their own bodies shaped by the prevailing body norm of the culture and, perhaps, by subcultures within the larger culture. If one's body image differs from the body norm, social and physical rationalizations come into play. Insofar as those rationalizations themselves are exaggerated from yet other norms, healthcare interventions may be required.

Intercultural differences exist in regards to body image norms (Hallinan, 1988). Body image and its related disturbances are influenced by sociocultural factors, and the conceptions of the perfect body changes from culture to culture over time. In Canada, for example, it may be commonly held belief that the body should look and act in certain ways, but even these dominant cultural perspectives can be challenged. Gittelsohn et al. (1996) studied Ojibwa-Cree members and found that larger body shapes and sizes were preferred. Though cultural studies may find differences in size acceptance and body image, it is important to avoid generalizations that all individuals attached to a particular cultural identity will see body image in the same way.

Body image is one's mental image of one's physical self. Individual body images may change over time, depending on life tasks such as learning one's gender role, performing a job or sport, creating a family, body or brain chemistry and structure, or aging. In chronic illness body image is both a modifier of, and is modified by, the illness. Chronic illness, in its capacity to change the body, typically necessitates revisitations to one's body image. These revisitations are modified by the psychology of the individual and his or her perceptions of the ideal. That is, the individual will need to decide, consciously or unconsciously, whether to persevere in meeting an ideal body image (the culturally defined perfect body), reformulate or readjust the ideal to conform to his or her own attributes, or reject the ideal.

Significant research in body image has occurred only recently, despite being a common subject in the literature since the late 1800s. In fact, since 2004 an entire journal, entitled *Body Image* (published by Elsevier), has been devoted to the subject. In nursing there appears to be a large gap between an initial spate of studies in the 1970s to those of the 1990s, with a substantial increase in research since 2000. Most of the literature examining body image is found in practice disciplines such as nursing, medicine (e.g., neurology), bioengineering, psychology, and vocational counselling. This literature focuses on neurological and psychological studies of person and gender, health studies on chronic illness (particularly, cancer), and, most recently, bariatric studies on obesity. In addition, some body image studies focus on plastic surgery or reconstruction, which are increasingly used by a number of persons for cosmetic reasons and/or as interventions for illness, accidents, obesity, or other treatments (Frederick, Lever, & Peplau, 2007).

DEFINITIONS OF BODY IMAGE

Body image is defined and referred to in two ways. The most prevalent definition of body image is the psychological view, in which body image is the mental image of one's physical self, including attitudes and perceptions of one's physical appearance, state of health, skills, and sexuality. Another term with the same definition is "body schema." Cash and Pruzinsky (2002) referred to body image as "people's subjective perceptions and attitudes about their own body, with an emphasis on physical appearance" (p. 397).

Body image is how one perceives one's own body, including its attractiveness, and how that body image influences interactions and others' reactions. Therefore, body image is not only the way people perceive themselves but, equally important, the way they believe others see them. Consequently, body image is a major delimiter of social interactions and as such has a profound effect on physical health, social interaction, psychological development, and interpersonal relationships. Moreover, because body image is conceptual, even if it is expressed inferentially, as in anorexia nervosa, most literature describes body image from information taken from cognitively intact, communicative human beings. Issues of profoundly developmentally disabled individuals and their body images, for example, are more likely examined from the perspective of others as they regard the person's body and whether it deviates from norms, as well as the reactions of others to the person.

The second way in which body image is defined is more neurological and technical. In this definition body image has been shown to relate to the association of brain areas, particularly the *motor cortex*, with portions of the body, such as the limbs or lips. Particular parts of the brain are also associated with the sense of the body in space and that the self is localized, or embodied, within body borders (Blanke, 2007). Embodiment is important to the models of the self or self-consciousness and, also more tangibly, of body parts properly belonging to one's person. Abnormalities in embodiment can lead to such distress as "amputation desire" or "amputation envy," in which persons are profoundly frustrated by their sense that one of their body parts (limbs) does not "belong" to them and actively seek its removal to satisfy their sense of body/ embodiment (Mueller, 2007–2008). Voluntary movement of body limbs and sensations, often of pain, have been shown to be linked to limbs, teeth, or breasts when certain brain areas or neurons are invoked. Thus, body image is defined and discussed in the theory, empiricism, and language of brain, neuropathology, neurology, anatomy, and/or physiology (Lewis, 1983; Mueller, 2007–2008; Ramachandran, 2004; Ramachandran & Rogers-Ramachandran, 2007).

It is interesting that the symptoms of the psychiatric diagnosis body dysmorphic disorder (BDD) also are characterized as both psychological and neuropathological. Persons with BDD, a chronic disorder, suffer distress and functional impairment due to a preoccupation with even a slight defect in their appearance. The preoccupation can progress to a delusional state. BDD is a fairly common disorder with an estimated prevalence of about 0.7% to 1.7% of the population, but it often goes unrecognized. Persons with BDD often seek plastic surgery or dermatological treatment for this "abnormality" but are never satisfied with the results and thus may seek repeated procedures (Feusner, Yaryura-Tobias, &

Saxena, 2008). In addition, they believe they are mocked by others for their defect and see themselves as generally less healthy and capable than the rest of the population (Didie, Kuniega-Pietrzak, & Phillips, 2010).

One can develop BDD in response to brain trauma or disease of the central nervous system, especially in the temporal lobe area. About 8% of persons with BDD can identify relatives with obsessive compulsive disorder or BDD, indicating inheritability. Phillips and Hollander (2008) suggested that persons with BDD have fundamental differences in visual processing with a focus on the specific rather than on an overall picture, both in consideration of the self and their environment. It is also speculated based on neuropsychological evaluation that emotional arousal may contribute to the attentional bias (concentration on defect) and social anxiety associated with the disorder.

Body image is referred to in two other ways in the literature. First, body image is conceptualized as a *final product* or end state—a state of being, such as, "Charles's body image is that of a muscular young man." Second, body image can be portrayed as a *process*—a continuous examination by the self or others, whereby one's body is defined and redefined. In both conceptualizations a number of factors influence body image. Furthermore, the attitudes and perceptions about one's body guide evaluation and investment in body image, which affect physical and psychosocial functioning. Attitudes about body image are related to one's self-esteem, interpersonal functioning, eating and exercise patterns, self-care activities, and sexual behaviours (Cash & Fleming, 2002; Peelen & Downing, 2007).

In summary, body image is theorized as conceptual and neurological, with each concept feeding into the other. Body image is one's perception of one's body and its interactions with others. It includes a sense of ownership and boundaries of one's body, the image of which is constructed psychologically and through the neurological system of the brain—through proprioception (the sense of the body in space), vision, and the vestibular system. Body image can be thought of as both a process and an end product, and one's body image affects physical and psychosocial functioning.

HISTORICAL FOUNDATIONS OF BODY IMAGE

Although body image has been discussed in the literature since the 1880s, it was not until Schilder presented his work in 1935 that a new understanding of this concept arose. In *The Image and Appearance of the Human Body*, Schilder (1950) explored the dimensions of body image: "The image of the human body means the picture of our own body which we form in our mind, that is to say the way in which the body appears to ourselves" (p. 11). He believed the perception of one's body is based on a three-dimensional image that comprises physiological, psychological, and social experiences. Schilder's work affected subsequent researchers, even into the 21st century. Critiquing Schilder's broad and complex theory, Cash and Pruzinsky (1990) claim that Schilder's chief contribution was not just the idea of body image but the idea that body image has "central pertinence not only for the pathologic but also everyday events of life" (p. 9). Later, Cash and Pruzinsky (2002) assert that Schilder "single handedly moved the study of body image beyond the exclusive domain of neuropathology" (p. 4).

Most current discussions now frame body image as having a perceptual component, a psychological component, and a social component (Cash & Fleming, 2002; Galagher, 2005;

Thompson & Gardner, 2002; Thompson & Van Den Berg, 2002). For example, with regard to eating and weight disorders, the perceptual component is the accuracy of the person's body size estimation, the psychological component is the person's attitudes or feelings toward his or her own body, and the social component might be the cultural context in which body image is assessed.

Like others, Thompson and Gardner (2002) and Cash and Fleming (2002) argued that body image is not a simple perceptual phenomenon but is highly influenced by cognitive, affective, attitudinal, and other variables. Thompson has been attributed as the impetus in the 1990s to a more clinically and physiologically based concept of body image, particularly in examining eating disorders (Cash & Pruzinsky, 2002). Building on his work, research later focused on cultural overlays, including feminist critiques of the 1990s and, later, the effects of family or ethnicity on body image. More recent work in the 2000s is refocusing on the physiological basis of body image, while attending to more evidence-informed interventions on body image and its effects (Cash & Pruzinsky, 2004).

Currently, major empirical analyses of body image focus on neurology, particularly those studies involving the brain and associated visual, vestibular, vascular, and proprioceptor stimuli. Important studies by Ramachandran and Rogers-Ramachandran (2007) indicated that body image can be shaped and changed by the brain. Using vision and proprioceptor cues, they were able to map where in the brain (somatosensory, motor, and parietal cortices) cues were received to fashion a virtual sense of body that did not correspond to actuality. The idea that body image can be so profoundly shaped by the brain has important implications for both theory and treatment. In a related set of studies Ramachandran (2004) indicated that when motor signals are sent to muscles, duplicate signals are sent to the brain's parietal lobes, giving a sense of real limbs when there are actually amputations, leading to the phenomenon of phantom limb syndrome. Therefore, as is known in the field of prosthetics, amputees who are unable to incorporate a change in body image that genuinely indicates a lost limb were shown to be unable to use prosthetics effectively.

Of particular importance to healthcare professionals in chronic illness is the empirically derived idea that the perceptual elements of body image are complex. Fisher (1986) found that people not only compartmentalized their body image but also differed in how they did so. Some localized their body image, whereas others had a more global view of their body. For instance, people with serious body defects might approach their bodies as separate regions, specifically isolating the defective region so that it does not influence their overall evaluation of self. Fisher believed this ability suggested "important defensive and maturational significance in how differentiated one's approach to one's body is" (p. 635). He also argued that the rubric of body image itself is vague, representing a number of dimensions of the same and different constructs. Newer neurological data (Ramachandran, 2004; Ramachandran & Rogers-Ramachandran, 2007) indicate that certain brain regions governing specific body parts play a role in whether body images can be sustained or demarcated as separate. For example, clients with left-sided hemiplegia caused by a stroke often experience dissociation from their paralyzed limbs.

FACTORS IN THE DEFINITION OF BODY IMAGE

Definitions of body image, although varied, share similarities. Common to many definitions is the belief that body image develops in response to multiple sensory inputs (visual, tactile, proprioceptive, and kinaesthetic). Therefore, although physicality is included in one's body image, body image is subjective and dynamic because it is influenced by multiple factors (Cash, 2002; Pruzinsky, 2004). Body image is brought into the immediate focus of the individual by pain, physical or psychological illness, age, or weight (Krueger, 2002). Kinaesthetic perceptions of function, sensation, and mobility are also part of our image. For example, children without sensation of body parts (e.g., spina bifida) often do not include in their art those body parts where they lack sensation.

Body image also includes feelings and thoughts. How one thinks and feels about one's body influences social relationships and other psychological characteristics. Furthermore, how people feel and think about their bodies influences the way they perceive the world (Cash & Fleming, 2002).

Nezlek (1999) found three factors were included in the definition of body image: body attractiveness, social attractiveness (how attractive people believed others found them to be), and general attractiveness. For both men and women self-perceptions of body attractiveness and social attractiveness were positively related to intimacy. Cash, Theirault, and Annis (2004) asserted that body image dysfunction for both genders was linked to less secure general interpersonal attachment and more anxious romantic relationships. According to Cash et al., core facets of body image attributes include evaluation (body satisfaction), investment (appearance self-schemas), and affect (body image emotions). Because body attractiveness is an important function of body image, this concept frequently is confused with body image itself; however, body image encompasses more than attractiveness.

Many definitions of body image today involve the notions of the real and the ideal. Theorists would argue that the ideal image of one's self and the real image must be compatible, or dissonance results. A discrepancy between the real and the ideal body image may lead to conflicts that adversely affect personality, interactions, and health. For example, "normative discontent" refers to the pervasive negative feelings women and girls experience when they negatively distort their appearance, experience body image dissatisfaction, or over-evaluate appearance in defining a sense of self (Striegel-Moore & Franko, 2002).

For the healthcare professional definitions of body image indicate the complexity of the concept but, more importantly, emphasize how significantly the client's cultural, social, historical, and biological factors affect body image. Perhaps even more important to healthcare professionals and their professionally derived norms is that body image and the factors affecting it are not merely cosmetic. A client's perceptions and attitudes about his or her body can affect health, social adjustment, interpersonal relationships, and general well-being. These perceptions are profoundly affected by chronic illness, as shown in this text.

Although body image is socially constructed, it is central to self-concept. Perhaps because body image is so vital to issues of ordinary health as well as chronic illness, it has come to be associated with, or even confused with, several other terms.. The terms "body image," "self-concept," and "self-esteem" are frequently used interchangeably. Body image is not the same as body attractiveness but is related to both attractiveness and self-esteem. Body image is a mental image of one's physical self, moderated by one's psychology and the social environment and, as is

being discovered, by certain physiological parameters of the brain. Body image thus is an integral component of self-concept. Self-concept is the total perception an individual holds of self—who one believes one is, how one believes one looks, and how one feels about one's self (Mock, 1993). Research extends self-concept to include not only ongoing perceptions of one's self but also the idea that self-concept so mediates and regulates behaviour that it is one of the most significant regulators of behaviour (Markus & Wurf, 1987). Self-concept also is used to describe roles in which one casts the self, which can further stretch, and perhaps muddy, the concept. Finally, self-esteem is related to "the evaluative component of an individual's self-concept" (Corwyn, 2000, p. 357).

FACTORS INFLUENCING ADJUSTMENT TO BODY IMAGE

Meaning and Significance

As critical as each influence may be to the individual's adaptation, it is most important the meaning of the event to the individual be understood. Knowing clients may compartmentalize both the meaning and the body's parts, the healthcare professional must recognize and accept how each client assesses the changes occurring in his or her body, their importance, and the way the client chooses to incorporate (or not) changes into the body image. Thus, treatment of chronic illness, and by association body image, functionality, or appearance, cannot be far removed from the meaning attributed to such by the client or significant other.

In most cultures body parts carry emotional attribution quite aside from functionality or appearance. The hands, for instance, are critical portrayals of the meanings and metaphysics of religions, whether shown invitingly open, in clasped position, or thumbs and forefingers together. Similarly, the mind is associated with the brain and all the significance attached to it in a knowledge society, whereas the heart is universally seen as the font of emotions. The heart is, to many, the symbol of love, courage, and life and the seat of joy, hate, and sorrow. Indeed, in some cultures the heart is seen as the location of the soul. Consider the emotional significance, then, that damage to the heart would engender in the body image of the affected client. Most nurses have been taught about clients who, after sustaining a myocardial infarction, are so anxious they become a "cardiac cripple" due to their fear of death from exercise or normal activity. Clearly, the self-image of such clients has sustained a serious insult. Dementia creates issues of self-image not only for the person undergoing the change but also for significant others in the interactions and subsequent reappraisals. How many times have nurses heard families say they "no longer know their loved one" as the disease progresses?

To counter the insult to body image and functionality and knowing likely prognoses, the healthcare professional must reassure the client and family about their perceptions of body image and help them reconcile to the present and future realities of the situation. That is, the healthcare professional should make efforts to reconcile the ideal body image of the client with the current attributes of the person and encourage the client to move toward a more realistic body image, while recognizing that, for the client, losing their desired body image can create a grieving process that must also be managed.

Body image and the insults to functionality from chronic illness cannot be isolated from the meaning and significance the client gives to them. Furthermore, the meaning and significance to family members or significant others can also play an important role in the client's response. For example, young and middle-aged women's body esteem was found to be positively related to their perceptions of their partner's approval of their appearance (McKinley, 1999). These are crucial factors to consider in offering and performing effective and sensitive care. Of all the aspects of body image in chronic illness, the appreciation and understanding of the meaning and significance to the client are areas to which nursing can most contribute. The client's meaning and significance of the change in body image must not be overlooked or downplayed. Nursing's empathic and holistic approach can be of great value in this arena of health care.

The cause of the person's chronic illness and associated insult to one's body image can be an important coping factor. If the change was caused by an accident, healthcare mismanagement, or personal negligence, the person may harbour unresolved anger, blame, and shame. The person may also be guarded about sharing and discussing such matters, which confounds recovery and makes it more difficult. On the other hand, if the cause was recommended or was a life-saving intervention, the person perceives the body image insult as an unavoidable consequence and a relatively small price to pay (Rybarczyk & Behel, 2002).

Another important factor the nurse must not forget is the "fifth vital sign," or pain. If pain is associated with the cause of the body image change, the meaning and significance of the altered body image can be negatively influenced.

Pain may also nourish a persisting and even worsening negative body image and impair recovery in functionality (Rybarczyk & Behel, 2002). Hence, it is essential to assess the person for pain and discomfort and to treat accordingly.

Influence of Time

The length of time during which body changes occur may influence one's body image and subsequent psychological adjustment (White, 2002). Changes in body image may occur slowly, over a lifetime, or quickly, within hours or days. Although some might argue that more time gives individuals greater opportunity to reformulate a body image, the fact remains that some individuals will never adapt their body image to the ideal they hold or their current attributes. A person with type 2 diabetes may have a slow progression of changes and ample time for denial and grief resolution, whereas trauma and sudden illness, such as head trauma, stroke, or certain surgeries, may lead to abrupt changes in the body and in body image. Individuals who experience sudden traumatic illnesses have no warning and thus little opportunity to adjust to the changes (Bello & McIntire, 1995). A classic example is the lag between limb amputations and phantom pain, where clients are confused about whether they still have the appendage. To adjust to rapid change the client must grieve the loss as well as physically adjust to the changes. The client who cannot cope with the dysfunction is at high risk for infection, noncompliance with therapeutic care, depression, social isolation, and obsession with or denial of the changes in body image (Dropkin, 1989).

The permanence of the change in appearance also affects adjustment to changes in body image. A person may better cope with changes in appearance that are temporary (i.e., temporary ileostomy) more so than those that are permanent (i.e., limb amputation). However, adjusting to body image changes depends partly on the meaning the individual ascribes to the changes and, in some cases, the length of time during which the change occurs (White, 2002).

Social Influences

Each sociocultural group establishes its own norms governing the acceptable, especially in terms of physical appearance and personality attributes (Jackson, 2002). Societies can hold a persistent, pervasive view with standards that dictate ideal physical appearance and role performance. These standards, although some with caveats, serve all members of that social group, including those who have chronic illness and those who do not.

Groups target their social influence and affect the self-images of individuals. Family relationships are often important to people with a chronic illness and can impact their initial perception of their own body image when they become chronically ill. Negative family reactions about appearance, behaviour, performance, and body image have been linked with recurrent poor body image consequences (Byely, Archibald, Graber, & Brooks-Gunn, 1999; Kearney-Cooke, 2002). Peers are also important mediating groups, particularly for those who are uncertain how to structure their lifestyles (e.g., adolescents). On one hand, peers can help shape conformance to a model. An example is the currently popular view of the muscle-bound, minimal-body-fat male model that is popular among young people (Olivardia, Pope, & Hudson, 2000). On the other hand, peer groups can call into question the appropriateness of such modelling for their own age group (e.g., older adults' perception of the aforementioned male model).

Persons with disfigurements are often, with little choice in the matter, forced to deal with their body image and the prevailing societal view. Depending on the visibility of the disfigurement and the coping of the disfigured person, sanctions such as staring, whispering, or shunning can negatively affect body image and personal value (Pruzinsky, 2002; Rumsey, 2002).

Untoward issues of body image often begin early in life. In North America and some European countries both girls and boys as young as 6 years old are overly conscious of their body weight and begin dieting in an attempt to meet social norms of idealized thin and handsome young men and women. These young children, especially girls, are reported to be influenced by parental models and fashion magazines toward a desired thinness (Fornari & Dancyge, 2006; Lowes & Tiggemann, 2003; McCabe, Ricciardelli, & Lina, 2005). Body image issues that begin in early years often persist throughout adolescence and into adulthood (Striegel-Moore & Franko, 2002).

The effect of society and environment on body image is reciprocal. Societal reactions can affect body image, but the individual is not entirely passive and so can react in opposition to such standards. Nevertheless, societal influences weigh heavily on behaviour and body image, frequently leading to stereotypical assignments that affect individual body image adjustments. For example, persons with craniofacial disfigurement or those who are chronically obese have been subjected to societal reactions and expectations of ideal beauty throughout their lives. Over the years, having been constantly compared with the "ideal" beautiful or thin person, individuals with chronic illness have had to manage their own responses as well as those of others in the obvious discrepancy between an ideal body and their own real bodies.

Cultural Influences

It is within the context of culture that body image develops, and therefore many aspects of culture affect body image. A cultural map has been suggested by Helman (1995) in which the members of a particular cultural or social group share a view of the body. This cultural map tells individuals how their body is structured and how it functions, includes ideal body definitions, and identifies "private" and "public" body parts as well as differentiating between a "healthy" and an "unhealthy" body (Helman, 1995).

Members of the Healthcare Team

The care given to persons with a chronic disease or disability has a direct influence on their ability to adapt to societal pressures. Members of the healthcare team, although subject to the norms of the larger society, also have perceptions of illness and certain disabilities shaped by such professional norms as objectivity, compassion, and moral judgment. When caring for an individual with chronic illness, reactions from the healthcare team are important in the clients' adjustment and acceptance of body image.

Healthcare team members must understand they are often the first person to see the changes engendered by the chronic illness or treatment. Their reactions often set the stage for body image expectations of their clients. Seeing their caregiver's reactions may reinforce body images for clients that continue for a long period of time, whether those images are positive or negative. Healthcare team members must therefore learn to manage their demeanour, voice, tone, and body reactions, avoiding any obvious rejections or trivialization of clients with chronic illness. One of the goals of the healthcare team should be to assist clients in having and/or maintaining a positive image and acceptance of self.

For example, the client who has recently undergone breast reconstructive surgery after a mastectomy may have problematic body image issues. The support and guidance by healthcare team members in helping the client with information about surgery, pain relief, self-care, positive reinforcement, family relationships, and emotional support are important to building a positive body image (Van Deusen, 1993). Assessing concerns related to appearance and allowing clients to express fears, beliefs, thoughts, and life experiences also contribute to adjustment to body image changes (White, 2002).

Age

Erik Erikson's classic developmental theory is useful in examining phases of psychosocial development, particularly as this theory examines various stages throughout the lifespan that encourage or inhibit body image and personal feelings of value (Erikson, 1963). In younger age groups conflicts about industry versus inferiority are changed into feelings of worth and competence (Cash & Pruzinsky,1990). If there were negative effects during early developmental stages, altered or poor body image may result.

It is thought that younger children may be able to adapt more easily to changing body images because they have not fully come to recognize or appreciate their body image, unlike an adolescent or adult. Because their bodies are constantly changing and because they are attending to their peers, adolescents can have an especially difficult time adapting to body image changes brought on by chronic illness. Patients with juvenile diabetes or adolescents with visible physical disfigurements, such as skin or neurological diseases, frequently act out their frustrations via risky behaviours, depression, or withdrawal.

In a qualitative study of young men (18–25 years of age) and body image, Bottamini and Ste-Marie (2006) found that males are often reluctant to acknowledge their investment in body image because they believe it is seen as a more appropriate preoccupation of women. Nevertheless, these young men see attractiveness and the resultant positive body image they project as important in the work world because they believe an employer would associate a good physique with the ability to persevere. The authors hypothesize that body image awareness in men has increased with the decline of males as breadwinners due to women's expanding roles and earning capacity. Muscularity is not typically attained by women (at least to the same degree), so muscularity is seen as a last bastion of male prowess.

Body image in an adult has likely been well established and serves as an identity base. Adaptation to changes in body image can be more difficult to accept in older age groups because illness challenges their fundamental identity. Older adults' acceptance of body image changes tends to be related more to the ability to be useful in society, loss of independence and health status, and, possibly, attractiveness to others (Krauss-Whitbourne & Skultety, 2002).

Older adults may still feel young at heart, but as their bodies age they are subject to changes in skin, hair, posture, strength, or speed of action, which are compounded by various chronic illnesses such as cardiac, respiratory, orthopaedic, visual, or hearing problems. They may feel young, but their outer appearances demonstrate their age and associated conditions in a culture that values the young. The elderly often want to maintain an accepted social body image, so it is important to consider these issues when possible body image disturbances arise.

Gender

The gender of a person may influence his or her response to a change in body image. Although both genders are subject to norms of beauty, women and girls are reported to be more affected by breaches of the norms of beauty than boys and men are (Emslie, Hunt, & Macintyre, 2001). Women with burns, for example, generally have a more negative body image than do men with burns, although the effect of burns on body image depends on the locus of the burn and the percentage of body surface involved (Orr, Reznikoff, & Smith, 1989; Thombs et al., 2008). It is important to note, however, that females in most cultures tend to have negative body image perceptions more often than males across age and cultures; therefore, women may experience more disturbances in body images than males when faced with a chronic illness (Ahmad, Waller, & Verduyn, 1994; Davis & Katzman, 1998; Striegel-Moore & Franko, 2002).

Typically, the male gender is associated with a "masculine, strong" appearance, and the female gender is associated with a "feminine, softer" appearance. Role behaviours are less strictly segregated now than in the 1950s, 1960s, and 1970s, yet many older clients were socialized to gender roles during those years and have strong expectations of clear role behaviours. Men were expected to be strong, active, rational, and silent, whereas women were expected to be indirect, passive, capable, and emotional. These views have an impact on their self-image and the differences engendered by chronic illness. Older men with chronic illness or widowers who need assistance in learning to cook or women learning to be more assertive even as their bodies are less conducive to these activities often must change their body image. Often they do so gracefully, as we hear in the admonition, "Growing old is not for sissies." However, it behoves healthcare professionals—many of whom were not born in the times generating the social norms governing the body

images of the older adults—to learn about the histories of those individuals whose chronic illnesses they treat. By doing so the healthcare professional can become more empathetic and understand the possible contributions to the body images of their clients. This is particularly important, for example, for older women with diabetes who feel the need to be good cooks to accommodate their self-image as competent women but whose diets must now be strictly managed. Another example is men with hypertension taking medication that limits libido or sexual performance.

Prior Experience and Coping Mechanisms

Body image is thought to be individually developed through each person's concept of his or her "ideal" perception and based on his or her previous experiences within society as well (Cash & Pruzinsky, 2002). Because past experiences, positive or negative, can substantially affect present circumstances, understanding how a client is likely to perceive an event and cope with it is one of the more important assessments performed by the healthcare professional. This awareness is particularly beneficial to the individual who has not had much exposure to the healthcare system and may require advocacy by the healthcare professional.

Coping mechanisms already developed by the individual through support from family, the healthcare team, or the client's social group are helpful in promoting adaptation to changes in body image during chronic illness. Understanding the individual's perception of body image before and during a diagnosis of chronic illness can be helpful to the healthcare professional in easing the client's adjustment to body image changes. Knowing that body image is an inferential health concern is helpful for the healthcare professional to discern whether clients are persevering, reformulating, or rejecting their body image.

The anxiety associated with the diagnosis of a chronic illness influences a person's coping style. Such crises can present the opportunity for personal growth or for overwhelming loss. Often, in the initial phase of chronic illness, clients display an over-reliance on their typical coping mechanisms, even if those methods are not particularly effective in the current circumstances. At the same time, early in the trajectory of chronic illness the person's ability to develop alternative coping mechanisms may be compromised. Identifying previously functional defences as well as new, potentially helpful coping styles can be the first step taken by the healthcare professional in the outgoing assessment and management of body image alterations in persons with chronic illness.

ASSESSMENT OF BODY IMAGE

Evidenced-informed practice guidelines are not yet available for the assessment or treatment of impaired body image. Yet, there are many assessment techniques from which the sensitive or skilled healthcare professional may derive interventions. Practice in psychological assessment is useful. The focus in this section is therefore on assessment.

Assessing the behaviours of individuals who have experienced an alteration in function or change leading to a disruption in body image is vital in planning appropriate interventions. This assessment leads to a determination of perceptions and meanings associated with the change that is unique to the client and allows recognition of barriers to health. Such an assessment requires the observation and interviewing of the client to determine the nature and meaning of the threat.

Only after such an assessment and validation of its correctness may the healthcare professional provide interventions.

A key to a successful assessment is a therapeutic relationship with the client. Trust, sensitivity to the client's thoughts and feelings, and provision of accurate and realistic support all help to build and strengthen the therapeutic relationship between the client and provider (Hayslip, Cooper, Dougherty, & Cook, 1997).

A complete assessment of a client's experience and meaning of change is facilitated by asking questions related to the client's perception of the experience, knowledge of the illness and its effects, and others' perceptions of the client's illness. Accounting for these factors in the assessment process creates a client-centred knowledge base for choosing appropriate interventions. In addition, assessing the client's psychosocial history and support systems allows the provider to elicit greater support for the client in areas already known to the client.

Assessing a client's unique influencing factors is essential in planning interventions. Knowing how much value is placed on the appearance or functioning of the body helps the healthcare professional determine the impact of the image disruption. Assessing self-esteem and the client's perceived attitudes of others is also important in discovering the meaning and impact of the disruption to the client. Ascertaining the phase of recovery of the client is essential and is particularly important in planning specific client-centred interventions. Knowing when to implement educational, supportive, or rehabilitative interventions makes these interventions most useful.

Questions that might help the healthcare professional assess whether a client has a poor body image, particularly because of illness or injury, might focus on hiding or denial. Denial of one's self, self-effacement, or denial of the injury's severity is one hint of a poor self-image. A more typical indication of poor self-image or self-esteem is hiding, physically or mentally, from others. Actions such as avoiding others, avoiding close contact (such as undressing in front of others or sexual intimacy), avoiding displays of the injury or scars, or feelings of shame or embarrassment when discussing the injury or illness, are important clues to self-image.

CASE STUDY

Mary Ellen is a 36-year-old single mother of two children, an 8-year-old girl and a 10-year-old boy. Mary Ellen is 5 feet 6 inches tall and weighs 137 kg (body mass index 48.7, which is considered very obese). Her mother and two sisters are also obese. Mary Ellen was never thin in childhood or adolescence and was occasionally teased at school, but more serious problems did not occur until adulthood. After her pregnancies and a painful divorce she progressively gained weight. She has tried numerous diets with limited success, subsequently regaining even more weight. She is becoming increasingly unhappy for a number of reasons, which include her daughter's burgeoning weight, her inability to keep up with her son's involvement in sports (climbing into the stands at games, long walks to the baseball field from parking), and hints that her son is ashamed of her appearance. She believes her obesity has also influenced her work life. She is an accountant with a public accounting firm, and she is no longer assigned the better projects that lead to promotion because those choice assignments involve going to client offices. On her last assignment she had difficulty fitting into the chairs at the client's site and was certain there was snickering by both the client and her coworker. Realizing these stresses trigger binge eating and additional guilt, Mary Ellen feels increasingly unable to manage her life. She has reluctantly decided to seek medical attention to learn about bariatric surgery. She dreads seeing a healthcare practitioner; in the past she has felt rejected by providers because of her lack of success in managing her weight.

Discussion Questions

1. In assisting patients like Mary Ellen, nurses must examine their own attitudes about obesity. Do you consider it a chronic disease, an unhealthy lifestyle choice, a sign of weakness or overindulgence, a socially constructed phenomenon (meaning that the categorization of weight difference comes from social and cultural understandings or norms of what bodies should look like), or a food addiction? Do you consider obesity with a "live and let live" attitude or some other conceptualization/belief about the condition? How do your views influence your approach and recommendations to Mary Ellen?
2. Do you believe you are obliged to tell Mary Ellen your views as you counsel her, because they inform your recommendations? That is, Mary Ellen may want to "consider the source" and actively choose to accept in whole or in part what you suggest. What are your obligations as a healthcare professional involved in Mary Ellen's care?
3. The stigmatization of obesity is often considered "the last acceptable prejudice." Because obese persons in our society are socialized the same as the rest of society, how might that influence body image for persons with obesity?
4. What are Mary Ellen's strengths? What opportunities do you see to assist her to improve her body image and perceptions of self-efficacy?

In some instances it may be necessary to use a standardized assessment tool to measure body disturbances and number and types of support systems. Many tools are available for this use (Cash & Pruzinsky, 2002). Tools about body disturbances generally have questions on general appearance, body competence, others' reaction to appearance, value of appearance, and so forth. These tools have incorporated related concepts to body image, such as self-esteem and self-concept, and are able to measure affective, cognitive, and behavioural components of body image (Thompson & Van Den Berg, 2002).

Incorporating families into assessment is encouraged. This can be done by interviewing, observing, and taking note of both verbal and nonverbal interactions within the family system (Wright & Leahey, 2000). Assessing family meanings of the chronic illness, perceived losses, and stresses placed on the family because of the illness is important in planning interventions.

BODY IMAGE ISSUES IMPORTANT TO CHRONIC ILLNESS

Chronic illness has many challenges, one of which includes the adaptation to changes in body image. The process of adaptation depends on many factors, but primary among those are the external changes to the person, functional limitations, the changes' significance and importance to the person, the time over which the changes (and losses) have occurred, social influences, and the impact of culture.

External Changes

Important external factors that influence body image are the visibility and functional significance of the body part involved, the importance of physical appearance to the individual, and the rate at which the change occurred (Rybarczyk & Behel, 2002). For example, epilepsy is a chronic disease that illustrates all these factors. Epileptic seizures, such as tonic–clonic seizures, can affect the entire body; the seizures are easily observed and happen suddenly. Epilepsy may also prevent the client from maintaining a job, driving a car, or engaging in sports or popular activities such as swimming. Typically, epilepsy's onset is acute. The person does not have time to prepare for accepting this chronic disease. A seizure occurs and the person's life is changed from that moment forward. This can make it more challenging to accept and live "normally" with the image of "being an epileptic" and potentially having a very visible, sudden, and dysfunctional (possibly dangerous) experience. The severity of insult to appearance and functional significance and the degree of importance to the person must be considered on an individual basis. For example, some persons may find epilepsy a minor nuisance, whereas others might find mild psoriasis traumatizing, because the latter is more visible. It is essential to assess the meaning and significance of the change to the person.

Another common example is the client dealing with obesity. Recent studies have indicated a worrisome increase in the prevalence of obesity in Canada, United States, and other Western countries (Ogden, Flegal, Carroll, & Johnson, 2002; Phipps, Burton, Osberg, & Lethbridge, 2006; Tremblay & Willms, 2000); because of its close ties to body image it deserves increased consideration in this discussion. Obesity is typically a nonacute, slowly progressing condition, which has come to be viewed as a major risk factor in several chronic illnesses, such as diabetes, heart disease, and osteoarthritis. Obesity is also considered déclassé in Western culture, often viewed as an indicator of overindulgence and sloth and frequently associated with lower socioeconomic status. Although the obesity risk has been challenged (Campos, 2005; Flegal, Graubard, Williamson, & Gail, 2007), most healthcare professionals still believe obesity must be medically managed. Today, there are public health campaigns to reduce obesity, beginning in childhood. Obese persons are reacting to the medicalisation and stigmatization of obesity.

The stigmatization of obesity is considerable in the United States, Canada, and throughout the developed world. There is evidence that weight is perhaps the most important factor in evaluating female attractiveness (Swami & Tovee, 2005; Tovee, Reinhardt, Emery, & Cornelissen, 1998). Fairburn and Brownell (2002) posited that the antiobesity sentiment originates in the Euro-American ideal of individualism in which the bad situations in which people find themselves are the result of their own doing. There is a widespread myth that obesity is the result of personal failings and a lack of self-discipline, although scientific evidence suggests that body weight is determined by a complex interaction of biological and environmental factors that are at best only partially controlled by the individual. There is also evidence that the greater the degree of deviation from the socially perceived ideal body weight, the greater the degree of stigmatization, suggesting that the more obese a person becomes the more he or she is stigmatized (Swami et al., 2008).

Mental illnesses can also influence body image, and yet many healthcare professionals overlook this aspect of chronic mental illness. For instance, a person with schizophrenia may have a negatively altered body image as part of the disturbed thinking caused by the illness and/or from the perceived change the illness has on the behaviour and presentation of the person. Furthermore, the medication used to treat schizophrenia can affect body image because of its neurological side effects (movement disorders), weight gain, and sexual dysfunction. Therefore, ignoring the potential side effects in treating individuals with mental illness is likely to affect not only medication compliance but also physical self-image.

External changes and their rapidity of change are important in assessing body image. Healthcare professionals should not assume, but verify with the client, what the current body image is and what it means to the client. Each person is unique, and therefore each experience with chronic illness and its impact on body image is unique.

Appearance

The physical appearance of a disease is frequently a change for which clients are unprepared. Given the possibility of perseverance, reformulation, or rejection of changes, further studies are needed of the ways in which body image and its accompanying variables affect acceptance by others. Empirical evidence and anecdotal data exist to guide us in considering suitable interventions. For example, when appearance also draws attention to a disease's underlying cause, clients and their significant others are often ostracized, particularly when the disease is one that carries a stigma. Many clients with AIDS develop Kaposi's sarcoma, a common and sometimes disfiguring tumour related to HIV. Because the skin is a common site for Kaposi's sarcoma, the characteristic purple hue of Kaposi's sarcoma is easily visible and is considered by many patients as a "public signa-ture" of HIV (deMoore, Hennessey, Kunz, Fer-rando, & Rabkin, 2000). In more severe cases of illness, in which the body is catastrophically de-bilitated, as in amyotrophic lateral sclerosis, Helman (1995) noted that the entire body image may accommodate the body as separated from the sense of self—that is, "It is my body that is diseased, but not me."

Visibility and Invisibility

Chronic illness and its treatment provide visible, outward changes in appearance and invisible, internal changes. Both types of change can sig-nificantly affect individuals' perceptions of themselves. In an adult it is suggested the more visible or extensive the body alteration, the more likely it is to be perceived as a threat to one's body image. Loss of hair, scarring, edema, amputations, and disfigurement are common examples in the body image literature. In reading the life accounts of severely disfig-ured persons, many choose to work at unusual times (nights) and in jobs in which they have lit-tle contact with others. In a meta-analysis of 12 articles that met their inclusion criteria, Bessel and Moss (2007) reported that truly efficacious interventions are lacking for adults with visible differences in appearance. In a related study, Thompson and Kent (2001) reported that per-sons with disfigurements shape their self-image by interactions with others in social contexts and that interventions are available. Like Bessel and Moss, they noted reports and interventions were not methodologically rigorous or informed by theory.

In another study of patients with severe burns and their adjustment to disfigurement,

Thombs and colleagues (2008) found that over time women, more than men, suffered dissatis-faction with body image, particularly with larger burns, and that their dissatisfaction inter-fered with psychological functioning over time. The findings of these studies argue a need for more research of a longitudinal and qualitative nature, toward a better understanding of the pro-cesses and outcomes of visible differences and their impact on body image.

The matter of body image and incorpora-tion of changes seems to be more ambiguous in children. Children are strongly subject to the norms imposed by their peers, with their self-image being readily influenced. A visible change or disfigurement in a child could ostracize the child from his or her peer group. Of particular strength and importance to children, especially for those with "stigmatized" body images, are the family members or healthcare professionals who can support the child's acceptance of the body image changes. Puberty is one time of life in normal development in which personal iden-tity and body image are strongly affected. It is during this time then that parents and adults who work with children should support healthy body images and intervene when a child begins to de-velop poor body images (see, for example, Fornari & Dancyge, 2006). The diagnosis of a chronic illness, with or without visible body changes, can profoundly affect the adolescent at this vulnerable time in his or her life.

When a change is not markedly visible, as when an ostomy is created or its treatment (e.g., colostomy appliances) is introduced, persons with chronic illness must take previously "invis-ible" body parts and make them "visible" (Hel-man, 1995). This dynamic is further compounded when the new intervention is preferentially hidden from others. Such procedures and the management of visible and hidden change likely lead to dramatic changes in an individual's lifestyle and self-image. For example, clients with a stoma must periodically empty the appliance bag, learn to change it, irrigate the stoma when needed, cope with social matters such as dressing to fit the appliance, and manage social etiquette with problems of leaking, odours, and the noises resulting from involuntary discharge into the appliance. The person dealing with such challenges may keep this hidden and limit social functioning to avoid possible embarrassment (Kirkpatrick, 1986). Nonetheless, the visibility or invisibility of an illness, injury, or treatment regimen must be managed, and in that management exists the potential to enhance or diminish body images held by the individual.

Functional Limitations

Functionality is something conceptualized as "external," in that functionality is usually a visible part of enactment of one's role—though some functions, such as sexual function, are carried out privately. Function is the ability of a body part to conduct its usual purpose. The ability to function in a meaningful way is essential to a sense of well-being; consequently, any limitation of functional ability may alter one's concept of body image. Most clients and their significant others are not prepared for the appearance and functional limitations associated with chronic illness.

The function of a body part and its importance and visibility are critical to one's body image. The leg, because of its functional importance in mobility and a person's life, is more likely to be a more important part of body image than, say, a toe (Brown, 1977). Loss of a toe, for example, is likely to be viewed as less problematic than loss of a leg, because more function can be retained by compensatory body parts and also because a toe is less visible. Therefore, one might expect different accommodations in body image to such amputations, even as it is recognized that perception of loss and its impact vary from person to person and culture to culture.

The roles of worker, gendered persona, and sexual being are three important facets of body image. Chronic illness or treatment can threaten the client's ability to perform each of these roles. Furthermore, the stage of one's life can make a major difference in the perception of the strength of the threat or its incorporation into one's body image. A teenager, perhaps, is likely to regard work or sexual function and his or her concomitant body image differently from a seasoned elder who has had different experiences and, usually, changed body appearance and function.

Loss of sexual function for most persons, particularly those who are sexually active, is often perceived as a profound loss. Women with breast removal from cancer or men and women with genital cancers frequently avoid sexual situations after treatments (Golden & Golden, 1986). The male client may feel especially vulnerable if he believes sexuality or provider role is compromised by chronic illness. Testicular cancer is the most common cancer in young men ages 18 to 35 and typically results in the removal of the diseased testicle. Older men with prostate cancer may require the removal of both testicles, with a resultant loss of libido and virility and compromised perception of "manhood."

Although implants can be used, the perception of functional loss can strongly persist. The nurse can be, and may often be, the main source of professional support and education and thus can assist clients with the sensitive issues involved with body image.

INTERVENTIONS

Interventions, particularly those of assessment, have been described throughout this chapter. Interventions are used to help clients manage their own reactions and the reactions of others to changes in body structure, function, or appearance as the result of chronic illness. These changes are frequently interpreted as setting one apart and as different from one's peers, leading to self-doubt, inhibited participation in social activities, and a disruption of perceptions of self. Finding appropriate interventions for clients experiencing an altered body image can aid the client in healing and adapting to changes in body image (Norris, Connell, & Spelic, 1998).

Adapting to changes in body image resulting from chronic illness is a dynamic process. On a daily basis clients are faced with thoughts and reminders of their illness and changes to their bodies. During periods of exacerbation, remission, and rehabilitation, clients are grieving the loss of their former selves, living with the uncertainty of their chronic illness, and learning to create new images of self (Cohen, Kahn, & Steeves, 1998). Knowing the process is continually changing, with steps forward and backward, helps the nurse to support clients as they adapt to changes in body image.

Interventions are chosen after careful assessment of the client. As mentioned previously,

a therapeutic relationship with the client is an essential beginning to the process. Before successful intervention can occur the following must be addressed: acknowledgment of barriers to communication, feelings about the illness, changes the illness caused, and personal biases on the part of the healthcare professional. Accurate knowledge about the disease process and the client's response are also necessary if the healthcare professional is to assist the client. In addition, the healthcare professional must be able to recognize that body image changes require a supportive, accepting, and consistent relationship that can withstand setbacks and emotional tension. It is important to be aware of the client's attitude and participation in the recovery process. This may involve professional rehabilitation, including physical and occupational therapy, or it may involve informal self- or family-directed interventions. The healthcare professional who is knowledgeable about evidence-informed practice, guidelines, and treatment regimens can be influential in acknowledging subtle progress that the client may or may not be aware of and supporting the benefit of rehabilitation as part of the overall recovery process. Through evidence-informed practice the knowledgeable healthcare professional can provide not only quality care in the chronic illness, but also begin helping the client toward forming a more balanced and realistic body image.

Communication

Providing opportunities for clients to express feelings and thoughts about the changes they are experiencing can be beneficial to both clients and healthcare professionals. It allows clients to speak and be heard and also allows careful assessment of the clients' thoughts and feelings. Assumptions should not be made about the meaning of experiences relating to changes in body image (Cohen et al., 1998). In addition, ensuring client comfort in expressing both positive and negative feelings and emotions helps strengthen the therapeutic relationship and facilitate the journey to wholeness. Allowing family members to express their thoughts, feelings, and concerns is also beneficial and should be incorporated into the recovery process.

Talk therapy, either individual or group, can be of much benefit in the recovery process. Cognitive-behavioural therapy has a proven record—that is, it is evidence-informed practice—in helping clients change their dysfunctional thinking and related behaviours associated with chronic illness and negative body image (Peterson et al., 2004; Rumsey & Harcourt, 2004; Rybarczyk & Behel, 2002; Veale, 2004).

There is some evidence that healthcare professionals who have had similar life experiences may be perceived as more credible sources of information and inspiration to clients experiencing difficulty coping with illnesses. In the substance abuse treatment system, providers often are in recovery themselves. In a qualitative study of self-perceptions of obesity, Thomas, Mosely, Stallings, Nichols-English, and Wagner (2008) found that obese women overwhelmingly preferred to work with healthcare professionals who had experienced weight problems themselves over those who were thin and had not had the personal experience of being overweight. The degree of self-disclosure by healthcare professionals is a matter governed by boundary considerations and personal choice; however, some degree of self-disclosure to those suffering from body image difficulties may enhance communication.

Self-Help Groups

Self-help groups for clients experiencing body image changes may help to buffer the stressors created by the changes. Providing clients with opportunities to share experiences with others in similar situations can be therapeutic for some individuals. Self-help or support groups offer important emotional, social, and spiritual fellowship as well as education about the focus of the support group. Before encouraging support groups as an intervention, it is important to assess the willingness of individuals to participate in a group setting. Support groups that are most helpful are those where the members are encouraged, but not forced, to share information and where the leader can lead the discussions to bring out salient points intelligently, empathetically, and fairly. Groups should be avoided that are unstable, promote products or purchases, or that charge inordinate fees. Groups that encourage gripe sessions, allow individuals to dominate a discussion, or that demand cult-like allegiances or sharing of information clients do not wish to share should also be avoided (Centers for Disease Control and Prevention, 2008).

Some individuals are not comfortable in a group setting, especially when they are dealing with a body image disruption. For those who find it helpful, the benefits are many. Seeing others on the road to recovery, helping those who are struggling, developing friendships, or finding where they themselves are in the journey can help with the healing process (Corey & Corey, 1997). Furthermore, these groups provide an opportunity for clients to begin socializing with others in a safe and nonthreatening environment.

Evidence-Informed Practice Box

Many women in all age groups harbour negative body images, especially related to weight and the self-perception of physical attractiveness (Frederick, Peplau, & Lever, 2006). Women suffer low self-esteem and even depression as a result of a negative body image. Arbour and Ginis (2008) recognized that exercise can positively influence body image and that walking was one of the most acceptable physical activities for adult women across the lifespan. Because of the multiple demands of family and home to women, they are particularly attracted to "lifestyle activity" as an exercise regimen. Lifestyle activities are those that can be incorporated into everyday life with minimal disruption. Arbour and Ginis (2008) conducted a randomized clinical trial to examine whether walking as a lifestyle activity, measured in the number of steps recorded on a pedometer during an 11-week period, would mediate change in the body image of previously sedentary women.

The women who participated and completed the assigned activities of the study were largely White and middle aged. In the control group ($n = 25$) the women simply self-monitored steps daily using a pedometer, whereas the experimental group ($n = 17$) monitored their steps but also developed an action plan. Defined as self-regulatory strategies that entail formation of strong mental associations between a situational cue and a specific behavioural response, action plans assist motivated individuals to generate specific regimens to move good intentions into actual behaviour (Gollwitzer, 1999).

Using the Adult Body Satisfaction Questionnaire (ABSQ), Arbour and Ginis measured two subscales of the ABSQ that represented two aspects of body image they speculated could be influenced by exercise. These included satisfaction with physical functioning and satisfaction with physical appearance. Measurements were done during the 1st and the 11th week of the intervention. The ABSQ is considered a reliable instrument to measure body image with an alpha of 0.85 in this study. Steps were measured using a standard pedometer.

Post-testing verified the intervention (action planning) predicted the mediator (the number of steps), which in turn was associated with higher scores on the satisfaction with physical functioning subscale of the ABSQ. Analysis indicated that 41% of the effect of the intervention on the satisfaction with physical functioning was mediated by the number of steps taken. However, results did not support a similar relationship among the variables related to satisfaction with physical appearance.

The authors noted the benefits of this relatively simple yet effective activity-enhancing intervention. Thus, exercise not only positively influences physical health in women but may support aspects of a more positive body image.

Sources: Arbour and Ginis (2008), Frederick et al. (2006), and Gollwitzer (1999).

Spiegel and colleagues' (2008) research indicated that breast cancer patients who participated in a support group lived, on average, 18 months longer than those who did not belong to a support group. Subsequent research could not duplicate those findings, but women who have joined support groups have shown other benefits, primarily experiencing less depression, distress, anxiety, and pain and, importantly, obtaining information about their disease and its treatment.

In another survey of 367 women with advanced breast cancer, almost as many clients got their information from the Internet (39%) as from their doctors (42%) (Y-ME National Breast Cancer Organization, 2007). These data indicate that healthcare professionals must find more meaningful ways to convey needed information to this group of patients. Because of the findings on support groups and because of the needs of clients with breast cancer, support groups have found a place in therapeutic regimens. Almost all oncology centres can direct patients to such groups, as patients increasingly find them a useful adjunct and information site as they manage work, family, sexuality, and uncertain cancer prognoses.

Nurses and other healthcare professionals can locate a variety of support groups or can even begin one as a therapeutic intervention. The Internet is an excellent tool for locating support groups and the resources needed to begin or maintain support groups; there are also many web-based support groups. Nurses, by virtue of their place in the healthcare delivery system, are poised to address both physical and psychosocial needs of patients and are able to deliver information in helpful ways: Support groups are one intervention that nurses can develop to help patients meet their needs for information and emotional support.

Education and Anticipatory Guidance

This intervention is effective only when the client has indicated a readiness to learn. Knowledge of disease processes, information about symptoms, and methods of treatment are important educational topics for the client. In providing education it is important to consider the preferred learning style (e.g., visual, auditory, and/or practice) of the client (Cohen et al., 1998). The benefits of client education and anticipatory guidance should be stressed to stimulate and support the client's readiness to learn.

Self-Care

Encouraging clients to participate in the activities of daily living that are meaningful to them helps restore feelings of normalcy. Whether engaging in personal grooming activities, such as applying cosmetics, jewellery, or hair accessories, caring for one's self can be an effective intervention. Self-care helps the client incorporate the change in body image into the normal functioning of daily living. This intervention may also help the client become less sensitive to physical appearances and learn to manage everyday activities (Norris et al., 1998). Regular exercise can be helpful to improve body image as well as support physical health and function (Wetterhahn, Hanson, & Levy, 2002).

Prostheses

The oldest prosthesis known of is a large wooden toe that was found attached by leather thongs to the foot of an ancient Egyptian female mummy. This well-carved prosthesis, unhidden by a sandal, aided the woman in walking and maintaining balance ("A Ticklish Matter," 2007). Prostheses vary in sophistication and availability. Most healthcare professionals are familiar with prosthetic eyes, hearing aids, various "limbs" (e.g., hand, foot, leg, arm), or breast, penile, or testicular implants. In amputations the age of the client presents unusual concerns. The prosthetic hand, foot, or knee of a child, for example, may require, for the child's adequate social development, that the prosthetic stand up to repeated use in play—for example, in swimming, it must withstand the effects of water, sand, chlorine, and/or salt. Adults may wish to maintain a physically normal appearance and avoid the functional "hook" hand prosthesis. In older adults whose gait problems may be exacerbated by joint problems, the "fit" of a prosthesis, as in a hip replacement, is a special concern. The rehabilitation required after hip replacement is particularly necessary, and its success has much to do with subsequent body image improvement related to increased mobility.

Spinal cord injury has sparked research that focuses on current knowledge of spinal cord treatment, electrical stimulation, mechanisms of secondary damage, and possibilities for regeneration of nerves. Bioengineering, electric-powered prostheses, invasive and noninvasive sensors to control prostheses, and use of brain waves or pupillary contraction to power computers for communication are currently being used or being tested. Their success is a huge event for the affected person, and this specialized area of knowledge typically requires focus and specialization by healthcare professionals.

The use of prostheses and the unique technologies to power these prostheses will continue to expand in the future. It is important to understand the field of prosthetics requires knowledge about the illness as well as the care with which clients implement and maintain their prosthetics and the impact of prosthetics on body image.

SUMMARY

Body image, the physical aspect of self-concept, is closely linked with the concept of self-esteem. Disturbances of self-concept along with personal identity disturbance, chronic low self-esteem, and situational low self-esteem are considered part of what Carpenito-Moyet (2008) globally calls disturbed self-concept. Alterations in self-concept can occur from an immediate problem, such as sudden disfiguration from surgery or burns; from long-term changes resulting from disease processes, therapies, dietary and medication management; or from lifestyle changes or an uncertain future.

Defining characteristics of alterations in self-concept can be multiple: denial, withdrawal of the individual, refusal to be part of the care required, refusal to look at the body part involved or let immediate family look at it, refusal to discuss rehabilitation efforts, signs and symptoms of grieving, self-destructive behaviour such as alcohol or drug abuse, and hostility toward healthy individuals. One's sense of femininity or masculinity may also be threatened, which can lead to difficulty in sexual functioning, and, combined, these changes can lead to social anxiety, self-consciousness, and depression (Carpenito-Moyet, 2008; White, 2002).

Indications of improving body image include use of the affected body part, patients' willingness to touch the affected body part, their satisfaction with body appearance or body function, and their willingness to use strategies to adjust to their new status and changes in bodily appearance or function. These adjustments can occur with bodily changes that result from injury, surgery, or life trajectories (e.g. adolescence, aging) (Moorhead, Johnson, Maas, & Swanson, 2008). The ultimate therapeutic goal for patients is successful adaptation to their own body appearance and function, and we argue that the definition of success should be defined by the patients themselves and supported by the healthcare professional.

STUDY QUESTIONS

1. What are the general themes of body image discourse? How did this chapter help you in furthering the discussion or in understanding everyday concerns about body image?
2. What elements would you include in an educational intervention for a patient group with body image issues? Justify your choices.
3. Name three concepts related to body image and explain their relationship.
4. Describe how you would assess a client with a changed body image.
5. Discuss how age, gender, and culture can affect body image.
6. How often in your own friendships do issues of body image come up in conversation?

INTERNET RESOURCES

Canadian Obesity Network. Obesity Canada: www.obesitynetwork.ca
Dietitians of Canada-Body Image: www.dietitians.ca
Daily Strength Support Group Resource: www.dailystrength.com
Kids Health: http://kidshealth.org/parent/general/body/overweight_obesity.html
National Eating Disorder Information Centre: www.nedic.ca
U.S. Department of Health and Human Services, Women's Health: http://womenshealth.gov/
Weight-control Information Network: www.win.niddk.nih.gov/publications/health_risks.htm

For a full suite of assignments and additional learning activities, use the access code located in the front of your book and visit this exclusive website: **http://go.jblearning.com/kramer-kile**. If you do not have an access code, you can obtain one at the site.

REFERENCES

A ticklish matter: Photograph and caption. (2007, July 28). *Pittsburgh Post-Gazette.*

Ahmad, S., Waller, G., & Verduyn, C. (1994). Eating attitudes and body satisfaction among Asian and Caucasian adolescents. *Journal of Adolescence, 17,* 461–470.

Altabe, M. (1998). Ethnicity and body image: Quantitative and qualitative analysis. *International Journal of Eating Disorders, 23,* 153–159.

Arbour, K., & Ginis K. (2008). Improving body image one step at a time: Greater pedometer step counts produce greater body image improvements. *Body Image, 5,* 331–336.

Bello, L., & McIntire, S. (1995). Body image disturbance in young adults with cancer. *Cancer Nursing, 18*(2), 138–143.

Bessel, A., & Moss, T. P. (2007). Evaluating the effectiveness of psychosocial interventions for individuals with visible differences: A systematic review of the empirical literature. *Body Image, 4*(3), 227–238.

Blanke, O. (2007). I and me: Self-portraiture in brain damage. *Frontiers of Neurology and Neuroscience, 22,* 14–29.

Bottamini, G., & Ste-Marie, D. (2006). Male voices on body image. *International Journal of Men's Health, 5*(2), 109–132.

Brown, M. S. (1977). The nursing process and distortions or changes in body image. In F. L. Bower (Ed.), *Distortions in body image in illness and disability* (pp. 1–19). New York, NY: Wiley.

Byely, L., Archibald, A., Graber, J., & Brooks-Gunn, J. (1999). A prospective study of familial and social influences on girls' body image and dieting. *International Journal of Eating Disorders, 28,* 155–164.

Campos, P. (2005). *The diet myth: Why America's obsession with weight is hazardous to your health.* New York, NY: Gotham.

Carpenito-Moyet, L. (2008). *Handbook of nursing diagnosis* (12th ed.). Philadelphia, PA: Lippincott Williams & Wilkins.

Cash, T. F. (2002). Cognitive behavioral perspectives on body image. In T. Cash & T. Pruzinsky (Eds.), *Body image: A handbook of theory, research, and clinical progress* (pp. 38–46). New York, NY: Guilford Press.

Cash, T. F., & Fleming, E. C. (2002). The impact of body image experiences: Development of the body image quality of life inventory. *International Journal of Eating Disorders, 31*, 455–460.

Cash, T. F., & Pruzinsky, T. (1990). *Body images: Development, deviance, and change.* New York, NY: Guilford Press.

Cash, T. F., & Pruzinsky, T. (2002). Understanding body image: Historical and contemporary perspectives. In T. Cash & T. Pruzinsky (Eds.), *Body image: A handbook of theory, research, and clinical progress* (pp. 30–37). New York, NY: Guilford Press.

Cash, T., & Pruzinsky, T. (2004). *Body image: A handbook of theory, research, and clinical practice.* New York, NY: Guilford Press.

Cash, T. F., Theirault, J., & Annis, N. M. (2004). Body image in an interpersonal context: Adult attachment, fear of intimacy and social anxiety. *Journal of Social and Clinical Psychology, 23*(1), 89–103.

Centers for Disease Control and Prevention. (2008). Chronic fatigue syndrome: Support groups. Retrieved from http://www.cdc.gov/cfs/-general/treatment/options.html

Cohen, M. Z., Kahn, D. L., & Steeves, R. H. (1998). Beyond body image: The experience of breast cancer. *Oncology Nursing Forum, 25*(5), 835–841.

Corey, M., & Corey, G. (1997). *Groups: Process and practice* (5th ed.). Boston, MA: Brooks/Cole.

Corwyn, R. F. (2000). The factor structure of global self-esteem among adolescents and adults. *Journal of Research and Personality, 34*, 357–379.

Davis, C., & Katzman, M. A. (1998). Chinese men and women in the United States and Hong Kong: Body and self esteem ratings as a prelude to dieting and exercise. *International Journal of Eating Disorders, 23,* 99–102.

deMoore, G. M., Hennessey, P., Kunz, N. M., Ferrando, S. J., & Rabkin, J. G. (2000). Kaposi's sarcoma: The scarlet letter of AIDS. The psychological effects of a skin disease. *Psychosomatics, 41*(4), 360–363.

Didie, E., Kuniega-Pietrzak, T., & Phillips, K. (2010). Body image in patients with body dysmorphic disorder: Evaluations of and investment in appearance, health, illness, and fitness. *Body Image, 7,* 66–69.

Dropkin, M. J. (1989). Coping with disfigurement and dysfunction after head and neck cancer surgery: A conceptual framework. *Seminars in Oncology Nursing, 5*(3), 213–219.

Emslie, C., Hunt, K., & Macintyre, S. (2001). Perceptions of body image among working men and women. *Epidemiology and Community Health, 55*, 406–407.

Erikson, E. (1963). *Childhood and society* (2nd ed.). New York, NY: Norton.

Fairburn, C., & Brownell K. (2002). *Eating disorders and obesity: A comprehensive handbook* (2nd ed.). New York, NY: Guilford Press.

Feusner, J., Yaryura-Tobias, J., & Saxena, S. (2008). The pathophysiology of body dysmorphic disorder. *Body Image, 5,* 3–12.

Fisher, S. (1986). *Development and structure of the body image* (Vol. 2). Hillsdale, NJ: Lawrence Erlbaum Associates.

Flegal, K. M., Graubard, B. I., Williamson, D. F., & Gail, M. H. (2007). Cause-specific excess deaths associated with underweight, overweight, and obesity. *Journal of the American Medical Association, 298*(17), 2028–2037.

Fornari, V., & Dancyge, I. F. (2006). Physical and cognitive changes associated with puberty. In T. Jaffa & B. McDermott (Eds.), *Eating disorders in children and adolescents* (pp. 57–69). Cambridge, England: Cambridge University Press.

Frederick, D. A, Lever, J., & Peplau, L. A. (2007). Interest in cosmetic surgery and body image: Views of men and women across the lifespan. *Plastic & Reconstructive Surgery, 120*(5), 1407–1415.

Frederick, D., Peplau, L., & Lever, J. (2006). The swimsuit issue: Correlates of body image in a sample of 52,677 heterosexual adults. *Body Image, 4,* 413–419.

Galagher, S. (2005). Dynamic models of body shematic processes. In H. De Preester & V. Knockaret (Eds.), *Body image and body schemas: Advances in consciousness research* (Vol. 62, pp. 233–250). Amsterdam, Netherlands: John Benjamins.

Gittelsohn, J., Harris, B. S., Thorne-Lyman, A. L., Hanley, A. J., Barnie, A., & Zimman, B. (1996). Body image concepts differ by age and sex in an Ojibway-Cree community in Canada. *Journal of Nutrition, 120*(12), 2990–3000.

Golden, J. S., & Golden, M. (1986). Cancer and sex. In J. M. Vaeth (Ed.), *Body image, self-esteem, and sexuality in cancer patients* (2nd ed., pp. 68–76). Basel, Switzerland: Karger.

Gollwitzer, P. (1999). Implementation intentions: Strong effects of simple plans. *American Psychologist, 54,* 493–503.

Hallinan, C. (1988). Muslim and Judaic-Christian perceptions of desirable body shape. *Perceptions and Motor Skills,* 67, 80–82.

Hayslip, B., Cooper, C. C., Dougherty, L. M., & Cook, D. D. (1997). Body image in adulthood: A projective approach. *Journal of Personality Assessment, 68*(3), 628–649.

Helman, C. G. (1995). The body image in health and disease: Exploring patients' maps of body and self. *Patient Education and Counseling, 26,* 169–175.

Jackson, L. A. (2002). Physical attractiveness: A sociocultural perspective. In T. Cash & T. Pruzinsky (Eds.), *Body image: A handbook of theory, research, and clinical progress* (pp. 13–21). New York, NY: Guilford Press.

Kearney-Cooke, A. (2002). Familial influences on body image development. In T. Cash & T. Pruzinsky (Eds.), *Body image: A handbook of theory, research, and clinical progress* (pp. 99–107). New York, NY: Guilford Press.

Kirkpatrick, J. R. (1986). The stoma patient and his return to society. In J. M. Vaeth (Ed.), *Body image, self-esteem, and sexuality in cancer patients* (2nd ed., pp. 24–27). Basel, Switzerland: Karger.

Krauss-Whitbourne, S., & Skultety, K. (2002). Body image development: Adulthood and aging. In T. Cash & T. Pruzinsky (Eds.), *Body image: A handbook of theory, research, and clinical progress* (pp. 83–90). New York, NY: Guilford Press.

Krueger, D. W. (2002). Psychodynamic perspectives on body image. In T. Cash & T. Pruzinsky (Eds.), *Body image: A handbook of theory, research, and clinical progress* (pp. 30–37). New York, NY: Guilford Press.

Lewis, J. (1983). *Something hidden: A biography of Wilder Penfield.* Halifax, Nova Scotia: Goodread Biographies.

Lowes, J., & Tiggemann, M. (2003). Body dissatisfaction, dieting awareness, and the impact of parental influence in young children. *British Journal of Health Psychology, 8,* 135.

Markus, H., & Wurf, E. (1987). The dynamic self-concept: A social psychological perspective. *Annual Review of Psychology,* 38, 299–337.

McCabe, M., & Ricciardelli, P., & Lina A. (2005). A prospective study of pressures from parents, peers, and the media on extreme weight change behaviours among adolescent boys and girls. *Behaviour Research and Therapy, 43,* 653–668.

McKinley, N. M. (1999). Women and objectified body consciousness: Mothers and daughters body experiences in cultural, developmental and familial context. *Developmental Psychology, 35,* 760–769.

Mock, V. (1993). Body image in women treated for breast cancer. *Nursing Research, 42*(3), 153–157.

Moorhead, S., Johnson, M., Maas, M., & Swanson, E. (Eds.). (2008). *Nursing outcomes classification (NOC)* (4th ed.). St. Louis, MO: Mosby.

Mueller, S. (2007–2008). Amputee envy. *Scientific American Mind, 18*(6), 60–65.

Nezlek, J. B. (1999). Body image and day-to-day social interaction. *Journal of Personality, 67*(5), 793–817.

Norris, J., Connell, M. K., & Spelic, S. S. (1998). A grounded theory of reimaging. *Advances in Nursing Science, 20*(3), 1–12.

Ogden, C., Flegal, K., Carroll, M., & Johnson, C. (2000). Prevalence and trends in overweight among US children and adolescents, 1999–2000. *Journal of the American Medical Association, 288,* 1728–1732.

Olivardia, R., Pope, H. J., & Hudson, J. I. (2000). Muscle dysmorphia in male weightlifters: A case control study. *American Journal of Psychiatry, 157,* 1291–1296.

Olmsted, M. P., & McFarlane, T. (2004). Report: Body weight and body Image. *BMC Women's Health 2004, 4*(Suppl. 1), 1–9.

Orr, D. A., Reznikoff, M., & Smith, G. M. (1989). Body image, self-esteem, and depression in burn-injured adolescents and young adults. *Journal of Burn Care and Rehabilitation, 10*(5), 454–461.

Peelen, M., & Downing, P. E. (2007). The neural basis of visual body perception. *Nature Reviews Neuroscience, 8*(8), 636–648.

Peterson, C. B., Wimmer, S., Ackard, D. M., Crosby, R., Cavanagh, L. C., Engbloom, S., & Mitchell, J. E. (2004). Changes in body image during cognitive-behavioral treatment in women with bulimia nervosa. *Body Image, 1*(2), 139–153.

Phillips, K., & Hollander, E. (2008). Treating body dysmorphic disorder with medication: Evidence, misperceptions, medication, and a suggested approach. *Body Image, 5,* 3–12.

Phipps, S. A., Burton, P. S., Osberg, L. S., & Lethbridge, L. N. (2006). Poverty and the extent of child obesity in Canada, Norway and the United States. *Obesity Reviews, 7*, 5–12.

Pruzinsky, T. (2002). Body image adaptation to reconstructive surgery for acquired disfigurement. In T. Cash & T. Pruzinsky (Eds.), *Body image: A handbook of theory, research, and clinical progress* (pp. 440–449). New York, NY: Guilford Press.

Pruzinsky, T. (2004). Enhancing quality of life in medical populations: A vision for body image assessment and rehabilitation as standards of care. *Body Image, 1*, 71–81.

Ramachandran, V. S. (2004). *A brief tour of human consciousness*. New York, NY: Pearson Education.

Ramachandran, V. S., & Rogers-Ramachandran, D. (2007). It's all done with mirrors. *Scientific American Mind, 18*(4), 16–18.

Rumsey, N. (2002). Body image and congenital conditions with visible differences. In T. Cash & T. Pruzinsky (Eds.), *Body image: A handbook of theory, research, and clinical progress* (pp. 226–233). New York, NY: Guilford Press.

Rumsey, N., & Harcourt, D. (2004). Body image and disfigurement: Issues and interventions. *Body Image, 1*, 83–97.

Rybarczyk, B., & Behel, J. (2002). Rehabilitation medicine and body image. In T. Cash & T. Pruzinsky (Eds.), *Body image: A handbook of theory, research, and clinical progress* (pp. 387–394). New York, NY: Guilford Press.

Schilder, P. (1950). *The image and appearance of the human body*. New York, NY: International Universities Press.

Spiegel D., Butler L. D., Giese-Davis J., Koopman C., Miller E., Dimiceli S., . . . Carlson, R. W. (2008). Reply to effects of supportive-expressive group therapy on survival of patients with metastatic breast cancer: A randomized prospective trial. *Cancer, 112*(2), 444.

Striegel-Moore, R., & Franko, D. (2002). Body image issues among girls and women. In T. Cash & T. Pruzinsky (Eds.), *Body image: A handbook of theory, research, and clinical progress* (pp. 183–191). New York, NY: Guilford Press.

Swami, V., Furnham, A., Amin, R., Chaudri, J., Jundi, S., Miller, R., . . . Tovee, M. J. (2008). Lonelier, lazier, and teased: The stigmatizing effect of body size. *Journal of Social Psychology, 148*(5), 577–593.

Swami, V., & Tovee, M. (2005). Female physical attractiveness in Britain and Malaysia: A cross cultural study. *Body Image, 2*, 115–128.

Thomas, A., Mosely, G., Stallings, R., Nichols-English, G., & Wagner, P. (2008). Perceptions of obesity. Black and white differences. *Journal of Cultural Diversity, 15*(4), 174–180.

Thombs, B. D., Notes, L. D., Lawrence, J. W., Magyar-Russell, G., Bresnick, M. G., Faurerbach, J. A. (2008). From survival to socialization: A longitudinal study of body image in survivors of severe burn injury. *Journal of Psychosomatic Research, 64*(2), 205–212.

Thompson, A., & Kent, G. (2001). Adjusting to disfigurement: Process involved in dealing with being visibly different. *Clinical Psychology Review, 21*(5), 663–682.

Thompson, J., & Gardner, R. (2002). Measuring perceptual body image in adolescents and adults. In T. Cash & T. Pruzinsky (Eds.), *Body image: A handbook of theory, research, and clinical progress* (pp. 142–154). New York, NY: Guilford Press.

Thompson, J., & Van Den Berg, P. (2002). Measuring body image attitudes among adolescents and adults. In T. Cash & T. Pruzinsky (Eds.), *Body image: A handbook of theory, research, and clinical progress* (pp. 155–162). New York, NY: Guilford Press.

Tovee, M., Reinhardt, S., Emery, J., & Cornelissen, P. (1998). Optimum body mass index and maximum sexual attractiveness. *Lancet, 352*, 548.

Trembley, M., & Willms, J. D. (2000). Secular trends in the body mass index of Canadian children. *Canadian Medical Association Journal, 163*, 1429–1433.

Van Deusen, J. (1993). *Body image and perceptual dysfunction in adults*. Philadelphia, PA: W. B. Saunders.

Veale, D. (2004). Advances in cognitive behavioural model of body dysmorphic disorder. *Body Image, 1*(1), 113–125.

Wetterhahn, K., Hanson, C., & Levy, C. (2002). Effect of participation in physical activity on body image of amputees. *American Journal of Physical Medicine and Rehabilitation, 81*(3), 194–201.

White, C. A. (2002). Body image issues in oncology. In T. Cash & T. Pruzinsky (Eds.), *Body image: A handbook of theory, research, and clinical progress* (pp. 379–386). New York, NY: Guilford Press.

Wright, L., & Leahey, M. (2000). *Nurses and families: A guide to family assessment and intervention* (3rd ed.). Philadelphia, PA: F.A. Davis.

Y-ME National Breast Cancer Organization. (2007). Survey underscores importance of emotional, educational needs among women with advanced breast cancer. Retrieved from http://www.sciencedaily.com/releases/2007/12/071216104300.htm

CHAPTER 8

Quality of Life

Original chapter by Victoria Schirm
Canadian content added by Marnie L. Kramer-Kile

INTRODUCTION

This chapter focuses on quality of life for individuals and their families who live with chronic illness around the world. Though the financial burden of chronic disease is great, the cost to the quality of life of people living with a chronic condition is immeasurable (Canadian Nurses Association, 2005). Nursing research throughout the world is at the forefront of developing nursing interventions for clients and their families that seek to understand and promote quality of life. The Canadian Nurses Association asks nurses to promote quality of life for clients living with chronic conditions by developing primary healthcare frameworks that focus on promoting health, collaborating with clients and their families, ensuring appropriate services are available, becoming aware of other therapeutic modalities that may be outside of the biomedical framework of care (i.e., complementary therapies), considering wider influences on health such as social determinants of health, and advocating for increased preventative care measures.

Nurses can achieve this through nursing research and the implementation of practice changes. This chapter includes theoretical conceptualizations and clinical research findings that demonstrate the unique contribution of nursing in assessment, intervention, and outcomes evaluation of quality of life in chronic illness.

Nursing practice and nursing research are well positioned to meet the challenge of identifying, testing, and applying interventions that promote quality of life for survivors of acute illness who are living with a chronic condition. Applying research findings to an individual's quality of life enables nurses and other healthcare professionals in clinical practice to plan and deliver evidence-informed care. Nursing interventions guided by the best available evidence can then be individualized to the values and preferences of the client, thereby ensuring better adherence to a plan that must be a lifelong commitment. Client participation in clinical decision making about the effect that treatments may have on quality of life can be used to monitor therapy over the long term.

Quality of life evaluations can also be used to scrutinize the appropriateness of treatments and show progress toward attainment of treatment goals and responses to therapy. Objective knowledge about desired treatment outcomes for chronic illness that incorporate quality of life domains (improved health and function, pain and symptom control, or prolonged life) can be considered against expected, negative treatment effects such as financial burdens, anxiety, and disrupted lives.

Quality of life assessments provide a way to evaluate the impact of chronic illness on clients and their families. The complex interrelationships of the associated burdens of chronic illness are appreciated more fully when the client's overall quality of life is known. In chronic illness research, quality of life is studied to identify and evaluate specific problems and needs of clients with illness or disability. In the larger arena of the healthcare system, quality of life evaluations are used to monitor the extent to which delivered services address client needs. Outcomes that promote quality of life are valued, particularly when positive results are achieved with efficiency and cost savings. This chapter demonstrates that managing the effects of chronic illness and enhancing quality of life is a multifaceted, complex endeavour.

DEFINING QUALITY OF LIFE _____

Defining quality of life has never been easy. Each individual's unique circumstances and experiences shape quality of life, and this subjective component is an important defining element in quality of life. At the same time objective indicators of what constitutes quality of life are needed to assess outcomes. The general or global meaning of quality of life and an overall sense of well-being may be anchored to an individual's social and economic conditions, living arrangements, and community environment as well as to culture, personal values, happiness, life satisfaction, and spiritual well-being.

The more specific health-related quality of life generally refers to perceived physical and mental health over time. Healthcare providers typically use quality of life measures to learn about an individual's illness and its effect on daily life. In the public health arena quality of life is evaluated to identify and track different population groups. This information can aid in supporting policies and in developing interventions that enhance quality of life (Centers for Disease Control and Prevention, 2010a).

Regardless of whether one is referring to global quality of life or health-related quality of life, the subjective or individual perspective is important to the definition. Rene Dubos's (1959, p. 228) definition addresses the subjective nature and the multidimensionality of quality of life:

> [People] naturally desire health and happiness. . . . The kind of health that [people] desire most is not necessarily a state in which they experience physical vigor and a sense of well-being, not even one giving them a long life. It is, instead, the condition best suited to reach goals that each individual formulates for [him- or herself].

The World Health Organization (WHO, 1948, p. 100) definition of health as "a state of complete physical, mental, and social well-being and not merely the absence of disease or infirmity" recognizes the multidimensionality of health that is inclusive of a personal evaluation of one's circumstances. Nurses and other healthcare professionals involved in chronic illness care have a stake in understanding distinctions and overlaps in quality of life, health-related quality of life, and self-perceived health.

CONCEPTUALIZING AND MEASURING QUALITY OF LIFE ____

The theoretical frameworks or models that influence the patient's and family's illness trajectory are key to understanding quality of life. Additionally, if increased or "better" quality of life is a patient outcome, the need to quantitatively measure quality of life is necessary.

Theoretical Frameworks

Theories, frameworks, or models in chronic illness explain the complex interrelationships among factors that influence the illness trajectory on quality of life. Such conceptualizations are important not only to generate new evidence for best nursing practice, but also to test and evaluate existing interventions that may affect quality of life in chronic illness. This section presents the literature on quality of life as a theoretical framework or conceptualization and quality of life as an outcome influenced by various factors depicted in an explanatory model. Examples from the nursing literature are given that use quality of life as a specific outcome of nursing interventions for persons with chronic illness.

Plummer and Molzahn (2009) conducted a critical appraisal of nursing theories to examine quality of life as embedded within theorists' original frameworks. They evaluated four attributes of quality of life as depicted by nurse theorists (Imogene King, Madeleine Leininger, Rosemarie Parse, Hildegard Peplau, and Martha Rogers): contextual, subjective, intangible, and health related. Plummer and Molzahn concluded there is merit in considering quality of

life as more useful to nursing than the term "health." In relation to nursing practice they proposed that quality of life is valuable because it considers connections between the intangible and subjective aspects of the client's environment. They recommended that further research be done to develop a better understanding of quality of life for differing client populations.

Naef and Bournes (2009) reviewed quality of life in a similar fashion, comparing and contrasting it with the lived experience of waiting. Their purpose was to derive knowledge for nursing practice and research. Although Naef and Bournes limited their study to clients awaiting lung transplantation, they concluded that the concept of waiting has commonalities with quality of life outcomes for other clients. To this end they noted the framework offers guidance to nursing practice as well as nursing research in that living in the context of waiting influences quality of life.

Understanding the theoretical underpinnings of quality of life in the context of chronic illness informs nursing research and nursing practice. For example, Weinert, Cudney, and Spring (2008) described their conceptual model of adaptation in chronic illness. Their evolving "women to women conceptual model for adaptation to chronic illness" consists of three constructs: environmental stimuli, psychosocial response, and illness management. Quality of life is a component of the model, defined and measured according to the WHO (1948) definition of physical health, psychological well-being, social relationships, and environment. The purpose of the model is to provide a conceptualization that increases understanding of adaptation to chronic illness and gives direction to development of appropriate nursing interventions. Weinert and colleagues noted that adaptation to chronic illness is related to psychosocial responses, self-management skills, and enhanced quality of life.

Some quality of life theoretical frameworks have been posited from an ethical perspective. Allmark (2005) suggested that ethical theories are relevant to answering moral questions, especially regarding issues of quality of life versus quantity of life. An ethical framework is useful in clinical nursing practice because it gives guidance to ways individuals' voices can be discerned, enhances development of decision making in routine clinical practice, and considers the client's beliefs, values, and preferences in the context of complex questions (Allmark, 2005).

Hirskyj (2007) considers ethical ramifications of resource allocations associated with the quality-adjusted life year (QALY) concept. QALY is an outcome measure that can be used to determine the efficacy of nursing care as measured by not only the quantity of life (length of life) but also the quality of life. The QALY framework provides a means to estimate and reveal client's values, beliefs, and preferences in relation to care outcomes. Although nurses may be hesitant to use formulas in providing holistic care, especially in the context of resource allocation, the QALY concept is supported by evidence that suggests better clinical outcomes are achieved with cost-effective care. QALY offers a systematic, evidence-informed model to practice nursing care and meet the individual needs of clients (Hirskyj, 2007). These frameworks provide a context in which to consider the ethical issues that surround quality of life outcomes in chronic illness.

Other researchers expanded the knowledge base and theory development in understanding quality of life in chronic illness by investigating

clients' priorities and perceptions. Carter, MacLeod, Brander, and McPherson (2004) found that clients' perspectives with regard to quality of life in terminal illness are important components. A framework that considers quality of life outcomes from clients' perspectives, as opposed to models developed by experts emphasizing a good death, can lead to interventions that are more client centred. For example, knowing that "being in charge" is more important to a dying person's quality of life than "having a good death" can support development of appropriate interventions that facilitate client control within the context of the illness.

Theoretical models have also been constructed to elicit variables that can significantly influence and predict quality of life for the many older adults who live with chronic illness (Low & Molzahn, 2007). Such models are helpful in understanding the complex interrelationships among physical functioning, perceived health, and emotional and mental well-being to quality of life as an outcome of nursing care. Low and Molzahn found that good health, financial stability, and meaning and purpose in life have substantial positive effects on the quality of life of older adults. This model provides conceptual links among several variables— financial resources, health, physical function, meaning and purpose in life, emotional support, and environment—to quality of life. The underpinnings of this model provide direction for improving the quality of life of older adults through development of nursing interventions that promote activities of daily living, provide emotional support, or enhance the environment.

The structure, process, and outcome framework originally developed by Donabedian (1988) to assess quality of healthcare delivery guided a randomized clinical trial of a discharge intervention for hospitalized older adults with hip fractures (Huang & Liang, 2005). A structured discharge plan that was systematically implemented by an advanced practice nurse was used to evaluate several outcomes, including quality of life, after hospital discharge of elders who had sustained a hip fracture as a result of a fall.

Suhonen, Välimäki, Katajisto, and Leino-Kilpi (2005) used a model of individualized nursing care to evaluate outcomes of satisfaction, autonomy, and health-related quality of life in hospitalized clients. This model testing demonstrated a positive association between clients' perceptions of care given by nurses and their ratings of satisfaction with care, ability to make decisions about care, and health-related quality of life. This affirmation of individualized nursing care as explicated in the model provides supporting data for evidence-informed nursing practice.

Saunders and Cookman (2005) explored the theoretical underpinnings of depression related to hepatitis C virus infection to gain a better understanding of quality of life in this client population where the illness is often chronic. The symptom experience, stigma associated with the illness, and uncertain illness trajectory were described as multidimensional components of hepatitis C–related depression. Saunders and Cookman proposed that the conceptualisation provides a model for developing nursing interventions that are likely to be effective for maximizing quality of life outcomes in this special population.

Theoretical frameworks also have been advanced to explain the changing dimensions of cancer care. Once viewed as an acute, life-limiting illness, cancer in most instances is now managed as a chronic illness. Cancer nursing with children is one area where the science

of nursing is embedded within the art of nursing practice (Cantrell, 2007). This conceptualization views quality of life as foundational to the experiences of children and adolescents with cancer. For good quality of life to be an outcome, the values, beliefs, and wishes of children and their families as well as the values and expertise of the oncology nurse must be acknowledged and applied with the best available scientific evidence. One without the other is not sufficient to produce health-related quality of life in paediatric oncology.

Clark (2004) used quality of life as the conceptual basis to determine how psychiatric nurses assess and provide care to clients with serious mental illness residing in community settings. Three themes emerged as ways in which quality of life influenced psychiatric nursing practice. One was that quality of life defined the goal of care in that it permeated everything nurses did. The second was that the nurse's concern for quality of life focused interventions on the person and away from the mental illness. The third theme was that quality of life formed the foundation of the nurse–client relationship, where the focus is the individual client's perspective as opposed to management of a disease or symptoms.

Measuring Quality of Life

As described in the previous section, theoretical frameworks provide a systematic approach to studying quality of life. Regardless of whether quality of life is conceptualized as a complex set of relationships that influence the chronic illness trajectory or as an outcome of the illness itself, an appropriate measure of quality of life is crucial. Valid and reliable measures are needed to capture accurately the elements or concepts that characterize quality of life. Quality of life has a subjective component as defined by the individual's unique situation that reflects happiness and life satisfaction (Centers for Disease Control and Prevention, 2010b). This general quality of life includes health as well as culture, values, beliefs, and environment. The more specific health-related quality of life is usually defined in relationship to health and physical function and emotional and mental well-being. Elements that contribute to the more general or global quality of life may not be considered in assessments about health-related quality of life. At the same time, reference to health-related quality of life may suggest illness or disease.

Nurses, in particular, have a stake in understanding the distinctions and the overlaps in the quality of life dimensions. When used as a framework, the dimensions of quality of life provide a context for assessing nursing's contribution to improved care outcomes for clients with chronic illness. In clinical practice nurses can use standardized quality of life assessments to plan, implement, and evaluate evidence-informed care for clients with chronic illnesses. Measurement is a first step in the process because accurate and appropriate assessment of symptom status has the potential for better care management and evaluation of nursing intervention effectiveness. To this end, Sousa, Ryu, Kwok, Cook, and West (2007) created a model and validated a measure to assess the impact of rheumatoid arthritis on quality of life. They found two factors, arthritic pain and general symptoms, to be confirmatory and predictive of quality of life evaluations. They surmised that nursing interventions aimed at assessing pain and managing overall symptoms have the most potential to enhance quality of life and function for individuals with rheumatoid arthritis.

The SF-36-v2 (1999) is a multipurpose short-form health survey that contains 36 questions addressing functional health and well-being as well as physical and mental health (a link to this form is provided at the end of the chapter). Respondents to the survey are asked to rate their perceptions of their health, reflect on how their current health influences their abilities to carry out activities, rate how their health influences their abilities to maintain relationships and interact with others, and assess if pain is interfering with their ability to carry out their functional roles or ability to interact with others. The SF-36-v2 is frequently used by nurse researchers as an indicator for quality of life measures. It has been found to detect changes in health within general populations and is being increasingly used in research related to chronic illness. However, as with all survey tools, the SF-36-v2 does have some limitations. A frequent critique is that it does not question respondents about their sleep patterns and amount of sleep; it also does not question sexual health and functioning, which is also often conceptualized as an indicator for quality of life. To address these gaps it may be helpful for nurse researchers to follow up the SF-36-v2 with further research methods to acquire a more accurate picture of individuals' perceptions of their quality of life.

The WHO (2004) developed a standardized tool to measure quality of life and health from the individual's perspective. The WHO quality of life measure has 26 items that assess an individual's feelings of satisfaction and enjoyment with life, limitations due to pain, capacity for work, ability to perform activities of daily living and to get around, access to health care, and satisfaction with relationships. Both the SF-36-v2 and the WHO tools have the common objective to quantify and standardize measurement of quality of life. These tools are intended to measure health and well-being in healthy populations and to detect illness conditions that could benefit from early intervention and treatment.

Increasingly, nursing as a discipline has recognized that it too needs to focus on measurable outcomes related to interventions. The measurement of quality of life, including health-related quality of life, has become one such standardized assessment as an indicator for outcomes of nursing care. Quality of life determinations that use consistent measures provide an objective assessment of clients' care needs. Measures that include appropriate determinants that contribute to or influence quality of life can be used by nurses to give care based on the best available evidence.

CONTEXT OF QUALITY OF LIFE IN CHRONIC ILLNESS _____

Quality of life in chronic illness can be viewed within the context of health and functioning, psychological and spiritual well-being, societal roles, and economic status. These multiple dimensions provide a practical way to discuss the background that contributes to quality of life for individuals living with chronic illness. Considerable overlap exists amongst these components. For example, health and function are multifaceted and may include perceived health, energy level, pain experiences, stress levels, independence, capacity to meet responsibilities, access to and use of health care, and usefulness to others. This view of health and function together as a quality of life component shows that reliance on any one clinical parameter may not capture the client's overall picture of health and well-being. People with chronic illness may report a good perceived quality of life but clinically have objective symptoms.

Thus, knowledge of how symptoms affect clients' health and function can lead to a better understanding of their quality of life in chronic illness. Typically, the presence of symptoms prompts an individual to seek health care—for example, weakness and poor coordination in the individual with multiple sclerosis. In addition, people with chronic illness are subjected to symptoms from the iatrogenic effects of their treatments. Regardless of the origin, physically distressing symptoms affect health and function and, ultimately, one's quality of life. Moreover, symptoms and the distress they cause result in varying reports about health and function as perceived by clients. Healthcare professionals and family members sometimes report conflicting views about a person's health and function, thereby producing quality of life ratings that may differ. Treatment decisions may be impacted by such ratings, demonstrating the importance of using quality of life assessments that consider clients' perspectives of their health and function.

The complexity of health and function in chronic illness suggests that neither good health nor optimal function is a necessary or sufficient condition for quality of life. Psychological and spiritual components are part of quality of life and include intangibles such as happiness, peace of mind, and a belief system. Considerable overlap exists between psychological and spiritual well-being. Psychological well-being may be thought of as an essential component of quality of life that influences overall adjustment to chronic illness. More directly, spirituality has been advanced as an important element in quality of life measurement across different cultures (Moreira-Almeida & Koenig, 2006). At the same time caution is urged—spirituality is different from religiosity and from meaning in life, hope, and peace. Most definitions take into consideration that spirituality affects all aspects of a person's well-being. Persons living with a chronic illness sometimes must make significant life changes to maintain quality of life. For many individuals with chronic illness, there may be an increased reliance on psychological and spiritual resources and on the social and emotional support offered by friends and confidantes. Spirituality that included components of life satisfaction, less stress, and meaning in life was the basis for a study of women with cancer (López, McCaffrey, Griffin, & Fitzpatrick, 2009). For these women family activities, listening to music, and helping others were the most frequently used spiritual practices. López and colleagues concluded that it is beneficial to support women in their ongoing spiritual practices as they deal with a chronic illness.

Supportive care or the lack of it influences how individuals manage and cope with stress. Indeed, most people know the positive effect of having "moral support" and companionship at times of difficulty. Family health and relationships are a large part of this aspect of quality of life. Any illness affecting a family member inevitably affects other family members, resulting in a changed quality of life for them as well. For example, when family members become primary caregivers of a member with chronic illness, there are role changes, additional responsibilities, and increased stressors that have varying effects on quality of life. Without a doubt the overwhelming nature of chronic illness affects the quality of life not only for the client, but also for family members. Therefore, nursing interventions to promote quality of life in chronic illness are frequently aimed at caregivers. It is reasonable to expect that when caregivers are helped to manage their stress and anxiety, both the caregiver and the client realize better quality of life.

The social and cultural contexts related to quality of life are far-reaching components, as is evidenced by the manner in which organizations such as the WHO define and measure quality of life. Unique cultural interpretations can influence perceived quality of life. Social conditions, expectations of individual behaviours, and cultural regulations affect and contribute to quality of life. Social support and cultural influences are intertwined frequently with economic aspects. Chronic illness affects the financial resources of individuals and their families. The negative impact causes psychological and emotional burdens and drains financial assets. The reasons for financial strain and its effects vary. Frequently, a chronic illness requires individuals to decrease, suspend, or end their work, leading to a reduction or loss of income. Furthermore, if the care recipient requires much assistance or supervision, the primary family caregiver may also have to terminate employment. Therefore, a family with a member with chronic illness faces an increased financial burden resulting from the unemployment of two members. These situations contribute to an adverse quality of life through decreased workforce participation and ultimately cause lost productivity, which further increases the overall cost of chronic illness.

Individuals with chronic illness also suffer financially because of the additional expenses incurred with medical insurance rates or out-of-pocket expenses for items not covered by insurance. Transportation to medical or treatment appointments, for example, or the extra cost of special dietary foods or supplements can add up quickly. The desperately ill person who has found little benefit from traditional therapies may spend large amounts of money on alternative forms of treatment to improve their health. The combined effect on quality of life associated with decreased income and increased expenses may not always be obvious. Therefore, nurses must be aware of how this financial burden may contribute to decreased quality of life. For example, clients may take fewer medications because they cannot afford to take the prescribed amount, or the family caregiver may be overtaxed by the caregiving burden because the family cannot afford assistance.

The following case study illustrates many aspects of quality of life in living with a chronic illness, including health and function, psychosocial elements, socioeconomic components, and the meaning of support from family and friends. The story narrative transitions across the many trajectories of living with a chronic illness.

CASE STUDY

Quality of Life in Multiple Phases of Chronic Illness

Terry, a 53-year-old wife and mother of two, received a diagnosis of breast cancer while already facing the challenges of living with multiple sclerosis (MS). She had made numerous adjustments in her life because of MS. She was aware of the progressive decline that accompanies her type of MS and had given up any notion of working outside the home when she received the MS diagnosis initially. She felt overwhelmed at the prospect of coping with the burden of another life-altering illness. This dual diagnosis truly required individualized treatment not only because of the symptom variability of MS but also because unexpected relapses may occur with the added stress of surgery, chemotherapy, and radiation for her breast cancer. Terry worked diligently to surround herself with support. Most of the time she was her best advocate for keeping all care providers informed of her situation. In a sense she was striving for health care that was person-centred, coordinated, comprehensive, and compassionate. This was no easy task in a healthcare delivery system dominated by a focus on acute, episodic, and fragmented care. MS has forced Terry to face undesirable challenges in her life, and she believed she was making great strides in living with it. She is concerned that her cancer diagnosis will now superimpose added stress on her and her family's ability to maintain quality of life.

Discussion Questions

1. What barriers do you see that may be factors in maintaining quality of life for Terry?
2. What nursing interventions could be used to promote self-care and provide educational resources to Terry?
3. Discuss the issues that Terry and her family face in dealing with the complexity of her situation.
4. Describe the process to promote collaboration among healthcare providers that could enhance quality of life for Terry.
5. What potential quality of life issues are likely to arise and what assessments and interventions would be appropriate?

Although chronic illness usually involves great financial costs, caution is warranted in assuming that a positive relationship exists between a good quality of life and an adequate income. The high degree of subjectivity in quality of life and the existence of many interrelated components suggest that other aspects may influence one's quality of life. The interrelatedness of these various quality of life aspects is evident in the literature that reports results of interventions in chronic illness conditions (Baird & Sands, 2006; Crone, 2007; Jonas-Simpson, Mitchell, Fisher, Jones, & Linscott, 2006).

EVIDENCE-INFORMED GUIDELINES

Clinical practice guidelines provide easily accessed and current, evidence-informed information about recommendations, strategies, or information for care and decision making in specific clinical conditions (Coopey, Nix, & Clancy, 2006). Guidelines about interventions specific to promoting quality of life are embedded in some guidelines, and many guidelines include nurses as the intended users. Four guidelines are presented in **Table 8-1**: self-management in chronic care, advance care planning with cancer patients, clinical practice for quality palliative care, and end-of-life care during the last days and hours. Guidelines can be used by nurses and other healthcare practitioners to evaluate quality of life as it is influenced by clinical decision making and intervening in chronic illness situations. For example, the evidence-informed guideline for chronic care self-management was developed for counselling, evaluation, and management of families who have children with chronic illnesses. This guideline, created by an expert panel at a major children's hospital,

specifically targets families of children with chronic illness. Intended users include advanced practice nurses, among others.

EVIDENCE-INFORMED INTERVENTIONS TO PROMOTE QUALITY OF LIFE

Evidence-informed nursing practice has the most potential to enhance quality of life in chronic illness. The best available research evidence combined with nursing expertise and consideration of individual values and preferences enables effectiveness and efficiency in nursing care. Nurses cannot afford to base practice solely on tradition or experience, or even on knowledge of experts or highly rated textbooks. Increasingly, nursing interventions are seen as having a direct impact on patient outcomes. In chronic illness care this pivotal nursing role raises the bar to practice nursing that is systematic, produces outcomes that contribute to cost effectiveness, and enhances quality care.

This section reviews nursing interventions in chronic illness that promote and evaluate quality of life as an outcome. Overall, a reasonable outcome of any nursing intervention is improved quality of life for clients. In chronic illness this goal is even more salient. Nurses as essential healthcare professionals to clients with chronic illness can be instrumental in planning, carrying out, and evaluating care that promotes quality of life. For clients, enhancing their quality of life amid the debilitating effects of a long-term illness becomes an especially relevant outcome. Moreover, quality of life from the client's context is a reasonable outcome measure of the effectiveness of clinical interventions. The review includes nursing and related investigations on quality of life outcomes for clients

Table 8-1 Comparison of Guidelines That Measure Quality of Life Outcomes

Guideline Title	Evidence-based care guideline for chronic care: Self-management (2007)	Advance care planning with cancer patients (2008)	Adult asthma guidelines for nurses: Promoting control of asthma (2004; revised 2007)	End-of-life care during the last days and hours (2011)
Guideline Developer(s)	Cincinnati Children's Hospital Medical Center	Program in Evidence-Informed Care	Registered Nurses Association of Ontario (RNAO)	Registered Nurses Association of Ontario (RNAO)
Disease/Condition(s)	Chronic illness/condition	Cancer	Asthma	Bereavement, palliative care
Clinical Specialty	Family practice, internal medicine, nursing, nutrition, paediatrics, physical medicine, rehabilitation, psychology	Oncology	Nursing	Nursing
Intended Users	Advanced practice nurses, allied health personnel, dietitians, healthcare providers, nurses, patients, pharmacists, physicians, psychologists/non-physician behavioral health clinicians, social workers	Advanced practice nurses, nurses, physician assistants, physicians	Advanced practice nurses, nurses	Advanced practice nurses, nurses
Guideline Objective(s)	To provide evidence-informed recommendations for self-management by families of children with chronic conditions to improve health outcomes and quality of life	To evaluate advance care planning (ACP) impact on cancer patient outcomes; key elements of ACP for cancer patients; and barriers to engaging in and following through on ACP with cancer patients	To provide nurses working in diverse settings with an evidence-informed summary of basic asthma care for adults; aims to assist nurses to work with their clients to help them make informed decisions to help improve their quality of life and health outcomes	To provide evidenced-informed recommendations for nurses caring for clients in their final days and hours of life

(continues)

Table 8-1 Comparison of Guidelines That Measure Quality of Life Outcomes *(continued)*

	Evidence-informed care guideline for chronic care: self-management (2007)	Advance care planning with cancer patients (2008)	Adult asthma guidelines for nurses: promoting control of asthma (2004; revised 2007)	End-of-life care during the last days and hours (2011)
Guideline Title	Evidence-informed care guideline for chronic care: self-management (2007)	Advance care planning with cancer patients (2008)	Adult asthma guidelines for nurses: promoting control of asthma (2004; revised 2007)	End-of-life care during the last days and hours (2011)
Client Population	Children with chronic conditions and their families	Cancer patients are the relevant population; noncancer patients with chronic or life-threatening illnesses	Adults 18 years and older who are living with asthma	Adults 18 years and older who have progressed to a terminal stage in their illness trajectory and are receiving care in their final days and hours of their life
Major Outcomes Considered	Self-efficacy; health-related quality of life; healthcare utilization; parent/patient satisfaction; missed days from usual activities; cost-specific disease measures	Meeting patient or substitute preferences; healthcare resource use	To improve quality of life and overall reduction in morbidity of adults living with asthma	Practice recommendations for nursing assessment, decision support, care and management, educational recommendations, and organization and policy for individuals at the end-of-life
Methods Used to Access the Quality and Strength of the Evidence	Not stated	Expert consensus	Weighting according to a rating scheme using the AGREE (Appraisal of Guidelines for Research and Evaluation) Instrument	Weighting according to a rating scheme using the AGREE (Appraisal of Guidelines for Research and Evaluation) Instrument
Methods Used to Formulate the Recommendations	Expert consensus (Delphi Expert consensus and nominal group techniques)	Available evidence from published literature, environmental scan, and expert opinion to reach consensus	Available evidence from published literature, previous best practice guidelines, expert opinion, stakeholder review of guidelines and feedback	Available evidence from published literature, previous best practice guidelines, expert opinion, stakeholder review of guidelines and feedback

Source: Agency for Healthcare Research and Quality (2011); Registered Nurses' Association of Ontario. (2011). End-of-life care during the last days and hours. Retrieved January 17, 2012, from http://www.rnao.org; Registered Nurses' Association of Ontario. (2004). Adult asthma guidelines for nurses: Promoting control of asthma. Retrieved from http://www.rnao.org/Storage/27/2206_Asthma_Guideline_and_Supplement_-_FINAL_20071.pdf

and families who have conditions that are the leading causes of death, such as heart disease and cancer. Also included are studies that address quality of life as an outcome in chronic conditions such as arthritis, mental illness, and functional decline associated with aging. A review of the quality of life research for those at end of life is presented as well. These investigations provide examples of ways that nurses can intervene effectively to promote quality of life for clients and their families living with a chronic illness, disability, or other conditions.

Clinical areas where children with chronic illness and their families are cared for are the practice areas in which these guidelines are most likely to be used. As an outcome, health-related quality of life is one measure that healthcare professionals can use to evaluate the effects of their interventions on client outcomes.

The accessibility and ease of use related to evidence-informed guidelines provide an efficient and effective manner for nurses to intervene and evaluate quality of life for clients and their families with chronic illness. At the same time it is important the user evaluate the relevance, currency, and validity of guidelines for measurement of intended outcomes. Consequently, along with guideline use, nurses must be aware of the recent quality of life research and measurement to apply the best available evidence at the client-care level. Therefore, it is important to consider specific practice characteristics that may influence guideline effectiveness and the time and effort that might be required to implement recommendations (Coopey et al., 2006). The guideline should reflect the nurses' clinical knowledge and experience as well as the clients' values and preferences (Clark, Donovan, & Schoettker, 2006).

Using clinical best practice guidelines ensures the recommendations, strategies, and information are based on systematic literature reviews and scientific evidence. Guidelines offer recommendations for practice that are based on a specified level of evidence. For example, Table 8-1 shows that expert consensus was the primary means to formulate the recommendations put forth in the guideline for advance care planning with cancer patients. A consensus process involving well-recognized palliative care organizations was used to evaluate the quality of the recommendations in application of these guidelines to palliative care, with quality of life for client and family, incidence of ethical/legal issues, and use of end-of-life support programs as outcomes. For application in clinical practice, nurses could review the guidelines and assess the methods and rating scheme that were used in development. A determination can be made that if a recommendation is strong, the intervention is always indicated and acceptable and, therefore, likely to positively influence quality of life for clients. On the other hand, nurses would need to use additional information in their decision-making process if the recommendation has a lower rating, such as "useful," "should be considered," or "not useful."

Interventions from the Research Literature to Promote Quality of Life

A review of nursing and health-related literature that report the effects of various interventions on quality of life as one outcome in chronic illness conditions is presented in this section. Much of the research is descriptive in nature; therefore, cause-and-effect relationships between nursing interventions and quality of life as an outcome are not well established. It is also difficult to collect data on outcomes that are sensitive and unique to nursing care interventions. Individuals with chronic illness are seen by a variety of healthcare professionals who may potentially affect their quality of life. Nevertheless, findings from many studies suggest that quality of life has usefulness as a nurse-sensitive quality indicator and as a measure of intervention effectiveness in chronic conditions. Doran and colleagues (2006) noted that linking outcomes to nursing interventions is necessary to determine and identify specific nursing interventions that improve health outcomes and provide the evidence base to improve nursing care in chronic illness.

Most reports view the quality of life of a client as an important outcome measure across several domains, and specific interventions have focused on outcomes such as stage of the disease, disability, and mortality rates. The view of outcomes in terms of morbidity and death discounts other aspects of health and function in chronic illness, such as the client's perceived health, pain experiences, stress levels, independence, capacity to meet responsibilities, access to and use of health care, and usefulness to others. These outcomes are important to clients who want to know how interventions are going to influence health and function. Clients also want guidance in choosing options that produce the best outcomes. In addition, regulatory bodies and manufacturers of pharmaceuticals and technological devices want guidance about product effectiveness on client outcomes, in particular how an individual's quality of life is affected. The results of the research and of the other literature reviewed here show the many facets of client quality of life outcomes in chronic illness care.

OVERVIEW OF NURSING

Interventions

Nursing interventions can empower clients to practice healthy behaviours and enable them to be self-directed in their care and thereby

contribute appreciably to quality of life. Feldman, Murtaugh, Pezzin, McDonald, and Peng (2005) found that use of an email reminder improved self-care management and health-related quality of life for clients with heart failure. The email reminders provided evidence-informed, condition-specific information to nurses as they cared for heart failure clients. These reminders were integrated into the assessment and routine teaching interventions that nurses carried out for clients. When compared with routine care, the basic email reminder to nurses that they should teach to the specific areas of medication knowledge, diet, and weight monitoring produced positive results in clients' quality of life. Moreover, Feldman and colleagues found that this basic teaching for heart failure generated results similar to that of a more intensive intervention that included more reminders and additional nursing time. The study is limited in that the sample was from one urban homecare agency. However, the results are useful in linking a nursing practice intervention to clients' quality of life and thereby add to a better understanding of nursing interventions that are appropriate as well as cost effective.

Nursing-led management and intervention in chronic disease care has been investigated and evaluated in relation to client quality of life outcomes. These investigations are hampered frequently by an inability to produce conclusive results regarding nursing impact on quality of life. Results of one study provide evidence that nurse-mediated interventions have the potential to yield positive quality of life outcomes for clients with implantable cardioverter-defibrillators (Dickerson, Wu, & Kennedy, 2006). However, establishing a link via statistically significant results is more complicated. This situation frequently occurs as the result of multiple factors that affect quality of life, inability to isolate a single nursing intervention, or failure in the adequacy of the measurement (Dickerson et al., 2006). At the same time the imperative to promote quality of life in chronic illness care requires continued nursing research. Taylor and colleagues (2005) acknowledged the urgency of the need for ongoing research in their systematic review of evidence effectiveness related to nursing's role in chronic obstructive pulmonary disease (COPD). As a chronic illness, COPD is a prime example of an escalating public health burden in terms of number of persons affected and the resources used. Nurses have been recognized as playing a critical role in chronic illness care of COPD. Taylor and colleagues called for reprioritization of nurse-led models of chronic illness care. The equivocal results of this study and many others investigating quality of life as a result suggest the need for more carefully designed nursing interventions as well as measurement of additional outcomes.

Health and Function

Health and function as determinants of quality of life are used frequently with traditional clinical and disease indicators to evaluate outcomes for older adults with chronic illness. In clinical practice these quality of life assessments can enhance understanding about treatment preferences and future care needs. For example, health-related quality of life was used as a predictor of potential need for future hospital care for older adults in a large primary care practice (Dorr et al., 2006). Dorr and colleagues found that consideration of quality of life may improve decision making about treatment preferences and intensity for care. Knowledge of an older person's capacity for self-care and functional abilities can maximize appropriate resources and need for care when critical situations arise.

Many times the needed information about quality of life addressing psychosocial aspects of chronic illness is missing from assessments. The assessment data can be used to plan, carry out, and evaluate treatments. In situations in which treatments are known to cause extreme debility, changes should be considered for older clients based on quality of life outcomes.

Nursing care for elderly cancer survivors is one area where information about potential effects on quality of life can be used in clinical practice. Quality of life and related symptoms in elderly women with breast cancer are entangled frequently with other chronic health conditions or are attributed to aging. Heidrich, Egan, Hengudomsub, and Randolph (2006) found that poor social situations, a pessimistic outlook on life, and not knowing the reason for many distressing symptoms further contribute to decreased quality of life. In these situations effective interventions may include helping older women better understand why they are experiencing symptoms and that depression, anxiety, or lack of energy may be caused by cancer and are not part of normal aging.

Clients need information about the reason for symptoms and to know that some symptoms are intertwined with chronic illness and compounded by the aging process. This knowledge can help older adults develop more effective coping strategies. Targeting intervention strategies also can be done more appropriately when quality of life outcomes are better identified. Awareness that women report worse quality of life compared with men because women tend to have a higher prevalence of chronic illness and related functional declines can lead to more proactive early detection and health promotion interventions (Orfila et al., 2006).

Frequently, lack of awareness about available help and treatments is an obstacle to better quality of life. In a study of bowel function and associated faecal incontinence among those older than 75 years of age, researchers found that decreased quality of life was influenced by the amount of dependence that symptoms caused (Stenzelius, Westergren, & Hallberg, 2007). Appropriate assessment of bowel symptoms and the extent of dependency along with nurses' encouragement of clients to seek appropriate care are straightforward interventions that can have a positive impact on quality of life for older adults with bowel dysfunction.

Cancer Care

Nursing research related to care of clients with cancer and their families provides an excellent illustration of the complexity of measuring, intervening, and evaluating quality of life in chronic illness. Cancer is increasingly recognized as a chronic illness because of better survival rates that have resulted from effective treatments. With the increased survival after a diagnosis of cancer, quality of life emerges as a predominant issue. Identification, prevention, and management of the long-term effects of cancer and related treatments have received attention by nurse researchers. Bender, Ergÿn, Rosenzweig, Cohen, and Sereika (2005) identified the prevalence of symptoms experienced by women across three phases of breast cancer treatment. They assessed global quality of life and evaluated how vasomotor, physical, psychosocial, and sexual components were experienced by women in the various phases of breast cancer care and treatment. Fatigue, cognitive impairments, and mood disturbances emerged as common symptoms experienced by the women, regardless of the phase of illness or treatment. Fatigue associated with cancer and

related treatments was an especially bothersome symptom, suggesting that nursing interventions focused on alleviating and managing fatigue may promote better quality of life for women with breast cancer.

The positive effect on quality of life produced by interventions that prevent or lessen fatigue associated with cancer has been given attention in the nursing literature. Cancer-related fatigue is frequently measured as a quality of life component, and various interventions have been proposed to reduce fatigue. Mitchell, Beck, Hood, Moore, and Tanner (2007) conducted a systematic review of the literature and used a rating scheme to support the efficacy of different interventions to reduce fatigue associated with cancer care and treatment. For many interventions effectiveness was not well established, due to insufficient or poor quality data. These interventions included alternative therapies, such as yoga, acupuncture, and nutritional supplements; drugs that may help alleviate fatigue; and psychotherapy. Strategies that teach clients to manage and balance activity, rest, and sleep were rated as likely to be effective, because the evidence is based on small, descriptive studies or expert consensus. Exercise was the one intervention that was recommended for practice because of the strength of the evidence and because the benefits outweighed the harm.

Other studies have also shown that exercise is a safe and effective intervention for reducing fatigue and promoting quality of life in cancer patients. Exercise combined with structured group sessions was effective, due in part to the group cohesion and atmosphere and the direct effects exercise has on reducing fatigue (Losito, Murphy, & Thomas, 2006). This understanding and awareness of the evidence supporting nursing interventions for cancer care promotes best practices interventions for clients and their families. In particular, the growing body of evidence that cancer clients reap many benefits from exercise provides substantial rationale for nurses to promote and use physical activity as a means of improving health and quality of life for many clients with cancer (Hacker, 2009).

Quality of Life in Terminal Illness

Nurses' involvement as researchers and clinicians in end-of-life care has created heightened interest in measuring, promoting, and maintaining quality of life as a nursing care outcome for clients at the end of life. Indeed, the primary objective of palliative and hospice care is to optimize quality of life for individuals and their families. In their review of the literature, Jocham, Dassen, Widdershoven, and Halfens (2006) found that research on nursing interventions in quality of life in palliative cancer care creates special challenges. A primary challenge is the methodological issues related to measurement of quality of life. Most often the aim of end-stage treatment is to control physical symptoms and promote psychological, social, and spiritual comfort. Hence, an individual's quality of life becomes anchored in other aspects of life, and traditional measures may not be accurate or appropriate. Despite the presence of a terminal illness, clients may continue to give rather favourable ratings to their situation, suggesting that other values, goals, and preferences are important to quality of life.

In older adults measuring quality of life at end of life, likewise, is beset by methodological issues because it is difficult to quantify the experiences of clients and families. Gourdji, McVey, and Purden (2009) conducted a qualitative study on the meaning of quality of life in 10 individuals receiving palliative care. Responses of these individuals showed a strong desire to overcome the negative aspects of their situation and to find ways to fully engage in life. Based on the findings, Gourdji and colleagues recommended interventions that enable patients with terminal illness to continue doing the things they want to do, being helpful to others, and sharing a caring environment.

The aging process alters responses to illness, and disease and symptoms may not manifest in ways in which nurses are familiar in younger adults. Evidence-informed activities that promote and maintain quality of life for terminally ill older adults include attention to age-related changes and the impact on sensory function and physiological responses. Particular consideration should be given to pain assessment, medication management, and assessments of depression and cognitive status (Amella, 2003). Others have shown that asking seriously ill clients what they view as quality of life is instructive in helping decide on treatment plans, making advance directives, or prioritizing activities (Vig & Pearlman, 2003).

Psychosocial and Other Supportive Interventions

Nursing studies have focused on interventions to promote quality of life when technology and other well-established treatments fail or when these tools and machinery are insufficient to maintain health and function. Facing suffering on a daily basis and the need to find meaning and purpose in living with a chronic disability challenges healthcare professionals to address a client's needs in other than physical ways. Psychosocial well-being, including health and functionality, contributes immensely to one's quality of life in chronic illness. This type of well-being can be characterized as the capacity to view oneself in a positive manner and to see the world as meaningful, manageable, and logical. The capacity to view self in a positive manner, despite serious physical symptoms that accompany chronic illness, has been shown to be moderated by a strong sense of coherence (Delgado, 2007). In some situations the simple act of listening to a client's burdens and feelings promotes quality of life. This response comes about through the contentment, respect, and nurturance shown by the nurse who listens without judgment (Jonas-Simpson et al., 2006). Interventions that enable better understanding and use of coping skills can be supportive of quality of life for clients and families experiencing chronic illness. Clients who were post-myocardial infarction and who reported quality of life improvements used optimistic, self-reliant, and confrontational coping strategies most frequently over a 1-year period (Kristofferzon, Löfmark, & Carlsson, 2005).

In addition to psychosocial-related activities that augment chronic illness care, evidence-informed alternative interventions can likewise be part of the client's care routine. Interventions such as guided imagery and relaxation therapy have the potential to supplement traditional medical and health care that chronically ill clients need. The combination of guided imagery and relaxation techniques improved health-related quality of life for women with osteoarthritis by alleviating pain intensity and increasing mobility. Moreover, this intervention is easily taught and readily available to clients (Baird & Sands, 2006).

Clients with chronic mental illness can also benefit from interventions that augment prescribed medication and counselling therapies.

Crone (2007) reported that physical activity programs enabled mentally ill individuals to have positive emotional experiences, increased social interaction, and enhanced well-being. Nurses can be instrumental in facilitating development and referral to programs that help increase physical activity for clients with mental illnesses and thereby promote quality of life. Individuals with other chronic conditions also have benefited from exercise programs. Knowing the stage of a client's readiness to engage in exercise is an additional factor that can give nurses information to tailor education more specifically (Lee, Chang, Liou, & Chang, 2006).

Interventions for Family Quality of Life

Nursing interventions to promote quality of life are, likewise, important to family members and others who are caregivers to clients living with a chronic illness. Consequently, it is important to know how caregivers experience quality of life. In general, chronic illness affects quality of life for the entire family. Therefore, family assessment and intervention are necessary. The level of the nurse's involvement with the family will determine the extent of the interventions. Most nurses can meet the basic need that families of clients with chronic illness have for factual information. This information may include education about the disease, treatments, and prognosis. Being available to answer questions and to give practical advice is important. Intervening at this fundamental level establishes trust with families that helps foster continued support. Nurses can invite family members to participate in care activities as appropriate. Families with complex problems may need referral to a specialist. Appropriate use of support groups can create an added network for clients and relieve some of the family burden that may be present (Sutton & Erlen, 2006). The nurse is often in a position to evaluate how such supportive interventions may affect quality of life. A safe and supportive environment can facilitate family sharing of feelings about the illness. Appropriate support groups can be suggested for clients and their family caregivers. The nurse is one member of a collaborative healthcare team that is needed to maintain and promote optimum quality of life for clients with chronic illness and their families.

The complex trajectory of chronic illness poses difficulties in making a strict separation of interventions for quality of life for both clients and family members. It is therefore reasonable to expect that nursing interventions with families can be as helpful as interventions that directly promote health and function in the individual with chronic illness. Moreover, inclusion of the family may strengthen the adjustments that clients with chronic illness must make during the course of illness. As family members increasingly are relied on to provide time-consuming health care, their health and well-being directly affect care outcomes for the chronically ill member. As a result, defining and assessing quality of life is not limited to the client but should include specific measures that enable nurses to assess and meet the needs of family caregivers (Kitrungrote & Cohen, 2006).

A study of the effects of mental illness on families offers insights into strategies that nurses can use to promote quality of life for caregivers (Walton-Moss, Gerson, & Rose, 2005). An important finding of the research is that nurses need to recognize the variability among families in how they respond to mental illness. All family members, regardless of where the relative with mental illness is within the illness trajectory, need to be listened to as they tell their stories and want help to communicate with their loved one. This nursing care is supportive of a family's quality of life when members are coping reasonably well or when they are overwhelmed by numerous challenges. Ultimately, the social and emotional support and financial resources of families impact quality of life. Knowledge about resources, services, and organizations for chronic illness conditions can help in making appropriate and timely referrals that better maintain quality of life and well-being of clients and families.

Individuals and families shift perspectives on their quality of life as they progress through the illness trajectory. At various points the illness may be primary; at other times wellness may predominate. When illness is at the centre, a situation that occurs most often with a new diagnosis, the focus is on suffering, loss, and burden. Families may become overwhelmed. When the focus is on wellness, this may provide an opportunity to refocus on aspects that engage the family and client to promote quality of life. The nurse who is aware of these shifts in chronic illness behaviour is better equipped to support clients through appropriate interventions.

Quality of Life and Technological Interventions

Nurses are becoming increasingly involved either directly as researchers or indirectly as research coordinators in clinical trials that evaluate quality of life as one outcome for clients receiving new products, devices, and drugs. Attention to and awareness of the effects that technological advances have on clients' quality of life therefore becomes important in nursing care.

Measurement of client-related outcomes is a particularly important evaluation component in clinical trials, with quality of life being one such aspect. This approach provides insight regarding treatment effectiveness that can be determined only by clients. An individual's perspective about a drug or treatment effect provides corroboration with observable clinical data. This confirmation is important, because enhanced clinical outcomes such as better glucose control or decreased blood pressure may not necessarily correspond to improvements in function or well-being if the individual is experiencing side effects of the new treatment or drug. In addition, many clinical trials are investigating therapies that are expensive and carry with them uncertain outcomes with regard to quality of life (Grusenmeyer & Wong, 2007). In these instances it is important for clinicians to understand that extraordinary economic costs may be at issue with minimal impact on an individual's quality of life. Clients with life-threatening chronic illnesses also are confronted with choosing life-extending treatments at the expense of quality of life, as these treatments may cause debilitating side effects. Periodic quality of life assessments throughout the course of treatment may offer a better discrimination between improvements versus deterioration in quality of life and allow client preferences to be included in the decision to continue or forgo the specific treatment (Bozcuk et al., 2006).

Another issue with technological interventions that extend life is deciding when to forgo continued treatment. For example, implantable cardioverter-defibrillators have become a well-accepted, evidence-informed practice for high-risk, life-threatening arrhythmias. Individuals with these devices do not only experience a better quality of life but also live longer. These issues bring to the forefront nurses' role in assessing and managing physical and psychological responses to the devices and what to do when an individual needs end-of-life care. Care of clients and families in these situations requires nursing knowledge about the efficacy and cost effectiveness of interventions to promote quality of life (Dunbar, 2005).

Similar issues confront those receiving hemodialysis for end-stage renal disease. Hemodialysis frequently impacts quality of life throughout the course of the disease, such that physical and mental well-being are negatively affected. The concern at hand becomes identification of indicators that offer realistic appraisals of outcomes associated with the quality as well as the quantity of life (Cleary & Drennan, 2005).

SUMMARY

Quality of life as an outcome of care is being increasingly addressed by all healthcare entities, including providers, payers, and consumers. In addition, the increased attention globally to chronic illness care makes it imperative that nurses address quality of life as a nurse-sensitive quality indicator.

Clearly, as an outcome of nursing care, quality of life can be influenced by appropriately designed care interventions. Nurses are in a position, through research and clinical application of interventions, to make a difference in the lives of clients and families. They can apply evidence-informed practices that relieve symptoms and provide comfort; these are actions that promote quality of life. Decision making to initiate, continue, modify, or withdraw treatments can be made by evaluating quality of life as an outcome. The efficacy of clinical nursing interventions and practice behaviours, likewise, can be evaluated based on their contribution to clients' quality of life. By evaluating the extent to which nursing interventions improve quality of life for clients and families, nurses are in a position to show the efficacy of what they do. That nurses can carry out interventions to promote quality of life becomes meaningful to cost-effective care as well.

Throughout this discussion repeated emphasis has been given to interrelatedness and overlap of interventions that promote and maintain quality of life in a variety of chronic illness conditions. Physical, functional, and psychosocial components are related, especially in the context of chronic illness. As such they are significant determinants of one's quality of life. In many instances these characteristics and the social and environmental context of the individual can influence quality of life negatively or positively, depending on the particular set of circumstances. The presence of resources, family support, and access to social and health services can have a powerful and affirming influence on quality of life, despite serious chronic illness disability.

Assessing outcomes of nursing interventions using quality of life as a measure contributes to a fuller description of the accountability nurses have in promoting quality care and outcomes. Knowledge of the individual circumstances that influence quality of life in chronic illness enables better care planning. This targeting of interventions to the specific quality of life for individuals can lead to successful preventive and therapeutic approaches in caring for people with chronic illness. With an ever-present awareness of the many components that influence quality of life in chronic illness, nurses can intervene more effectively.

STUDY QUESTIONS

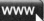

1. What elements are a part of quality of life evaluations in chronic illness? Discuss how the perceptions of individual clients and healthcare professionals contribute to quality of life evaluations.

2. Identify a theoretical or conceptual framework that addresses quality of life as an outcome for clients and families with a chronic illness. Describe an intervention using that framework that demonstrates how nursing can make a difference in quality of life.

3. Describe the importance of quality of life as a nurse-sensitive quality indicator.

4. As an outcome of care, how is quality of life viewed by healthcare providers, consumers, agencies, and third-party payers?

5. Describe how nurses can use guidelines to promote evidence-informed quality of life care to clients and families with chronic illness.

6. What interventions can nurses use to promote client and family quality of life at end of life?

7. Describe outcomes that indicate a good quality of life. How might quality of life outcomes change over time?

8. What potential ethical dilemmas arise when evaluating quality of life in chronic illness?

INTERNET RESOURCES

SF-36-v2 link: http://www.healthmeasurement
.org/pub_pdfs/_questionnaire_sf-36,%20
version%202.pdf

For a full suite of assignments and additional learning activities, use the access code located in the front of your book and visit this exclusive website: **http://go.jblearning.com/kramer-kile**. If you do not have an access code, you can obtain one at the site.

REFERENCES

Agency for Healthcare Research and Quality. (2011). National guideline clearinghouse. Retrieved from www.guidelines.gov

Allmark, P. (2005). Can the study of ethics enhance nursing practice? *Journal of Advanced Nursing, 51*(6), 618–624.

Amella, E. J. (2003). Geriatrics and palliative care: Collaboration for quality of life until death. *Journal of Hospice and Palliative Nursing, 5*(1), 40–48.

Baird, C. L., & Sands, L. P. (2006). Effect of guided imagery with relaxation on health-related quality of life in older women with osteoarthritis. *Research in Nursing & Health, 29(5)*, 442–451.

Bender, C. M., Ergÿn, F. S., Rosenzweig, M. Q., Cohen, S. M., & Sereika, S. M. (2005). Symptom clusters in breast cancer across 3 phases of the disease. *Cancer Nursing, 28*(3), 219–225.

Bozcuk, H., Dalmis, B., Samur, M., Ozdogan, M., Artac, M., & Savas, B. (2006). Quality of life in patients with advanced non-small cell lung cancer. *Cancer Nursing, 29*(2), 104–110.

Canadian Nurses Association. (2005). Chronic disease and nursing: A summary of the issues. Retrieved from http://www2.cna-aiic.ca/CNA/documents/pdf/publications/BG3_Chronic_Disease_and_Nursing_e.pdf

Cantrell, M. A. (2007). The art of pediatric oncology nursing practice. *Journal of Pediatric Oncology Nursing, 24*(3), 132–138.

Carter, H., MacLeod, R., Brander, P., & McPherson, K. (2004). Living with a terminal illness: Patients' priorities. *Journal of Advanced Nursing, 45*(6), 611–620.

Centers for Disease Control and Prevention. (2010a). Health-related quality of life. Retrieved from http://www.cdc.gov/hrqol/

Centers for Disease Control and Prevention. (2010b). Health-related quality of life: Methods and measures. Retrieved from http://www.cdc.gov/hrqol/methods.htm

Clark, E., Donovan, E. F., & Schoettker, P. (2006). From outdated to updated, keeping clinical guidelines valid. *International Journal for Quality in Health Care, 18*(3), 165–166.

Clark, E. H. (2004). Quality of life: A basis for clinical decision-making in community psychiatric care. *Journal of Psychiatric and Mental Health Nursing, 11*, 725–730.

Cleary, J., & Drennan, J. (2005). Quality of life of patients on haemodialysis for end-stage renal disease. *Journal of Advanced Nursing, 51*(6), 577–586.

Coopey, M., Nix, M. P., & Clancy, C. M. (2006). Translating research into evidence-based nursing practice and evaluating effectiveness. *Journal of Nursing Care Quality, 21*(3), 195–202.

Crone, D. (2007). Walking back to health: A qualitative investigation into service users' experiences of a walking project. *Issues in Mental Health Nursing, 28*, 167–183.

Delgado, C. (2007). Sense of coherence, spirituality, stress and quality of life in chronic illness. *Journal of Nursing Scholarship, 39*(3), 229–234.

Dickerson, S. S., Wu, Y. B., & Kennedy, M. C. (2006). A CNS-facilitated ICD support group: A clinical project evaluation. *Clinical Nurse Specialist, 20*(3), 146–153.

Donabedian, A. (1988). Quality assessment and assurance: Unity of purpose diversity and means. *Inquiry, 25*, 173–192.

Doran, D. M., Harrison, M. B., Laschinger, H. S., Hirdes, J. P., Rukholm, E., Sidani, S., . . . Cranley, L. (2006). Nursing-sensitive outcomes data collection in acute care and long-term-care settings. *Nursing Research, 55*(2S), S75–S81.

Dorr, D. A., Jones, S. S., Burns, L., Donnelly, S. M., Brunker, C. P., Wilcox, A., & Clayton, P. D. (2006). Use of health-related, quality-of-life metrics to predict mortality and hospitalizations in community-dwelling seniors. *Jour-nal of the American Geriatrics Society, 54*(4), 667–673.

Dubos, R. (1959). *Mirage of health: Utopias, progress, and biological change.* Garden City, NY: Doubleday.

Dunbar, S. B. (2005). Psychosocial issues of patients with implantable cardioverter defibrillators. *American Journal of Critical Care, 14*(4), 294–303.

Feldman, P. H., Murtaugh, C. M., Pezzin, L. E., McDonald, M. V., & Peng, T. R. (2005, June). Just-in-time evidence-based e-mail "reminders" in home health care: Impact on patient outcomes. *HSR: Health Services Research, 40*(3), 865–885.

Gourdji, I., McVey, L., & Purden, M. (2009). A quality end of life from a palliative care patient's perspective. *Journal of Palliative Care, 25*(1), 40–50.

Grusenmeyer, P. A., & Wong, Y. (2007). Interpreting the economic literature in oncology. *Journal of Clinical Oncology, 25*(2), 196–202.

Hacker, E. (2009). Exercise and quality of life: Strengthening the connections. *Clinical Journal of Oncology Nursing, 13*(1), 31–39.

Heidrich, S. M., Egan, J. J., Hengudomsub, P., & Randolph, S. M. (2006). Symptoms, symptom beliefs, and quality of life of older breast cancer survivors: A comparative study. *Oncology Nursing Forum, 33*(2), 315–322.

Hirskyj, P. (2007). QALY: An ethical issue that dare not speak its name. *Nursing Ethics, 14*(1), 72–82.

Huang, T., & Liang, S. (2005). Care of older people: A randomized clinical trial of the effectiveness of a discharge planning intervention in hospitalized elders with hip fracture due to falling. *Journal of Clinical Nursing, 14,* 1193–1201.

Jocham, H. R., Dassen, T., Widdershoven, G., & Halfens, R. (2006). Quality of life in palliative care cancer patients: A literature review. *Journal of Clinical Nursing, 15,* 1188–1195.

Jonas-Simpson, C. M., Mitchell, G. J., Fisher, A., Jones, G., & Linscott, J. (2006). The experience of being listened to: A qualitative study of older adults in long-term care settings. *Journal of Gerontological Nursing, 32*(1), 46–53.

Kitrungrote, L., & Cohen, M. Z. (2006). Quality of life of family caregivers of patients with cancer: A literature review. *Oncology Nursing Forum, 33*(3), 625–632.

Kristofferzon, M., Löfmark, R., & Carlsson, M. (2005). Issues and innovations in nursing practice: Coping, social support, and quality of life over time after myocardial infarction. *Journal of Advanced Nursing, 52*(2), 113–124.

Lee, P., Chang, W., Liou, T., & Chang, P. (2006). Issues and innovations in nursing practice: Stage of exercise and health-related quality of life among overweight and obese adults. *Journal of Advanced Nursing, 53*(3), 295–303.

López, A., McCaffrey, R., Griffin, M., & Fitzpatrick, J. (2009). Spiritual well-being and practices among women with gynecologic cancer. *Oncology Nursing Forum, 36*(3), 300–305.

Losito, J. M., Murphy, S. O., & Thomas, M. L. (2006). The effects of group exercise on fatigue and quality of life during cancer treatment. *Oncology Nursing Forum, 33*(4), 821–825.

Low, G., & Molzahn, A. E. (2007). Predictors of quality of life in old age: A cross-validation study. *Research in Nursing & Health, 30,* 141–150.

Mitchell, S. A., Beck, S. L., Hood, L. E., Moore, K., & Tanner, E. R. (2007). Putting evidence into practice: Evidence-based interventions for fatigue during and following cancer and its treatment. *Clinical Journal of Oncology Nursing, 11*(1), 99–113.

Moreira-Almeida, A., & Koenig, H.G. (2006). Retaining the meaning of the words religiousness and spirituality: A commentary on the WHOQOL-SRPB group's "A cross-cultural study of spirituality, religion, and personal beliefs as components of quality of life." *Social Science & Medicine, 63,* 843–845.

Naef, R., & Bournes, D. (2009). The lived experience of waiting: A Parse method study. *Nursing Science Quarterly, 22*(2), 141–153.

Orfila, F., Ferrer, M., Lamarca, R., Tebe, C., Domingo-Salvany, A., & Alonso, J. (2006). Gender differences in health-related quality of life among the elderly: The role of objective functional capacity and chronic conditions. *Social Science & Medicine, 63,* 2367–2380.

Plummer, M., & Molzahn, A. (2009). Quality of life in contemporary nursing theory: A concept analysis. *Nursing Science Quarterly, 22*(2), 134–140.

Saunders, J. C., & Cookman, C. A. (2005). A clarified conceptual meaning of hepatitis C-related depression. *Gastroenterology Nursing, 16*(46), 123–130.

Sousa, K. H., Ryu, E., Kwok, O., Cook, S. W., & West, S. G. (2007). Development of a model to measure symptom status in persons living with rheumatoid arthritis. *Nursing Research, 56*(6), 434–440.

Stenzelius, K., Westergren, A., & Hallberg, I. R. (2007). Bowel function among people over 75 years reporting faecal incontinence in relation to help seeking, dependency and quality of life. *Journal of Clinical Nursing, 16*, 458–468.

Suhonen, R., Välimäki, M., Katajisto, J., & Leino-Kilpi, H. (2005). Provision of individualized care improves hospital patient outcomes: An explanatory model using LISREL. *International Journal of Nursing Studies, 44*, 197–207.

Sutton, L. B., & Erlen, J. A. (2006). Effects of mutual dyad support on quality of life in women with breast cancer. *Cancer Nursing, 29*(6), 488–498.

Taylor, S. J. C., Candy, B., Bryar, R. M., Ramsay, J., Vrijhoef, H. J. M., Esmond, G., . . . Griffiths, C. J.. (2005). Effectiveness of innovations in nurse led chronic disease management for patients with chronic obstructive pulmonary disease: Systematic review of evidence. *British Medical Journal, 331*(7515), 485.

Vig, E. K., & Pearlman, R. A. (2003). Quality of life while dying: A qualitative study of terminally ill older men. *Journal of the American Geriatrics Society, 51*(11), 1595–1601.

Walton-Moss, B., Gerson, L., & Rose, L. (2005). Effects of mental illness on family quality of life. *Issues in Mental Health Nursing, 26*, 627–642.

Weinert, C., Cudney, S., & Spring, A. (2008). Evolution of a conceptual model for adaptation to chronic illness. *Journal of Nursing Scholarship, 40*(4), 364–372.

World Health Organization. (1948). WHO definition of health. Retrieved from https://apps.who.int/aboutwho/en/definition.html

World Health Organization. (2004). The World Health Organization quality of life (WHOQOL)–BREF. Retrieved from http://www.who.int/substance_abuse/research_tools/en/english_whoqol.pdf

CHAPTER 9

Uncertainty

Original chapter by Faye I. Hummel

> *The words of the radiologist, "it's breast cancer," rang through my head over and over again as I sat in silence, alone, trying to make sense of this dreadful news. I couldn't believe my body had forsaken me. I felt betrayed. Why me? Would I survive? Could this be true? What if . . . ? Uncertainty built inside me, like a violent thunderstorm on a hot summer day. Uncertainty drenched me to my very core. That dark cloud of uncertainty follows me, even on the sunniest of days.*
>
> —Rita, 59-year-old woman with breast cancer

INTRODUCTION

Uncertainty in chronic illness is pervasive. Chronic illness is marked by unpredictable changes in physical, cognitive, social, and lifestyle functions. Chronic illness restricts the terrain of the sufferer to local and familiar territory where one is least likely to be exposed to the gaze and questions of others (Goffman, 1963). With chronic illness the timing, duration, and severity of symptoms are erratic. Misgivings about what one may be able to achieve in the present or in the future persist. Doubt about the success of treatment to slow disease progression and modify the disease course erodes self-confidence and generates stress and anxiety.

Chronic illness brings a prolonged state of impending adversity. The legend of Damocles' sword illuminates the insidious nature of uncertainty and chronic illness. In this tale Damocles spoke of his sovereign's wealth and happiness, and as a result Dionysius invited him to a great banquet at which Damocles was seated beneath a sharp sword suspended by a single hair (*Encyclopedia Britannica*, 2011). Damocles' sword symbolizes the precarious nature of everyday life for persons with chronic illness. On any given day an individual with chronic illness may need to forgo cherished or longed for activities, experience loss of freedom due to limitations and special needs, or be unable to purchase prescribed treatments and pharmaceuticals. Everyday life changes dramatically and is filled with unknowns. Uncertainty in chronic illness has been described as a cognitive stressor marked by a loss of control and a perception of doubt. Uncertainty impedes coping and adjustment to chronic illness, increases psychological and emotional distress, and diminishes quality of life.

NATURE OF UNCERTAINTY

Uncertainty arises when details of situations are "ambiguous, complex, unpredictable, or uncertain, probabilistic; when information is unavailable or inconsistent; and when people feel insecure in their own state of knowledge or the state of knowledge in general" (Brashers, 2001, p. 478). Uncertainty is derived from one's self-perception of cognition. Thus, a person who believes him- or herself to be uncertain is uncertain. Further, uncertainty may be experienced in relation to probability of an event. When the likelihood of an event is 0% or 100%, uncertainty is lowest. If there are multiple alternatives with equal probability, then uncertainty is highest (Brashers, 2001). Attributes of probability, perception, and temporality are present in every situation of uncertainty (McCormick, 2002).

Uncertainty is a hallmark of acute and chronic illness. Uncertainty is experienced by those with chronic illness who may fear rejection and social isolation; some may be concerned with diagnosis and treatment, whereas others may worry about recurrence of their illness even with improved physical health. An understanding of the nature of uncertainty enhances one's ability to describe and explain influences on behaviour and to develop interventions to improve people's lives (Brashers, 2001).

UNCERTAINTY IN CHRONIC ILLNESS IS CERTAIN

The dynamic nature of chronic illness makes uncertainty a part of life (Mishel, 1999). In acute illness individuals act to decrease uncertainty, whereas individuals with chronic conditions seek to manage uncertainty. Even though uncertainty is experienced in the present, uncertainty is based on past experiences and assumptions for the future (Penrod, 2001). Embedded within the illness experience are ambiguity, inconsistency, vagueness, unpredictability, unfamiliarity, and the unknown, all creating uncertainty (Mishel, 1984). Persons with chronic illness experience

situations and symptoms for which they have no experience or knowledge, thus triggering uncertainty. Uncertainty is a psychological state in which individuals initially perceive it and respond relative to how they believe it will impact them. As such, uncertainty is a neutral experience, neither good nor bad (Brashers, 2001; Mishel, 1988). The assessment of uncertainty as beneficial or harmful determines one's affective response to uncertainty (Mishel, 1988).

Uncertainty is the inability of an individual to understand the meaning of illness-related events such as disease process or treatment (Mishel, 1988) and one's perception of ambiguity, complexity, inconsistency, and unpredictability associated with illness and illness-related events (Mishel, 1984, 1990). Vague prognosis, lack of illness-related information, and unpredictability of symptoms and complications lead to uncertainty (Mishel, 1984, 1988).

When certainty exists, the future is taken for granted. When uncertainty exists, the future becomes the focus, with attempts to capture a clear vision of what was never clear to begin with (McCormick, 2002). Persons with chronic conditions do not know how their chronic illness will impact the future. They may feel good one day and incapacitated the next. They receive inconsistent information from healthcare providers and information sources about disease management and necessary lifestyle changes. Uncertainty clouds one's ability to determine if aches and pains are associated with the disease process or are benign.

Building on Mishel's (1981, 1988, 1990) theoretical work on uncertainty in acute and chronic illnesses, scholars have identified similar experiences of uncertainty in many chronic illnesses. Uncertainty is a universal phenomenon among chronic illnesses, including cancer (Clayton, Mishel, & Belyea, 2006; Sammarco &

Konecny, 2010), peritoneal dialysis (Madar & Bar-Tal, 2009), Parkinson's disease (Sanders-Dewey, Mullins, & Chaney, 2001), multiple sclerosis (McNulty, Livneh, & Wilson, 2004), chronic pain (Johnson, Zautra, & Davis, 2006), organ transplantation (Lasker, Sogolow, Olenik, Sass, & Weinrieb, 2010; Martin, Stone, Scott, & Brashers, 2010), and HIV/AIDS (Brashers et al., 2003). Uncertainty influences the way in which individuals respond to a diagnosis, deal with illness symptoms, manage treatment regimens, and maintain social relationships.

Illness uncertainty influences coping with and adapting to fibromyalgia. Johnson and colleagues (2006) examined the role of uncertainty in coping with pain in 51 women with fibromyalgia. They found women who were experiencing greater pain levels and high illness uncertainty had more difficulty coping with their disease. Women with endometriosis reported uncertainty and emotional distress as a result of the complexity and impact of endometriosis on their lives (Lemaire, 2004). In persons undergoing home peritoneal dialysis, uncertainty was positively associated with self-rated illness severity (Madar & Bar-Tal, 2009).

Uncertainty is present across the illness trajectory, during events of diagnosis, treatment, and prognosis (Mishel, 1981, 1984, 1988). A longitudinal study examined uncertainty and anxiety in 127 women with suspected breast cancer during the diagnostic period. Results demonstrated that uncertainty and anxiety were significantly higher before the diagnosis than after the diagnosis. Uncertainty and anxiety were significantly lower for women diagnosed with benign disease than for those women with malignant diagnosis (Liao, Chen, Chen, & Chen, 2008).

Uncertainty was measured in three groups of adolescents and young adults with cancer at specific times in their cancer experience: newly diagnosed, diagnosed 1 to 4 years, and diagnosed 5 or more years. Overall level of uncertainty remained unchanged among the three groups, although differences did exist in the specific concerns related to uncertainty (Decker, Haase, & Bell, 2007). Women who had undergone surgery for ovarian malignancies reported that anxiety and depression played an important role in uncertainty throughout their illness (Schulman-Green, Ercolano, Dowd, Schwartz, & McCorkle, 2008).

Martin and colleagues (2010) identified sources of uncertainty across the transplantation trajectory. Thirty-eight participants who were waiting for or who had received an organ transplant were interviewed. During all phases of the transplant experience participants reported medical, personal, and social forms of uncertainty. Denny (2009), in a qualitative study of 31 women with endometriosis, found uncertainty exists around diagnosis, disease course, and the future. In a longitudinal, descriptive study of persons with an implantable cardioverter-defibrillator, 21 male participants—who were educated, married, and White—demonstrated that uncertainty did not change significantly over time (Mauro, 2010).

Uncertainty is pervasive and can persist for long periods of time even after life-saving procedures and treatments are complete (Martin et al., 2010; Mauro, 2010). Persson and Hellstrom (2002) reported uncertainty as a theme that emerged from interviews with nine patients after ostomy surgery. Similarly, uncertainty of cancer recurrence was highlighted by persons with colorectal cancer (Simpson & Whyte, 2006). For breast cancer survivors, survivor uncertainty persists long after treatment completion due to fear of recurrence (Dirksen & Erickson, 2002) and erodes quality of life (Sammarco & Konecny, 2008). Gil and colleagues (2004) examined the sources of uncertainty in 244 older African American and White long-term breast cancer survivors. They found the most important triggers for uncertainty were hearing about someone else's cancer and their own new aches and pains. Among breast cancer patients, uncertainty affects the illness experience, adaptation, quality of life, and sense of hope (Sammarco, 2001).

> From the moment of my diagnosis of breast cancer to this very day two years later, uncertainty has been constant and consistent. First it was doubt about surgery and treatment. Were my healthcare providers competent? Did I have enough information to make the right decisions? Would I be able to handle all that was ahead of me? Even during the first year of being "cancer free," I always felt as though the other shoe was going to drop. And sure enough, results from a follow-up mammogram fueled my cancer fears. The biopsy showed no further breast cancer, I was relieved but . . . I simply can't subdue the nagging doubt and fear that cancer will return at any time. Uncertainty, a constant reminder there simply is no guarantee with cancer.
>
> —*Rita*

Older adults report less intolerance of uncertainty compared with their younger counterparts (Basevitz, Pushkar, Chaikelson, Conway, & Dalton, 2008). Uncertainty appears to decrease with age. Older people in Taiwan report less illness uncertainty than when they were younger (Lien, Lin, Kuo, & Chen, 2009). Younger Taiwanese women with breast cancer reported higher uncertainty due to concerns with changes in their physical condition, careers, and family roles (Liao et al., 2008).

Other uncertainty differences were noted in the literature. Sammarco and Konecny (2010)

reported higher levels of uncertainty in Latina breast cancer survivors compared with White breast cancer survivors. Level of education affects uncertainty and stress; for example, in one study (Madar & Bar-Tal, 2009) educated patients were better able to manage levels/feelings of uncertainty. The ability of patients to process information influences uncertainty.

Current research supports a positive association between symptom severity and uncertainty in chronic illness. Mullins and colleagues (2001) found a relationship between illness intrusiveness and uncertainty among persons with multiple sclerosis. Kang (2006) reported similar findings with adults diagnosed with atrial fibrillation. Those with greater symptom severity perceived more uncertainty. Wolfe-Christensen, Isenberg, Mullins, Carpentier, and Almstrom (2008) found a similar relationship among college students with asthma. Mullins, Chaney, Balderson, and Hommel (2000) found with increased illness severity, uncertainty had a significant effect on depression in young adults with long-standing asthma.

UNCERTAINTY AND SOCIAL NETWORKS

Illness uncertainty affects the individual with chronic illness as well as those within his or her social network, including caregivers, family members, and friends. Members of a social network of someone with a chronic illness face their own feelings and fears of uncertainty and unpredictability (Donovan-Kicken & Bute, 2008; Mitchell, Courtney, & Coyer, 2003; Northouse et al., 2002) and may experience discomfort and anxiety about how to act and what to say to the person with chronic illness. Adults with a parent with probable Alzheimer's disease reported uncertainty about the medical aspects of Alzheimer's disease, including etiology, symptoms, treatment, and prognosis. They reported uncertainty about their own predisposition for Alzheimer's disease as well as conflicting caregiver roles and their financial responsibilities. Social sources of uncertainty experienced by these families included unpredictability of social reactions and social interactions, including family dynamics (Stone & Jones, 2009).

In a qualitative study investigating the experiences of informal caregivers, including spouses and adult children of stroke survivors, Greenwood, Mackenzie, Wilson, and Cloud (2009) reported uncertainty as a central theme. Reich, Olmsted, and van Puymbroeck (2006) reported uncertainty significantly impacted the partner relationships of patients with fibromyalgia. Uncertainty among family and friends of someone with a chronic illness is managed by seeking information from a variety of sources, including the Internet, professional and mainstream publications, healthcare providers, support groups, and other members in their social network (Donovan-Kicken & Bute, 2008).

SOURCES OF UNCERTAINTY

Uncertainty permeates all aspects of diagnosis, treatment, and prognosis. Medical uncertainty has been associated with insufficient information about diagnosis, ambiguous symptoms and disease trajectory, and complex treatments and interventions (Mishel, 1988, 1990). In research conducted with persons with HIV disease, Brashers and colleagues (2003) extended Mishel's (1990) model of uncertainty in illness to include not only medical uncertainty but also personal and social sources of uncertainty. Sources of medical uncertainty identified by persons with HIV disease were ambiguity about their HIV diagnosis and associated diagnostic tests as well as unpredictability and multiplicity of opportunistic infections. Personal sources of uncertainty were related to the invisibility of their chronic illness, social roles, and precarious financial situations due to the expense of necessary medications (Brashers et al., 2003). Families coping with Alzheimer's disease reported similar sources of uncertainty. Interviews with participants in Sammarco and Konecny's (2010) examination of the experiences of adult children of a parent with Alzheimer's disease revealed medical, personal, and social sources of uncertainty.

CASE STUDY

Jim, age 70, lives with his wife, Nancy, age 68. Both Jim and Nancy are retired. They have been married for 25 years and have no children. Both are in excellent physical health. They have many friends and have been active in social and community organizations and events. They enjoy sports and travel frequently. Two years ago, with little notice, Jim began having difficulty remembering minor things, such as where he put his keys or what he had for breakfast. He thought these changes were probably just a sign of "old age." But with time Jim experienced even more difficulty with his memory, and after a number of tests and physician visits

(continues)

CASE STUDY   (Continued)

he was diagnosed with Alzheimer's disease. This devastating news was confusing and overwhelming. Jim and Nancy were consumed with questions, worries, and stress. Jim began pharmacological treatment for his Alzheimer's disease. When one drug failed to slow his symptoms, he tried another. As Jim's cognitive abilities continued to slowly erode, he experienced more frustration, anxiety, and depression with associated fatigue and loss of appetite. Nancy has been very attentive to Jim's needs and provides psychological and behavioural support. She has cut back on her social activities to minimize the time Jim is home alone. They now see their friends less frequently and often decline invitations for social gatherings. Nancy and Jim are reluctant to travel despite a long-planned trip to Mexico.

Discussion Questions

1. Discuss how uncertainty is manifested in Alzheimer's disease for Jim. Discuss for Nancy.
2. Explore the issue of uncertainty for a chronic illness using the four constructs of uncertainty (ambiguity, complexity, inconsistency, and unpredictability).
3. How is uncertainty different and similar for the person with chronic illness compared with the caregiver? Compared with others in the social network?
4. Design an action plan to assist persons with chronic illnesses and their families to manage uncertainty and promote quality of life.

THEORETICAL UNDERPINNINGS OF UNCERTAINTY

Early work on uncertainty distinguished clinical from functional uncertainty (Davis, 1960). McIntosh (1974, 1976) examined uncertainty in persons with cancer and other chronic conditions. Mishel (1981) posited uncertainty as one's inability to form a cognitive schema, which is created when stimuli are recognized and classified, a process that gives meaning to an event. Based on Lazarus and Folkman's (1984) stress and coping framework, Mishel (1988) developed a middle range theory of uncertainty to explain how people with illness cognitively process illness-related stimuli to construct meaning for illness events. This theory purports that

uncertainty occurs when there is difficulty constructing a cognitive schema—a person's subjective interpretation—of illness events. Mishel subsequently extended her theory to uncertainty in chronic illness. Mishel (1990) recognized those with acute illness experienced time-limited uncertainty, whereas those with chronic conditions experienced uncertainty throughout their lives. Mishel's theory progressed from predicting, controlling, and eliminating uncertainty to include managing and accepting uncertainty as a way of life in chronic illness.

Mishel (1988) identified the primary antecedent of uncertainty as stimuli frame. Stimuli frame has three components: symptom pattern, event familiarity, and event congruence. Symptom pattern is the consistency of symptoms to form a pattern. Event familiarity is the degree to which a situation is habitual, repetitive, or contains recognizable cues and is determined by time and experience in a healthcare environment (Mishel, 1988). Event congruence is the consistency between the expected and actual experience with an illness-related event. Events are reliable and stable, subsequently facilitating interpretation and understanding. These three components of the stimuli frame reduce uncertainty (Mishel, 1988).

The stimuli frame is influenced by two variables: cognitive capacity and structure providers. Cognitive capacity is the ability of the person to process information. Limited cognitive capacity due to information overload, ability of a person to process information, and the physiological factors that may impair cognitive ability diminishes the ability to recognize the symptom pattern, event familiarity, and event congruence. The second variable, structure providers, is the resources used to interpret the stimuli frame. Structure providers reduce uncertainty by assisting in the interpretation of an illness event or by helping identify symptom patterns, event familiarity, and event congruence. Structure providers include credible authority, social support, and education (Mishel, 1988). Credible authority is the degree to which a person has trust and confidence in his or her healthcare provider. Social support is the ability of the person to express his or her thoughts and feelings with those (e.g., family, social network) who are also experiencing the disease. Together these variables support development of a cognitive schema for interpretation of illness events and thus reduce uncertainty (Mishel, 1988).

Persons with chronic illness cannot assign a definite value to objects or events or predict outcomes with accuracy (Bailey et al., 2009). If one does not have sufficient cues to structure or categorize an illness event, uncertainty arises. Inconsistent symptom patterns, lack of familiarity with healthcare providers and procedures, and unanticipated illness experiences contribute to one's uncertainty. Further, one's stimulus frame is influenced by his or her cognitive capacity and structure providers such as education, social support, and credible authority that assist the individual in interpreting the stimulus frame. One's cognitive capacity may be impaired by illness-related factors such as pain or medication, creating difficulty in constructing meaning from the stimuli cues. On the other hand, receiving assurance from a trusted and competent healthcare provider about some aspect of his or her chronic condition can diminish uncertainty.

Illness uncertainty has four forms: (1) ambiguity about the illness, (2) complexity of the treatment and healthcare system, (3) inadequate information about the disease and its seriousness, and (4) unpredictability about the disease and its trajectory (Mishel, 1988). Uncertainty may lead to psychological distress if coping responses are insufficient to resolve or manage uncertainty.

Uncertainty is neutral until it is assessed to be a danger or an opportunity. Illness events perceived as a danger imply harm. Uncertainty is perceived as a threat to well-being based on previous personal experiences. With perceived harm, coping strategies are implemented to reduce uncertainty. Uncertain events evaluated as opportunity imply a positive outcome. Appraisal of uncertainty as an opportunity is explained as construction of a positive meaning for an event based on one's personal beliefs or purposeful misrepresentation (Mishel, 1990). In the case of uncertainty as an opportunity, strategies to maintain uncertainty are initiated. If coping strategies are effective, adaptation occurs (Mishel, 1988).

Mishel and Braden (1988) tested the theoretical variables of uncertainty with 61 women with gynaecological cancer. Their research found that these women had low levels of uncertainty. Further, they found significant relationships between uncertainty and theory variables, symptom patterns, event familiarity, credible authority, social support, and education. Mast (1998) explored the antecedents of uncertainty in research with 109 survivors of breast cancer. As a result, antecedent variables proposed by Mishel (1988) were modified to include symptom distress, concurrent illness, and fear of recurrence. Wallace (2005) conducted research to examine the antecedents associated with uncertainty in 19 men with prostate cancer who were undergoing watchful-waiting management. Study results revealed significant relationships between level of education, length of illness, and uncertainty, lending support to Mishel's (1988) uncertainty in illness model and enhancing understanding of factors that influence uncertainty.

Ambiguity and subsequent uncertainty can generate stress and inhibit effective coping (Lazarus & Folkman, 1984). Uncertainty is one of the greatest challenges in successfully adapting to chronic illness. Individuals with a variety of chronic illnesses experiencing increased levels of uncertainty experience diminished levels of adjustment (McNulty et al., 2004). In a sample of 50 individuals with multiple sclerosis, researchers examined the contributions of illness uncertainty and spiritual well-being to psychosocial adaptation. Spiritual well-being influenced adaptation to multiple sclerosis and mitigated the impact of uncertainty on adaptation (McNulty et al., 2004).

Bailey and colleagues (2009) examined the constructs of ambiguity, complexity, inconsistency, and unpredictability in 126 persons undergoing a watchful-waiting protocol for individuals with chronic hepatitis C. Ambiguity was identified as a primary construct of illness uncertainty having the strongest relationships with depressive symptoms, quality of life, and fatigue. Persons with chronic hepatitis C responded to ambiguity by limiting their investment of energy in future activities, acting on information they perceived important, and favouring nonthreatening explanations of symptoms. These results give healthcare providers parameters for assisting persons with chronic illness self-management interventions.

UNCERTAINTY AS OPPORTUNITY

Mishel (1988) proposed reconceptualisation of uncertainty from a deficit to a source of personal growth. Uncertainty outcomes are not always negative. Uncertainty can be a useful coping mechanism for persons with chronic illness. Sometimes not knowing is better than knowing (Greenwood et al., 2009).

> March was our "ignorance is bliss" month. Radiation and chemotherapy were over in February, and although the effects of the treatment had been brutal, we felt that better days surely were coming. R's next PET scan wasn't scheduled until mid-April, giving us 6 weeks of respite from treatment, albeit uncertainty as well as respite. However, it served as a healing time for us mentally. The future might be bright or bleak, as we were uncertain what the PET scan would show, but somehow, not knowing was OK. We were able to move cancer to the side for awhile.
>
> *—Jenny, wife of a 63-year-old man*
> *with stage III oesophageal cancer*

Uncertainty can provide the opportunity for persons with chronic illness to reevaluate their lives and establish priorities. The literature reflects evidence of positive reappraisal including increased tolerance and appreciation for others, greater self-acceptance, increased optimism and joy in life (McCormick, 2002), getting a second chance in life, and enjoying the simple pleasures and small things in life. In the case of a potentially negative outcome, uncertainty can be more desirable than certainty. Maintaining a level of uncertainty can help an individual with a chronic illness to preserve hope (Brashers, Goldsmith, & Hsieh, 2002; Mishel, 1988).

UNCERTAINTY AS HARM

The chronic illness experience can trigger perceptions of harm that increase illness uncertainty. Factors that promote uncertainty are discussed in this section.

Stress and Uncertainty

Uncertainty is a significant psychological stressor, particularly in a cultural context that values predictability and control (Mishel, 1990). It is also associated with decreased quality of life (Mishel, 1983, 1999) and diminished coping with illness symptoms (Johnson et al., 2006). Other psychological dimensions of chronic illness are fear and anxiety, coping, and worry. Chronic psychological stress of living with a chronic illness is associated with anticipation of an unwanted decline. The inability to make a prediction about one's disease course is stressful. For example, uncertainty is significantly associated with decreased perceived control and increased psychological distress in adolescents with type 1 diabetes (Hoff, Mullins, Chaney, Hartman, & Domek, 2002). This can result in

psychological distress if coping responses are not sufficient to resolve the uncertainty.

A high degree of uncertainty is related to increased emotional distress, anxiety, and depression (McCormick, 2002). Persons with multiple sclerosis who reported greater uncertainty about their chronic illness were less hopeful and had more negative moods (Wineman, Schwetz, Zeller, & Cyphert, 2003). In 44 dyads composed of individuals with Parkinson's disease and their caregivers, uncertainty in illness did not predict distress for persons with the disease; however, uncertainty emerged as a significant predictor of distress for their caregivers. Caregivers reported stress as they faced an uncertain future regarding their caregiver responsibilities and tasks (Sanders-Dewey et al., 2001). Addressing psychological issues in chronic illness is vital to diminishing uncertainty and increasing quality of life (Lasker et al., 2010).

Anxiety

Increased illness uncertainty was associated with greater anxiety in a sample of 56 older adolescents with childhood-onset asthma (Hommel et al., 2003). Fifty research studies were examined to synthesize the state of the science on uncertainty in relation to women undergoing diagnostic evaluation for suspected breast cancer. All studies reported anxiety persisting throughout the diagnostic period until the final diagnosis (Montgomery, 2010).

Loss of Control

One's perception of self-control impacts illness uncertainty (Mishel, 1997). A decline in self-efficacy and sense of mastery may contribute to a lack of confidence in making decisions about treatment and daily activities. Because of uncertainty, persons with chronic conditions frequently put their lives on hold. Loss of control is a component of uncertainty. Mishel (1988) hypothesized that persons with high internal locus of control would be more likely to perceive uncertainty as an opportunity, but people with an external locus of control would appraise uncertainty as a threat or danger. If the person's external locus of control is related to a strong belief in a higher power, then uncertainty may not necessarily be viewed as a threat or danger by the individual (McCormick, 2002).

Waiting

Waiting is a hallmark of the healthcare system. Waiting creates a loss of control for those who must wait for treatment decisions, test results, appointments, and so forth. Waiting produces anxiety, depression, panic, and uncertainty (Bailey, Wallace, & Mishel, 2007; Mishel, 1999; Wallace, 2003). Waiting is "a grueling experience of unsure stillness" (Bournes & Mitchell, 2002, p. 62). For women suspected of having breast cancer, waiting is limbo (Montgomery, 2010). In a qualitative research study with 21 women and 5 men who had been affected by cancer, waiting emerged as a theme. Waiting was described by many of the informants "as the worst part of the cancer experience: waiting for diagnosis, waiting for treatment, waiting for remission, and waiting for relapse" (Mulcahy, Parry, & Glover, 2010, pp. 1065–1066). Waiting became a feature of the cancer experience, exacerbating the constant uncertainty at each stage of the cancer journey.

McCormick, McClement, and Naimark (2005) explored the experience of waiting for coronary artery bypass surgery. Telephone interviews were conducted with 25 participants. The study authors concluded that lengthy waits resulted in significant psychological disturbance, including anxiety and uncertainty about the future.

Watchful waiting is a protocol often used in chronic conditions. Watchful waiting is observation, expectant management, active monitoring, or deferred treatment (Wallace, Bailey, O'Rourke, & Galbraith, 2004). Watchful waiting provokes uncertainty. Without active treatment many persons with chronic conditions are left worrying about how their illness will unfold in the future; for example, the person may wonder, "Is the cancer growing while we wait?" As such, these persons must not only manage their lives with a chronic illness but deal with uncertainty about disease progression (Bailey et al., 2009).

Lack of Information

Information may increase or decrease uncertainty. Information about a particular chronic illness may or may not be readily available to clients and their social network. Information from various sources may lack consistency and may be contradictory. Additionally, individuals who seek information may not have the cognitive abilities to comprehend, integrate, and apply the information. Health information can be challenging and difficult to understand. Frequently, health information contains medical jargon that is not easily understood. Healthcare providers may provide unsolicited and unwanted advice to individuals in an attempt to manage the uncertainty.

Compounding these issues with the availability of information, outcomes in chronic illness are difficult to predict. Clear milestones in the chronic illness trajectory do not exist due to individual differences and responses to the illness and treatment. Because of this unpredictability it is challenging for the healthcare provider to provide an accurate progression of disease or timeline, thus adding to uncertainty.

In a correlational study with 71 patients undergoing peritoneal dialysis, Madar and Bar-Tal (2009) examined factors of severity and duration of disease, credible authority of healthcare providers, social support and education, and levels of uncertainty and stress. Patients' self-rated health, level of education, and their perception of their doctors as credible authorities contributed significantly to explaining patients' uncertainty. Uncertainty and stress were influenced by the patient's level of education. Factors associated with a patient's ability to process information most influenced his or her uncertainty.

Patients need healthcare providers to deliver the desired level and amount of information to them as well as to assess the psychological and physical qualities that potentially contribute to uncertainty. The level of education of the person with chronic illness affects the time needed for that individual to construct meaning and context for the events in chronic illness. Persons with more education, more social support, and more trust in healthcare providers experience less uncertainty (Mishel, 1988).

Evidence-Informed Practice Box

Illness uncertainty continues long after cancer diagnosis and treatment. Older women who have survived breast cancer experience ongoing illness uncertainty, fears about cancer recurrence, and symptoms from treatment side effects. Vicarious experiences such as hearing about cancer in a friend, having unfamiliar aches and pains, and media coverage about cancer can trigger feelings of uncertainty. Based on the theory of uncertainty in illness (Mishel, 1988, 1997), an uncertainty management intervention for older long-term breast cancer survivors was developed. The intervention consisted of cognitive-behavioural messages delivered by audiotapes and a self-help manual. Four hundred eighty-three recurrence-free women (342 White and 141 African American women) were randomly assigned to either the intervention or usual care (control) group. Nurses guided women through the intervention during four weekly telephone sessions and focused on one of four skills: relaxation, pleasant imagery, calming self-talk, and distraction. The nurses guided the women through the self-help manual that contained educational material and resources. Results indicated that the intervention in uncertainty management resulted in improvements in cognitive reframing (viewing their situation in a more positive light), cancer knowledge, and a variety of coping skills. At 20 months post-intervention, women continued to demonstrate benefits from the intervention in terms of decline in illness uncertainty and improved personal growth. Cognitive-behavioural interventions are beneficial to women with chronic illness. These interventions improve knowledge and behavioural skills and help foster a more positive appraisal of illness. This research supports the importance of nurses to assist persons with chronic illness in identifying appropriate sources of information and in developing behavioural skills.

Sources: Gil et al. (2005, 2006).

INTERVENTIONS

Certainty and predictability of outcomes are valued in Western society. When persons face chronic conditions with uncertain outcomes, they search for a cure (Mishel, 1990). The goal of nursing interventions is to reduce uncertainty in persons with chronic illness and promote self-confidence in their abilities, thus increasing certainty in their daily lives. A number of factors have been demonstrated to enhance self-confidence and promote certainty. Social support that enables the person with a chronic illness to rely on others, including family members, friends, or healthcare professionals, enhances self-confidence and certainty. Education and information given at the right time, at the right place, and at the right educational level are essential to enhancing certainty. Trust and confidence in one's healthcare provider are essential in managing chronic illness.

Chronic illness is complex and often poorly understood because there are no cures and treatment effectiveness varies. Predicting outcomes is difficult and increases uncertainty. Despite extensive research and practice knowledge about the trajectory of chronic illness, individual characteristics and diversity of symptom experiences produce unpredictability. Uncertainty looms large with limited information about the course of the disease and treatment options. Negative effects of uncertainty can be ameliorated by anticipating and understanding patients' individual needs along their illness trajectory.

Managing uncertainty is complex and dynamic and requires thoughtful and vigilant assessment by the healthcare provider. For some, lack of information may stimulate uncertainty. Others may embrace uncertainty and not desire more information, because more information might bring bad news. Some may embrace a watch-and-wait perspective rather than seek information about the future. Negative effects of uncertainty can be ameliorated by anticipating and understanding a patient's needs along their illness trajectory.

Strategies to maximize perceptions of confidence and control are essential to the management of uncertainty. Cognitive, emotive, and behavioural strategies act in concert to alter a patient's perception of uncertainty. First, however, an assessment of the psychological and physical factors that potentially contribute to uncertainty is essential. Persons experiencing chronic illness need healthcare professionals to provide the desired level and amount of information to them and their social network. Interventions to manage uncertainty across the chronic illness trajectory include strategies to control emotion, to restructure life to incorporate the unpredictability of symptoms and promote normalization of life, and to understand the illness to better formulate an illness schema (Mishel, 1999). The strategies for management of illness uncertainty discussed in this section are based on Mishel's (1988) uncertainty theory (**Figure 9-1**).

Cognitive Strategies

Uncertainty can be reduced by cognitive strategies that provide and process facts, assist with problem solving, and address knowledge deficits. Uncertainty can be diminished by providing clients and families with information and skills needed to alter their perception of stress. Meaning can be enhanced through personalized plans of care and appropriate educational interventions. Nurses can reduce uncertainty with "structural resources" that include education, social support, and care from healthcare providers who are credible sources of confidence and authority (Donovan-Kicken & Bute, 2008; Mishel, 1988, 1999).

Education

Increased availability of education that adds to patient and family knowledge reduces uncertainty (Clayton et al., 2006; Donovan-Kicken & Bute, 2008). Information reduces uncertainty and facilitates understanding of the chronic disease (Mishel, 1988). However, it is important to note individual differences. For some persons with chronic illness their uncertainty can be reduced by seeking out information and taking action based on that information. Others use avoidance to protect themselves from undesirable information.

Education for clients and their social support network has long been the hallmark of quality health care. Regardless of the inevitability of disease progression and physical deterioration intrinsic to chronic illness, education is an effective tool to promote a sense of control and manage uncertainty. Unfortunately, it is often difficult to ascertain the amount of information that individuals want or can process. As healthcare providers we often provide more information, particularly in the beginning of a disease process, than the person with chronic

illness and family can absorb. More is not always better. A thorough assessment of the needs of the individual and family, taking into account their educational background, past life experiences, and cultural beliefs, forms the basis for educational interventions.

The healthcare provider should be aware that for some patients, health information does not decrease uncertainty. Not knowing may be less threatening and less stressful than potentially bad news (Brashers et al., 2002; Brashers, Neidig, & Goldsmith, 2004). For other persons, having adequate information enables them to cope, participate in healthcare decisions, and deal with illness uncertainty. The premise that individuals with chronic illness and their families desire information and options for their treatment and care is a valued feature of Western healthcare practice. However, for many in diverse social groups healthcare decisions are within the purview of others, whether they are family members or healthcare providers. Healthcare providers must assess when informational support is appropriate. The role of education in reducing uncertainty is complex (Clayton et al., 2006).

The literature on treatment decision making suggests those who resist assuming this active

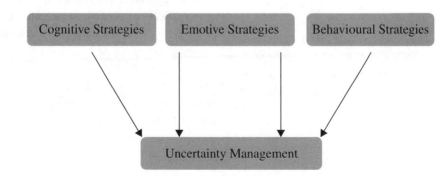

FIGURE 9-1 Adaptation to uncertainty.

role may be overwhelmed, misinformed as to the treatment options, and, in general, lack the capacity to participate. In a qualitative study with five women diagnosed with breast cancer, in-depth interviews revealed patients' ambivalence in making treatment decisions were efforts to recast identities and positions of patients and physicians in the cancer care organization. Patients seek not only information but interpretation of information by their oncologists (Sinding et al., 2010).

Cultural values and beliefs must be considered in education. Persons from family-centred cultures may be reluctant to assume responsibility for seeking information about their chronic disease and treatment and rely on family members to take charge. In family-centred cultures families interact with healthcare providers to seek information and may handle information in such a manner as to shield the person with the chronic illness from negative information that may result in the loss of hope (Brashers et al., 2002).

Nurses play a pivotal role by providing the right education in the right manner and at the appropriate point in the illness trajectory. Nurses may assist individuals in identifying credible sources of information that match the cognitive processing ability of the client. Healthcare providers need to be aware of local and national sources of information and support related to chronic conditions. Many chronic conditions have voluntary agencies with resources that provide information and other social support. Professional organizations are excellent resources for persons with a chronic condition and also for healthcare providers.

Know Thy Illness

Knowledge of self-management programs that incorporate information about the chronic disease is essential for the individual and family.

Identification of triggers that exacerbate illness symptoms and the activities that help modify and manage those symptoms are also important aspects of self-management.

Persons with chronic illness experience uncertainty when making decisions regarding treatment options and subsequent interventions. Nurses need to be aware of this uncertainty and provide support and information to help make informed decisions (Guadalupe, 2010).

Symptom Management

Individuals often have difficulty managing chronic illness symptoms (O'Neill & Morrow, 2001). Nursing assessment and intervention must include attention to symptom management. Individuals may need assistance in setting priorities for activities of daily living, strategies to diminish illness symptoms such as fatigue or pain, and fostering a plan of care that engenders confidence and normalcy to the highest degree possible. Interventions need to focus on physiological and emotional response to illness.

Designing and Adapting Routines

Individuals with chronic illness are unable to make predictions about the impact of illness on their lives. To help facilitate predictability, healthcare providers can assist the client and family to focus on planning for the short term and for events with immediate consequences. Individuals can make decisions and plans despite uncertainty. People can cushion the effects of uncertainty by developing a structure or routine that encourages familiar and recognizable patterns of behaviour.

Social Support

Social support plays an important role in uncertainty and adaptation. Social support can provide stable relationships where people can openly express emotions and feelings and find reassurance of their humanness and worthiness. Supportive others assist those with chronic conditions to reappraise uncertainty as opportunity or inconsequential and to incorporate uncertainty as a normal part of life. Social support directly and indirectly reduces uncertainty (Lien et al., 2009; Mishel, 1988) and promotes coping with chronic illness. Social support facilitates information seeking and avoidance and encourages reappraisal of uncertainty (Brashers et al., 2004). When persons with chronic illness have the opportunity to discuss and reflect on their illness, they gain insight and clarity about their situation and achieve more certainty (Bar-Tel, Barnoy, & Zisser, 2005). Active and reflective listening by nurses are key strategies to promote opportunity for persons with chronic illness to reflect and gain understanding of their illness experience.

Healthcare providers must be aware of the importance of social support in not only reducing uncertainty but enhancing quality of life. In Latina breast cancer survivors perceived social support and uncertainty played a pivotal role in managing and maintaining quality of life. Perceived social support promoted quality of life, whereas uncertainty diminished quality of life (Sammarco & Konecny, 2008). Sammarco and Konecny (2010) examined the differences between Latina and White breast cancer survivors and their perceived social support, uncertainty, and quality of life. Whites reported significantly higher levels of perceived social support and quality of life than their Latina counterparts. Healthcare providers must be aware of these differences and integrate cultural values and demographic differences into their plans of care in addressing quality of life.

Advice giving is a form of social support that may or may not be helpful. Advice giving is an effective support intervention when the advice is appropriate, relevant, and presented in a positive manner. However, when giving advice to persons with chronic illness, healthcare providers need to assess whether the individual wants their advice. If the individual is not receptive to advice, then other forms of support such as active listening or emotional support may be more appropriate (Thompson & O'Hair, 2008).

The nurse may need to assist the client in establishing a helpful social network. In addition to family members and friends, nurses and other healthcare providers are an important source of social support. Brashers and colleagues (2004) examined the effect of social support on management of uncertainty in persons living with HIV or AIDS. They found social support helps people with HIV and AIDS through information gathering and avoiding; providing instrumental support, skill development, acceptance, and validation; allowing venting; and encouraging shifts in perspective.

Emotive Strategies

Emotive intervention strategies alter feelings of uncertainty. Management programs that enhance coping and improve overall well-being are effective in persons with chronic illness (Gil et al., 2006).

Normalization

An emotive method to manage uncertainty in chronic illness is to restructure life to incorporate the unpredictability of chronic illness symptom onset, severity, and duration. Living in the present, one day at a time, reduces uncertainty. Activities of daily living are designed to incorporate realistic expectations and include a contingency plan.

Control Emotion

Strategies to control emotion are used by persons with chronic illnesses to control uncertainty. Healthcare professionals must assist clients and their families with viewing uncertainty as an opportunity. Uncertainty can be used to move from a perspective of limited choice to that of multiple opportunities (Mishel, 1990).

Formulate Cognitive Schema

Mishel (1999) suggested forming illness schema as a management method for uncertainty. Nurses can work with clients with chronic illness to construct personal scenarios of their illness that include the beginning of the illness, the progression of the illness, and how recovery will occur. This provides clients with an opportunity to integrate incongruent events into an individualized illness framework that provides meaning and understanding. Promoting self-care behaviours facilitates redefining an uncertain situation into one that is manageable.

Trust and Confidence in Healthcare Providers

Chronic illness requires attention to issues of life and death and wellness and illness, as well as daily management of symptoms and treatment. Trust and confidence in healthcare providers play a significant role in reducing uncertainty in persons with chronic illness (Madar & Bar-Tal, 2009).

Becoming Engaged

Becoming engaged in support groups and other support resources allows persons with chronic illness to have a sense of control over their illness. When people are engaged in the decisions regarding the management of their condition and are more informed about their options, they have a greater sense of control. However, patients may experience obstacles in becoming engaged in support services and groups because of fatigue, illness, or lack of confidence and resources. Nurses need to assess the client for the capability and desire to become engaged. Available and appropriate resources need to be identified and referred to the client and family.

Mindfulness

Mindfulness is an attribute of consciousness associated with psychological well-being. Brown and Ryan (2003) reported a relationship between mindfulness and positive emotional states. Mindfulness-based stress reduction uses techniques that help individuals cope with clinical and nonclinical problems (Grossman, Niemann, Schmidt, & Walach, 2004) and mitigate the negative effects of illness uncertainty. An intervention study of persons with cancer demonstrated that increased mindfulness over time resulted in decreases in mood disturbances and stress (Brown & Ryan, 2003). Mindfulness techniques are accessible to everyone and do not require financial resources or special equipment. Nurses can assist their clients with chronic illness to identify appropriate and acceptable mindfulness strategies to incorporate in their activities of daily living. These activities focus on outcomes such as acceptance and living in the present and recognition and acknowledgment of negative thoughts, feelings, or coping difficulties. Mindfulness exercises to reduce the negative effects of uncertainty include meditation, deep breathing exercises, and listening to music.

Cognitive Reframing

Cognitive reframing techniques are powerful tools that assist clients with chronic illness to deal with and manage symptoms, reduce uncertainty, and find meaning in life as it changes. Cognitive reframing seeks to alter one's cognitive schema and identify other ways of interpreting present and future situations and circumstances. Cognitive reframing in essence puts a new perspective on a situation while acknowledging the reality of the situation.

Bailey, Mishel, Belyea, Stewart, and Mohler (2004) evaluated the effectiveness of an intervention to help men cognitively reframe and manage the uncertainty of watchful waiting. Those in the intervention group received weekly calls from a nurse and those in the control group received usual care. Intervention participants reported greater improvement in the quality of their life and their future quality of life compared with the control group, thus documenting the effectiveness of cognitive reframing in reducing uncertainty.

Nurses can teach clients reframing strategies by helping them examine their expectations and exploring ways to set realistic expectations for themselves. Nurses can assist clients with acknowledging their changing needs and making modifications, substitutions, and adaptations when necessary and appropriate to accommodate their changing needs. Cognitive reframing requires ongoing attention and repetition; thus, nurses must provide ongoing encouragement and support for clients to use this technique successfully. Cognitive reframing techniques help persons with chronic illness rethink their perceptions of uncertainty and can impact mood and hopefulness.

Behavioural Strategies

Healthcare providers must be alert to expressions of uncertainty. These expressions can be ascertained in language and in behaviour such as withdrawing from self-care activities or social interaction.

Activities of Daily Living

A focus on daily routines and expectations reduces uncertainty and diminishes anxiety. Living in the present with a "today focus" rather than a "tomorrow focus" helps reduce uncertainty (Greenwood et al., 2009).

Managing Unpredictability: Anticipatory Guidance

In anticipation of progressive disability, nurses may refer persons to rehabilitative therapies for interventions designed to enhance and prolong independence in their daily activities, occupation, and relationships. Members of the interdisciplinary team should be used to help the client and family deal with financial or vocational issues that may contribute to uncertainty. Individuals may seek out advice from others who had the same condition to assist them in anticipating an effective way to engage in health promotion and maintenance activities.

SUMMARY

Uncertainty is chronic and persists over the trajectory of disease. Accepting uncertainty is an adaptive mechanism (Mishel, 1990). Negative effects of uncertainty can be ameliorated by anticipating and understanding individual needs across the disease course. Nurses and other healthcare professionals can work with persons with chronic illness to modify negative outcomes of the illness experience and promote positive perceptions of uncertainty.

Nurses are valuable partners of persons with chronic conditions and their families in assisting them to cope with uncertain experiences by providing positive communication and support. Nursing assessments and interventions directed toward reducing uncertainty can improve quality of life and adaptation to living with chronic conditions (Elphee, 2008). Assessment of uncertainty needs to be included as an element of all nursing assessments of persons with chronic illness. Theory-based nursing interventions designed to educate and support persons with chronic illness to integrate and manage uncertainty across their disease trajectory are essential. Unacknowledged and unaddressed uncertainty can erode quality of life for those with chronic conditions and for those in their social network.

> For a full suite of assignments and additional learning activities, use the access code located in the front of your book and visit this exclusive website: **http://go.jblearning.com/kramer-kile**. If you do not have an access code, you can obtain one at the site.
>
> **www**

STUDY QUESTIONS

www

1. Describe the social and cultural factors related to uncertainty in chronic illness.
2. Apply Mishel's theory of uncertainty to one of your clients with a chronic condition.
3. How does cognitive reframing assist a client with uncertainty?
4. Describe how one would assess a patient and family for educational/informational needs.
5. The primary antecedent of Mishel's theory is the stimuli frame. Describe its components and how they influence uncertainty.
6. Seeing uncertainty as "harm" is understandable, but how can uncertainty be seen as an opportunity?

REFERENCES

Bailey, D. E., Landerman, L., Barroso, J., Bixby, P., Mishel, M. H., Muir, A. J., . . . Clipp E. (2009). Uncertainty, symptoms, and quality of life in persons with chronic hepatitis C. *Psychosomatics, 50*(2), 138–146.

Bailey, D. E., Mishel, M. H., Belyea, M., Stewart, J. L., & Mohler, J. (2004).Uncertainty intervention for watchful waiting in prostate cancer. *Cancer Nursing, 27*(5), 339–346.

Bailey, D. E., Wallace, M., & Mishel, M. H. (2007). Watching, waiting and uncertainty in prostate cancer. *Journal of Clinical Nursing, 16*(4), 734–741.

Bar-Tel, Y., Barnoy, S., & Zisser, B. (2005). Whose informational needs are considered? A comparison between cancer patients and their spouses' perceptions of their own and their partners' knowledge and informational needs. *Social Science & Medicine, 60*(7), 1459–1465.

Basevitz, P., Pushkar, D., Chaikelson, J., Conway, M., & Dalton, C. (2008). Age-related differences in worry and related processes. *International Journal of Aging and Human Development, 66*(4), 283–305.

Bournes, D. A., & Mitchell, G. J. (2002). Waiting: The experience of persons in a critical care waiting room. *Research in Nursing & Health, 25*, 58–67.

Brashers, D. E. (2001). Communication and uncertainty management. *Journal of Communication, 51*, 477–497.

Brashers, D. E., Goldsmith, D. J., & Hsieh, E. (2002). Information seeking and avoiding in health contexts. *Human Communication Research, 28*, 258–271.

Brashers, D. E., Neidig, J. L., & Goldsmith, D. J. (2004). Social support and the management of uncertainty for people living with HIV or AIDS. *Health Communication, 16*, 305–331.

Brashers, D. E., Neidig, J. L., Russell, J. A., Cardillo, L. W., Haas, S. M., Dobbs, L. K., . . . Nemeth, S. (2003). The medical, personal, and social causes of uncertainty in HIV illness. *Issues in Mental Health Nursing, 24*, 497–522.

Brown, K. W., & Ryan, R., M. (2003). The benefits of being present: Mindfulness and its role in psychological well-being. *Journal of Personality and Social Psychology, 84*(4), 822–848.

Clayton, M. F., Mishel, M. H., & Belyea, M. (2006). Testing a model of symptoms, communication, uncertainty and well-being in older breast cancer survivors. *Research in Nursing and Health, 29*, 18–39.

Davis, F. (1960). Uncertainty in medical prognosis clinical and functional. *American Journal of Sociology, 66*, 41–47.

Decker, C. L., Haase, J. E., & Bell, C. J. (2007). Uncertainty in adolescents and young adults with cancer. *Oncology Nursing Forum, 34*(3), 681–688.

Denny, E. (2009). "I never know from one day to another how I will feel": Pain and uncertainty in women with endometriosis. *Qualitative Health Research, 19*(7), 985–995.

Dirksen, S., & Erickson, J. (2002). Well-being in Hispanic and non-Hispanic Caucasian survivors of breast cancer. *Oncology Nursing Forum, 29*, 820–826.

Donovan-Kicken, E., & Bute, J. J. (2008). Uncertainty of social network members in the case of communication-debilitating illness or injury. *Qualitative Health Research, 18*(1), 5–18.

Elphee, E. E. (2008). Understanding the concept of uncertainty in patients with indolent lymphoma. *Oncology Nursing Forum, 35*(3), 449–454.

Encyclopedia Britannica. (2011). Damocles. Retrieved from http://www.britannica.com/EBchecked/topic/150566/Damocles

Gil, K., Mishel, M. Belyea, M., Germino, B., Porter, L., & Clayton, M. (2006). Benefits of the uncertainty management intervention for African American and Caucasian older breast cancer survivors: 20-month outcomes. *International Journal of Behavioral Medicine, 13*, 286–294.

Gil, K. M., Mishel, M. H., Belyea, M., Germino, B., Porter, L. S., Carlton-LaNey, I., & Stewart, J. (2004). Triggers of uncertainty about recurrence and long-term treatment side effects in older African American and Caucasian breast cancer survivors. *Oncology Nursing Forum, 31*(3), 633–639.

Gil, K. M., Mishel, M. H., Germino, B., Porter, L. S., Carlton-LaNey, I., & Belyea, M. (2005). Uncertainty management intervention for older African American and Caucasian long-term breast cancer survivors. *Journal of Psychosocial Oncology, 23*, 3–21.

Goffman, E. (1963). *Stigma: Notes on the management of spoiled identity.* New York, NY: Simon and Schuster.

Greenwood, N., Mackenzie, A., Wilson, N., & Cloud, G. (2009). Managing uncertainty in life after stroke: A qualitative study of the experiences of established and new informal carers in the first 3 months after discharge. *International Journal of Nursing Studies, 46*, 1122–1133.

Grossman, P., Niemann, L., Schmidt, S., & Walach, H. (2004). Mindfulness-based stress reduction and health benefits: A meta-analysis. *Journal of Psychosomatic Research, 57*(1), 35–43.

Guadalupe, K. (2010). Understanding a meningioma diagnosis using Mishel's theory of uncertainty in illness. *British Journal of Neuroscience Nursing, 6*(2), 77–82.

Hoff, A. L., Mullins, L. L., Chaney, M. J., Hartman, V. L., & Domek, D. (2002). Illness uncertainty, perceived control, and psychological distress among adolescents with type 1 diabetes. *Research and Theory for Nursing Practice, 16*(4), 223–236.

Hommel, K. A., Chaney, J. M., Wagner, J. L., White, M. M., Hoff, A. L., & Mullins, L. L. (2003). Anxiety and depression in older adolescents with long-standing asthma: The role of illness uncertainty. *Children's Health Care, 32*(1), 51–63.

Johnson, L. M., Zautra, A. J., & Davis, M. C. (2006). The role of illness uncertainty on coping with fibromyalgia symptoms. *Health Psychology, 25*(6), 696–703.

Kang, Y. (2006). Effect of uncertainty on depression in patients with newly diagnosed atrial fibrillation. *Progress in Cardiovascular Nursing, 21*(2), 83–88.

Lasker, J. N., Sogolow, E. D., Olenik, J. M., Sass, D. A., & Weinrieb, R. M. (2010). Uncertainty and liver transplantation: Women with primary biliary cirrhosis before and after transplant. *Women & Health, 50*, 359–375.

Lazarus, R. S., & Folkman, S. (1984). *Stress, appraisal, and coping.* New York, NY: Springer.

Lemaire, G. S. (2004). More than just menstrual cramps: Symptoms and uncertainty among women with endometriosis. *Journal of Obstetric, Gynecologic, and Neonatal Nursing, 33*, 71–79.

Liao, M. N., Chen, M. F., Chen, S. C., & Chen, P. L. (2008). Uncertainty and anxiety during the diagnostic period for women with suspected breast cancer. *Cancer Nursing, 31*(4), 274–283.

Lien, C. Y., Lin, H. R., Kuo, I. T., & Chen, M. L. (2009). Perceived uncertainty, social support and psychological adjustment in older patients with cancer being treated with surgery. *Journal of Clinical Nursing, 18*, 2311–2319.

Madar, H., & Bar-Tal, Y. (2009). The experience of uncertainty among patients having peritoneal dialysis. *Journal of Advanced Nursing, 65*(8), 1664–1669.

Martin, S. C., Stone, A. M., Scott, A. M., & Brashers, D. E. (2010). Medical, personal, and social forms of uncertainty across the transplantation trajectory. *Qualitative Health Research, 20*, 182–196.

Mast, M. E. (1998). Survivors of breast cancer: Illness uncertainty, positive reappraisal and emotional distress. *Oncology Nursing Forum, 25*, 555–562.

Mauro, A. M. (2010). Long-term follow-up study of uncertainty and psychosocial adjustment among implantable cardioverter defibrillator recipients. *International Journal of Nursing Studies, 47*(9), 1080–1088.

McCormick, K. M. (2002). A concept analysis of uncertainty in illness. *Journal of Nursing Scholarship, 34*(2), 127–131.

McCormick, K. M., McClement, S., & Naimark, B. J. (2005). A qualitative analysis of the experience of uncertainty while awaiting coronary artery bypass surgery. *Canadian Journal of Cardiovascular Nursing, 15*(1), 10–22.

McIntosh, J. (1974). Processes of communication, Information seeking and control associated with cancer: A selective review of the literature. *Social Science & Medicine, 8*, 167–187.

McIntosh, J. (1976). Patients' awareness and desire for information about diagnosed but undisclosed malignant disease. *Lancet, 2*, 300–303.

McNulty, K., Livneh, H., & Wilson, L. M. (2004). Perceived uncertainty, spiritual well-being, and psychosocial adaptation in individuals with multiple sclerosis. *Rehabilitation Psychology, 49*(2), 91–99.

Mishel, M. H. (1981). The measurement of uncertainty in illness. *Nursing Research, 30*(5), 258–263.

Mishel, M. H. (1984). Perceived uncertainty and stress in illness. *Research in Nursing and Health, 7*(3), 163–171.

Mishel, M. H. (1988). Uncertainty in illness. *Image: Journal of Nursing Scholarship, 20*, 225–232.

Mishel, M. H. (1990). Reconceptualization of the uncertainty in illness theory. *Image: Journal of Nursing Scholarship, 22*, 256–262.

Mishel, M. H. (1997). Uncertainty in acute illness. *Annual Review of Nursing Research, 15*, 57–80.

Mishel, M. H. (1999). Uncertainty in chronic illness. *Annual Review of Nursing Research, 17*, 269–294.

Mishel, M. H., & Braden, C. J. (1988). Finding meaning: Antecedents of uncertainty. *Nursing Research, 37*, 98–103.

Mitchell, M. L., Courtney, M., & Coyer, F. (2003). Understanding uncertainty and minimizing families' anxiety at the time of transfer from intensive care. *Nursing and Health Sciences, 5*, 207–217.

Montgomery, M. (2010). Uncertainty during breast diagnostic evaluation: State of the science. *Oncology Nursing Forum, 37*(1), 77–83.

Mulcahy, C. M., Parry, D. C., & Glover, T. D. (2010). The "patient patient": The trauma of waiting and the power of resistance for people living with cancer. *Qualitative Health Research, 20*(8), 1062–1075.

Mullins, L. L., Chaney, J. M., Balderson, B., & Hommel, K. A. (2000). The relationship of illness uncertainty, illness intrusiveness, and asthma severity to depression in young adults with long-standing asthma. *International Journal of Rehabilitation and Health, 5*(3), 177–185.

Mullins, L. L., Cote, M. P., Fuemmeler, B. F., Jean, V. M., Beatty, W. W., & Paul, R. H. (2001). Illness intrusiveness, uncertainty, and distress in individuals with multiple sclerosis. *Rehabilitation Psychology, 46*(2), 139–153.

Northouse, L. L., Mood, D., Kershaw, T., Schafenacker, A., Mellon, S., Walker, J., . . . Decker, V. (2002). Quality of life of women with recurrent breast cancer and their family members. *Journal of Clinical Oncology, 20*, 4050–4064.

O'Neill, E. W., & Morrow, L. L. (2001). The symptom experience of women with chronic illness. *Journal of Advanced Nursing, 33*, 257–268.

Penrod. J. (2001). Refinement of the concept of uncertainty. *Journal of Advanced Nursing, 34*, 238–245.

Persson, E., & Hellstrom, A. (2002). Experiences of Swedish men and women 6 to 12 weeks after ostomy surgery. *Journal of Wound, Ostomy and Continence Nursing, 29*(2), 103–108.

Reich, J. W., Olmsted, M. E., & van Puymbroeck, C. M. (2006). Illness uncertainty, partner caregiver burden and support, and relationship satisfaction in fibromyalgia and osteoarthritis patients. *Arthritis & Rheumatism, 55*(1), 86–93.

Sammarco, A. (2001). Perceived social support, uncertainty, and quality of life of younger breast cancer survivors. *Cancer Nursing, 24*(3), 212–219.

Sammarco, A., & Konecny, L. (2008). Quality of life, social support and uncertainty among Latina breast cancer survivors. *Oncology Nursing Forum, 35,* 844–849.

Sammarco, A., & Konecny, L. M. (2010). Quality of life, social support, and uncertainty among Latina and Caucasian breast cancer survivors: A comparative study. *Oncology Nursing Forum, 37*(1), 93–99.

Sanders-Dewey, J. E. J., Mullins, L. L., & Chaney, J. M. (2001). Coping style, perceived uncertainty in illness, and distress in individuals with Parkinson's disease and their caregivers. *Rehabilitation Psychology, 46,* 363–381.

Schulman-Green, D., Ercolano, E., Dowd, M., Schwartz, P., & McCorkle, R. (2008). Quality of life among women after surgery for ovarian cancer. *Palliative Support Care, 6*(3), 239–247.

Simpson, M. F., & Whyte, F. (2006). Patients' experiences of completing treatment for colorectal cancer in a Scottish district general hospital. *European Journal of Cancer Care, 15*(2), 172–182.

Sinding, C., Hudak, P., Wiernikowski, J., Aronson, J., Miller, P., Gould, J., . . . Fitzpatrick-Lewis, D. (2010). "I like to be an informed person but . . .": Negotiating responsibility for treatment decisions in cancer care. *Social Science & Medicine, 71,* 1094–1101.

Stone, A. M., & Jones, C. L. (2009). Sources of uncertainty: Experiences of Alzheimer's disease. *Issues in Mental Health Nursing, 30,* 677–686.

Thompson, S., & O'Hair, H. D. (2008). Advice-giving and the management of uncertainty for cancer survivors. *Health Communication, 23,* 340–348.

Wallace, M. (2003). Uncertainty and quality of life of older men who undergo watchful waiting for prostate cancer. *Oncology Nursing Forum, 30,* 303–309.

Wallace, M. (2005). Finding more meaning: The antecedents of uncertainty revisited. *Journal of Clinical Nursing, 14,* 863–868.

Wallace, M., Bailey, D., O'Rourke, M., & Galbraith, M. (2004). The watchful waiting management option for older men with prostate cancer: State of the science. *Oncology Nursing Forum, 31*(6), 1057–1064.

Wineman, N. M., Schwetz, K. M., Zeller, R., & Cyphert, J. (2003). Longitudinal analysis of illness uncertainty, coping, hopefulness, and mood during participation in a clinical drug trail. *Journal of Neuroscience Nursing, 35*(2), 100–107.

Wolfe-Christensen, C., Isenberg, J. C., Mullins, L. L., Carpentier, M. Y., & Almstrom, C. (2008). Objective versus subjective ratings of asthma severity: Differential predictors of illness uncertainty and psychological distress in college students with asthma. *Children's Health Care, 37,* 183–195.

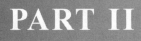

PART II

Impact on the Client and Family

CHAPTER 10

Sexuality

Original chapter by Margaret Chamberlain Wilmoth
Canadian content added by Joseph C. Osuji

INTRODUCTION

Humans are sexual beings from birth until death. Sexuality is an integral aspect of our personalities and is more than sexual contact and the ability to reach sexual satisfaction. It is a fundamental part of a full and healthy life that is central to human self-concept, self-esteem, and body image. Sexuality includes views of ourselves as a particular gender, feelings about our bodies, and the ways we communicate verbally and nonverbally our comfort about ourselves to others. It also includes the ability to engage in satisfying sexual behaviours alone or with another. Sexuality does not end when one reaches a certain age, and it does not end with the diagnosis of a chronic illness. In the presence of chronic illness, sexuality is considered as an important determinant for health and quality of life (Clayton & Ramamurthy, 2008). In fact, sexuality and intimacy may become *more* important after such a diagnosis as a way of reaffirming human connection, aliveness, and continued desirability and caring. Sexuality is a critical aspect of quality of life that, unfortunately, is often ignored by healthcare professionals.

This chapter briefly reviews standards of nursing practice as they relate to sexuality, sexual physiological functioning, alterations in sexuality caused by common chronic illnesses and their treatments, and nursing interventions. This chapter also provides nurses with suggestions for ways to incorporate discussions of sexuality into their practice.

DEFINITIONS

Sexuality is a multidimensional concept that affects and determines individual identity. It is a complex construct with terminology that has yet to be defined in a manner accepted by all. Sexuality, sexual behaviours, and attitudes vary greatly from culture to culture and on an individual basis. Contextual features that impact human sexuality include education, laws, ethnicity, family, peer groups, personal experiences. and religion (Esmail, Esmail, & Munro, 2002). When discussing sexuality with other professionals or with clients it is important to ensure everyone has the same frame of reference for the many descriptors used for aspects of sexuality.

Nurses also are encouraged to know the more "scientific" terms yet remember these are not the words used by most clients when they talk about their sexuality. Nurses need to find out what terms their clients use, clarify the meaning to ensure understanding, then use words the client knows and understands when discussing the impact of chronic illness on sexuality. Nurses should avoid using the term "sexual dysfunction" because this is a psychiatric diagnosis most nurses are not qualified to make. The American Psychiatric Association (2000) has identified sexual dysfunctions that are a result of chronic medical conditions and that have specific diagnostic criteria. **Table 10-1** lists the definitions used in discussing sexuality in this chapter.

STANDARDS OF PRACTICE

Standards of practice confer both a legal standard of practice and an ethical responsibility that nurses adhere to in their practice of nursing (Andrews, Goldberg, & Kaplan, 1996). Across the globe different nursing and health organizations have developed standards of practice that incorporate sexuality. Standards of practice for the profession, published by the American Nurses Association (2010), include six standards of care that encompass significant actions taken by nurses when providing care to their clients. These standards include the components of the nursing process and also assume that all relevant healthcare needs of the client will be assessed and appropriate care provided, including needs regarding sexuality. The Canadian Nurses Association does not mention sexuality specifically but states that nurses should help clients meet all their healthcare needs. Specialty organizations have derived standards of nursing practice from those published by the American Nurses Association that are specific to their practice. For example, the Oncology Nursing Society (2004) published nursing practice standards

Table 10-1 Sexuality Terms and Definitions	
Term	**Definition**
Sexuality	Everything that makes one human, including the need for touch, feelings about one's body, the need to connect with another human in an intimate way, interest in engaging in sexual behaviors, communication of one's feelings and needs to one's partner, and the ability to engage in satisfying sexual behaviors
Sexual behaviors	Specific activities used to obtain release of sexual tension alone or with another to achieve sexual satisfaction; refers also to the multiple ways one verbally and nonverbally communicates sexual feelings and attitudes to others
Sexual functioning	The physiological component of sexuality, including human sexual anatomy, the sexual response cycle, neuroendocrine functioning, and life cycle changes in sexual physiology
Sexual dysfunction	Characterized by disturbances in the processes of the sexual response cycle or by pain associated with sexual intercourse; is a psychiatric diagnosis (American Psychiatric Association, 2000) and should not be used by nurses unless they are specially trained in treating sexual dysfunctions

Sources: American Psychiatric Association (2000) and Wilmoth (2009).

that specifically identified sexuality as one potential area of client concern. These standards include both assessment criteria and outcome criteria. Nurses who care for cancer patients then are expected to follow each of these standards in the provision of patient care (**Table 10-2**).

Nurses and physicians are legally obligated to ensure clients have the necessary information to make decisions regarding treatment. The provision of informed consent also requires that all risks, benefits, and side effects of diseases and their treatments are provided to clients as they choose treatments for any illness. This includes information about potential sexual side effects of proposed treatments. Failure to provide this information could potentially lead to legal action by the client.

Table 10-2   Oncology Nursing Society Statement on the Scope and Standards of Oncology Nursing Practice

Standard I Assessment

The oncology nurse systematically and continually collects data regarding the health status of the patient.

Measurement Criteria

The oncology nurse collects data in the following 14 high-incidence problem areas that may include but are not limited to sexuality.

1. Past and present sexual patterns and expression.
2. Effects of disease and treatment on body image.
3. Effects of disease and treatment on sexual function.
4. Psychological response of patient and partner to disease and treatment.

Standard III Outcome Identification

The oncology nurse identifies expected outcomes individualized to the patient.

Measurement Criteria

The oncology nurse develops expected outcomes for each of the 14 high-incidence problem areas within a level consistent with the patient's physiology, psychosocial and spiritual capacities, cultural background, and value system. The expected outcomes include but are not limited to sexuality. The patient and/or family:

1. Identifies potential or actual changes in sexuality, sexual functioning, or intimacy related to disease and treatment.
2. Expresses feelings about alopecia, body image changes, and altered sexual functioning.
3. Engages in open communication with his or her partner regarding changes in sexual functioning or desire, within cultural framework.
4. Describes appropriate interventions for actual or potential changes in sexual function.
5. Identifies other satisfying methods of sexual expression that provide satisfaction to both partners, within cultural framework.
6. Identifies personal and community resources to assist with changes in body image and sexual functioning.

Source: Oncology Nursing Society (2004).

SEXUAL RESPONSE CYCLE AND SEXUAL PHYSIOLOGY

Two frameworks are commonly used to describe what is called the "sexual response cycle." The first, proposed by Dr. William Masters and Virginia Johnson (1966), is a four-stage model of sexual response of the male and female. The four phases of the Masters and Johnson (1966) model are excitement, plateau, orgasm, and resolution. The excitement stage causes an increase in the heart rate and vasocongestion to the penis. This is accompanied by lengthening and widening of the vagina, elevation of the cervix and uterus, and initial swelling of the labia minora (Guyton & Hall, 2006; Masters & Johnson, 1966). These changes are caused by vasocongestion and are secondary to a parasympathetic response mediated to S2 and S4 through the pudendal nerve and sacral plexus (Guyton & Hall, 2006). The second stage is the plateau stage, which is an increased state of arousal, causing the heart rate and blood pressure to increase, with a subsequent increase in respiratory rate (Katz, 2007).

The third stage is the orgasm, the phase of maximal muscular contraction (male ejaculation and female pelvic muscle contraction), with a peak of respirations and heart rate and a subjective feeling of intense pleasure that radiates throughout the body (Katz, 2007). Impending orgasm is determined by the presence of an intense colour change in the labia minora in women and full elevation of the scrotal sac to the perineal wall in men, all a result of intense vasocongestion (Masters & Johnson, 1966). Orgasm is mediated by the sympathetic nervous system and is the physical release and peak of pleasurable expression, followed by relaxation (Guyton & Hall, 2006). The sympathetic nerves between T12 and L2 control ejaculation (Koukouras et

al., 1991). The intensity of orgasm in women depends on the duration and intensity of sexual stimulation.

The final stage is resolution, when vasocongestion resolves and the body returns to its normal nonaroused state (Katz, 2007). Men also have what is referred to as a "refractory period," which is the period within which the male is unable to achieve an erection satisfactory for penetration. This period of time is age and health-status dependent (Masters & Johnson, 1966).

Physical changes that occur in both men and women as a result of sexual stimulation are vasocongestion and myotonia. Vasocongestion occurs in the penis in men and in the labia in women and is an essential requirement for orgasm and subsequent sexual satisfaction. Myotonia refers to the involuntary muscular contractions that occur throughout the body during sexual response (Kolodny, Masters, Johnson, & Biggs, 1979).

The second framework is from Kaplan. Kaplan's (1979) modification of the sexual response cycle includes aspects of sexual physiology involving the prelude to sexual activity as well as the consequences of sexual activity. These three phases are desire, arousal, and orgasm. Desire is the prelude to engaging in satisfying sexual behaviours and is the most complex component of the sexual response cycle. Desire is often affected by factors such as anger, pain, and body image as well as by disease processes and medications (Kaplan, 1979). When sexual stimuli are perceived by women, they are processed physiologically and physically, leading to subjective feelings of arousal and a responsive feeling of desire (Katz, 2007). This may explain why psychogenic factors can be a determinant cause of male and female sexual dysfunction.

Arousal, manifested by erection in males, is mediated by the parasympathetic nervous system and is the result of either psychic or somatic sexual stimulation (Masters & Johnson, 1966). Alternately, activation of the sympathetic nervous system leads to loss of an erection through vasoconstriction. It was previously thought that an analogous process of parasympathetic nervous system stimulation led to arousal in women. However, evidence suggests it is stimulation of the sympathetic nervous system that is responsible for female arousal (Meston, 2000). Data also suggest that stimulation of the sympathetic nervous system may enhance arousal in women with low sexual desire (Meston & Gorzalka, 1996) and that induction of relaxation may negatively affect arousal (Meston, 2000).

Although many women suggest the Gräfenberg spot (G-spot) plays an important role in their sexuality, the existence of this sensitive area remains open for verification (Hines, 2001). The G-spot is purportedly located in the anterior wall of the vagina, about halfway between the back of the pubic bone and the cervix along the course of the urethra (Ladas, Whipple, & Perry, 1982). When stimulated, this tissue swells from the size of a bean to greater than a half dollar (Ladas et al., 1982). Stimulation of this area appears to cause a different orgasmic sensation, and it is hypothesized that this response is mediated by the pelvic nerve, causing the uterus to contract and descend against the vagina rather than elevate, as with stimulation mediated by the pudendal nerve (Ladas et al., 1982). Approximately 40% of women experience expulsion of a fluid upon orgasm caused by G-spot stimulation (Darling, Davidson, & Conway-Welch, 1990). Research suggests this is a prostatic-like fluid that is released during orgasm (Zaviacic & Ablin, 2000; Zaviacic & Whipple, 1993). Belief that this is not urine but a normal release of fluid that occurs during sexual response may lead to a reduction in embarrassment for many women.

The neurohormonal system influences sexual functioning through its effect on hormone production. The hypothalamic–hypophysial portal system plays an important role in sexual functioning in both genders through production of gonadotrophin-releasing hormone and subsequent stimulation of gonadotrophin production by the anterior pituitary gland. The anterior pituitary gland secretes six hormones, two of which play an essential role in sexual functioning. Follicle-stimulating hormone and luteinizing hormone control growth of the gonads and influence sexual functioning. In men luteinizing hormone influences production of testosterone by the Leydig cells in the testes through a negative feedback loop (Guyton & Hall, 2006). Production of gonadotrophin-releasing hormone is reduced, once a satisfactory level of testosterone has been attained. A negative feedback loop also exists in the woman, although it is much more complex, given the concurrent production of oestrogen and progesterone by the ovary and the production of androgens by the adrenal cortex.

Psychic factors appear to play a larger role in the sexual functioning of women than men, particularly in relation to sexual desire. Multiple neuronal centres in the brain's limbic system transmit signals into the arcuate nuclei in the mediobasal hypothalamus. These signals modify the intensity of gonadotrophin-releasing hormone release and the frequency of the impulses (Guyton & Hall, 2006). This may explain why desire in women is more vulnerable to emotions and distractions than it is in men.

Aging affects the sexual response cycle in predictable ways, but it does not signal the end of sexuality. In fact, the old adage "use it or lose it" is applicable to continued sexual activity throughout life (Masters & Johnson, 1981). The general impact of aging on the sexual response cycle is a slower, less intense sexual response (Lindau et al., 2007). The frequency of sexual activity in earlier years is predictive of frequency as one ages. The quality of the sexual relationship appears to be the greatest influence on the frequency and satisfaction of sexual activity (Masters & Johnson, 1981). As in younger adults, the quality of communication in a relationship, degree of mutual intimacy, and level of commitment to the relationship are vital to a satisfying sexual relationship and to achieving sexual satisfaction.

In clients aged 60 or older, organic factors are the most important determinant of erectile dysfunction (ED) (Corona et al., 2007). The frequent comorbidity of multiple metabolic and hemodynamic abnormalities in aging clients can substantially increase the incidence and progression of atherosclerotic lesions, leading to vascular forms of ED (Corona et al., 2007). Masters and Johnson (1966) found that in men between 51 and 90 years of age, the time to achieve erection was two to three times longer than in younger men. Achieving erection also required more tactile stimulation than in younger years. However, once achieved, older men can maintain a full erection for a longer period before ejaculation. Scrotal vasocongestion is reduced, with a subsequent decrease in testicular elevation. Basal and dynamic peak cavernosal velocity was shown to be reduced in older patients via Doppler ultrasound penile examination (Corona et al., 2007). The ability to attain orgasm is not impaired with aging, but there is an overall decrease in myotonia and fewer penile and rectal sphincter contractions.

There is an increase in time from hours to days before older men can achieve another erection once they have ejaculated and achieved an orgasm (refractory period).

Women also experience sexual response cycle changes as they age, primarily after completing the menopausal transition. Common complaints include decreased desire, dry vagina, and difficulty attaining orgasm (Lindau et al., 2007). Vaginal changes include a thinning of the mucosa, with a decrease in vaginal lubrication. In women who abstain from sexual intercourse, narrowing and stenosis of the introitus and vaginal vault can occur (Leiblum & Segraves, 1989). Older women experience a decrease in the vasocongestion of the labia and other genitalia analogous to the decrease in penile tumescence experienced by men. Orgasm in sexually active women is not impaired; however, there is some decrease in the degree of myotonia experienced. Intense orgasm may lead to involuntary distension of the external meatus, leading to an increase in frequency of urinary tract infections in older women.

SEXUALITY AND CHRONIC ILLNESS

The presence of a chronic illness affects all aspects of an individual's life, including sexuality. There are numerous chronic illnesses, and discussion of the impact of each on sexuality is beyond the scope of this chapter. Therefore, this chapter is limited to a brief discussion of the effects of coronary artery disease, diabetes mellitus, cancer, and multiple sclerosis on sexuality. For a more detailed conceptual framework on chronic diseases and their impact on sexuality, see Verschuren, Enzlin, Dijkstra, Geertzen, and Dekker (2010).

Coronary Artery Disease

The heart is linked to romance and to the soul, so any threat to cardiac functioning is emotionally linked to matters of the self, sexuality, and intimacy. Cardiovascular disease, including coronary artery disease and stroke, is the second leading cause of death in Canada (Statistics Canada, 2012) and number one cause of death in the United States in both genders and all racial and ethnic groups (Centers for Disease Control and Prevention, 2004). More men and women than ever before are living longer and continue to lead productive lives after experiencing a myocardial infarction (MI); however, recent data suggest women experience a lower degree of quality of life than men (Agewall, Berglund, & Henareh, 2004; Svedlund & Danielson, 2004).

Erectile disorders occur in 60% of all patients diagnosed with cardiovascular disorders (Archer, Gragasin, Webster, Bochinski, & Michelakis, 2005). Kazemi-Saleu et al. (2008) found that poorer sexual relations and adjustment manifested more in women than men after coronary artery disease diagnosis, whereas fear of sexual activity was more pronounced in men than women. Therefore, adequate and accurate knowledge about sexuality after diagnosis may have a positive impact crucial to individuals' self-concept, sexuality, and sexual relationships.

The consensus study from the Second Princeton Consensus Conference collaborates and clarifies the risk stratification algorithm that was developed by the first Princeton Consensus Panel to evaluate the degree of cardiovascular risk associated with sexual activity for men with varying degrees of cardiovascular disease (Kostis et al., 2005). The algorithm emphasizes the importance of risk factor evaluation and management for all patients with ED.

The relative safety in which clients can engage in sexual activity depends on their degree of cardiac disease. This panel recommended a classification system that would stratify clients into a risk category based on the extent of their cardiac disease. These categories and management recommendations are found in **Table 10-3**. Patients with less than three major risk factors for cardiovascular disease (age, hypertension, diabetes mellitus, cigarette smoking, dyslipidaemia, sedentary lifestyle, and family history of premature coronary artery disease) are generally at low risk for significant cardiac complications from sexual activity or the treatment of sexual dysfunction (Kostis et al., 2005). Clients whose cardiac conditions are uncertain and those with multiple risk factors require further testing or evaluation before resuming sexual activity (Kostis et al., 2005). Patients with a history of MI (>2 weeks and <6 weeks) may be at somewhat greater risk for coitus-induced ischemia and reinfarction as well as malignant arrhythmias (Kostis et al., 2005). The level of risk associated within this time period post-MI can be assessed with an exercise stress test.

Counselling of all clients regarding lifestyle changes and activity restrictions should begin as soon as the client is stabilized. Discussions regarding sexual activity should be included in the counselling. Potential fear of cardiac arrest during sexual activity should be eradicated as soon as possible by assuring clients and their partners that this risk is only 1.2% and that sex accounts for only 0.5% to 1.0% of all acute coronary incidents (DeBusk, 2000).

Reports continue to validate the appropriateness of the stair-climbing tolerance test for successful return to sexual activity after 6 weeks post-MI. Sexual activity conceptualized simply as arousal is unassociated with physical exertion.

Table 10-3 Management Recommendations Based on Graded Cardiovascular (CV) Risk Assessment		
Grade of Risk	**Categories of CVD**	**Management**
Low risk	Asymptomatic, 6 weeks; mild valvular disease, LVD/CHF (NYHA class I); patients with pericarditis, mitral valve prolapse, or atrial fibrillation with controlled ventricular response should be managed on an individualized basis	Primary care management; consider all first-line therapies; reassess at regular intervals
Intermediate risk	Three major risk factors for CAD; moderate, stable angina; recent MI (>2 weeks, <6 weeks); LVD/CHF (NYHA class II); noncardiac sequelae of atherosclerotic disease (e.g., CVA, PVD)	Specialized CV testing; restratification into high or low risk based on results of CV testing
High risk	Unstable or refractory angina; uncontrolled hypertension; LVD/CHF (NYHA class III/IV); recent MI (<2 weeks), CVA; high-risk arrhythmias; obstructive hypertrophic and other cardiomyopathies; moderate–severe valvular disease	Priority referral for specialized CV management; treatment for sexual dysfunction deferred until cardiac condition stabilized and dependent on specialist recommendations; sexual activity should be deferred until a patient's cardiac condition has been stabilized by treatment or a decision has been made by a specialist

CAD, coronary artery disease; CHF, congestive heart failure; CVA, cerebrovascular accident (stroke); CVD, cardiovascular disease; LVD, left ventricular dysfunction; NYHA, New York Heart Association; PVD, peripheral vascular disease.
Sources: From DeBusk et al. (2000) and Kostis et al. (2005).

It is not until exertion is coupled with arousal that energy expenditure occurs. Data indicate that the man in the top position results in greater responses of heart rate and maximum volume of oxygen (VO_2) and thus greater energy expenditure that may or may not reflect both heightened arousal and exertion. If sexual activity is conceptualized as exertion, then the capacity to climb two flights of stairs without limiting symptoms is a clinical benchmark of exercise tolerance and subsequent ability to engage in sexual activity without symptoms (DeBusk, 2000).

Depression has been indicated as a psychological cause of sexual dysfunction and may increase the risk of cardiac mortality in both genders (Roose & Seidman, 2000). A discrepancy between male and female sexual desire, which could disturb relationships, can be observed in many aging couples (Corona et al., 2007). Roose and Seidman (2000) indicated that the male client with ischemic heart disease who is depressed is also likely to have erectile difficulties. This is also a predisposing factor for other adverse cardiac events. Therefore, it appears prudent that all post-MI clients be evaluated for depression and receive appropriate therapy. A wide body of evidence supports the hypothesis of a strong association between depression and ED (Corona et al., 2007). The age-dependent increased use of psychotropic drugs such as antidepressants and antipsychotics may play an important role in ED in older clients (Corona et al., 2007).

Clients should be counselled regarding the effects of medications on sexuality. Calcium channel inhibitors, nonselective beta-blockers, angiotensin II antagonists, and diuretics may increase the risk of ED. ED does not seem to be a problem in men using organic nitrates, angiotensin-converting enzyme inhibitors, selective beta-blockers, or serum lipid-lowering agents (Shril et al., 2007). Counselling and education about return to preinfarct activities, including sexual activities, should be a part of a comprehensive cardiac rehabilitation program. Age and marital status should not be a factor in determining who receives information about resuming sexual activity. If clients have a spouse or regular partner, they should be included in education and counselling sessions unless the clients request otherwise. Discussions about sexual activity should include talking about anxieties concerning resumption of sexual activities with one's partner, scheduling sexual encounters after periods of rest, avoiding sex after heavy meals or alcohol ingestion, and keeping nitroglycerin at the bedside as a form of reassurance (Steinke, 2000). An integral part of successful resumption of sexual activity is engaging in regular exercise based on physician recommendations. Partners of cardiac clients also experience distress because the disease may manifest as decreased intimacy and may require intervention to assist them in adjusting to disease-related stressors (O'Farrell, Murray, & Hotz, 2000).

Diabetes Mellitus

The incidence of diabetes mellitus around the world is on the increase and is estimated to have reached 285 million cases (Canadian Diabetes Association, 2012). In Canada approximately 2 million individuals were living with diabetes in 2006–2007, and the number of new cases has continued to rise (Public Health Agency of Canada, 2012). Therefore, nurses must be prepared to assist these individuals with the multiple life changes they will experience because of this disease, including changes in sexual functioning.

Diabetes mellitus has serious effects on sexual functioning in men. Prevalence of ED in diabetic males ranges from 33% to 75% depending on age, glycaemic control, and presence of other behaviours such as smoking (Jackson, 2004). There is great variability in reports on the effect of diabetes on the sexual response cycle in women (Sarkadi & Rosenquist, 2004), with one report indicating that 25% of sexually active diabetic women report low overall sexual satisfaction (Enzlin et al., 2009).

Men with diabetes typically experience minimal changes in their desire for sexual activity. Any changes in desire may be attributable to difficulties in achieving satisfactory arousal. Arousal difficulties are manifested by the lack of adequate penile erection typically referred to as ED. The term "impotence" has multiple negative psychological connotations and is no longer used by healthcare professionals. An estimated 50% to 75% of diabetic men have ED to some degree, a rate about fourfold higher than in non-diabetic men (Consortium for Improvement in Erectile Dysfunction, 2007). Acute onset of ED may reflect poor glycaemic control of the disease; however, ED may be reversible if control is regained. Acute onset of ED reflects accumulation of sorbitol and water in autonomic nerve fibres and is generally a temporary condition. ED can result from vasculogenic, neurogenic, hormonal, and/or psychogenic factors as well as alterations in the nitric oxide/cyclic guanosine monophosphate pathway or other regulatory mechanisms (Qaseem et al., 2009). A report from a large randomized controlled trial of 761 men with type 1 diabetes who were assigned to either intensive or conventional diabetic therapy reported that decreased libido was the most common form of sexual dysfunction reported (55%), rather than ED (34%) (Penson, Wessells, Cleary, Rutledge, & DCCT/EPI Group, 2009).

Treatment options for ED in diabetic men include use of sildenafil or similar medications, intracavernosal injection therapy, or placement of a penile prosthesis (Jackson, 2004). Men who experience ED should be referred to a urologist for workup before making a decision about treatment options (**Table 10-4**). In addition, because clients' responses to therapy vary according to risk factors, the more difficult to treat patients (e.g., those with conditions such as hypertension or diabetes) will most likely have a lower response rate and need more frequent follow-up visits than those with fewer risk factors (Consortium for Improvement in Erectile Dysfunction, 2007).

Men with diabetes are capable of experiencing orgasm and ejaculation even after developing ED, because the disease has lesser effects on the sympathetic autonomic nervous system. Men may experience a retrograde ejaculation due to autonomic system disruption of the internal vesical sphincter (Tilton, 1997). Fertility may also be impaired in diabetic men secondary to ED, low semen volume, and lowered sperm counts. Couples should be referred to a counsellor to help them adjust to the relationship strains of chronic illness, and those desiring children should be referred to a fertility specialist.

Despite recent efforts in identifying and quantifying the prevalence of sexual problems in women with diabetes, data continue to be inadequate (Bhasin, Enzlin, Coviello, & Basson, 2007; Enzlin et al., 2009). What evidence is available, however, suggests that female sexual dysfunction (FSD) is an issue in about 35% of women with type 1 diabetes (Enzlin et al., 2009). Other prevalence data suggest that all phases of the sexual response cycle are negatively affected in women with insulin-dependent diabetes mellitus, with diabetic women reporting 27% dysfunction as compared with 15% of those in a control group (Enzlin et al., 2002). More recent reports suggest that FSD is found in 35% of women with type 1 diabetes, with a greater incidence in married women who report depression (Enzlin et al., 2009). In a sample of 424 women with type 1 diabetes, of those who met the criteria for FSD, 57% reported decreased desire, 51% reported difficulty achieving orgasm, 47% reported inadequate lubrication, 38% reported decreased arousal, and 21% reported dyspareunia (Enzlin et al., 2009). Data are scarce in comparing levels of desire between women with insulin-dependent diabetes mellitus and non–insulin-dependent diabetes mellitus. Reports suggest a correlation between sexual dysfunction and depression in women with diabetes (Bhasin et al., 2007; Enzlin et al., 2009).

Vaginal lubrication is a manifestation of sexual arousal and can be viewed as analogous to erection in men. As such, women may experience alterations in vaginal capillary dilation and loss of transudate formed in the vagina. The most common hormonally related problem associated with diminished sexual arousal is oestrogen, because sexual arousal is influenced by levels of this chemical. Women experiencing oestrogen deficiencies at menopause are often impacted by changes in vaginal structure and function (Grandjean & Moran, 2007). Women with diabetes may be at higher risk for sexual

Table 10-4 Treatments for Erectile Dysfunction

Treatment	Mechanism of Action	Side Effects	Pro/Con
Sildenafil citrate (Viagra), tadalafil (Cialis), vardenafil (Levitra)	Blocks enzyme phosphodiesterase type 5 and allows for persistent levels of cyclic GMP. This chemical is produced in the penis during sexual arousal and leads to smooth muscle relaxation in the penis and increases blood flow, leading to erection.	Headache, flushing of face, gastrointestinal irritability, nasal congestion, muscle aches	*Pro:* Allows for some degree of spontaneity *Con:* Cannot be taken if the client also takes nitrates for cardiac disease
Intraurethral prostaglandin	Relaxes smooth muscle of ductus arteriosus. Produces vasodilation, inhibits platelet aggregation, and stimulates intestinal and uterine smooth muscle. Induces erection by relaxation of trabecular smooth muscle and by dilation of cavernosal arteries.	Flushing, bradycardia, diarrhoea, urethral pain, haematoma, back pain, and pelvic pain	*Pro:* Allows for some degree of spontaneity
Intracavernosal injections	Medications act on sinusoidal smooth muscle to induce relaxation and enhance corporal filling.	Penile pain during injection; priapism in 1%; haematoma in 8%	*Pro:* Allows for some degree of spontaneity *Con:* Requires office visits to ensure proper technique; can use only every other day; expensive
Vacuum extraction device (VED)	Places negative pressure on corporal bodies of the penis to allow for blood flow into the penis and to cause an erection. A constriction band is placed around the base of the penis to prevent loss of erection until the sex act is completed.	Penile haematoma; injury to erectile tissue or penile skin necrosis may lead to permanent penile deformity Painful erections due to impairment of blood flow by the constriction band at the base of the penis	*Pro:* Allows for penile–vaginal penetration *Con:* Loss of spontaneity; erection only involves a part of the penis
Inflatable penile prosthesis	Inflate erectile cylinders from reservoir. As fluid moves from the reservoir into corporal bodies, the penis becomes erect.	Infection in first few months after implanted; may have failure of device, requiring removal and replacement	*Pro:* Allows intercourse to continue *Con:* Reports of sexual dissatisfaction caused by loss of girth and length of erection; surgical procedure
External prosthetic penis	A strap-on dildo made of silicone rubber. Shaft of dildo is mounted at angle on flanged base, which holds it in the harness. Cleaning: soap/water.	No physiological implications; may require counselling with partner to overcome hesitancy	*Pro:* Allows intercourse to continue; enhances partner satisfaction *Con:* Personal inhibition may make this appear as a nonlegitimate option

GMP: guanosine monophosphate

dysfunction because of vaginal dryness, dyspareunia, decreased arousal or desire, and psychological factors. Treatment modalities are discussed for each of these specific problems (Grandjean & Moran, 2007). Women also reported that it took longer to reach a level of arousal necessary to be orgasmic but that there were no discernible changes in their orgasms since the onset of diabetes. Other research reported varying frequencies of orgasmic difficulties. Kolodny (1971) found that 35% of his sample reported complete loss of orgasm, Jensen (1981) had 10% of his subjects report decreased or absent orgasm, and Enzlin et al. (2009) reported that 51% of women with symptoms of FSD reported difficulty with orgasm. Clearly, much more research is needed in this area.

Although the data cannot pinpoint the exact percentage of women and men diagnosed with diabetes with sexual difficulties or identify exactly when in the course of the disease sexual problems occur, nurses still have an obligation to address this aspect of care. Factors influencing sexual dysfunction in women with diabetes include depression, marital dissatisfaction, difficulty adjusting to the diagnosis, and low satisfaction with diabetic treatment options. Sexual dysfunction in men also appears to be related to depression and poor adjustment to the diagnosis and negative appraisal of the disease (Enzlin, Matieu, & Demytteanere, 2003). Nurses should assume that all clients with diabetes will experience sexual difficulty at some point in time and *routinely* assess the sexual concerns of their clients. Women who report vaginal dryness can be encouraged to use over-the-counter, water-soluble vaginal lubricants. Eating yogurt with active cultures may help in reducing the frequency of yeast infections. Maintaining close control over fluctuations in blood glucose levels will also reduce the frequency of yeast infections. Couples should be referred to counselling as issues arise related to the strains of living with a chronic illness so that better communication may occur about these issues.

Cancer

Cancer occurs in people of all ages. Cancer happens to an individual, a couple, and a family. A complete discussion of the multiple ways cancer can have an impact on sexuality is beyond the scope of this chapter. For more detailed information the reader is referred to any of the major cancer nursing textbooks and other journal publications. This discussion is limited to the general ways cancer and cancer treatments affect sexuality.

In general, surgical treatments for cancer have an impact on body image and the ability to function sexually. Surgical procedures for cancers of the gastrointestinal system can lead to sexual difficulties secondary to damage to nerves that enervate sexual organs or cause alterations in body image that affect sexuality. Other procedures may involve removal of or alterations in organs that directly impact the ability to function sexually. Radical hysterectomy renders a woman unable to bear children and leads to a surgically induced menopause if oophorectomy (removal of the ovaries) is included in the procedure. Because of removal of the upper portion of the vagina, women and their partners may be concerned that having a shortened vagina precludes satisfactory sexual intercourse. Postoperative discussions should include positions that might reduce dyspareunia. On the other hand, diagnosis and treatment of breast cancer in women can have significant impact on a woman's sexuality. According to

Katz (2011), in addition to feelings of loss in feminine identity and alteration in body image, during treatment and sometimes long after treatment these women may experience "fatigue, loss of libido, decreased physiological signs of arousal in response to sexual stimulation, and pain with penetration (dyspareunia), resulting from vaginal dryness secondary to decreased estrogen" (p. 63).

Men also experience sexual side effects from surgical intervention. According to Gurevich, Bishop, Bower, Malka, and Nyhof-Young (2004), men that have undergone surgery after testicular cancer reported it as "alternately inhibiting and enhancing masculinity" (p. 1597), because what is being removed "is not only an anatomical structure, but a signifier of masculinity and normalcy" (p. 1601). Characteristics associated with postoperative sexual recovery after radical prostatectomy include younger age, use of nerve-sparing techniques, smaller prostate at time of surgery, pretreatment erectile ability, presence of a sexually functional partner, and absence of androgen deprivation (Hollenbeck, Dunn, Wei, Sandler, & Sanda, 2004). **Table 10-5** provides specific information regarding the effects of other surgical procedures on sexual functioning.

Radiation therapy can cause alterations in organ functioning, primary organ failure resulting in either permanent or temporary alterations in fertility, as well as side effects that are not directly related to sexual functioning (**Table 10-6**). Fertility may be preserved by the use of modern

Table 10-5	**Effects of Cancer Surgery on Sexual Functioning**	
Type of Surgery	**Effects on Sexual Functioning**	**Client Education**
Colorectal surgery with colostomy	Varies; depends on type and extent of surgical procedure; major impact on body image and self-concept	Encourage expression of feelings and communication with partner.
Abdominoperineal resection	*Females*: shortening of vagina; vaginal scarring may cause dyspareunia; decreased lubrication if ovaries also are removed	Use water-soluble lubricant before intercourse; allow more time for pleasuring before attempting penetration; with shortened vagina, use coital positions that decrease depth of penetration (e.g., side-to-side lying, man on top with legs outside the woman's, woman on top).
	Males: erectile dysfunction; decrease in amount/force of ejaculate or retrograde ejaculation because of interruption of sympathetic and parasympathetic nerve supply. Amount of rectal tissue removed appears to determine degree of dysfunction. Capacity for orgasm not altered	ED may be temporary or permanent; encourage use of touch, other means of communication.
Transurethral resection of bladder/partial cystectomy	Mild pain or dyspareunia	Encourage more time for pleasuring.

(Continues)

Table 10-5   Effects of Cancer Surgery on Sexual Functioning *(continued)*

Type of Surgery	Effects on Sexual Functioning	Client Education
Radical cystectomy	*Females:* surgery usually includes removal of bladder, urethra, uterus, ovaries, fallopian tubes, and anterior portion of vagina. *Males:* surgery involves removal of bladder, prostate, seminal vesicles, pelvic lymph nodes, and possibly urethra. May cause retrograde or loss of ejaculation and decrease in or loss of erectile ability.	Vaginal reconstruction is possible; use water-soluble lubricant; encourage self-pleasuring and use of dilators; encourage use of touch and other means of sexual communication. Explore possibility for penile implant.
Radical prostatectomy	Involves removal of prostate, seminal vesicles, and vas deferens. Damage to autonomic nerves near prostate may cause loss of erectile ability; loss of emission and ejaculation.	Desire, penile sensations, and orgasmic abilities not altered. Explore possibility for penile prosthesis.
Transurethral resection of prostate	Causes retrograde ejaculation because of damage to internal bladder sphincter.	Reassure that erection and orgasm will still occur but that ejaculate will be decreased or absent; urine may be cloudy.
Bilateral orchiectomy	Results in low levels of testosterone; causes sterility, decreased libido, impotence, gynaecomastia, penile atrophy, and decreased growth of body hair and beard.	Discuss option of sperm banking before surgery; discuss optional ways of expressing sexuality with patient and partner.
Retroperitoneal lymph node dissection	Damages sympathetic nerves necessary for ejaculation; results in temporary or permanent loss of ejaculation; patient maintains potency and orgasmic ability.	Discuss option of sperm banking.
Total abdominal hysterectomy with bilateral salpingo-oophorectomy	Loss of circulating oestrogens; decrease in vaginal elasticity, decrease in vaginal lubrication; some women report decreased desire, orgasm, and enjoyment.	Use water-soluble lubricants; intercourse may be resumed after 6-week post-op check; encourage discussion about meaning of loss of uterus to self-identity.
Mastectomy	Decrease in arousal associated with nipple stimulation; affects body image, self-concept.	Encourage communication with partner.
Radical vulvectomy	Removal of labia majora, labia minora, clitoris, bilateral pelvic node dissection; loss of sexually responsive tissue with concomitant loss of vasocongestive neuromuscular response.	Possibility of perineal reconstruction with split-thickness skin graft or gracilis muscle grafts. Intercourse is still possible; explore ways of achieving arousal other than genital stimulation. Preoperative and postoperative counselling are essential.
Penectomy	Degree of sexual limitation depends on length of remaining penile shaft. Glands are removed; remainder of shaft of penile tissue will respond with tumescence and will allow ejaculation and orgasm.	Discuss possibility of artificial insemination if children are desired.

Table 10-6	Site-Specific Effects of Radiation Therapy on Sexuality	
Radiated Site	**Effect on Sexuality**	**Client Education**
Testes	Reduction in sperm count begins in 6–8 weeks and continues for 1 year. Doses of 2 Gy* result in temporary sterility for about 12 months. Doses ≥5 Gy result in permanent sterility. Libido and potency will be maintained.	Discuss sperm banking before therapy and continued use of contraceptives.
Prostate	*External beam:* temporary or permanent ED because of fibrosis of pelvic vasculature or radiation damage of pelvic nerves. *Interstitial:* less incidence of impotency.	Age is variable—men older than age 60 have higher incidence of impotence. ED—may experience pain during ejaculation because of irritation of urethra. Potency preserved in 70–90% of men who were potent before treatment.
Cervix/vaginal canal	*External beam:* vaginal stenosis and fibrosis, fistula, cystitis. *Intracavitary:* vaginal stenosis, dry, friable tissue, loss of lubrication. Both result in decreased vaginal sensation and dyspareunia.	Use of water-soluble lubricant; empty bladder before and after sex; encourage pleasuring before attempting penetration; use dilators or frequent intercourse to lessen amount of stenosis. Explore new positions for intercourse to allow woman control over depth of penile penetration.
Pelvic region	*Women:* temporary or permanent sterility dependent on dose of radiation, volume of tissue irradiated, and woman's age; the closer to menopause, the more likely permanent sterility will result. A single dose of 3.75 Gy causes complete cessation of menses in women older than age 40. *Men:* temporary or permanent ED secondary to vascular or nerve damage.	Oophoropexy and shielding may help to maintain fertility in women; continue use of contraceptives; use of water-soluble lubricant. Both genders: encourage alternate means to express sexuality, such as touch.
Breast	Skin reactions, changes in breast sensations.	Explore alternate pleasuring techniques and good communication techniques; breastfeeding should occur on nonradiated side.

*Gy (gray) is the International System (SI) unit of radiation dose expressed in terms of absorbed energy per unit mass of tissue (Health Physics Society, 2011). Retrieved from http://hps.org/publicinformation/radterms/radfact79.html

Source: Wilmoth (2009).

radiation therapy techniques and lead shields to protect the testes. Women diagnosed with invasive cervical cancer are frequently treated by a combination of external and internal radiation therapy. Side effects include fatigue, diarrhea, vaginal dryness, and vaginal stenosis (Maher, 2005). Vaginal dryness will definitely occur; however, vaginal stenosis can be prevented. A patent vagina is important in maintaining sexual function as well as allowing for adequate follow-up evaluations. Women must be educated about the need to either use a vaginal dilator or have vaginal intercourse on a regular basis (Wilmoth & Spinelli, 2000). In women older than 40 years, infertility may occur at lower doses of radiation. Women may undergo surgery to protect the ovaries by moving them out of the field of radiation (National Cancer Institute, 2007). Likewise, men who receive either external beam or brachytherapy for prostate cancer are at increased risk for sexual dysfunction (Hollenbeck et al., 2004). Current techniques such as conformal external-beam radiation therapy are reported to lead to ED in as many as 40% to 60% of men with prostate cancer (Wiegner & King, 2010). These rates of ED are also reported in newer delivery techniques of radiation therapy such as intensity-modulated radiation therapy.

Chemotherapy treatments frequently cause temporary or permanent infertility. These side effects are related to a number of factors, including the client's gender, age at time of treatment, the specific type and dose of radiation therapy and/or chemotherapy, the use of single therapy or multiple therapies, and the length of time since

treatment (National Cancer Institute, 2007). The extent of the impact on fertility varies according to the patient's gender, type of cancer, and the type and dosage of chemotherapy. Primary factors related to altered fertility appear to be combination chemotherapy that includes alkylating agents and female gender and age older than 35 years. In addition to altered fertility, chemotherapy can lead to altered ovarian function and subsequent menopause (McInnes & Schilsky, 1996). Menopausal symptoms such as hot flashes, vaginal dryness, and skin changes in addition to chemotherapy side effects can be traumatic for women, particularly if they are not aware of the potential for menopause (Wilmoth, Coleman, Wahab, & Kneisl, 2009). The nurse could suggest using vitamin E and water-soluble vaginal lubricants and doing Kegel exercises to reduce symptoms (Wilmoth, 1996).

The use of alkylating agents in men has a major impact on their sexuality and fertility. Men who receive cumulative doses greater than 400 mg are always azoospermic, as are those treated with cisplatin (Krebs, 2005). Adult men, regardless of age, are likely to experience long-term side effects of chemotherapy. However, age, total dose, and time since therapy are essential to recovery of fertility. If fertility is to recover, normal sperm counts should return to normal within 3 years after completion of treatment. As demonstrated in this section, the effects of treatment for cancer on sexual functioning may be devastating. Before beginning treatment clear communication with the patient and family about potential effects on sexual function is needed.

CASE STUDY

You are the nurse in charge of the outpatient cancer clinic in the community. Your next patient is Carol, a 43-year-old breast cancer survivor, 4 years post-diagnosis. Carol was diagnosed at age 39 with a stage IIb, ER/PR negative tumour and had a lumpectomy followed by chemotherapy. Her chief complaint after chemotherapy has been hot flashes.

You begin the visit asking Carol about how things are going with work and her husband. Carol noticeably tenses when she talks about her husband. You probe a little and reflect that you noticed some tension; you ask how things are between her and her husband. Have they been able to go away on any vacations? What has he said about how well she is doing after completing chemotherapy?

When Carol provides some vague responses, you talk about the menopause chemotherapy has caused and ask Carol if she thought that this, most likely permanent, problem was a source of stress between her and her husband. Carol begins to cry and says she just hasn't felt like being intimate, and when she has it has been painful.

You take a short sexual health history to get a comprehensive background on her sexual functioning, both before and after diagnosis. You learn that Carol and her husband had a healthy sexual relationship before her diagnosis, were active three to four times weekly, and had been trying to become pregnant when Carol was diagnosed with cancer. Carol has been taking fluoxetine (Prozac), a selective serotonin reuptake inhibitor, since diagnosis to help cope with some mild depression. About midway during chemotherapy Carol began having hot flashes, mood swings, and complained of lack of interest, dyspareunia, and inability to reach orgasm whenever she and her husband were intimate. Finally, you refer Carol and her husband to a sex therapist to help them work through some of their sexual and relationship challenges.

Discussion Questions

1. What might you include in a more focused sexual assessment? What type of chemotherapy agents cause either a temporary or permanent menopause? Is infertility an area of concern?

2. How do selective serotonin reuptake inhibitors affect sexuality in women? Are there any antidepressants with a lesser impact on sexuality?

3. What factors do you need to consider when recommending herbal remedies for menopausal symptoms to women with breast cancer?

4. What other specific suggestions might you make to Carol about ways to enhance her sexuality and reduce dyspareunia?

Multiple Sclerosis

Multiple sclerosis (MS) has the potential to have a profound impact on the sexual relationships of couples due to the resulting motor, sensory, and cognitive alterations. The prevalence of sexual difficulties ranges between 60% and 80% in men and 20% and 60% in women (McCabe, 2002). Sexual difficulties in persons with MS can be classified as primary, secondary, or tertiary in origin (Lowden, O'Leary, & Stevenson, 2005). Primary sexual problems are those that are caused by the pathological damage to the central nervous system and hormonal issues (Lowden et al., 2005). Secondary problems arise from symptoms including bladder dysfunction, fatigue, pain, cognitive dysfunction, and mobility issues (Lowden et al., 2005). Tertiary causes are psychological in nature and are primarily related to attitudes and feelings about sexuality that are compounded by the interaction of the disease process and societal norms about sexuality (Lowden et al., 2005).

Neurological changes caused by MS can affect sexual feelings as well as sexual response. There are common issues that affect both men and women in achieving sexual response—most prominent are changes in sensation that lead to sexual stimuli and the ability to achieve orgasm (Lowden et al., 2005). Counselling for underlying emotional concerns as well as depression may affect treatment of desire problems as well. Changes in genital sensations can be troubling, because something that used to feel good may now be noxious. Teaching couples to communicate about these changes and to try new techniques may be helpful (Kalb, 2008). Vaginal dryness can be improved with the use of water-soluble lubricants. Unfortunately, treatment of ED in men is not as easily remedied. Treatment options for ED in MS are the same as those for men with other chronic illnesses (see Table 10-4).

Secondary sexual alterations caused by MS are a result of the physical symptoms that accompany the disease. Spasticity during sexual activity appears to affect women more than it does men and may be controlled by baclofen, chemical nerve blocks, and surgery. Bowel and bladder problems can cause significant alterations in sexuality and can severely impair spontaneity of sexual activity. Engaging in sexual activity successfully requires open communication as well as aggressive symptom management. Limiting fluid intake for several hours before sexual activity and urinating immediately before sexual activity can help with bladder control. Medications are available for incontinence; however, these medications may also increase vaginal dryness. Intermittent catheterization or taping a permanent catheter out of the way can allow successful activity. Bowel problems may be constipation, no control, or lack of predictability of function. A regular bowel regimen consisting of laxatives, enemas, or disimpaction can allow stress-free sexual interactions.

Fatigue is a pervasive symptom of MS as well as other chronic illnesses. In MS, fatigue can be managed with several pharmacological agents and energy-conserving techniques. Medications include amantadine or pemoline. Use of wheelchairs or motorized carts or regular naps during the day can allow clients to conserve energy for activities they enjoy, including sexual activity. Cognitive impairment can also have a pervasive impact on a relationship. Memory loss, impaired judgment, and other problems can impair the interpersonal communication that is integral in any intimate relationship.

The psychosocial changes that accompany MS cause tertiary sexual dysfunction. Decreased self-concept, grieving for loss of self, and role changes affect both the client and the partner. Persons with MS report lower levels of sexual activity, sexual satisfaction, and relationship satisfaction than those without MS (McCabe, McKern, McDonald, & Vowels, 2003). Ongoing counselling and participation in support groups can help couples deal with these sexual and relationship issues caused by MS (McCabe, 2002). The MS Society published a pamphlet on intimacy and sexuality for persons with MS. This pamphlet provides both permission to continue being sexual and limited information for both the person with MS and their partner (Kalb, 2008).

INTERVENTIONS

Many healthcare providers are hesitant to ask patients about their sexuality, fearing privacy issues. However, sexuality is a part of one's quality of life. Assessing sexuality and responding to issues is essential in caring for the whole patient.

Sexual Assessment

Sexual assessment should be a routine part of every physician- or nurse-initiated assessment for nearly every client diagnosed with a chronic illness (Wilmoth, 2000, 2006). Assessing sexuality as routinely as other body systems serves two purposes. First, it decreases embarrassment on the part of the client and practitioner if it is accepted as a normal aspect of health care. Second, routine inclusion gives the client permission to mention sexual difficulties to the practitioner and gives the practitioner permission to ask specific questions when it is suspected the client might be experiencing a sexually related side effect of the disease or treatment.

The clinician should keep the same principles in mind when discussing sexuality with a client and/or partner as with any other topic. Clients need reassurance about the safety of treatments for issues with sexuality. These instances again reinforce the importance of the clinician as an educator, emphasize the professional nature of these discussions, clarify the content component of communications, and reinforce permission to include sexuality in the plan of care. An example of a bridge question is, "Has anyone talked with you about how your (injury/illness/treatments) can affect your ability to have sex?" *Unloading* a topic is another technique that is useful in discussing sexuality and can ease a client's concern once he or she learns that others have experienced this problem (Woods, 1984). An example of unloading is, "Many women who have received chemotherapy have had problems with vaginal dryness. What problems have you had with this?"

The inclusion of questions on sexuality in the admission assessment is an excellent way to legitimize the role of the nurse in addressing sexuality. Woods (1984) suggested that such questions should proceed from less intimate questions, such as role functioning, to more personal ones on sexual functioning. Closed (yes/no) questions should be avoided because they eliminate opportunities for further discussion. Questions for an initial assessment include the following (Wilmoth, 1994a; Woods, 1984):

- How has (diagnosis/treatment) affected your role as wife/husband/partner?
- How has (diagnosis/treatment) affected the way you feel about yourself as a woman/man?

- What aspects of your sexuality do you believe have been affected by your diagnosis/treatment?
- How has your (diagnosis/treatment) affected your ability to function sexually?

A more medically focused sexual evaluation might include determination of chief complaint, sexual status, medical status, psychiatric status, family and psychosexual history, relationship assessment, and summary with recommendations (Krebs, 2007). A complete sexual history is not usually indicated unless initial assessment indicates the presence of a sexual problem. Most nurses are not adequately prepared to conduct a full sexual assessment; therefore, referral to a more appropriate practitioner is appropriate.

Including Sexuality in Practice

Four areas of competency must be achieved for nurses to successfully incorporate sexuality into practice to attain the published standards of practice: comfort with one's own sexuality and comfort in discussing sexuality with others, excellent communication skills, a knowledge base about sexuality in health and illness, and role models that demonstrate integration of sexuality into practice (Wilmoth, 1994b; Woods, 1984).

Participation in each of the aforementioned processes will add to the nurse's knowledge base about normal sexual functioning. Professional nurses should also engage in independent study within their specialty regarding the effects that the illnesses, treatments, and medications have on sexuality. Engaging in discussions with other healthcare providers, such as physicians or pharmacists, or participating in interdisciplinary journal clubs and research projects can add depth to the nurses' knowledge. Such interdisciplinary efforts will have large payoffs for clients and their partners.

Nurses who are comfortable with their own sexuality, are proficient communicators, and have knowledge about sexuality possess the foundation necessary to incorporate sexuality into their practice. However, many are still reluctant to do so. Peers who can role model the incorporation of sexuality into nursing practice may be influential in helping others incorporate it into their practices. Role models can assist in this process by relating positive experiences with clients about discussions surrounding sexuality, by role playing ways of initiating discussions about sexuality, and by acting as a resource for staff. However, there is little research documenting the effectiveness of role models in teaching others to incorporate sexuality into practice.

Grand rounds and presentations of individual cases that exemplify typical sexual concerns associated with a particular treatment, medication, or diagnosis are other strategies for enhancing comfort in including sexual discussions in practice. Physicians and pharmacists could discuss a particular disease process and treatment options, including medications and their effect on sexual functioning. A social worker or clinical nurse specialist skilled in assessing and educating about sexual issues could lead practitioners through the sexual assessment and educational process. Finally, a clinician or sex therapist could discuss interventions most practitioners could use in their counselling of persons with sexual issues.

Comfort with sexuality and enhancement of communication skills can be attained through reading, values clarification exercises, and participation in courses on sexuality. Some options include semester-long college courses related to sexuality or shorter weekend courses, often referred to as "SARs" or *sexual attitude reassessments*. These programs combine explicit films with small group discussions over a 2- or 3-day period to allow for analysis of one's personal values surrounding sexuality. Knowing one's own values and attitudes toward a variety of other sexual practices and sexual orientations is the first step in becoming comfortable with sexuality (Wilmoth, 1994a). Values clarification exercises can assist in this process. The outcome of clarifying one's values about sexuality is knowing what one believes is acceptable sexual behaviour. It is important to remember there is no right or wrong set of behaviours or values, just different ones.

Comfort in discussing sexuality and enhancing the ability to communicate clearly about sexuality can be achieved through a variety of methods. One option is to form a discussion group or journal club among colleagues. This group could engage in discussion of values clarification exercises or articles related to human sexuality in general or disease-focused articles on sexuality. Sharing with a peer group, particularly an interdisciplinary peer group, is a nonthreatening way in which to become comfortable

talking about sexuality. This approach also assists with increasing knowledge about a variety of illnesses, their treatments, and their effects on sexuality.

Nurses are skilled communicators, but they initially may find initiating discussions with clients about sexuality anxiety provoking. Nurses should assume their clients have some form of sexual experience rather than none at all and that they have questions about the impact of their disease or its treatments on their sexuality. Experience has shown that patients are most appreciative when asked about this part of life in relation to their chronic illness. Nurses should use terminology, including slang, their clients understand. Many health professionals use the PLISSIT model (Annon, 1976) to assist them in their sexual assessments. In this model P stands for *permission*, LI for *limited information*, SS for *specific suggestions*, and IT for *intensive therapy* (**Table 10-7**). All nurses should be able to intervene at all levels except for provision of

Table 10-7 PLISSIT Model	
Permission (P)	(Assessment) Actions taken by the nurse to let the patient/partner know that sexual issues are a legitimate aspect in providing nursing care. This could include questions about sexuality that are incorporated into the general admission assessment or questions specifically related to their disease process or treatment.
Limited Information (LI)	(Education) Sharing of information regarding the effects of disease, treatments, and medications. Examples of limited information include discussing when sexual intercourse may be resumed after surgery, the possibility of menopause occurring in conjunction with chemotherapy, or medications leading to ED.
Specific Suggestions (SS)	(Counselling) This level of care requires specialized knowledge about specific conditions and their relationship to sexual functioning. Various techniques, positions, and alternate techniques useful in achieving sexual satisfaction are examples of counselling concerns.
Intensive Therapy (IT)	(Referral) Treatment of sexual dysfunction requires specialized training in psychotherapy, sex therapy techniques, crisis intervention, and behavior modification.

Source: Annon (1976).

intensive therapy. If assessment suggests a problem beyond the level of needing specific suggestions, the client and partner should be referred to a sex therapist.

SUMMARY

The following are the desired client and partner outcomes that may be anticipated after nursing intervention (American Nurses Association/Oncology Nursing Society, 2004):

- The ability to identify potential/actual changes in sexuality, sexual functioning, or intimacy related to disease and treatment
- The ability to express feelings about alopecia, body image changes, and altered sexual functioning
- The ability to engage in open communication with his or her partner regarding changes in sexual functioning or desire, within a cultural framework
- The ability to describe appropriate interventions for actual or potential changes in sexual function
- The ability to identify personal and community resources to assist with changes in body image and sexuality

STUDY QUESTIONS   www

1. Why is it important for nurses and other healthcare professionals to include a sexual assessment and sexual education when providing care?
2. What are key changes in sexual response that should be expected to occur with healthy aging?

STUDY QUESTIONS (Cont.)   www

3. In general, what changes in sexuality are caused by chemotherapy in women? In men?
4. What do men and their partners need to know about the pathophysiology of diabetes mellitus on erectile ability and options to continue sexual intercourse?
5. What should be discussed about sexuality with a patient newly diagnosed with multiple sclerosis?
6. What are some methods a nurse manager could implement with a nursing staff to increase comfort and knowledge regarding the impact of disease on sexuality?

Evidence-Informed Practice Box

The Consortium for Spinal Cord Medicine published clinical practice guidelines in 2010 drawn from a clinical and epidemiological evidence-informed model from the Agency for Healthcare Research and Quality. The committee conducted a systematic review of the literature on the topic of spinal cord injury and sexuality and reproductive health published between 1995 and September 2007. The thorough methodology used for this review is outlined. Evidence-informed guidelines for sexual assessment after spinal cord injury are provided as well as education guidelines for educating the individual and his or her partner on ways to maintain sexual functioning after injury. The guidelines also provide the professional with evidence-informed suggestions on how to manage a variety of health problems that occur frequently in men and women with spinal cord injury that may negatively impact sexual functioning. Recommendations for further research are also provided.

Source: Consortium for Spinal Cord Medicine (2010).

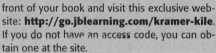

For a full suite of assignments and additional learning activities, use the access code located in the front of your book and visit this exclusive website: **http://go.jblearning.com/kramer-kile**. If you do not have an access code, you can obtain one at the site.

REFERENCES

Agewall, S., Berglund, M., & Henareh, L. (2004). Reduced quality of life after myocardial infarction in women compared with men. *Clinical Cardiology, 27*(5), 271–274.

American Nurses Association. (2010). *Nursing: Scope and standards of practice* (2nd ed.) Washington DC: Author.

American Nurses Association/Oncology Nursing Society. (2004). *Statement on scope and standards of oncology nursing practice.* Washington DC: Author.

American Psychiatric Association. (2000). *Diagnostic and statistical manual of mental disorders* (4th ed., text revision). Washington DC: Author.

Andrews, M., Goldberg, K., & Kaplan, H. (Eds.). (1996). *Nurse's legal handbook* (3rd ed.). Springhouse, PA: Springhouse Corporation.

Annon, J. S. (1976). *The behavioral treatment of sexual problems: Volume I: Brief therapy.* New York. NY: Harper & Row.

Archer, L. S., Gragasin, S. F., Webster, L., Bochinski, D., & Michelakis, D. E. (2005). Aetiology and management of male erectile dysfunction and female sexual dysfunction in patients with cardiovascular disease. *Drugs Aging, 22*(10), 823–844.

Bhasin, S., Enzlin, P., Coviello, A., & Basson, R. (2007). Sexual dysfunction in men and women with endocrine disorders. *Lancet, 369*(9561), 597–611.

Canadian Diabetes Association. (2012). The prevalence and cost of diabetes. Retrieved from http://www.diabetes.ca/diabetes-and-you/what/prevalence/

Centers for Disease Control and Prevention, Office of Minority Health. (2004). Eliminate disparities in cardiovascular disease. Retrieved from http://www.cdc.gov/omhd/AMH/factsheets/cardio.htm

Clayton, A., & Ramamurthy, S. (2008). The impact of physical disease on sexual dysfunction. *Advanced Psychosomatic Medicine, 29,* 70–88.

Consortium for Improvement in Erectile Dysfunction. (2007). *Collaborative for advancement of urological, sexual, and endocrine education.* Retrieved from http://causeeducation.org/

Consortium for Spinal Cord Medicine. (2010). Sexuality and reproductive health in adults with spinal cord injury: A clinical practice guideline for health-care professionals. *Journal of Spinal Cord Medicine, 33*(3), 281–336.

Corona, G., Mannucci, R., Mansani, R., Petrone, L., Bartolini, M., Giommi, R., . . . Maggi, M. (2007). Aging and pathogenesis of erectile dysfunction. *International Journal of Impotence Research, 16*(5), 395–402.

Darling, C. A., Davidson, J. K., & Conway-Welch, C. (1990). Female ejaculation: Perceived origins, the Grafenberg spot/area, and sexual responsiveness. *Archives of Sexual Behavior, 19,* 29–47.

DeBusk, R. (2000). Evaluating the cardiovascular tolerance for sex. *American Journal of Cardiology, 86*(2A), 51F–56F.

DeBusk, R., Drory, Y., Goldstein, I., Jackson, G., Kaul, S., & Kimmel, S. E. (2000). Management of sexual dysfunction in patients with cardiovascular disease: Recommendations of the Princeton Consensus Panel. *American Journal of Cardiology, 86*(2), 175–181.

Enzlin, P., Matieu, C., & Demytteanere, K. (2003). Diabetes and female sexual functioning: A state-of-the-art. *Diabetes Spectrum, 16,* 256–259.

Enzlin, P., Mathieu, C., Van den Bruel, A., Bosteels, J., Vanderschueren, D., & Demyttenaere, K. (2002). Sexual dysfunction in women with type 1 diabetes: A controlled study. *Diabetes Care, 25*, 672–677.

Enzlin, P., Rose, R., Wiegel, M., Brown, J., Wessells, H., Gatcomb, P., . . . Clearly, P. A. (2009). Sexual dysfunction in women with type I diabetes. *Diabetes Care, 23*(5), 780–785.

Esmail, S., Esmail, Y., & Munro, B. (2002). Sexuality and disability: The role of health care professionals in providing options and alternatives for couples. *Sexuality and Disability, 19*(4), 267–282.

Grandjean, C., & Moran, B., (2007). The impact of diabetes mellitus on female sexual well-being. *Nursing Clinics of North America, 42*(4), 581–592.

Gurevich, M., Bishop, S., Bower, J., Malka, M., & Nyhof-Young, J. (2004). (Dis)embodying gender and sexuality in testicular cancer. *Social Science and Medicine, 58*(9), 1597–1607.

Guyton, A. C., & Hall, J. E. (2006). *Textbook of medical physiology* (11th ed.) Philadelphia, PA: Elsevier Saunders.

Hines, T. M. (2001). The G-spot: A modern gynecologic myth. *American Journal of Obstetrics and Gynecology, 185*(2), 359–362.

Hollenbeck, B. K., Dunn, R. L., Wei, J. T., Sandler, H. M., & Sanda, M. G. (2004). Sexual health recovery after prostatectomy, external radiation or brachytherapy for early stage prostate cancer. *Current Urology Reports, 5*, 212–219.

Jackson, G. (2004). Sexual dysfunction and diabetes. *International Journal of Clinical Practice, 58*(4), 358–362.

Jensen, S. B. (1981). Diabetic sexual dysfunction: A comparative study of 160 insulin-treated diabetic men and women and an age-matched control group. *Archives of Sexual Behavior, 10*, 493–504.

Kalb, R. C. (2008). *Intimacy and sexuality in MS*. New York, NY: MS Society.

Kaplan, H. S. (1979). *Disorders of sexual desire and other new concepts and techniques in sex therapy*. New York. NY: Simon & Schuster.

Katz, A. (2007). *Breaking the silence on cancer and sexuality. A handbook for healthcare providers*. Pittsburgh, PA: Oncology Nursing Society.

Katz, A. (2011). Breast cancer and women sexuality. *American Journal of Nursing, 11*(4), 63–67.

Kazemi-Saleh, D., Pishgou, B., Farrokhi, F., Assari, S., Fotros, A., & Naseri, H. (2008). Gender impact on the correlation between sexuality and marital relation quality in patients with coronary artery disease. *Journal of Sexual Medicine, 5*(9), 2100–2106.

Kolodny, R. C. (1971). Sexual dysfunction in diabetic females. *Diabetes, 20*, 557–559.

Kolodny, R., Masters, W., Johnson, V., & Biggs, M. (1979). *The textbook for human sexuality for nurses*. Boston, MA: Little, Brown.

Kostis, J. B., Jackson, G., Rosen, R., Barrett-Connor, E., Billups, K., Burnett, A. L., . . . Shabsigh, R. (2005). Sexual dysfunction and cardiac risk, the second Princeton consensus conference. *American Journal of Cardiology, 96*(12B), 85M–93M.

Koukouras, D., Spiliotis, J., Scopa, C. D., Dragotis, K., Kalfarentzos, F., Tzoracoleftherakis, E., . . . Androulakis, J. (1991). Radical consequence in the sexuality of male patients operated for colorectal carcinoma. *European Journal of Surgical Oncology, 17*, 285–288.

Krebs, L. U. (2005). Sexual and reproductive dysfunction. In C. H. Yarbro, M. H. Frogge, M. Goodman, & S. L. Groenwald (Eds.), *Cancer nursing: Principles and practice* (6th ed., pp. 841–869). Sudbury, MA: Jones & Bartlett.

Krebs, L. U. (2007). Sexual assessment: Research and clinical. *Nursing Clinics of North America, 42*(4), 515–529.

Ladas, A. K., Whipple, B., & Perry, J. D. (1982). *The G-spot*. New York, NY: Dell.

Leiblum, S. R., & Segraves, R. T. (1989). Sex therapy with aging adults. In S. R. Leiblum & R.C. Rosen (Eds.), *Principles and practice of sex therapy: Update for the 1990s* (2nd ed., pp. 352–381). New York, NY: Guilford Press.

Lindau, S. T., Schumm, L. P., Gaumann, E. O., Levinson, W., O'Muircheartaigh, C. A., & Waite, L. J. (2007). A study of sexuality and health among older adults in the United States. *New England Journal of Medicine, 357*(8), 820–822.

Lowden, D., O'Leary, M., & Stevenson, B. (2005). Sexuality issues in patients with MS. *Multiple Sclerosis Counseling Points, 1*, 1–9.

Maher, K. (2005). Radiation therapy: Toxicities and management. In C. H. Yarbro, M. H. Frogge, & M. Goodman (Eds.), *Cancer nursing: Principles and practice* (6th ed., pp. 283–314). Sudbury, MA: Jones & Bartlett.

Masters, W. H., & Johnson, V. E. (1966). *Human sexual response.* Philadelphia, PA: Lippincott-Raven.

Masters, W. H., & Johnson, V. E. (1981). Sex and the aging process. *Journal of the American Geriatrics Society, 24*(9), 385–390.

McCabe, M. P. (2002). Relationship functioning and sexuality among people with multiple sclerosis. *Journal of Sex Research, 39*(4), 302–309.

McCabe, M. P., McKern, S., McDonald, E., & Vowels, L. M. (2003). Changes over time in sexual and relationship functioning of people with multiple sclerosis. *Journal of Sex & Marital Therapy, 29*(4), 305–321.

McInnes, S., & Schilsky, R. L. (1996). Infertility following cancer chemotherapy. In B. A. Chabner & D. L. Longo (Eds.), *Cancer chemotherapy and biotherapy* (2nd ed., pp. 31–44). Philadelphia, PA: Lippincott-Raven.

Meston, C. M. (2000). Sympathetic nervous system activity and female sexual arousal. *American Journal of Cardiology, 86*(2 Suppl. 1), 30–34.

Meston, C. M., & Gorzalka, B. B. (1996). The differential effects of sympathetic activation on sexual arousal in sexually functional and dysfunctional women. *Journal of Abnormal Psychology, 105*, 582–591.

National Cancer Institute. (2007). Sexual and reproductive issues. Retrieved from http://www.cancer.gov /cancertopics/pdq/supportivecare/sexuality/Patient /page1

O'Farrell, P., Murray, J., & Hotz, S. B. (2000). Psychologic distress among spouses of patients undergoing cardiac rehabilitation. *Heart and Lung, 29*(2), 97–104.

Oncology Nursing Society. (2004). *Statement on the scope and standards of oncology nursing practice.* Pittsburgh, PA: Author.

Penson, D. F., Wessells, H., Cleary, P., Rutledge, B. N., & DCCT/EDI Group. (2009). Sexual dysfunction and symptom impact in men with long-standing type I diabetes in the DCCT/EDIC study. *Journal of Sexual Medicine, 6*(7), 1969–1978.

Public Health Agency of Canada. (2012). Report from the national diabetes surveillance system: Diabetes in Canada, 2009. Retrieved from http://www.phac-aspc .gc.ca/publicat/2009/ndssdic-snsddac-09/2-eng.php

Qaseem, A., Snow, V., Denburg, T. D., Casey, D. E., Forcica, M. A. Owens, D. K., . . . Shekelle, P. (2009). Hormonal testing and pharmalogic treatment of erectile dysfunction: A clinical practice guideline from the American College of Physicians. *Annals of Internal Medicine, 151*, 1–11.

Roose, S. P., & Seidman, S. N. (2000). Sexual activity and cardiac risk: Is depression a contributing factor? *American Journal of Cardiology, 86*(2A), 38F–40F.

Sarkadi, A., & Rosenquist, U. (2004). Intimacy and women with type 2 diabetes: An exploratory study using focus group interviews. *Diabetes Educator, 29*(4), 641–652.

Shril, R., Koskimaki, J., Hakkien, A., Auvinen, T., Tammela, J., & Hakama, M. (2007). Cardiovascular drug use and the incidence of erectile dysfunction. *International Journal of Impotence Research, 19*(2), 208–212.

Statistics Canada. (2012). Leading causes of death. Retrieved from http://www.statcan.gc.ca/daily-quotidien/111101/dq111101b-eng.htm

Steinke, E. E. (2000). Sexual counseling after myocardial infarction. *American Journal of Nursing, 100*(12), 38–44.

Svedlund, M., & Danielson, E. (2004). Myocardial infarction: Narrations by afflicted women and their partners of lived experiences in daily life following an acute myocardial infarction. *Journal of Clinical Nursing, 13*(4), 438–446.

Tilton, M. C. (1997). Diabetes and amputation. In M. L. Sipski & C. J. Alexander (Eds.), *Sexual function in people with disability and chronic illness: A health professional's guide* (pp. 279–302). Rockville, MD: Aspen.

Verschuren, J. E., Enzlin, P., Dijkstra, P. V., Geertzen, J. H., & Dekker, R. (2010). Chronic disease and sexuality: A generic conceptual framework. *Journal of Sex Research, 47*(2–3), 153–170.

Wiegner, E. A., & King, C. R. (2010). Sexual function after stereotactic baby radiotherapy for prostate cancer: Results of a prospective clinical trial. *International Journal of Radiation Oncology, Biology, Physics, 78*(2), 442–448.

Wilmoth, M. C. (1994a, Spring). Strategies for becoming comfortable with sexual assessment. *Oncology Nursing News*, pp. 6–7.

Wilmoth, M. C. (1994b). Nurses' and patients' perspectives on sexuality: Bridging the gap. *Innovations in Oncology Nursing, 10*(2), 34–36.

Wilmoth, M. C. (1996). The middle years: Women, sexuality and the self. *Journal of Obstetric, Gynecologic, and Neonatal Nursing, 25*, 615–621.

Wilmoth, M. C. (2000). Sexuality patterns, altered. In L. J. Carpenito (Ed.), *Nursing diagnosis: Application to clinical practice* (8th ed., pp. 837–857). Philadelphia, PA: Lippincott.

Wilmoth, M. C. (2006). Life after cancer: What does sexuality have to do with it? The 2006 Mara Mogenson Flaherty Memorial Lectureship. *Oncology Nursing Forum, 33*(5), 905–910.

Wilmoth, M. C. (2009). Sexuality. In C. Burke (Ed.), *Psychosocial dimensions of oncology nursing care* (2nd ed., pp. 101–124). Pittsburgh, PA: Oncology Nursing Press.

Wilmoth, M. C., Coleman, E. A., Wahab, H. T., & Kneisl, J. (2009). Preliminary work in validating the symptom cluster of fatigue, weight gain, psychological distress and altered sexuality. *Southern Online Journal of Nursing Research, 9*(13), Article 13.

Wilmoth, M. C., & Spinelli, A. (2000). Sexual implications of gynecologic cancer treatments. *Journal of Obstetric, Gynecologic and Neonatal Nursing, 29*, 413–421.

Woods, N. F. (1984). *Human sexuality in health and illness* (3rd ed.). St. Louis, MO: Mosby.

Zaviacic, M., & Ablin, R. J. (2000). The female prostate and prostate-specific antigen. Immunohistochemical localization, implications for this prostate marker in women, and reasons for using the term "prostate" in the human female. *Histology Histopathology, 15,* 131–142.

Zaviacic, M., & Whipple, B. (1993). Update on the female prostate and the phenomena of female ejaculation. *Journal of Sex Research, 30*, 48–151.

CHAPTER 11

Powerlessness

Original chapter by Faye I. Hummel
Canadian content added by Joseph C. Osuji

> *This was the first time. . . . When I woke up the other morning I couldn't get out of bed. I couldn't believe it . . . my body, my legs, they just wouldn't move. I was terrified. I thought I'd had a stroke or something. I called for John, but he didn't hear me. I just had to lie there, staring at the ceiling, trying to calm myself. I felt so helpless, so powerless. There was nothing I could do but wait for John to come . . . he helped me into the bathtub where the warmth of the water soothed my aching body. I've always been able to handle my never ending pain . . . the stiffness and rigidity of my body, but that morning . . . that morning was different . . . and now I wonder.*
>
> —Anne, 62-year-old woman with
> fibromyalgia and Parkinson's disease

INTRODUCTION

Chronic illness changes one's sense of self and sense of time. Living with chronic illness requires one to adapt to a continuous changing of outlooks in which the existence of dualities, such as hope and despair, self-control and loss of power, dependence and independence, can elicit feelings of ambiguity, anxiety, and frustration (Delmar et al., 2006). Chronic illness creates threats to well-being and produces multidimensional changes and challenges for the individual and family. Whether these changes occur suddenly or over a long period, chronic illness requires that individuals and families deal with and adapt to an unrelenting altered reality.

Managing real and perceived powerlessness is significant. Lack of control and the incapacity to act and change may dominate everyday life for persons with chronic illnesses. Accepting and acknowledging one's limitations as a result of chronic illness may result in a sense of helplessness and loss, as evidenced in the case of Anne:

Last week I watched John working in our garden . . . we have planted a garden for years together. I can't work outside anymore. . . . I miss getting my hands in the dirt. I had to quit my job too. I was an accountant for years. . . . I really miss my work, my friends; we shared so much. Now . . . now my body is just not able. I have so much pain . . . constant . . . pain is ever with me. My body seems foreign to me. . . . I'm losing control of my body. It takes me the better part of the day to get around, to take care of myself. . . . I try to cook for us and keep house. I try to plan ahead but I'm just not able to do what needs to be done. . . . I don't have a choice. John has to do more around the house now. . . . I'm not much help.

PHENOMENON OF POWERLESSNESS IN CHRONIC ILLNESS

The diagnosis of a chronic illness comes with uncertainties about the future, feelings of vulnerability and lack of control, and sometimes resignation to fate. At some point in the course of chronic illness individuals experience powerlessness. Powerlessness in the absolute sense is the inability to affect an outcome; the inability to have agency in one's own life (Miller, 2000). Powerlessness may be a real loss of power or a perceived loss of power. For some persons the feelings of powerlessness may be short lived, whereas for others they are persistent.

What and who determines powerlessness and what factors facilitate powerlessness? The natural history of chronic illness is highly variable and does not conform to a predictable course of events. The uncertainty of chronic illness, exacerbation of symptoms, failure of therapy, physical deterioration despite adherence to treatment regimens, side effects of drugs, iatrogenic influences, depletion of social support systems, and the disintegration of the client's psychological stamina can all contribute to powerlessness (Miller, 2000). Chronic illness results in a pronounced loss of functioning over time, disrupts social roles and activities, and limits fulfilment of role expectations (Beal, 2007). Fatigue and inability to participate and engage in social activities contribute to social withdrawal (Asbring, 2001; Beal, 2007) and loss of relationships. Loss of employment, social contacts, and physical and mental function can contribute to disempowerment of individuals with chronic illness. The quintessence of ill health is powerlessness (Strandmark, 2004).

Powerlessness occurs when an individual is controlled by the environment rather than the individual controlling the environment. Therefore, powerlessness is a situational attribute (Miller, 2000). In Anne's story she experiences powerlessness in part because of the degenerative nature of her disease. Despite her previous life successes Anne now feels powerless over her own circumstances. Although Anne experienced physical limitations associated with her chronic conditions for a number of years, she was able to successfully adapt and respond to the slow progressive deterioration of her physical condition. Anne maintained power and control over her daily life. When she began to experience the crushing effects of her illness symptoms and physical limitations, Anne felt a loss of control, a sense of powerlessness. No longer was Anne able to maintain her veneer of normalcy, and she was not able to sustain her work and home obligations. Anne resigned from her job and struggled to keep up with her household demands. When Anne begins to consider herself without worth in terms of social norms and expectations, feelings of powerlessness arise. Her autonomy and existence are threatened. Over time, Anne becomes exhausted from fatigue and grief and feels powerless over her life situation (Strandmark, 2004).

Dorothy Johnson was one of the first individuals to explore the concept of powerlessness in nursing. Johnson (1967) defined powerlessness as a "perceived lack of personal or internal control of certain events or in certain situations" (p. 40) and urged nurses to take into account the concept of powerlessness as nursing interventions would not be effective, particularly health education, if the client felt powerless. The work of Miller (1983, 1992, 2000) has also been instrumental in the development of the concept of powerlessness in chronic illness. Miller (1983, 1992, 2000) differentiated powerlessness from similar constructs, including helplessness, learned helplessness, and locus of control. Helplessness and locus of control are based on a reinforcement paradigm, whereas powerlessness is an existential construct (Miller, 2000). Miller (2000) categorized locus of control as a personality trait as opposed to powerlessness, which is situationally determined. Locus of control refers to the degree to which people attribute accountability to themselves (internal control), such as personal behaviour or characteristics, versus uncontrollable forces (external control), such as fate, chance, or luck (Rotter, 1966). The physical and psychosocial outcomes of seeking and gaining control over chronic illness have been the focus of research by social scientists for decades. Locus of control and the beliefs of individuals about whom and what controls their lives are linked to physical and psychological health (Bandura, 1989).

Chronic illness erodes individual control, and this loss of personal control results in powerlessness. Progressive physiological changes resulting from chronic illness may limit mobility and/or diminish cognitive abilities. The progressive nature of chronic illness limits possibilities and opportunities to exert control over daily life events as well as plans for the future. Chronic illness sharply delineates the nature and quality of control, often resulting in a sense of powerlessness in individuals and their families.

Chronic illness disrupts personal control and changes life activities and expectations. Maintaining personal control is important for persons with chronic illness; lack of self-management and inability to predict the course of their disease can be distressing. Decision making to manage and control everyday life with a chronic illness is complex and bound to individually constructed lives (Thorne, Paterson, & Russell, 2003). According to Strandmark (2004), the essence of ill health is powerlessness, which is made manifest by a "self image of worthlessness, a sense of being imprisoned in one's life situation and emotional suffering" (p. 135). Perceptions of control are associated with greater levels of psychosocial well-being, whereas perceptions of powerlessness are associated with poorer health and psychosocial outcomes (Hay, 2010). Persons with inflammatory bowel disease reported personal control required maintaining a balance between what one could control versus what one needed to control for everyday life (Cooper, Collier, James, & Hawkey, 2010). Using grounded theory methodology, Pihl-Lesnovska, Hjortswang, Ek, and Frisman (2010) interviewed 11 persons with Crohn's disease. Dominant themes that emerged from their analysis of the data included quality of life, self-image, confirmatory relations, powerlessness, attitude toward life, and a sense of well-being.

Rånhein and Holand (2006) conducted a hermeneutic-phenomenological study of women's lived experience with chronic pain and fibromyalgia. Themes of powerlessness, ambivalence, and coping emerged from interviews with 12 women with fibromyalgia. The stories of these women revealed their struggles to manage and control the severe symptoms of their disease and their efforts to reduce their feelings of powerlessness that surfaced with pain, fatigue, and immobility. Individuals with chronic illness who develop effective systems for controlling their most severe symptoms have a more positive outlook and a lessened sense of powerlessness. The main challenge of women with chronic pain is to maintain a sense of control of self and pain to avoid becoming discouraged. In a theory synthesis Skuladöttir and Halldorsdöttir (2008) postulated that women with chronic pain face multiple challenges and the threat of demoralization. However, interactions with healthcare providers may be either positive or negative. Positive interactions can result in empowerment in which a sense of control is maintained. Negative interactions can disempower clients and eliminate a sense of control over self and the situation.

Persons with health failure experience increasing powerlessness (Falk, Wahn, & Lidell, 2007). A systematic review of 14 qualitative research studies conducted with older adults found that living with chronic heart failure was characterized by physical limitations and stressful symptoms, feelings of powerlessness and hopelessness, and social and role interruptions (Yu, Lee, Kwong, Thompson, & Woo, 2008). Aujoulat, Luminet, and Deccache (2007) conducted interviews with 40 individuals with various chronic conditions and asked them to discuss their experiences of powerlessness. They found that powerlessness extends beyond medical and treatment issues to feelings of insecurity and threats to their social and personal identities. They found an overwhelming feeling of powerlessness among these individuals, which participants described in terms of loss of control over one's body, loss of control over one's emotions, loss of control in the context of transgenerational transmissions, loss of control over time, loss of control over one's environment, and above all, loss of one's social and personal identities. Desperation and powerlessness were also expressed by women with long-term urinary incontinence. Women who lacked control of their urinary incontinence reported their autonomy was threatened, which promoted a sense of powerlessness to control their own bodies (Hägglund & Ashlström, 2007).

The phenomenon of powerlessness in chronic illness is a dynamic and complex issue. Powerlessness in chronic illness can be triggered by individual attributes and perceptions or stimulated by the evolving nature of the chronic disease. Powerlessness is inherent and impending in chronic illness. However, feelings of powerlessness recede and advance throughout the course of the chronic illness as individuals negotiate between control and loss and navigate the changing landscape of their daily realities. Variables such as the degree of physical limitation, anticipated prognosis, and ability to manage symptoms of chronic illness can also influence an individual's experience with powerlessness.

PARADOX OF POWERLESSNESS IN CHRONIC ILLNESS

The paradox of powerlessness in chronic illness is that power and powerlessness exist simultaneously. Power takes for granted powerlessness and vice versa (Kuokkanen & Leino-Kilpi, 2000). Power is defined as the "ability to act or produce an effect" and "possession of control, authority, or influence over others" (*Merriam-Webster*, 2011). Power can be enabling and enhance one's autonomous ability and capacity. Despite the limiting effects of chronic illness and feelings of powerlessness, individuals continue to exert power and control in areas of their lives through adaptation and accommodation to their evolving abilities and selves.

Power is an individual psychological characteristic (McCubbin, 2001), a personal resource inherent in all individuals, and is the ability to influence what happens to one's self (Miller, 2000). Seeking, getting, and preserving power are a dynamic process that reflects a human being's ability to achieve a desired goal in the face of personal, social, cultural, and environmental facilitators and barriers (Efraimsson, Rasmussen, Gilje, & Sandman, 2003).

In the individual-oriented societies of the world such as Canada, the United States, and most of Western Europe, power is associated with independence and self-determination. Although we may think of power as an individual quality, in reality power is a relational attribute. Power has no meaning in the absence of relationships with others and the context of the interaction. Power is developed and maintained in relationships. Power can restrict self-determination with forcefulness or authority by restricting the autonomy of another in personal relationships as well as hierarchical organizations (Moden, 2004). Power is a "social, political, economic, and cultural phenomenon, since all these dimensions of human societies determine who has power and what kind" (McCubbin, 2001, p. 76).

Individual power resources include physical strength and physical reserve, psychological stamina and social support, positive self-concept, energy, knowledge, motivation, and hope (Miller, 2000). Chronic illness can diminish these power resources. When power resources are significantly altered and affected, an individual with chronic illness may experience feelings of powerlessness. To deal with this powerlessness persons with chronic illness should direct their energy toward their intact power resources. Power resources facilitate coping with chronic illness. Accordingly, when one power resource becomes depleted, other power components may need to be developed to avert or reduce powerlessness (Miller, 2000).

THEORETICAL PERSPECTIVES OF POWERLESSNESS AND POWER

Persons with chronic illness live in a dual world, that of wellness and sickness, of control and powerlessness, and of hope and despair. The shifting perspectives model of chronic illness (Paterson, 2001a, 2003) describes chronic illness as a complex dialectic between the individual and his or her world. This model posits that persons with chronic illness shift between the perspective of wellness in the foreground and illness in the background and vice versa. Furthermore, this model suggests the experience of living with a chronic illness is a dynamic process that reflects the elements of both wellness and illness that comprise chronic illness. A perspective shift is a cognitive and affective strategy to negotiate the effects of chronic illness and to make sense of the experience. The perspectives of wellness and illness are not mutually exclusive; rather, there is a fluctuation of the degree to which illness or wellness is in the foreground or background (Paterson, 2001a).

Rather than a static outlook, there is a continual shifting of perspectives (Paterson, 2003). Persons living with chronic illness have a preferred perspective that is assumed most frequently. Therefore, persons with an illness perspective in the foreground focus on their illness, their symptoms, and the negative impact their chronic condition has on them and others. Conversely, from a perspective of wellness in the foreground, the individual views the chronic illness at a distance and focuses on his or her abilities to navigate daily life and to perform roles and responsibilities; the negative aspects of the chronic illness recede to the background. In addition to illness and wellness this shifting perspectives model acknowledges parallel and simultaneous contradictions in the chronic illness experience such as loss and gain, control, and powerlessness (Paterson, 2003). Hence, persons with a wellness perspective will likely exert power and control over their daily routines and social interactions.

The illness and wellness perspective is dynamic, so it can be interrupted and changed at a moment's notice. Such a shift in perspective can be stimulated by physiological changes, events, fears, and other individuals (Paterson, 2003). Social support, competent care providers, hope, and humour are factors that influence a shift from illness in the foreground to wellness in the foreground (Freeman, O'Dell, & Meola, 2003; Haluska, Jessee, & Nagy, 2002). Exacerbations of symptoms and other forms of illness intrusiveness such as pain, decreased physical function and mobility, low self-worth, and feelings of loss of life goals and aspirations (Mullins, Chaney, Balderson, & Hommel, 2000) may shift an individual's perspective to the disease state, and feelings of loss of control and powerlessness may arise. The "relative importance of the illness, physical experiences with the illness, and biomedical uncertainties" (Sutton & Treloar, 2007, p. 338) can also trigger a shift in perspective. Clinical indicators of chronic disease progression may not be congruent with individual perceptions of health and illness in that health and illness views are constructed within the individual's physical, emotional, and social spheres and may not be compatible with healthcare priorities (Sutton & Treloar, 2007). Although the focus of illness in the foreground can be self-absorbing, this perspective may provide the individual with an opportunity to learn more about his or her illness and effective strategies to treat and manage symptoms. **Figure 11-1** illustrates the shift of perspectives in chronic illness.

Self-Determination Theory

Self-determination theory highlights the psychological processes that promote optimal functioning and health. This theory posits three basic, innate psychological needs that are the basis for optimal functioning and personal well-being. These psychological needs—competence, relatedness, and autonomy—are universal and must be satisfied for all people to achieve

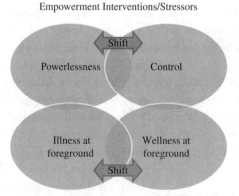

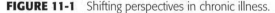

FIGURE 11-1   Shifting perspectives in chronic illness.
Source: Paterson, B. L. (2001a). The shifting perspectives model of chronic illness. *Journal of Nursing Scholarship, 33,* 21–26A; and Paterson, B. L. (2003). The koala has claws: Applications of the shifting perspectives model in research of chronic illness. *Qualitative Health Research, 13*(7), 987–994.

optimal health. These basic psychological needs provide a framework that specifies the conditions in which people can maximize their human potential. The need for competence results in an individual's ability to adapt to new challenges in a changing context; it stimulates unique talents of individuals and produces adaptive competencies and flexible functioning in the context of changing demands. The need for relatedness is the integration of the individual into the social world in which the individual seeks attachments, security, and a sense of belonging and intimacy with others. The tendencies of relatedness are to cohere to one's group and to feel connection with and care of others. However, the need for relatedness can compete or conflict with autonomy. Autonomy, according to self-determination theory, refers to self-organization and self-regulation and conveys adaptive advantage. Autonomous individuals function and respond effectively within changing contexts and circumstances. When behaviour is regulated by outside pressures and expectations, holistic functioning is precluded. Therefore, autonomous individuals are better able to regulate their actions in accordance with their perceived needs and available capacities as well as coordinate and prioritize courses of action that will maximize self-maintenance (Deci & Ryan, 2000; Ryan & Deci, 2000).

Self-determination theory distinguishes between autonomous and controlled behaviour regulation. Behaviours are autonomous when persons experience a sense of choice to act out of personal importance of the behaviour. Controlled behaviours, on the other hand, are those performed when persons feel pressured by external forces (Deci & Ryan, 1985, 1991). Autonomous regulation, or the choice to do what is important and relevant to the individual,

is associated with subjective experiences of vitality and energized behaviour and differentiated controlled and autonomous choice (Moller, Deci, & Ryan, 2006). Adjustment to chronic illness is influenced by the extent to which individuals believe themselves to be the source of their actions, that is, their feelings of autonomy (Igreja et al., 2000).

Patient-centred care is grounded in self-determination theory. In *Crossing the Quality Chasm,* the Institute of Medicine (2001) recognized the patient as the source of control. Patient-centred care focuses on the patient rather than the disease and gives the responsibility for disease management to the patient along with the resources and support needed to assume that responsibility. This becomes particularly important in the management of chronic illness because it encourages clients to take control of their lives and illness and empowers them toward autonomy and self-determination.

Cognitive Adaptation Theory

Cognitive adaptation theory posits that an individual's attempt to maintain or regain a sense of personal control may be heightened or activated by the psychological challenge that can arise out of an unpredictable illness. This theory is based on the assumption that individuals exhibit sometimes unrealistically positive views of themselves to enhance their well-being. This heightened sense of personal control may be used as a way to maintain positive adaptation to chronic illness. An enhanced perception of control may facilitate coping with an illness-related stressor such as exacerbation of symptoms or disease progression (Taylor, 1983), whereas absence of self-control promotes dependency, powerlessness, and erodes client autonomy

(McCann & Clark, 2004). Taylor (1983) argued that the adaptive process to a chronic illness, such as cancer, centres around three themes: a search for meaning, an attempt to regain mastery, and an effort to restore self-esteem. Taylor (1983) concluded that "when individuals experience personal tragedies or setbacks, they respond with cognitively adaptive efforts that may enable them to return to or exceed their previous level of psychological functioning" (p. 1170). These cognitive restructurings, according to Taylor, are in large parts based on illusions that may have no factual basis.

PROBLEMS AND ISSUES ASSOCIATED WITH POWERLESSNESS

A number of issues are associated with powerlessness. Issues discussed here are examples of what individuals and their families may experience; however, it is not an all inclusive list.

From a medical viewpoint, chronic illness comprises physical symptoms and limitations. From a broader perspective, chronic illness brings multiple losses for individuals and their families on the physical side but perhaps even more so on a psychological level. The diagnosis of a chronic illness may, in and of itself, represent a loss to the individual, and for some the diagnosis of a chronic illness may be as significant as a death. The diagnosis of the chronic illness may represent the loss of hopes and dreams, income, sexual ability, physical and mental ability, quality of life, or independence (Clarke & James, 2003). The loss of mobility and agility as a result of chronic illness affects one's ability to participate in social activities and to maintain social ties (Beal, 2007). Loss of paid employment due to chronic illness has a

significant impact on one's life. Leaving work not only results in the loss of income and daily routines but triggers a loss of positive social identity (Walker, 2010).

Persons with chronic illness have restrictions in their daily lives, experience social isolation, believe they are discounted, and fear becoming a burden to others (Charmaz, 1983). Loss of self is felt by many persons with chronic illness (Charmaz, 1983), in which the serious debilitating effects of chronic illness erode the former self-image of the individual. Over time, accumulated loss of self-image can result in diminished self-concept. Loss of self is a result of chronic illness that diminishes control over lives and futures (Charmaz, 1983). Lack of self-confidence and disrupted identity are two major factors of powerlessness. In-depth interviews with clients with various chronic conditions revealed numerous losses, including their loss of self-control and confidence as their environment and possibilities become diminished (Aujoulat et al., 2007). Ahlstrom (2007) reported that all persons with chronic illness experience repeated physical, emotional, and social losses, with the most common being "loss of bodily function, loss of relationships, loss of autonomous life, loss of the life imagined and loss of identity" (p. 76).

Uncertainty

Chronic illness generates a wide array of emotions and reactions and engenders anxiety and uncertainty. The uncertainty of chronic illness promotes feelings of loss of control and a sense of powerlessness in individuals and families (Mishel, 1999). Narratives of persons diagnosed with multiple sclerosis revealed concerns about the unpredictable progression of the disease and fear and anxiety relative to the unknown (Barker-Collo, Cartwright, & Read, 2006). Severity of the illness, the erratic nature of symptomatology, and the ambiguity of symptoms promote uncertainty in persons with chronic illness (Mishel, 1999). Anticipating and planning for the future becomes complicated. The unpredictability of physical symptoms and capabilities interferes with the individual's ability to schedule activities and events in the future and may result in an unwillingness to plan in advance. The uncertainty of the chronic illness raises salient concerns for persons about their future, their ability to control their illness and symptoms, and their capacity to garner necessary personal and financial resources to manage their illness.

Chronic Illness Management

Chronic illness management often entails a multifaceted self-management regimen. The complexity of chronic illness has the potential to strip away a client's sense of self-worth and confidence. Clients who lack confidence often are unable to assess their needs accurately and consequently are at risk of being manipulated or coerced by others and may capitulate to the wishes of family members or healthcare professionals. Self-management of complex chronic disease is often difficult to achieve and is reflected in low rates of adherence to treatment guidelines (Newman, Steed, & Mulligan, 2004). Although some healthcare professionals believe they can motivate persons with chronic illness to follow a treatment regimen, the impetus to follow a plan of care is internal.

Healthcare professionals must acknowledge the personal context of the chronic illness and assess the individual motivators to follow a plan of care (Singleton, 2002). Persons with a chronic illness may not be willing to or capable of carrying out the complex tasks and activities to manage their chronic illness, and a simple "pep talk" from one's healthcare professional simply does not suffice. Clients' realization that their days are built around their healthcare regimen—that is, specific treatments they must perform every day, doctor visits, lab tests, body scans, consults with other healthcare providers, physical therapy—and not other aspects of their lives can be unbearable. The power to dictate how individuals with chronic illness want to spend their day is gone. For example, Mrs. Jones, an elderly widow with end-stage renal disease, must spend 3 days a week at the local dialysis unit to manage her chronic illness. Even though she has accepted the time involved to adhere to her treatment regimen and has accommodated her lifestyle accordingly, she yearns to visit her extended family that lives some distance from her. At her peril Mrs. Jones chooses to spend time with her family, to forgo prescribed treatment, and to bear the consequences of her decision. In the end, although Mrs. Jones was able to continue her dialysis treatments, her decision was motivated by her personal desire and familial priority, not the prescribed treatment.

Mr. Smith, a young man with AIDS, experiences difficulties adhering to a complex pharmacological regimen because of financial constraints. Mr. Smith finds himself consumed with an ongoing process of seeking resources to maintain his prescribed treatment, which takes away his ability to participate in other areas of his life. The lives of the elderly woman (Mrs. Jones) and young man centre around their chronic illness and treatment-regimen activities. Both experience a loss of control over time management, personal choice, and quality of life. Their chronic illness and treatment regimens consume their daily lives to the detriment of other activities, and feelings of powerlessness arise. What was true for Mrs. Jones and Mr. Smith is also true for other persons dealing with chronic illness. The lack of self-control inherent in their disease and treatment fosters feelings of dependence and powerlessness and undermines client autonomy (McCann & Clark, 2004).

In contrast, the ability to control one's treatment plan, choose services, and avoid coercion diminishes powerlessness (Nelson, Lord, & Ochocka, 2001). Support is essential to meet the demands and expectations of complex management regimens of chronic illness. Necessary supports include good communication with healthcare professionals, adequate financial resources, time and ability to perform care tasks, and spiritual support (Singleton, 2002).

> Can we just have one day when we do not see a healthcare provider? It's a doctor appointment, re-checking lab results, radiation therapy, out-patient IV antibiotics, a port that is clogged, etc. This is a life? Where is our relationship of old when we used to talk about things other than "lab results," how much you've vomited, when the next appointment is? Why is every day of the weekend filled with an ER visit or an outpatient procedure of some type?
>
> *—Jenny, wife of a newly*
> *diagnosed cancer patient*

Another key element to adherence to treatment regimens is meaningful participation in healthcare organizations (Nelson et al., 2001). Choice of treatment regimen and control of that regimen are central to self-determination in persons with chronic conditions. To provide appropriate information the nurse must listen to the needs, wants, and desires of the client. Clients who believe they are unheard and have no voice feel invalidated, dismissed, and powerless (Courts, Buchanan, & Werstlein, 2004). As a result of this powerlessness the opportunity for the nurse to enhance client outcomes diminishes greatly.

Lack of Knowledge

Knowledge about chronic illness is essential for disease management and control. Lack of knowledge or skills about the disease may impact the dynamics of the disease. Often, information and education about the chronic illness occur during the acute phase of the illness or during hospitalization— overwhelming periods when the client and family may not have been able to grasp the concepts. Unfamiliar surroundings coupled with the insecurities of new or recurrent chronic illness diagnosis impact learning. Although the client may have listened intently to the instructions and education, he or she may not have been able to internalize and actualize the content. As a result, after discharge from the acute care setting the client may lack sufficient knowledge to effectively manage issues and problems that arise from the chronic condition. Lack of information to successfully meet the challenges of daily living further reinforces feelings of powerlessness.

Healthcare professionals frequently assume that once individuals have been provided with information about their chronic illness, they have adequate knowledge and skills to adopt necessary changes to effectively manage their chronic condition. However, Bodenheimer, Lorig, Holman, and Grumbach (2002) estimated that approximately 50% of clients leave a primary care setting with little or no understanding of what was said. Healthcare professionals must ensure clients have a clear understanding of health information related to management of their chronic illness.

Marginalization/Vulnerability

Knowledge alone is insufficient for management and control of chronic illness. The contextual determinants of health must also be acknowledged. Social determinants of vulnerability include low income, low education, fragile social identity, and limited social networks (Crossley, 2001). Lack of resources contributes to powerlessness. Persons who experience a marginalized sociocultural status and have limited access to economic resources have a greater than average risk of developing health problems and have higher rates of morbidity and mortality associated with chronic illness (Aday, 2001).

The burden of chronic illness disproportionately affects vulnerable populations (Sullivan, Weinert, & Cudney, 2003). Vulnerable clients are the most powerless and the least able to identify and express their needs and desires beyond the completely obvious (Niven & Scott, 2003). Chronic conditions are a significant healthcare challenge, and one's vulnerability is often brought into sharp focus by a chronic disease.

Clients identify the way healthcare professionals relate to them as the cause for their vulnerability, not their chronic illness (Mitchell & Bournes, 2000). Some clients are viewed as having less social value than others (Glaser & Strauss, 1968). Social value is subjective and influenced by such factors as age, marital status, income, living conditions, hygiene, and behaviour. Some clients with chronic illnesses may be perceived as having low moral worth. The nurse may believe the client's illness or condition is the result of poor or risky behaviours chosen by the client. Clients who do not behave within the prescribed norms and expectations of the institution or agency may be erroneously labelled as undesirable or noncompliant and may not have the opportunity to engage in decision making and control over their healthcare regimen.

Stigma

Persons with chronic illnesses are at risk for stigma based on the negative perceptions held by society. Stigma is a response to any physical or social attribute or characteristic that devalues a person's social identity and disqualifies him or her from full social acceptance (Goffman, 1963). This stigma and the associated stereotypes and misconceptions about chronic illness lead to a lack of inclusion and feelings of powerlessness. Confusion and misinformation about chronic illness can lead to discrimination and stigma and result in unintended, harmful effects for persons with a chronic condition. For example, family and friends of persons with hepatitis C may be fearful and lack knowledge about the virus. For the individual with hepatitis C, the ignorance of others may stimulate feelings of helplessness and infectiousness (Zickmund, Ho, Masuda, Ippolito, & LaBrecque, 2003) or fear of judgment and stigma from those around them (Sutton & Treloar, 2007). In this way external societal pressures can create and perpetuate feelings of powerlessness in individuals with chronic illness.

Culture

The concepts of powerlessness and power are grounded in the context of cultural values, beliefs, and practices of persons with chronic illness and their families. The traditional power and control culture in the healthcare setting may conflict with cultural customs and beliefs of an individual with a chronic illness. Many cultural groups view the individual as embedded in social relationships; thus, the role of the individual in decision making is not recognized. For group-oriented persons or families power and control may reside within the family rather than with the individual (Davis, Konishi, & Tashiro, 2003). For example, in some aboriginal families healthcare decisions are made by the matriarch of the family rather than the individual with chronic illness. Failure to include the family matriarch in the decision-making process diminishes adherence to prescribed treatment regimens. In some cultures the oldest male holds the power and control to make decisions. Cultural conflicts may arise when families are not consulted before an intervention or staff interferes with rituals deemed necessary by the client's family to promote healing.

Conversely, when a client chooses to go against his or her cultural norm or custom, the client must have the power to do so. In situations where families are in disagreement with the client about compliance with cultural customs, the nurse must support the client and give him or her the resources for self-determination (Zoucha & Husted, 2000). The desires and wishes of the individual client supersede the cultural values, beliefs, and practices of the culture in which the individual and family are in disagreement (Tang & Lee, 2004).

Culture is the context in which individuals, families, and groups make healthcare decisions. Power and control in Western society are based on the concept of individualism—a society consisting of autonomous individuals. Western societies promote the actualization of the individual self as the goal, yet other cultures do not. The Western principle of autonomy is self-determination. In other cultures the principle of autonomy is family-determination, that is, the family is the autonomous social unit in which the entire family, not the individual, has real authority in decision making. For Chinese cancer patients living in Hong Kong, emphasizing the Chinese cultural beliefs of loyalty to family, letting go, harmony with the universe, and the cycles of life and nature was essential to the development of feelings of empowerment (Mok, Martinson, & Wong, 2004).

Values, beliefs, practices, and responses to chronic illness vary by culture and within culture. Culture impacts and dictates one's responses to normal events of everyday life and is a driving force in the decisions and choices that individuals and families make about health and care (Salas-Provance, Erickson, & Reed, 2002). Some individuals experiencing chronic illness may remain silent about their experiences and issues with chronic illness. This is not an indicator of indifference or incompetence but a reflection of cultural differences in the use of silence. Culturally appropriate care can only occur when cultural care values, expressions, or patterns are known and used appropriately (Leininger, 1995). Life experiences and situations of the past influence the present. Knowledge of cultural values, beliefs, and practices provides an invaluable blueprint for healthcare providers in caring for diverse clients with chronic illness. Furthermore, the promotion of cultural values can help clients with chronic illness mitigate their experiences of powerlessness.

Healthcare System and the Community

Healthcare systems are based on the assumption that patient safety and system integrity depend on the expertise and authority of the healthcare professional. Although this type of complex process is essential for those with acute illness who lack expertise to make appropriate decisions, this system is counterproductive for those with chronic illness who develop competency and expertise with regard to management of their chronic conditions (Thorne, 2006). The healthcare system is designed for acute, episodic treatment and strives for efficient and cost-effective care. This fast-paced and impersonal care system leaves little time and individual focus for the person with a chronic condition, who requires a more long-term, illness-management approach. Thus, clients and their families are vulnerable and powerless in the healthcare power structure (Davis et al., 2003). Upon entry into the healthcare system the client relinquishes control over his or her life, loses self-identity and initiative, and becomes distant from supportive networks. The client's voice may be ignored by healthcare professionals or quieted by dwindling energy levels that come from the disease process itself or the side effects of treatment.

Power is inherent in the healthcare system. Education and professional status are sources of power for healthcare providers in the nurse–client relationship. The procedures and language used by healthcare professionals are foreign and strange to the client and leave many persons with chronic conditions unable or unwilling to be an active participant in their own care. The healthcare system provides fragmented care for persons with chronic illness and leaves individuals feeling isolated and left to care for themselves with inadequate knowledge and resources. Frustration and inability to overcome obstacles in accessing, receiving, and in some instances paying for services add to feelings of powerlessness.

The healthcare system perpetuates client vulnerability. It has the potential to restrict the autonomy of people and to disable and dominate them by virtue of its bureaucracy, scientific expertise, and technology. Clients surrender their independence to the healthcare system, where the physician is omniscient and clients begin the process of learned helplessness and an inability to speak for themselves (Hewitt, 2002). In the United States and other countries where health care in privately run and funded, most decisions in the healthcare system are made by power brokers who are neither providers nor consumers of health care (Sheridan-Gonzalez, 2000). These types of healthcare systems have the potential to marginalize both clients and healthcare practitioners and perpetuate their feelings of powerlessness, with subsequent negative impacts on care and patient empowerment.

> Powerlessness can be seen in the context of becoming a patient, the expectations of individuals, and the ways in which they play by the rules. It is also a key to understanding the ways in which their horizons change, both as facts—the loss of mobility and contact—and as metaphor—acceptance, control, and changing outlook. It is a response to the limits of the conditions itself, and to the power which is perceived to be vested in the health care system. (Gibson & Kenrick, 1998, p. 743)

> My life is like a roller coaster . . . some days my life is full of light and joy . . . but those up days are becoming fewer and fewer now that my fibromyalgia and Parkinson's are so much a part of my life. What can I do? The uncertainty of every day makes me so angry, so confused, so sad. I want to escape from all of this but where would I go? You know, I really thought I could beat this. I've

done it before but now . . . my pain is relentless! My body is unwilling! What choice do I have?

—Anne

INTERVENTIONS

Persons with chronic illness feel overwhelmed, exhausted, and discouraged at times. Therefore, one of the most important challenges for nurses working with these clients is to help them overcome feelings of powerlessness. Factors that impact powerlessness in persons with chronic illness are complex and multidimensional. Nursing interventions to address powerlessness in chronic illness should be equally multifaceted and require attention to the complex nature of the healthcare situation. Appropriate and relevant nursing interventions are based on ongoing assessments and observations of the client with chronic illness in his or her environment, the context in which the person manages and copes with chronic illness. This includes not only the physical surroundings but also the psychosocial dimensions of life.

Because of the dynamic nature of chronic illness, continuing evaluation of interventions with subsequent modifications to meet the current needs of the client are required. The goals of nursing interventions are to assist the client to manage the realities of his or her limitations and illuminate strengths to reduce a sense of powerlessness and loss and to create new boundaries for one's changed life.

Persons with chronic illness seek a sense of normalcy and a sense of dignity by focusing on personal strengths and remaining engaged in family and social activities to diminish isolation and loneliness (Skuladöttir & Halldorsdöttir, 2011). According to Mattsson, Moller, Stamm, Gard, and Bostrom (2011), although multifaceted uncertainty is the hallmark of chronic illnesses such as systemic lupus erythematosus, positive aspects and opportunities for strength could be possible. This highlights the "importance of health care professionals of gaining a better understanding of patients' uncertainty to enable them to support patients, allowing them to focus on health and opportunities" (Mattsson et al., p. 1).

CASE STUDY

WWW

Maria, a widowed 73-year-old Ukrainian-Canadian, lives independently in her small home in a rural community. She is a devout Catholic, attends mass daily, and is a member of the church's women's group. She works part time in the kitchen at the local nursing home to supplement her old age security income. Maria attended school in Ukraine and completed 8th grade equivalent. She speaks and reads limited English. Maria's only living child lives out of province and, because of finances and family commitments, is not able to visit frequently. During a recent hospitalization for influenza Maria was diagnosed with type 2 diabetes. When learning of her chronic illness Maria was overcome with emotion and anxiety about what her future would hold. Would she be able to continue to work to support herself? Would she lose her legs like her mother? Would she die like her son? Maria felt overwhelmed with all the

CASE STUDY   (Continued)   `www`

information the nurses and doctors were telling her about her treatment plan. They used words and language she didn't understand. She was reluctant to ask questions or tell them her concerns and needs. She was silent. She prayed.

Upon discharge, despite all the discharge instructions and papers she was given, Maria didn't know how to manage her care at home. She didn't feel well enough to return to work, and she stopped going to church and slept most of the day. At an office visit the diabetic nurse noted that Maria was having difficulty managing her diabetes and ordered home health visits. During her first visit, Sara, the home care nurse, told Maria exactly what she needed to do to get her diabetes under control. Sara wrote out detailed instructions for Maria about her medications, diet, and exercise. Yet again, Maria was unable to express her fears and wishes. At each subsequent visit Sara reinforced the treatment plan. When Maria was unsuccessful in maintaining glucose control, she was labelled a difficult patient and became discouraged, despondent, and overcome with feelings of hopelessness and powerlessness.

Discussion Questions

1. How do the physical and psychosocial challenges experienced by Maria contribute to her feelings of lack of control and sense of powerlessness?
2. How do theoretical perspectives of power and powerlessness guide a plan of care for Maria?
3. If you were the home care nurse, what nursing interventions would you implement to restore power and control to Maria? How would you prioritize her plan of care?
4. How would you ensure culturally appropriate restoration of power and control for Maria? How would you address issues of vulnerability and power?

Nursing interventions to restore client control and increase power resources in clients with chronic illness are discussed in this section. The following are summary strategies and tools to strengthen the client's power base but are in no means exhaustive.

Empowerment

Empowerment is a health-enhancing process. The outcome of client empowerment is self-efficacy, mastery and control, and a renewed and valued sense of self. Key issues to empowerment are self-awareness and self-determination. Self-determination is the ability to make choices and accept responsibility for one's choices (Aujoulat, d'Hoore, & Deccache, 2007). Client empowerment in chronic illness is the personal transformation through a dialectic process of "holding on" to former self-representations and roles and learning to manage the disease and treatment to differentiate one's self from the illness and "letting go" or relinquishing control to integrate the chronic illness into a reconciled self. "Holding on" is linked to efforts to gain control and maintain a sense of mastery, whereas the process of "letting go" is linked to a search for meaning and an acceptance that chronic illness is not always controllable (Aujoulat, Marcolongo, Bonadiman, & Deccache, 2008). The nurse–client relationship emphasizes the primacy of the client's own ideas, emotions, and beliefs about the chronic illness. Within this relationship the nurse must provide information and opportunities for choice and negotiation regarding treatment-related issues. The nurse must be attentive to individual beliefs and desires with regard to choice and control. Empowerment may not be a desirable outcome or process for all clients, because clients differ in their desire to participate in their own healthcare decisions (Loft, McWilliam, & Ward-Griffin, 2003) and rely on others such as family members or healthcare professionals to make decisions for them.

Empowerment strategies and efforts increase power and strengthen individual life circumstances. Two dimensions of empowerment emerge from the literature. One dimension is psychological, which includes self-esteem and self-efficacy. The other dimension of empowerment is social, action oriented, and comprises power, involvement, and control over individual life circumstances (Hansson & Bjorkman, 2005). Key features of empowering provider–client relationships include continuity of care, patient-centredness, and mutual acknowledgement and relatedness (Aujoulat et al., 2007).

Empowerment is important for clients with chronic illness because it increases perceived quality of life and promotes self-esteem. For empowerment, clients need access to information, resources, support, and opportunity (Laschinger, Gilbert, Smith, & Leslie, 2010). Empowerment results when individual perception of needs for care has been met (Roth & Crane-Ross, 2002).

Healthcare providers can promote client empowerment by providing access to relevant, timely, and appropriate information about an illness or treatment. Ongoing information can be provided through the use of information technology including email and vetted Internet sites. Client access to necessary support and resources further enhances empowerment. Nurses can assist clients with identifying sources of social support and introduce them to alternative resources within the family or community systems (Laschinger et al., 2010).

Health Coaching

Patient-centred strategies such as incorporating lifestyle changes, engaging in prevention strategies, and making decisions to promote self-management of chronic illness can be developed. Although not a new idea in the practice of nursing, the reemergence of the idea of client-centred care is reflected in health coaching. Health coaching is client centred, and clients are actively involved in determining what is important and what they want to accomplish relative to the management of their chronic illness. Health coaching motivates behaviour change in clients through collaboration, open-ended inquiry, and questions and reflection (Huffman, 2007).

Discharge Planning

Effective discharge planning is another strategy of empowerment. Discharge planning strengthens the client's position and role in social and healthcare systems. A client-tailored and well-orchestrated discharge plan enhances coping with relocation from one healthcare setting to another. Open and clear communication among all participants including the client, family, and healthcare professionals is essential for mutual understanding and successful discharge. Nurses may think of discharge planning simply from the acute healthcare setting to another care setting. However, the concept of long-range discharge planning is essential when dealing with clients with chronic illness, where the client transitions from one setting to another.

Collaboration

Successful management of chronic illness and optimal wellness is based on collaboration and partnership with clients to establish mutually negotiated and established healthcare and treatment goals. Collaboration is promoted when the client is encouraged and expected to participate in his or her own care and make decisions based on the client's self-determined needs (Laschinger et al., 2010). Standardized approaches to empowering and improving the quality of life in persons with chronic illness are not appropriate. If the healthcare professional's interventions do not match the patient's readiness, the patient may not adhere to the prescribed treatment regimen. Adherence is a dynamic process that is compromised by barriers usually related to different aspects of the chronic illness. Such barriers include social and economic factors, healthcare team and system, characteristics of the disease, therapies, and client-related factors. Solving problems related to each of these is necessary to promote client adherence (World Health Organization, 2003). In Canada the Interdisciplinary Chronic Disease Collaboration is made up of a team of researchers whose primary objective is to improve the health care of clients at risk of or living with chronic illness (see www.ICDC.ca).

The client with a chronic illness must be a full partner with the healthcare professional in decision making. Imparting knowledge and information to clients is an exchange process and requires active client participation. However, at times the client may not desire information because of fear, information overload, or inability to understand. The nurse needs to assess client readiness for information by acknowledging the client's concerns, listening to his or her perspectives, and respecting his or her desire for new information. Disempowering relationships result from discounting experiential knowledge and provision of inadequate resources (Paterson, 2001b).

Self-Management

Persons with chronic illness must be empowered to be managers of their own care within their own realities and settings. The opportunities to manage self-control depend on the context in which the clients live their everyday lives (Delmar et al., 2006). Psychological, behavioural, environmental, social, and socioeconomic factors determine one's ability to self-manage one's chronic illness and adhere to a complex treatment regimen (Granger, Moser, Germino, Harrell, & Ekman, 2006). In an institutional setting (acute or long-term care), clients with a chronic illness may be highly motivated to manage their own care. However, the clients' environment dictates the parameters of activities of daily living and may severely limit the opportunity to fully operationalise self-management despite ability and desire. In this instance nurses can be instrumental in altering the institutional structure to accommodate the self-control goals of clients.

Self-management is more than adherence to a treatment regimen; it also takes into account the psychological and social management of living with a chronic illness. (See the literature review on chronic disease self-management, prepared by The Elisabeth Bruyere Research Institute for the Chaplain Local Health Integration Network, Ontario, Canada, at http ://www.ontla.on.ca/library/repository/mon /24006/302504.pdf.) Chronic illnesses vary in how they intrude on the psychological and social worlds of individuals. The outcome of empowerment is self-management of chronic illness through the reinforcement of self-determination and control (Aujoulat et al., 2007). Self-management interventions for persons with chronic conditions need to be developed to assist them to better manage their illnesses and to take increasing responsibility for their disease. Healthcare providers must take into account the shifting nature of chronic conditions and offer self-management strategies appropriate for the problems and issues that may be encountered at a particular phase of the illness. Granger and colleagues (2006) proposed the use of trajectory theory to ensure interventions are patient-centred and relevant to an illness phase the client is experiencing or may encounter in the future. Further, healthcare providers must be aware that some persons with chronic illness may not have the physical or mental abilities for self-management. Assessment of the client to determine if self-management is attainable, realistic, and desired is necessary.

The difficulty in managing complex treatment schedules of chronic illnesses has led to the development of self-management interventions (SMIs). The key feature of these SMIs is to increase clients' involvement and control in their treatment and to improve the subsequent impact on their lives (Newman et al., 2004). The skills necessary for clients to develop an SMI

are problem solving and goal setting. Even with these skills in place, most persons with chronic illnesses are likely to encounter barriers to care that create major challenges in compliance with SMIs. Those who experience increased barriers are less likely to adhere to plans of care. Barriers include time constraints, knowledge deficits, limited social support, inadequate resources, limited coping skills, poor client–provider relationship, and low self-efficacy. Patient-centred, collaborative nursing strategies reinforce client strengths and ameliorate the impact of these barriers. The nurse becomes a partner with the client to facilitate collaboration in the development of a realistic self-management program and to identify resources and support systems to reach the goal of self-management. Failure of the nurse to identify or adequately estimate barriers to and resources for self-management will negatively impact adherence to the treatment regimen (Nagelkerk, Reick, & Meengs, 2006).

Control

Aujoulat and colleagues (2008) posited that "the process of relinquishing control is as central to empowerment as is the process of gaining control" (p. 1228). Perceived control is an antecedent to function, a mediator between social support and psychological well-being, and is useful for effective disease self-management (Jacelon, 2007). Perceived control is related to better adjustment to chronic illness. Nurses need to be aware of two dimensions of perceived control (Rotter, 1966). First, one can believe one is personally able to control one's outcomes. Second, one can believe that more powerful others control one's outcomes. The latter, vicarious control can be exerted by physicians, parents, God, or family. To assist the client in achieving optimal functioning, the nurse must assess the client's belief about the source of control, whether within self or from others.

When the professional nurse exerts too much control, the client may totally relinquish control and put his or her life in the hands of the professional to the detriment of his or her empowerment (Delmar et al., 2006). Client power is a fundamental element in the client–provider relationship because clients, due to their chronic illness, may become dependent and thus subordinate to healthcare professionals (Efraimsson et al., 2003). Independence, self-control, and self-responsibility are important elements for increasing patient empowerment. The ability to ask for assistance may be an indicator of self-control and self-management (Delmar et al., 2006).

Self-Determination

Self-determination is a basic human right of individual choice and control. Self-determination ensures an individual has the autonomy and support to make decisions and to reach personal goals. Self-determination must be balanced with safety and risk of the client and family. Self-determination restores power of choice to the client.

Fostering self-control is integral to promoting wellness in persons with chronic illness, and this control is central to self-determination. To be self-determined clients must have knowledge and resources to deal with illness-related issues as they arise (McCann & Clark, 2004). Good choices are the result of good options from which to choose. Nurses can give persons with chronic illness adequate and appropriate knowledge as a foundation for making the good choice (Delmar et al., 2006). To manage self-control

and live with dignity involves support from healthcare professionals and significant others in the decision-making process. Other people can help provide knowledge and expertise as a foundation for making the right choice. Clients with significant physical or mental impairments may be unable to engage in social discourse and may require additional resources to promote self-management. The nurse should provide the client with appropriate and relevant resources and work with the client and his or her family to obtain connections and referrals to appropriate community-based services.

Establishing a Sense of Mastery

Powerlessness is reduced and empowerment is facilitated by the development of a sense of mastery. Mastery is helping clients to focus on how they can affect their chronic conditions and can foster a sense of control in an otherwise uncontrollable illness course. Intervention techniques encourage clients to identify strengths and shift the focus away from uncontrollable aspects of chronic illness, such as use of a wheelchair or dialysis treatments, to the controllable aspects, such as decision making or self-care activities, which can imbue patients with a sense of mastery over their condition (Cvengros, Christensen, & Lawton, 2005). The World Health Organization (2003) published guidelines for healthcare professionals to facilitate client identification of strategies to reduce barriers to mastery and facilitate integration of self-care into daily activities.

Client and Family Education

Persons with chronic illnesses and their families need information, understanding, and competent interventions to help them reformulate their lives, assimilate their losses, and adjust to the changes brought about by their illnesses (Sullivan-Bolyai, Sadler, Knafl, & Gillis, 2003). Information about chronic disease management provides clients with a sense of control and thus increases empowerment (Sommerset, Campbell, Sharp, & Peters, 2001; Wollin, Dale, Spenser, & Walsh, 2000).

Over their lifetimes persons with chronic illness and their families must shoulder the burden of coordinating medical information and treatment regimens. The need for information must be tailored to meet the needs of the individual client relative to the disease course. The client may not be able to take in information at the time of the diagnosis of a chronic illness; therefore, information should be available to the client and his or her family at a follow-up visit to ensure understanding of information and available services (Barker-Collo et al., 2006). The time of diagnosis of a chronic disease is overwhelming and confusing for clients and their families. The expectation that clients will be able to assimilate the information given to them about their chronic illness may be unrealistic.

In addition to information and knowledge about the chronic illness, the client needs information about available, accessible, appropriate, and affordable resources and services within his or her community. The nurse is the client's link to these resources (Falk-Rafael, 2001). Therefore, it is necessary for the nurse to maintain current information about community resources and services. The nurse assesses the client's needs and preferences, selects appropriate resources for the client, and evaluates the effectiveness and acceptability of the resources to the client. The nurse may also link the client and his or her family to support groups, which can promote empowerment through the expression of shared experiences.

Many clients may also seek information about their chronic illness on the Internet. The ability to obtain this information independent of a healthcare professional can give the client a sense of control and self-determination. As a result many visit their healthcare providers with requests for specific tests or medications (Corbin & Cherry, 2001). However, this information should be evaluated by the nurse to determine the appropriateness of the suggestion. Online communication and Internet support groups have become not only sources of information for individuals with chronic illness but also sources of social support (Laschinger et al., 2010; van Uden-Kraan, Drossaert, Taal, Seydel, & van de Laar, 2009). Women are more likely to use the Internet for health information and illness-related support than are their male counterparts (Pandey, Hart, & Tiwary, 2003).

Healthcare System Navigation

The concept of patient navigation first appeared in the literature in the 1990s as a means to improve access to health care for medically underserved populations. Patient navigation moves beyond advocacy to identify barriers and challenges to healthcare access and focuses on individual well-being. It is a process in which clients are guided through the bureaucracy of the healthcare system by a nurse advocate to complete a specific diagnostic procedure or therapeutic task. Assisting underserved individuals to "navigate" the complex healthcare system reduces barriers to healthcare access and treatment. Patient navigators also mobilize appropriate resources for the client. In a U.S. study of low-income women of colour with breast abnormalities, patient navigation was shown to improve the timeliness of diagnosis, compliance with follow-up treatment (Psooy, Schreuer, Borgaonkar, & Caines, 2004), and diagnostic resolution follow-up by healthcare providers (Ell, Vourlekis, Lee, & Xie, 2007). Furthermore, patient navigation has been successful in reducing barriers to care and improving health outcomes in persons with HIV (Bradford, Coleman, & Cunningham, 2007).

Patient navigators promote self-determination in their clients as a means of empowering them. Although patient navigators are charged with helping clients obtain necessary healthcare services, clients must be afforded the respect to choose regarding their individual welfare. The role of patient navigators reveals the essential elements of nursing functions such as liaison and resource coordinator. Patient navigators also have potential utility for serving at-risk women with high incidences of powerlessness (Ell et al., 2007). All healthcare practitioners should be able to perform this role of patient navigator to a much or lesser degree, especially those caring for clients living with chronic illness.

Advocacy

In addition to patient navigation, advocacy is an important tool for increasing empowerment in clients with chronic illness. Advocacy activities seek to redistribute power and resources to people (individuals or groups) who demonstrate a need. Although the ideal of nursing advocacy is to empower clients within the healthcare system, often institutional, social, political, economic, and cultural constraints prevent clients from accessing health care. When such constraints are present, an advocate is necessary to facilitate procurement. The manner in which the nurse advocate intercedes to increase the client's power depends on the underlying values and beliefs held by the nurse regarding the advocate role. No one wants to depend on others, to inconvenience others, or to be a burden to others. Dignity and respect are linked with individual independence. The nurse must take care to ensure the client is still authoritative in his or her own life and is able to maintain responsibility and self-determination. Even when these elements are present, situations may arise in which clients need help from an advocate to regain dignity and integrity.

Decision Making

When clients make their own decisions and act on them, there may be a difference between the client's choices and those that would have been made by family members or healthcare professionals. Consequently, clients may not only experience disapproval from others regarding their decisions but also may encounter resistance when attempting to implement them. As previously discussed, Mrs. Jones made a decision to interrupt her dialysis treatments for several days to connect with her family despite protests from her primary care nurse and physician. Upon learning of Mrs. Jones's decision to discontinue treatment for a short time, the primary care nurse contacted the children of Mrs. Jones to persuade them to exert control and interrupt Mrs. Jones's plans. In the end, the sons and daughters of Mrs. Jones agreed to honour the choice and decision made by their mother. This example provides the foundation for further discussions among nurses engaged in client-empowered health care. How much control belongs to the client, the healthcare professional, or family members? How do control issues affect the nurse–client, the nurse–family, and the client–family relationships? What are the guiding principles in this approach to nursing care of clients with chronic illness?

Nurses must provide clients all information necessary to make a decision. Providing information about the illness and the services that are available will facilitate informed decisions (Aylett & Fawcett, 2003). As clients come to know the nature and meaning of their illnesses, their power tends to be restored and their vulnerability is reduced.

Anticipatory Guidance

Anxiety is triggered by an uncertain future. Uncertainty of the illness trajectory suggests the need for the nurse to offer anticipatory guidance to persons with chronic illnesses. Anticipatory guidance is based on identifying expected future needs and can begin weeks, months, or years before any actual help is required. Future needs can have a profound effect on clients' lives because major life decisions can be influenced by them. Clients need a coach to help them chart an anticipated course throughout their chronic illness (Courts et al., 2004). Anticipating future dependency needs allows clients with progressive chronic illnesses to express their own wishes and preferences for care options. Informed anticipation lacks certainty, but it facilitates greater rational future planning for clients and their families, minimizing potentially difficult decisions made during a time of crisis.

Cultural Competence

Cultural competence is a process in which the nurse integrates cultural awareness, cultural knowledge, cultural skills, cultural encounters, and cultural desire to provide care (Campinha-Bacote, 2002). This model assumes variation among persons of different ethnic and cultural groups. For example, in collectivist culture people may resonate to group norms to experience relatedness and autonomy. In individualist cultures acting in accordance with the group norm may be viewed as lack of individuality and a threat to autonomy (Ryan & Deci, 2000). It is imperative for nurses to explore potential differences and similarities among clients and their beliefs to ensure culturally competent care (Leininger & McFarland, 2002). This is of particular significance in countries such as Canada, where multiculturalism is encouraged and promoted. Leininger (1995) asserted, "clients who experience nursing care that fails to be reasonably congruent with the client's beliefs, values, and care life ways will show signs of cultural conflicts, noncompliance, stresses, and ethical or moral concerns" (p. 45). When nurses acknowledge and incorporate the client's cultural perspective, an environment of communication and understanding increases feelings of power and control in the client and family.

SUMMARY

Outcomes associated with powerlessness in clients with chronic conditions can be measured from three perspectives: self, relationships with others, and client behaviours. From the first perspective, changes in self are evaluated by measures such as increased self-confidence and self-esteem, which facilitate coping with and management of chronic illness. The best outcomes for persons with chronic illness occur when clients learn to self-manage their chronic illness. The client must monitor and make adjustments in the management of the chronic illness, just as a driver of a car turns the wheel, monitors speed, and applies the brakes while driving a car. Self-management presumes the client is given the opportunity to communicate effectively, seek information, collect data, analyze options, and make decisions. Clients need to have information and resources available to them when the need arises, as opposed to when it may be convenient for the healthcare provider to give the information to the client. Healthcare providers must recognize the limits of science for self-management of chronic illness and respect the inherent expertise and primary authority of the client in matters pertaining to living with a chronic illness. In doing so, healthcare providers become consultants and resource brokers within the context of shared care (Thorne, 2006).

The second outcome of measured change of powerlessness is relationships with others. Changes in relationships include improved relationships with family, friends, and healthcare professionals. Relationships are reciprocal in nature. That is, family, friends, and healthcare professionals must play an active role in providing social support and positive interaction with the client with chronic illness. Positive relationships have a powerful impact on the health and well-being of healthcare clients.

The last measurable outcome of reduced powerlessness is behaviour. Changes in behaviour include healthcare and goal-oriented decisions that promote personal responsibility for health (Falk-Rafael, 2001). Positive changes in behaviour can result in increased treatment-regimen adherence, better management of symptoms, and decreased feelings of powerlessness.

Evidence-Informed Practice Box

As chronic illness moves from a medical model of treatment and cure to one of self-management of illness with or without professional health care, the literature reveals a variety of strategies designed to enhance and promote patient empowerment. One such approach, face-to-face support groups, is an effective resource for information and support for persons with chronic illness. However, barriers such as geography, distance, time, and physical limitations can exclude persons with chronic conditions from participating in these support groups. As the Internet has become accessible and available to more and more people, online support groups have become a viable alternative to in-person support groups. Research suggests that persons with chronic conditions who participate in online support groups are empowered and report a sense of well-being.

Van Uden-Kraan and colleagues (2009) conducted a quantitative research project with 528 individuals who were active in online support groups for persons with breast cancer, fibromyalgia, and arthritis. Results of the online questionnaire found respondents were empowered in several ways by their participation in online support groups. The most significant empowering outcomes were "being better informed" and "enhanced social well-being" (p. 64). Participants had a better understanding of their illness from

(continues)

the personal experience of others and more information about what to expect in the future as a result of peer support. Study participants indicated that the on-line support group provided more social contacts for them and decreased their loneliness. Further, this research did not note any differences between the diagnostic groups with regard to empowering processes and outcomes. The authors concluded that empowerment is a generic mechanism among persons with chronic illness. Online patient support groups enhance empowerment in persons with chronic conditions. Healthcare providers need to become aware of online support groups as a resource for information and empowerment for their healthcare clients.

Source: van Uden-Kraan et al. (2009).

Recommendations for Further Conceptual and Data-Based Work

Chronic illness research with a focus on empowerment interventions is essential not only at the micro-level but at the macro-level. Continued development of knowledge and understanding of the experiences and needs of individuals with serious, chronic, progressive, and largely uncontrollable illnesses is essential to the development of effective strategies for greater perception of power and control. As we move away from the medical model to a sociological model of care, client and family empowerment are essential. The process of empowerment interventions at the social level would benefit clients with chronic illness, their families, and healthcare professionals.

STUDY QUESTIONS

www

1. Using the theoretical perspectives presented, design nursing interventions to reduce powerlessness in persons with chronic illness.
2. Critique the potential strengths and limitations of nursing interventions to reduce powerlessness.
3. Discuss the relationship between chronic illness and powerlessness.
4. Compare and contrast the concepts of power and powerlessness.
5. Discuss the factors that promote powerlessness in clients with chronic illness.
6. Examine the association between physiological and psychosocial factors and powerlessness.

For a full suite of assignments and additional learning activities, use **www** the access code located in the front of your book and visit this exclusive website: **http://go.jblearning.com/kramer-kile**. If you do not have an access code, you can obtain one at the site.

REFERENCES

Aday, L. (2001). *At risk in America*. San Francisco, CA: Jossey-Bass.

Ahlstrom, G. (2007). Experiences of loss and chronic sorrow in persons with severe chronic illness. *Journal of Clinical Nursing, 10*(3A), 76–83.

Asbring, P. (2001). Chronic illness: A disruption of life-identity-transformation among women with chronic fatigue syndrome and fibromyalgia. *Journal of Advanced Nursing, 34*, 312–319.

Aujoulat, I., d'Hoore, W., & Deccache, A. (2007). Patient empowerment in theory and practice: Polysemy or cacophony? *Patient Education and Counseling, 66*(1), 13–20.

Aujoulat, I., Luminet, O., & Deccache, A. (2007). The perspective of patients on their experience of powerlessness. *Qualitative Health Research, 17*, 772–785.

Aujoulat, I., Marcolongo, R., Bonadiman, L., & Deccache, A. (2008). Reconsidering patient empowerment in chronic illness: A critique of models of self-efficacy and bodily control. *Social Science & Medicine, 66*(5), 1228–1239.

Aylett, E., & Fawcett, T. N. (2003). Chronic fatigue syndrome: The nurse's role. *Nursing Standard, 17*(35), 33–37.

Bandura, A. (1989). Human agency in social cognitive theory. *American Psychologist, 44*, 1175–1184.

Barker-Collo, S., Cartwright, C., & Read, J. (2006). Into the unknown: The experiences of individuals living with multiple sclerosis. *Journal of Neuroscience Nursing, 38*(6), 435–446.

Beal, C. C. (2007). Loneliness in women with multiple sclerosis. *Rehabilitation Nursing, 32*(4), 165–171.

Bodenheimer, T., Lorig, K., Holman, H., & Grumbach, K. (2002). Patient self-management of chronic disease in primary care. *Journal of the American Medical Association, 288*(19), 2469–2475.

Bradford, J. B., Coleman, S., & Cunningham, W. (2007). HIV system navigation: An emerging model to improve HIV care access. *AIDS Patient Care and STDs, 21*, S49–S58.

Campinha-Bacote, J. (2002). The process of cultural competence in the delivery of health care services: A model of care. *Journal of Transcultural Nursing, 13*(3), 180–184.

Charmaz, K. (1983). Loss of self: A fundamental form of suffering in the chronically ill. *Sociology of Health & Illness, 83*(2), 168–195.

Clarke, J. N., & James, S. (2003). The radicalized self: The impact on the self of the contested nature of the diagnosis of chronic fatigue syndrome. *Social Science and Medicine, 57*(8), 1387–1395.

Cooper, J. M., Collier, J., James, V., & Hawkey, C. J. (2010). Beliefs about personal control and self-management in 30–40 year olds living with inflammatory bowel disease: A qualitative study. *International Journal of Nursing Studies, 47*, 1500–1509.

Corbin, J. M., & Cherry, J. C. (2001). Epilogue: A proactive model of health care. In R. B. Hyman & J. M. Corbin (Eds.), *Chronic illness research and theory for nursing practice* (pp. 294–299). New York, NY: Springer.

Courts, J. F., Buchanan, E. M., & Werstlein, P. O. (2004). Focus groups: The lived experience of participants with multiple sclerosis. *Journal of Neuroscience Nursing, 36*(1), 42–47.

Crossley, M. (2001). The "Armistead" project: An exploration of gay men, sexual practices, community health promotion and issues of empowerment. *Journal of Community and Applied Social Psychology, 11*, 111–123.

Cvengros, J. A., Christensen, A. J., & Lawton, W. J. (2005). Health locus of control and depression in chronic kidney disease: A dynamic perspective. *Journal of Health Psychology, 10*(5), 677–686.

Davis, A. J., Konishi, E., & Tashiro, M. (2003). A pilot study of selected Japanese nurses' ideas on patient advocacy. *Nursing Ethics, 10*(4), 404–413.

Deci, E. L., & Ryan, R. M. (1985). *Intrinsic motivation and self-determination in human behavior.* New York, NY: Plenum.

Deci, E. L., & Ryan, R. M. (1991). A motivational approach to self: Integration in personality. In R. Dienstbier (Ed.), *Nebraska symposium on motivation: Perspectives on motivation, 38* (pp. 237–288). Lincoln, NE: University of Nebraska Press.

Deci, E. L., & Ryan, R. M. (2000). The "what" and "why" of goal pursuits: Human needs and the self-determination of behavior. *Psychological Inquiry, 11*(4), 227–268.

Delmar, C., Bøje, T., Dylmer, D., Forup, L., Jakobsen, C., Møller, M., Sonder, H., & Pedersen, B. D. (2006). Independence/dependence—a contradictory relationship? Life with a chronic illness. *Scandinavian Journal of Caring Sciences, 20*(3), 261–268.

Efraimsson, E., Rasmussen, B. H., Gilje, F., & Sandman, P. (2003). Expressions of power and powerlessness in discharge planning: A case study of an older woman on her way home. *Journal of Clinical Nursing, 12*, 707–716.

Ell, K., Vourlekis, B., Lee, P. J., & Xie, B. (2007). Patient navigation and case management following an abnormal mammogram: A randomized clinical trial. *Preventive Medicine, 44*, 26–33.

Falk, S., Wahn, A. K., & Lidell, E. (2007). Keeping the maintenance of daily life in spite of chronic heart failure. A qualitative study. *European Journal of Cardiovascular Nursing, 6*, 192–199.

Falk-Rafael, A. (2001). Empowerment as a process of evolving consciousness: A model of empowered caring. *Advances in Nursing Science, 24*(1), 1–16.

Freeman, K., O'Dell, C., & Meola, C. (2003). Childhood brain tumors: Children's and siblings' concerns regarding the diagnosis and phase of illness. *Journal of Pediatric Oncology Nursing, 20*(3), 133–140.

Gibson, J. M. E., & Kenrick, M. (1998). Pain and powerlessness: The experience of living with peripheral vascular disease. *Journal of Advanced Nursing, 27*(4), 737–745.

Glaser, B. G., & Strauss, A. L. (1968). *Time for dying.* Chicago, IL: Aldine.

Goffman, E. (1963). *Notes on management of spoiled identity.* Englewood Cliffs, NJ: Prentice Hall.

Granger, B. B., Moser, D., Germino, B., Harrell, J., & Ekman, I. (2006). Caring for patients with chronic heart failure: The trajectory model. *European Journal of Cardiovascular Nursing, 5*, 222–227.

Hägglund, D., & Ahlström, G. (2007). The meaning of women's experience of living with long-term urinary incontinence is powerlessness. *Journal of Clinical Nursing, 16*(10), 1946–1954.

Haluska, H. B., Jessee, P. O., & Nagy, M. C. (2002). Sources of social support: Adolescents with cancer. *Oncology Nursing Forum, 29*, 1317–1324.

Hansson, L., & Bjorkman, T. (2005). Empowerment in people with a mental illness: Reliability and validity of the Swedish version of an empowerment scale. *Scandinavian Journal of Caring Sciences, 19,* 32–38.

Hay, M. C. (2010). Suffering in a productive world: Chronic illness, visibility, and the space beyond agency. *American Ethnologist, 37*(2), 259–274.

Hewitt, J. (2002). A critical review of the arguments debating the role of the nurse advocate. *Journal of Advanced Nursing, 37*(5), 439–445.

Huffman, M. (2007). Health coaching: A new and exciting technique to enhance patient self-management and improve outcomes. *Home Healthcare Nurse, 25*(4), 271–275.

Igreja, I., Zuroff, D. C., Koestner, R., Saltaris, C., Bropuillette, M. J., & LaLonde, R. (2000). Applying self-determination to the prediction and well-being in gay men with HIV and AIDS. *Journal of Applied Psychology, 30*(4), 686–706.

Institute of Medicine. (2001). *Crossing the quality chasm. A new health system for the 21st century.* Washington, DC: National Academies Press.

Jacelon, C. S. (2007). Theoretical perspectives of perceived control in older adults: A selective review of the literature. *Journal of Advanced Nursing, 59*(1), 1–10.

Johnson, D. (1967). Powerlessness: A significant determinant in patient behavior? *Journal of Nursing Education, 6*(2), 39–44.

Kuokkanen, L., & Leino-Kilpi, H. (2000). Power and empowerment in nursing: Three theoretical approaches. *Journal of Advanced Nursing, 31*(1), 235–241.

Laschinger, H. K. S., Gilbert, S., Smith, L. M., & Leslie, K. (2010). Towards a comprehensive theory of nurse/patient empowerment: Applying Kanter's empowerment theory to patient care. *Journal of Nursing Management, 18*, 4–13.

Leininger, M. L. (1995). *Transcultural nursing: Concepts, theories, research and practice.* Columbus, OH: McGraw-Hill College Custom Series.

Leininger, M. L., & McFarland, M. R. (2002). *Transcultural nursing: Concepts, theories, research and practices* (2nd ed.). New York, NY: McGraw-Hill.

Loft, M., McWilliam, C., & Ward-Griffin, C. (2003). Patient empowerment after total hip and knee replacement. *Orthopedic Nursing, 22*(1), 42–47.

Mattsson, M., Moller, B., Stamm, T., Gard, G., & Bostrom, C. (2011). Uncertainty and opportunities in patients with established systemic lupus erythematosus: A qualitative study. *Musculoskeletal Care, 10*(1), 1–12.

McCann, T., & Clark, E. (2004). Advancing self-determination with young adults who have schizophrenia. *Journal of Psychiatric and Mental Health Nursing, 11*, 12–20.

McCubbin, M. (2001). Pathways to health, illness and well-being: From the perspective of power and control. *Journal of Community and Applied Social Psychology, 11*, 75–81.

Merriam-Webster. (2011). Power. Retrieved from http ://www.merriam-webster.com/dictionary/power

Miller, J. F. (Ed.). (1983). *Coping with chronic illness: Overcoming powerlessness.* Philadelphia, PA: F. A. Davis.

Miller, J. F. (Ed.). (1992). *Coping with chronic illness: Overcoming powerlessness* (2nd ed.). Philadelphia, PA: F. A. Davis.

Miller, J. F. (Ed). (2000). *Coping with chronic illness: Overcoming powerlessness* (3rd ed.). Philadelphia, PA: F. A. Davis.

Mishel, M. H. (1999). Uncertainty in illness. *Annual Review of Nursing Research, 19*, 269–294.

Mitchell, G. J., & Bournes, D. A. (2000). Nurse as patient advocate? In search of straight thinking. *Nursing Science Quarterly, 13*(3), 204–209.

Moden, L. (2004). Power in care homes. *Nursing Older People, 16*(6), 24–26.

Mok, E., Martinson, I., & Wong, T. K. (2004). Individual empowerment among Chinese cancer patients in Hong Kong. *Western Journal of Nursing Research, 26*(1), 59–75.

Moller, A. C., Deci, E. L., & Ryan, R. M. (2006). Choice and ego-depletion: The moderating role of autonomy. *Personality and Social Psychology Bulletin, 32*(8), 1024–1036.

Mullins, L., Chaney, J., Balderson, B., & Hommel, K., (2000). The relationship of illness uncertainty, illness intrusiveness and asthma severity to depression in young adults with long-standing asthma. *International Journal of Rehabilitation and Health, 5*, 177–186.

Nagelkerk, J., Reick, K., & Meengs, L. (2006). Perceived barriers and effective strategies to diabetes self-management. *Journal of Advanced Nursing, 54*(2), 151–158.

Nelson, G., Lord, J., & Ochocka, J. (2001). Empowerment and mental health in community: Narratives of psychiatric consumer/survivors. *Journal of Community and Applied Social Psychology, 11*, 125–142.

Newman, S., Steed, L., & Mulligan, K. (2004). Self-management interventions for chronic illness. *Lancet, 364*(9444), 1523–1537.

Niven, C. A., & Scott, P. A. (2003). The need for accurate perception and informed judgment in determining the appropriate use of the nursing resource: Hearing the patient's voice. *Nursing Philosophy, 4*, 201–210.

Pandey, S. K., Hart, J. J., & Tiwary, S. (2003). Women's health and Internet: Understanding emerging trends and implications. *Social Science and Medicine, 56*, 179–191.

Paterson, B. L. (2001a). The shifting perspectives model of chronic illness. *Journal of Nursing Scholarship, 33*, 21–26.

Paterson, B. L. (2001b). Myth of empowerment in chronic illness. *Journal of Advanced Nursing, 34*(5), 574–581.

Paterson, B. L. (2003). The koala has claws: Applications of the shifting perspectives model in research of chronic illness. *Qualitative Health Research, 13*(7), 987–994.

Pihl-Lesnovska, K., Hjortswang, H., Ek, A. C., & Frisman, G. H. (2010). Patients' perspective of factors: Influencing quality of life while living with Crohn's disease. *Gastroenterology Nursing, 33*(1), 37–44.

Psooy, B. J., Schreuer, D., Borgaonkar, J., & Caines, J. S. (2004). Patient navigation: Improving timeliness in the diagnosis of breast abnormalities. *Canadian Association of Radiologists Journal, 55*(3), 145–150.

Rånhein, M., & Holand, W. (2006). Lived experience of chronic pain and fibromyalgia: Women's stories from daily life. *Qualitative Health Research, 16*(6), 741–761.

Roth, D., & Crane-Ross, D. (2002). Impact of services, met needs and service empowerment on consumer outcomes. *Mental Health & Mental Health Services Research, 4*, 43–56.

Rotter, J. P. (1966). Generalized expectancies for internal versus external control of reinforcement. *Psychological Monographs, 80*, 1–28.

Ryan, R. M., & Deci, E. L. (2000). Self-determination theory and the facilitation of intrinsic motivation, social development, and well-being. *American Psychologist, 55*(1), 68–78.

Salas-Provance, M., Erickson, J. G., & Reed, J. (2002). Disability as viewed by four generations on one Hispanic family. *American Journal of Speech-Language Pathology, 11*, 151–162.

Sheridan-Gonzalez, J. (2000). It's not my patient. *American Journal of Nursing, 100*(1), 13.

Singleton, J. K. (2002). Caring for themselves: Facilitators and barriers to women home care workers who are chronically ill following their care plan. *Health Care for Women International, 23*, 692–702.

Skuladöttir, H., & Halldorsdöttir, S. (2008). Women in chronic pain: Sense of control and encounters with health professionals. *Qualitative Health Research, 18*, 891–901.

Skuladöttir, H., & Halldorsdöttir, W. (2011). The quest for well-being: Self-identified needs of women in chronic pain. *Scandinavian Journal of Caring Science, 25*(1), 81–91.

Sommerset, M., Campbell, R., Sharp, D. J., & Peters, T. J. (2001). What do people with MS want and expect from health care services? *Health Expectations, 4*, 29–37.

Strandmark, M. K. (2004). Ill health is powerlessness: A phenomenological study about worthlessness, limitations and suffering. *Scandinavian Journal of Caring Science, 18*, 135–144.

Sullivan, T., Weinert, C., & Cudney, S. (2003). Management of chronic illness: Voices of rural women. *Journal of Advanced Nursing, 44*(6), 566–574.

Sullivan-Bolyai, S., Sadler, L., Knafl, K. A., & Gillis, C. L. (2003). Great expectations: A position description for parents as caregivers: Part 1. *Pediatric Nursing, 29*(6), 457–461.

Sutton, R., & Treloar, C. (2007). Chronic illness experiences, clinical markers and living with Hepatitis C. *Journal of Health Psychology, 12*(2), 330–340.

Tang, S. T., & Lee, S. C. (2004). Cancer diagnosis and prognosis in Taiwan: Patient preferences versus experiences. *Psycho-Oncology, 13*, 1–13.

Taylor, S. E. (1983). Adjustment to threatening events: A theory of cognitive adaptation. *American Psychologist, 38*, 1161–1173.

Thorne, S. (2006). Patient-provider communication in chronic illness: A health promotion window of opportunity. *Family and Community Health, 29*(1S), 4S–11S.

Thorne, S., Paterson, B., & Russell, C. (2003). The structure of everyday self-care decision making in chronic illness. *Qualitative Health Research, 13*(10), 1337–1352.

Van Uden-Kraan, C. F., Drossaert, C. H. C., Taal, E., Seydel, D. R., & van de Laar, M. A. F. J. (2009). Participation in online patient support groups endorses patients' empowerment. *Patient Education and Counseling, 74*, 61–69.

Walker, C. (2010). Ruptured identities: Leaving work because of chronic illness. *International Journal of Health Services, 40*(4), 629–643.

Wollin, J., Dale, H., Spenser, N., & Walsh, A. (2000). What people with newly diagnosed MS (and their families and friends) need to know. *International Journal of MS Care, 2*, 4–14.

World Health Organization. (2003). *Adherence to long-term therapies: Evidence for action.* Retrieved from http://www.who.int/chp/knowledge/publications/adherence_report/en/

Yu, D. S. F., Lee, D. T. F., Kwong, A. N. T., Thompson, D. R., & Woo, J. (2008). Living with chronic heart failure: A review of qualitative studies of older people. *Journal of Advanced Nursing, 61*(5), 474–483.

Zickmund, S., Ho, E., Masuda, M., Ippolito, L., & LaBrecque, D. (2003). "They treated me like a leper": Stigmatization and the quality of life of patients with hepatitis C. *Journal of General Internal Medicine, 18*, 835–844.

Zoucha, R., & Husted, G. L. (2000). The ethical dimensions of delivering culturally congruent nursing and health care. *Issues in Mental Health Nursing, 21*, 325–340.

CHAPTER 12

Self-Care and Self-Management

Original chapter by Judith E. Hertz
Canadian content added by Marnie L. Kramer-Kile

INTRODUCTION

On the surface self-care is simply taking care of one's self to remain healthy. However, self-care within the context of living with a chronic illness is more complex. Self-care is required for successful management and control of chronic illnesses such as arthritis (McDonald-Miszczak & Wister, 2005; Yip, Sit, & Wong, 2004), heart disease (Burnette, Mui, & Zodikoff, 2004; Chriss, Sheposh, Carlson, & Riegel, 2004; Inglis et al., 2006; Washburn, Hornberger, Klutman, & Skinner, 2005), diabetes (Berg & Wadhwa, 2007), HIV/AIDS (Mendias & Paar, 2007), asthma (Cortes, Lee, Boal, Mion, & Butler, 2004), and fecal incontinence (Bliss, Fischer, & Savik, 2005).

Self-care is also viewed as a pivotal concept in health promotion, disease prevention, and disease-screening programmes (Haber, 2002; Potempa, Butterworth, Flaherty-Robb, & Gaynor, 2010; Resnick, 2001, 2003). Furthermore, self-care has been viewed as essential to health in persons with chronic illnesses who receive care in nursing homes (Bickerstaff, Grasser, & McCabe, 2003), home care (Sharkey, Ory, & Browne, 2005), and rehabilitation (Singleton, 2000) and

during transitions from one healthcare setting to another (Coleman et al., 2004). Finally, self-care is applicable globally and transculturally when discussing health status in persons with chronic illnesses (Borg, Hallberg, & Blomqvist, 2006; Cortes et al., 2004; Inglis et al., 2006; Leenerts, Teel, & Pendleton, 2002; McDonald-Miszczak & Wister, 2005; Wang, Hsu, & Want, 2001; Yip et al., 2004).

Despite the widespread belief that self-care is integral to persons living with chronic illness, there is little agreement about the meaning of self-care. Sometimes self-care is defined as adherence/compliance with treatment regimens (Chriss et al., 2004), whereas other times it is referred to as having the functional ability to carry out activities of daily living (ADLs) and instrumental activities of daily living (IADLs) (Burnette et al., 2004). Other definitions imply that self-care is the belief that one can implement disease-treatment regimens (i.e., self-efficacy) (McDonald-Miszczak & Wister, 2005; Yip et al., 2004) or that one can manage and report symptoms associated with an illness (Chriss et al., 2004; Edwardson & Dean, 1999; Musil, Morris, Haug, Warner, & Whelan, 2001). The ability to meet basic holistic human needs and achieve self-actualization provides yet another perspective (Hertz & Rossetti, 2006; Mendias & Paar, 2007; Potempa et al., 2010). The meaning of self-care becomes even more complex, because often it is equated solely to independent behaviours to care for self (Borg et al., 2006; Burnette et al., 2004); therefore, if one depends on others for assistance, as often happens when living with chronic illnesses, then it is implied that self-care cannot exist. However, Naik and colleagues recognized this situation in their analyses and recommendations for assessing two aspects of autonomy related to self-care: decisional and executive autonomy (Naik, Dyer, Kunik, & McCullough, 2009a, 2009b; Naik, Teal, Pavlik, Dyer, & McCullough, 2008). Decisional autonomy centres on the ability of the client to deliberate and make treatment decisions while executive autonomy refers to the capacity of the client to execute the treatment plan. Furthermore, Naik et al. (2009) argue that healthcare practitioners should assess both of these areas of autonomy when completing clinical assessments and working with the client toward achieving self-care of their chronic condition.

Even with lack of agreement about the definition of self-care, there is implicit and explicit agreement that self-care is vital to individual health maintenance, disease prevention, and health promotion. When persons are living with chronic illnesses, the importance and need to care for self is further underscored.

KEY ISSUES AND FRAMEWORKS FOR VIEWING SELF-CARE WITHIN CHRONIC ILLNESS _____

The focus of this section is to compare and contrast the many definitions of self-care (or lack of self-care) with evidence to support each view,

followed by a working definition of self-care. The framework and key issues set the stage for application of the nursing process by highlighting important considerations for nurses to address when promoting self-care in clients.

Perspectives on Self-Care

Diverse perspectives of self-care are provided via research on self-care in various populations living with chronic illnesses. Self-care means (1) to comply or adhere to prescribed medical treatments for chronic illnesses, (2) to have a personal belief that one is capable of following disease treatment regimens, (3) to have the functional abilities to carry out ADLs and IADLs independently, and (4) to self-determine how to meet one's unique, personal basic human and self-actualization needs. Still others have addressed self-care as being multidimensional. Each perspective is discussed.

Self-Care as Adherence to Medical Treatments

Haber's (2002) critical analysis of federal initiatives regarding health promotion and aging emphasized physical aspects and a medical orientation toward self-care and health promotion. Self-care is implied as adherence to recommended secondary prevention interventions through disease risk reduction (e.g., smoking cessation) and screening practices (e.g., mammograms).

Edwardson and Dean (1999) explored how selected demographic, social, situational, and symptom-experience factors influence the "appropriateness" of self-care responses to symptoms. In other words, the way persons manage symptoms is influenced by many factors. In this study self-care was equated to medical management of symptoms. Healthcare professionals (HCPs) judged clients' responses to symptoms as either "appropriate" or "inappropriate" using an evidence-informed algorithm. If persons did not seek professional care, used "unsafe" remedies, or did not follow guidelines from professionals, their response was considered "inappropriate."

Sharkey and coworkers (2005) studied homebound older persons receiving meal delivery in North Carolina to identify the extent to which older persons use strategies to reduce out-of-pocket medication expenses when self-managing their medications. From this perspective lack of self-care was assumed to include noncompliance with medical treatment regimens. Twenty percent admitted to using one or more of the following behaviours to restrict medication use and costs: (1) taking less medicine than the prescribed amount, (2) going without the medication because of cost, (3) getting free drug samples from physicians, (4) obtaining a partial refill of a prescription, (5) taking the drug only when "needed," or (6) buying only the most important medications. Although these results seem to be "anti–self-management" or "anti–self-care," they highlight the need to address the concerns and perceptions of patients when trying to promote self-care. Sometimes caring for one's self conflicts with recommended treatment regimens.

In reviewing the literature regarding health outcomes in persons living with chronic illnesses (diabetes, chronic obstructive pulmonary disease, or chronic heart disease), self-care was equated to self-management of the person's disease state as well as adherence to medical treatment (Scollan-Koliopoulos & Walker, 2009; Sutherland & Hayter, 2009). The purposes of these reviews differed. Scollan-Koliopoulos and Walker examined studies on the effects of previous exposure to diabetes in family members on

self-care, referred to as a multigenerational timeline. Sutherland and Hayter's review was focused on self-care as an outcome of nurse-managed care. Nonetheless, both review teams limited their perspective on self-care to self-management of a disease process according to recommended medical treatments.

Others differentiate self-care from self-management (Ryan & Sawin, 2009). Self-care was linked primarily to carrying out ADLs without the advice of HCPs. Barlow, Sturt, and Hearnshaw (2002) also identified tasks performed by healthy people at home, including preventative strategies, as self-care. Self-management was viewed as daily tasks carried out at home by individuals to control or reduce the impact of disease on physical health. According to Ryan and Sawin these behaviours must be learned and require assistance from health providers. After reviewing the literature on self-management programmes for arthritis, asthma, and diabetes, Barlow and colleagues made recommendations for development of programmes to promote self-management of other chronic health conditions.

In summary, self-care has been linked to compliance with recommended medical treatment. However, sometimes self-initiated behaviours may be in conflict with those recommendations. Learning to live with chronic illness most certainly involves following medical recommendations to reduce exacerbations. However, in some situations self-care is not the same as self-management of an illness or compliance with medical recommendations.

Self-Care as Belief in Ability to Self-Manage

Typical disease self-management programmes for arthritis, chronic heart disease, HIV/AIDS, diabetes mellitus, and asthma focus on monitoring and reporting symptoms as well as monitoring adherence to medical regimens. Research on self-management programmes often attempts to identify how self-efficacy beliefs (i.e., belief that one is capable of self-managing one's treatment regimen); other psychological characteristics such as locus of control, perceived threat, or a sense of well-being; and situational variables such as demographics, living arrangements, and overall health influence the ability to self-manage a health condition. Outcomes from these studies often look at symptom relief, functional ability status, changes in self-efficacy beliefs, and laboratory values indicative of "disease control."

An arthritis self-management programme with older persons in Hong Kong introduced Tai Chi as a self-management technique. In this study self-efficacy was greater, pain decreased, and motor strength increased in the intervention group (Yip et al., 2004) when compared with the control group receiving "usual care." Self-efficacy beliefs were linked to self-care approaches in disease self-management and to positive health outcomes.

A longitudinal study (McDonald-Miszczak & Wister, 2005) with a national Canadian sample also linked self-efficacy to the 11 arthritis self-management "self-care" behaviours of diet, exercise, sleep, self-help group participation, use of alternative remedies, modifications of environment, reading, stress reduction, meditation/prayer, consulting family/friends, and consulting others with the same condition. Self-efficacy beliefs did not predict the use of these 11 behaviours to manage arthritis. However, previous use of these behaviours (i.e., past experience) was a strong predictor of these prescribed self-care behaviours and supplemented self-efficacy beliefs.

Similarly, at the end of 3 months, previous use of self-care behaviours was a significant predictor of self-care in monitoring symptoms, following medical guidelines, reporting symptoms, and seeking help in a self-management programme designed for persons with heart failure in a study conducted in the southwestern United States (Chriss et al., 2004). Other characteristics such as social support, education, gender, age, income, comorbidities, and symptom severity were not predictive of this type of self-care.

A descriptive correlational study was conducted with persons living with heart failure (Britz & Dunn, 2010). The relationship between self-care abilities (maintenance, management, and confidence) and multiple dimensions of quality of life was explored. Self-care confidence, similar to the concept of self-efficacy, was significantly related to physical, emotional, and overall quality of life.

These studies illustrate that previous lifestyle and experiences are predictive of how persons will manage chronic illnesses in terms of adhering to prescribed behaviours. Although some personal demographic characteristics, emotional state, and personal beliefs about being able to take control and manage a disease on a daily basis had some effect on following the prescribed behaviours, the strongest predictor was previous experience in using the behaviours. Life experiences and personal values may be very important in determining each individual's self-care behaviours.

Self-Care as Functional Abilities and Independence

Burnette and colleagues (2004) used functional abilities as an indicator of self-care in their study with a national sample of 597 persons diagnosed with coronary heart disease compared with those without coronary heart disease. These researchers proposed that most of the everyday work of managing coronary heart disease relied on self-care as opposed to professional care. They defined self-care as the active role persons play in determining outcomes resulting from professional care. The coping strategies of behavioural change, environmental adaptations, and medical equipment use represented self-care strategies in their study. These strategies were also linked to functional abilities related to ADLs, IADLs, and mobility. Impaired functional abilities indicated a lack of self-care.

Borg and colleagues (2006) proposed that "older persons who are not able to manage daily life by themselves may have a different view of life satisfaction than those with preserved self-care capacity" (p. 608). Self-care capacity was defined as having functional abilities to carry out activities independently. This study's findings imply that functional limitations are linked to self-care and that those limitations, more so than the presence of a chronic illness, can affect holistic health outcomes. Persons with functional limitations might need special assistance

and attention to support their self-care practices to promote health.

Self-neglect is the inability to meet basic needs and is viewed as the opposite of self-care (Dyer, Goodwin, Pickens-Pace, Burnett, & Kelly, 2007). In older clients receiving adult protective services in the United States, the prevalence of self-neglect is 50.3% nationally (Dyer et al., 2007, p. 1671). Dyer and colleagues developed a case definition of self-neglect based on characteristics of 538 cases. The mean age of these clients was 75.6 years, and 70% were women. Executive dysfunction, or the inability to execute specific complex tasks such as ADLs and IADLs independently, was at the root of self-neglect. Executive dysfunction was also associated with several chronic illnesses, including dementia, depression, diabetes, psychiatric illness, cardiovascular disease, and nutritional deficiency. Self-neglect—seemingly the converse of the definition of self-care—links self-care to the functional ability of acting independently.

CASE STUDY

You are employed in an ambulatory healthcare clinic in a rural healthcare system. One of your clients is Mrs. Smith, an 82-year-old widow who lives alone in a mobile home. Mrs. Smith was diagnosed with osteoarthritis more than 10 years ago and recently was diagnosed as being in the early stages of congestive heart failure. Mrs. Smith's 55-year-old daughter and family live 50 miles from her home, and her 45-year-old son lives with his wife and four teenage children 10 miles away. Mrs. Smith recently fell on the steps leading into her home. She was transported by ambulance to the closest emergency department located within the healthcare system at which you are employed, about 40 miles from Mrs. Smith's home. Luckily, Mrs. Smith did not fracture any bones when she fell. She was discharged but is now unable to drive a car and must use a walker because of severe leg pain. She has been taking five medications for her arthritis and heart condition, but her current pain is unrelieved. She has an appointment at your clinic 2 days after her discharge from the emergency department.

(continues)

CASE STUDY   (Continued)   www

Discussion Questions

1. How do you begin your assessment of Mrs. Smith? Why?
2. Identify at least one self-care goal related to each of Mrs. Smith's diagnosed chronic illnesses.
3. What intervention strategies should be used to help Mrs. Smith achieve each self-care goal? Why did you choose these strategies?
4. List at least three self-care outcomes related to the identified self-care intervention strategies.

Self-Care as Self-Determined Behaviours That Meet the Individual's Unique Needs

Singleton (2000) traced the history of self-care from Florence Nightingale to the present in an eloquent analysis of self-care. The analysis provided a framework for her study on how nurses encourage rehabilitation clients to care for themselves. She emphasized that self-care should be defined by how clients actually care for themselves and that greater understanding is needed regarding the methods used by nurses to encourage clients to care for themselves in ways that meet their unique needs.

In a nurse-led, home-based multidisciplinary intervention with older persons after hospitalization for heart failure in South Australia, Inglis and colleagues (2006) incorporated unique self-determined behaviours in their definition of self-care. Although interventions were aimed at promoting adherence to medical treatments as a means of promoting self-care, the researchers also included special interventions to empower older persons to facilitate their self-determination. Thus, self-determination of self-care was emphasized.

The self-care practices of older persons with faecal incontinence who were enrolled in one health maintenance organization were investigated by Bliss and colleagues (2005). On average, these persons reported 2.3 chronic conditions (range, 0–10) and 1.9 specific self-care practices (range, 0–7). Self-care activities included diet modifications, use of panty liners, reduction in activities, and use of medications to stop diarrhea. Only 43% reported discussing this problem and their self-care practices with their HCPs. Only the self-care practice of diet changes was routinely discussed with providers. This emphasizes that sometimes the self-care carried out by persons with chronic illnesses truly is unique to meet personal needs and that often these self-care practices are not discussed with HCPs.

In a 27-month longitudinal study with 387 randomly selected older community-dwelling adults (Musil et al., 2001), arthritis and cardiopulmonary symptoms were assessed for consistent recurrence and their effects on well-being and symptom management with self-care. Self-care was defined as the use of home remedies, over-the-counter medications, or changes in lifestyle but did not include deciding when to seek professional help. There were differences in the use of self-care for persons with each diagnosis. Persons with arthritis and chronic pain complaints across time used self-care, whereas those with cardiopulmonary symptoms did not. It was concluded that patterns differ by the type of symptom and illness and that managing chronic illness is a complex phenomenon.

Essential dimensions of self-care and an integrated model were proposed after reviewing research on self-care conducted in Sweden and Finland (Leenerts et al., 2002). In the model it was emphasized that self-care activities were related to the individual person's unique view of health and the individual's self-concept. The authors recommended that nurses incorporate the client's personal beliefs about health into their teaching about self-care activities and partner with clients to support meeting their personal needs. They also identified evidence-informed outcomes of health promotion in aging individuals as connectedness to others, resource use, transcendence, and well-being. Self-care activities or skills were classified as communication, healthy lifestyle, building meaning in life, and socializing. They added that self-care takes place within the context of internal and external human environments.

In another study Bickerstaff and colleagues (2003) identified activities that help nursing home residents transcend difficulties and live with contentment and satisfaction. In this study self-care meant activities that promoted holistic health. The 95 respondents, with an average age of 82.2 years, had lived in the nursing home from 3 to 177 months (mean, 35.6 months) and reported a variety of self-care activities: (1) generative activities through helping or reaching out to others and involving family; (2) introjective activities such as hobbies, travel, and life-long learning; (3) temporal integration activities that were past-, present-, and future-based behaviours; (4) body-transcendence activities that incorporated flexibility and making changes in

life; and (5) spiritual activities to develop relationships with self, others, and a higher being. These self-care activities encompassed more than a physical orientation to health and well-being and were based on the individual's perception of needs.

Likewise, Wang and colleagues (2001) used focus groups to explore the perceptions of health-promoting self-care in community-dwelling Taiwanese older adults. All but 4 of the 21 men and women participants were living with some type of chronic illness. The investigators identified five types of self-care activities used by these older adults in caring for themselves: (1) balancing or adjusting one's health, (2) initiating or purposefully using self-care activities, (3) regularizing or maintaining a daily rhythm over time, (4) socializing or involving and connecting with society, and (5) sublimating or seeing the positive side and transcending their situations. They concluded that older adults in Taiwan viewed health and self-care activities as mind–body connections with holistic harmony rather than merely as physical health.

Maddox (1999) conducted a 3-year qualitative study of older women in three different age groups to identify their self-care activities and the meaning they assigned to health. The groups comprised (1) twelve nuns ages 72 to 104, (2) eight 55- to 76-year-old women who lived in single-family dwellings and worked in blue-collar occupations, and (3) five 55- to 86-year-old residents of an urban retirement community who were previously employed as domestic help or worked on farms or in factories. Their reported self-care activities included (1) interactions with a being greater than one's self, (2) acceptance of self, (3) humour, (4) flexibility, and (5) quality of being other-centred. These self-care activities incorporated more than the traditional physical self-care activities of nutrition, exercise, and relaxation to include holistic, spiritual, social, and emotional behaviours.

Hertz and Rossetti (2006) also found that self-care actions or activities were unique for older persons with chronic illness who lived independently in apartments. Common themes and patterns were identified from the activities reported by the 14 male and female respondents. These themes represent the following types of self-care activities: (1) adapting to life as an older adult by using coping strategies, assistive devices, and avoiding hassles; (2) meeting needs for affiliated individuation by balancing activities that meet needs for independence and time alone with those that meet needs for dependence and socialization; (3) using self-care knowledge to promote and strive for holistic health by using personal beliefs and values to promote quality of life and self-actualization; (4) self-managing health problems through seeking medical and alternative treatments and by sometimes avoiding medical intervention or treatment; and (5) preventing health problems and issues by following recommendations for screenings and health promotion and by taking safety precautions. The diversity of these individually determined self-care activities also reflect the multidimensionality of self-care.

Self-Care as a Multidimensional Concept

Beattie, Whitelaw, Mettler, and Turner (2003) proposed a model that used community-based organizations such as area agencies on aging, faith-based organizations, and public health departments to promote health. The dimensions of self-care were implied to include reducing risks to illnesses, managing illnesses, and coping with functional limits.

Lubben and Damron-Rodriguez (2003) analyzed the World Health Organization's Kobe Centre model for organizing health care at the community level for the older adult population. Within this model self-care was differentiated from professional care (i.e., disease management) and social network care. The authors viewed self-care as multiple activities that prolonged active life and prevented functional declines. Recommendations were made initially to foster the individual's self-care capacity by encouraging productive roles and self-direction, followed by building social network support that accommodates the diverse needs of older adults, and finally engaging community professional services for health care of older adults. Enhancing home and community environments is important because those environments are the contexts in which persons live.

Summary and Working Definition of Self-Care

In summary, there are diverse perspectives about what self-care means, and evidence exists to support each perspective. Therefore, the working definition of self-care for this chapter incorporates these diverse perspectives.

Self-care has multiple dimensions, is self-determined, and is unique to each individual based on that person's life experiences, values, beliefs, and personal characteristics and abilities, including biopsychosocial-spiritual and functional abilities. Self-care influences each individual's holistic health. Self-care includes a variety of activities such as following prescribed medical treatments and lifestyle recommendations for chronic illnesses (e.g., take medications, monitor and report symptoms, smoking cessation, diet modifications), carrying out daily activities including ADLs, IADLs, and mobility (e.g., hygiene, dressing, toileting), adhering to recommended guidelines for disease prevention and health promotion (regular screenings, dietary guidelines, exercise), meeting basic needs (e.g., food, shelter, safety, socializing, individuation), and pursuing personal interests that promote spiritual well-being and self-actualization (e.g., meditation, prayer, hobbies, learning).

Self-care includes performing activities both independently and dependently. Furthermore, self-care can be supported and nurtured by nurses and other HCPs. The following framework provides guidelines for promoting self-care in persons living with chronic illnesses.

Self-Care: A Framework for Assessment and Intervention

In nursing, Orem's (2001) theory and perspective on self-care is frequently cited. The original focus of this theory was on patients' self-care deficits or the inability to carry out self-care tasks required for physical health. Conversely, self-care agency is the capability to care for one's self and emphasizes physical abilities. It is implied that HCPs, including nurses, define for clients what self-care is needed and then carry out those activities for the client if the client lacks the capability to do so. Within this definition there is logical incongruence. If self-care is caring for one's self, then it makes sense that the client, rather than the nurse or other HCP, should be the expert regarding what is needed. Therefore, a theory that is more congruent with the working definition of self-care is presented.

The self-care model (Hertz & Baas, 2006) from modelling and role-modelling (MRM) nursing theory (Erickson, 2006; Erickson, Tomlin, & Swain, 1988) provides a more congruent framework for addressing assessment, interventions, and outcome evaluations of self-care in persons living with chronic illnesses.

This perspective takes into account the unique, self-determined, multidimensional nature of self-care based on individual biology, values, and life experiences. It also recognizes that self-care is possible when persons are living with chronic illnesses and when they might depend on others for assistance. Finally, the overriding framework of MRM theory provides a focus for interventions that are self-care supportive via the five aims of intervention.

Figure 12-1 illustrates the MRM self-care model. In this model self-care has three components: self-care knowledge, self-care resources, and self-care actions. Self-care knowledge is the individual's personal knowledge regarding his or her personal needs and goals. Those personal needs can include basic and higher level human needs as described by Maslow (1962) and others (see Erickson et al., 1988; Erickson, 2006) as well as the need for affiliated individuation. This concept is unique to MRM theory and represents one's need for separateness and independence from others as well as the need for connectedness and reliance on others. Self-care knowledge also incorporates knowledge, either at a conscious or subconscious level, regarding what may have caused a health problem/issue and what will help resolve that issue. This personal knowledge includes perceptions of availability of resources and stressors in the individual's life. Self-care knowledge is the foundation for each individual's unique "model" or view of one's own world or life situation. Self-care knowledge is interrelated to self-care resources.

Self-care resources are internal and external to the individual. Internal resources include genetic makeup; physical, mental, and cognitive functioning; and psychosocial and spiritual characteristics and traits developed over the person's lifetime and as a result of need satisfaction.

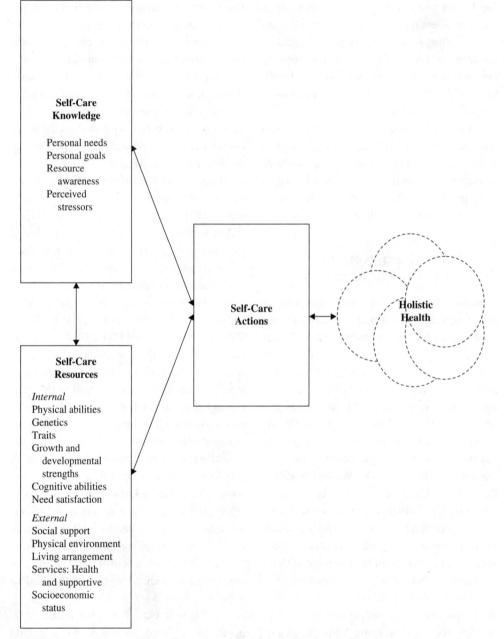

FIGURE 12-1 Framework for self-care in persons living with chronic illnesses.

External resources include persons who provide social support, the physical environment (e.g., geography, urban vs. rural, climate, community design), living arrangements (e.g., type of housing, accessibility, safety, neighbours, living alone), service availability (e.g., health care, transportation, social services), and socioeconomic status. These self-care resources are interdependent on self-care knowledge. For example, each person must recognize social support as such; an outsider's view of the presence of social support is less valid than the individual's view of the support. Although support may be available, the client may perceive the behaviours of those support persons as not helpful. Both self-care knowledge and resources are interrelated with self-care actions.

Self-care actions are those activities undertaken by persons to influence health status. Self-care actions require using one's personal self-care knowledge and mobilizing self-care resources to do what is best for one's self. Therefore, self-care actions require that each person perceive a sense of autonomy (Hertz, 1996). To some extent self-care actions are unique for each individual.

For example, all persons have a need for love and belonging and to affiliate with others. One person might meet this need by purposefully participating in social activities such as a family reunion where one feels he or she belongs and is loved as a member of a family unit; likely, this approach is based on life experiences within the family unit when that person previously felt love and belonging. Another person with different experiences and who has not experienced those feelings within the family unit might have personal needs for love and belonging met through the caring behaviours of a nurse. For that person self-neglect of a health problem might lead to reestablishment of a relationship with a nurse, which, in turn, could meet that person's need for love and belonging. In both instances persons are meeting needs for love and belonging and therefore are influencing their holistic health status. Obviously, the person who acted in a self-neglectful mode to meet those needs might eventually deplete his or her resources (physical and other coping resources). Therefore, the nurse can use nursing knowledge of health processes to assist this person to find other means for meeting those needs to build up rather than deplete resources over the long term.

According to this model of self-care health is holistic, meaning it is more than the absence of physical and mental illness. It incorporates aspects of biopsychosocial-spiritual well-being, quality of life, and self-actualization in addition to addressing and reducing the harmful effects of illnesses. This definition of health is applicable to persons living with chronic illnesses. A high level of health and chronic illness can coexist. Nurses can facilitate and nurture self-care through unconditionally accepting the person and that person's unique view or "model" of the world and then by "role-modelling" interventions that fit with that person's model.

There are five aims of interventions in MRM that guide the nurse with each person:

- Build trust with each client in the nurse–client relationship so that the client trusts others.
- Promote a positive orientation to one's self as a person of worth and to foster hope for the future.
- Facilitate client control so that each person feels and perceives a sense of control over the environment (internal and external) and the person's life situation.

- Build on strengths in terms of building on the person's capabilities and life experiences even in the presence of an illness.
- Set mutual health-directed goals based on the client's model of the world.

Structuring interventions around these aims is supportive of self-care.

STRATEGIES TO SUPPORT SELF-MANAGEMENT IN CHRONIC CONDITIONS

Self-management defines the tasks "individuals must undertake to live well with one or more chronic conditions" (Registered Nurses' Association of Ontario [RNAO], 2010, p. 73). It may be interchanged with self-care to describe behaviours that help to maintain physiological stability. Clients work with HCPs to assume greater responsibility for their healthcare decisions. The RNAO (2010) recently completed a clinical best practice guideline focused specifically on strategies to support self-management for chronic conditions. Practice recommendations emerging from this document are discussed in detail within this section. Recommendations within the guideline are based on key assumptions that clients are inevitably in charge of their self-management decisions, that each client requires different types of support, and collaborative relationships between clients and their families are essential for the success of self-management programmes. Information provided to clients by HCPs should always be evidence informed. Self-management options should focus on resources that are available to the client (RNAO, 2010).

According to the RNAO (2010), the tasks in self-managing a chronic condition or conditions may involve the following:

- Monitoring and managing the signs and symptoms of disease

- Engaging in health and lifestyle behaviours and taking medications appropriately
- Maintaining regular contact with HCPs

HCPs can encourage self-management for clients through educative and supportive interventions that increase clients' skills and confidence in managing their complex health issues. The goal, then, is to increase the client's confidence in his or her ability to change rather than focusing on compliance with the HCP's advice. According to the RNAO (2010), HCPs can support self-management through two main approaches: by developing and delivering self-management programmes and by providing clients information about behavioural strategies to help them to become effective self-managers. When using these approaches HCPs should apply the "5 A's" of behavioural change, which encourage the practitioner to assess, advise, agree, assist, and arrange client supports for self-management (RNAO, 2010).

The following section focuses on the 5 A's of behaviour change outlined within the RNAO clinical best practice guideline and provides a brief summary of the key practice recommendations for nurses outlined in each of these areas.

ASSESS: Beliefs, Behaviour, and Knowledge

It is important that HCPs working with clients living with chronic conditions adhere to the principles of the therapeutic relationship and take the time to establish trust and rapport with the client. Part of this process is to assess and address feelings of anger or frustration the client may be feeling related to coping with and caring for the chronic illness (RNAO, 2010). Depression has been identified as one of the most common complications of chronic illness and is a factor in a client's abilities to self-manage his or her condition. In some cases depression has been linked to increased rates in morbidity and mortality and increased rates of noncompliance to medical therapies (DiMatteo, Lepper, & Croghan, 2000). Therefore, it is the role of the HCP to screen for depression and to refer clients for treatment if appropriate.

It is imperative that HCPs work with the client and his or her family to construct an agenda for each visit. This provides an opportunity to address all the concerns of the members present and to focus the discussion. The client can take the time to go over the agenda and prioritize topics he or she wishes to discuss (RNAO, 2010, p. 29). This promotes collaborative planning and ensures the client has control over his or her care. Although the client may guide the discussion of self-management and outline goals, the HCP must also consistently assess the client's readiness for change. The *Stages of Change Model* (Prochaska, DiClemente, & Norcross, 1992, as cited in RNAO, 2010) is commonly used by HCPs to assess readiness for behaviour changes. Stages within this model include precontemplation, contemplation, preparation, action, maintenance, and relapse.

In the first stage, *precontemplation*, the client may not yet be thinking about the changes needed or may feel out of control, denying or believing the consequences of his or her behaviours are not serious. The second stage, *contemplation*, involves the client weighing the benefits and costs of behaviour to his or her health. They may develop proposed changes. In the third stage the client is *preparing to change* by making small changes, whereas in the fourth stage, *action*, the client takes definitive action to change. Over time, clients learn to *maintain* their changes or new behaviours; this is described as the fifth stage within the model. Finally, in the sixth stage they may *relapse* in

their efforts, and although this is a normal part of the change process, the client may feel frustrated and demoralized (Prochaska et al., 1992, cited in RNAO, 2010, p. 30).

Sometimes HCPs need to assist clients in determining what constitutes a risk to their health. In this case HCPs may use tools called health risk appraisal instruments to help clients obtain independent and objective information about their health. The role of the HCP is to provide interventional support when required after the client has identified his or her health concerns.

ADVISE: Provide Specific Information About Health Risks and Benefits of Change

The RNAO (2010) recommends that HCPs combine behavioural, psychosocial, and self-management education as part of delivering self-management support. Behavioural strategies may include involving the client in his or her own care. Clients who are knowledgeable and active in their care have improved health outcomes. The HCP achieves this by encouraging active learning and teaching clients the skills needed to manage their health. The HCP should integrate psychosocial strategies to address the feelings and attitudes of the client toward his or her condition. All educational interventions should be aimed at the developmental level, age, culture, and health literacy of the client.

The Canadian Public Health Association (2008) described health literacy as the "skills to enable access, understanding and use of information for health" (para.1). These skills may range from making healthy choices to accessing health information or locating health services. The Canadian Public Health Association (2008) reported that 60% of Canadians do not have the necessary skills to manage their health properly. The website www.ccl-cca.ca/ccl/Reports/Health Literacy.html includes a "Health Literacy Map for Canada" that summarizes health literacy levels throughout Canada.

HCPs can help to promote clients' health literacy by teaching them to use different methods to monitor their chronic conditions. These methods may include diaries, logs, or their personal health records (RNAO, 2010, p. 39). Part of this process is teaching clients to interpret and use the information gained from these self-monitoring techniques. For example, a client may need to learn how to take and keep track of blood glucose levels, but he or she must also learn what to do with these results to manage diabetes. The client needs to understand the rationale behind blood glucose monitoring, be able to interpret the results, and determine appropriate interventions to foster his or her health.

AGREE: Collaboratively Set Goals Based on Client's Interest and Confidence in the Ability to Change Behaviour

HCPs should collaborate with clients to establish goals for self-management, develop action plans, and monitor their progress toward their goals (RNAO, 2010, p. 40). Collaborative goal planning helps to move the client toward improving his or her clinical outcomes and in turn promotes self-efficacy, which manifests as the client's confidence to carry out behaviours necessary to meet desired goals. Strategies to increase self-efficacy include *action plans*, which are agreements between the clinician and the client to help clients work toward small behaviour changes (Handley et al., 2006). An action

plan must be something the client wants to achieve, be reasonable, and be behaviour specific (RNAO, 2010).

ASSIST: Identify Personal Barriers, Strategies, Problem-Solving Techniques, and Social/ Environmental Support

Motivational interviewing is a strategy used to facilitate behaviour change by helping clients explore their ambivalence to changing their health behaviours. Although the HCP may help clients to identify and resolve their issues toward behaviour change during these interviews, it is not a method that intends to "tell the client what to do" or coerce the client into new health behaviours the HCP believes the client should adopt. Instead, it is client centred and intends to elicit solutions from the client rather than providing answers or prescriptive approaches to care. Motivational interviewing is an advanced skill and requires practice to increase proficiency (RNAO, 2010).

In addition, it is also recommended that nurses teach and assist clients in developing problem-solving techniques. This involves helping clients to define their problems, generate possible solutions, implement these solutions, and then evaluate their effectiveness (RNAO, 2010). An integral role of the HCP in this process is to provide the client with access to community self-management programmes in a variety of settings.

ARRANGE: Specify Plan for Follow-Up

In addition to linking clients to self-management programmes, it is also the role of the HCP to arrange regular and sustained follow-up for clients based on their preference and availability

(RNAO, 2010). The HCP should integrate innovative delivery models such as electronic support systems, printed materials, telephone contacts, face-to-face interactions, and any new modalities or programmes in to the plan for the client (RNAO, 2010). These recommendations should also take into account the client's cultural, social, and economic contexts. Finally, the HCP should facilitate a collaborative practice team approach to ensure that self-management support for the client is effective (RNAO, 2010).

This section examined some of the practice recommendations from the RNAO pertaining to self-management support in chronic conditions. The HCP plays a role in supporting and collaborating with the client to meet his or her self-care goals. It is also the responsibility of HCPs to integrate these approaches into their educational programmes and advocate for them within their organizations. It is important that policies surrounding self-management and self-care focus on collaborative efforts with the client at the centre of this process. The remainder of this chapter examines research on self-management programmes and identifies some possible outcomes resulting from these interventions for chronic illness management.

SELF-MANAGEMENT PROGRAMMES

Lorig (2001), a nursing leader in self-management programme development and testing, comprehensively summarized findings from more than 20 years of research studies testing self-management programmes for arthritis. Characteristics of the programmes tested in sequential studies were analyzed to isolate the most important factors when designing programmes to support self-care in terms of disease self-management,

one aspect of self-care. First, programmes must be focused on the problems and concerns of clients. In other words, modelling the client's world is a key factor. Programmes should also be designed for a particular target population. The process of implementing the programme is as important as the content to be addressed. Written materials must be included as a reference and for additional reading. Programmes should promote self-efficacy by building on the client's strengths; congruent with the self-care model, positive aspects of abilities should be recognized and nurtured. Problem solving and decision making by the client should be emphasized rather than relying solely on professional judgment. Skills for communicating with HCPs should be incorporated. Other important aspects include providing a structure for the programme that is followed during each of its segments, encouraging sharing of ideas and feelings among group members attending the programme, employing lay instructors, and recognizing that other education and health teaching are valuable as well. A popular self-management training programme for HCPs is the Flinders Programme (formally known as the Flinders model). The Flinders Programme is an approach to help enable HCPs to empower their clients to become active partners in their care and more effective self-managers. The goals of this approach are to improve the partnership between clients and HCPs, identify specific problems in order to develop targeted interventions, and to provide motivation and support for sustained health behaviour change. This occurs at the levels of the client and HCP as well as within wider organizational and systemic levels of healthcare. For more information about the Flinders Programme please see the following link: http://www.flinders.edu.au/medicine/sites/fhbhru/self-management.cfm.

Chodosh and colleagues (2005) identified similar characteristics through a meta-analysis of 53 randomized trials testing chronic disease self-management programmes for older adults with diabetes, osteoarthritis, and hypertension. Although they did not find statistically significant elements of these programmes, they extrapolated that self-care, in the form of self-management, requires active participation in decision making and self-monitoring. In addition, programmes should be tailored to meet needs, be offered in group settings, provide feedback to participants, and emphasize psychological aspects of self-management in addition to medical management.

Rogers, Kennedy, Nelson, and Robinson (2005) identified the importance of the physician–patient relationship style in promoting self-management. Physicians and the health systems in which they practice need to be responsive to patient needs and preferences, and decision making must be shared with the patient. Indeed, the idea of responsiveness to client needs is essential to MRM interventions that promote self-care.

Likewise, the notion of active involvement and participation is also compatible with the self-care model. However, for some clients active participation might take the form of dependence on others as a self-care action. For example, the person with limited self-care resources might need to depend on others for aspects of self-care to preserve, rather than deplete, his or her limited resources.

Comprehensive Self-Care Programmes

Lynch, Estes, and Hernandez (2005) compared three types of chronic care initiatives for older adults. These comprehensive programmes are viewed as alternatives to the traditional medical model of care. The first is the integrated medical, home, and community-based services model that focuses on providing holistic, integrated health services to persons with complex, chronic care needs in their homes. This approach has many client-centred aspects. Research on this model of care indicates that clients rate the quality of healthcare services highly (Boyd et al., 2010). An example of this in Canada is the "Living Well with a Chronic Condition" programme created by Alberta Health Services (to view this programme online, see www.calgary healthregion.ca/cdm). This programme has three parts: education classes, exercise classes, and a self-management workshop called "Row Your Own Boat." Spouses, support persons, and caregivers are all invited to attend the classes alongside the person living with a chronic condition.

The second type of chronic care initiatives is the disease management programmes offered by a variety of providers. An example is the Kaiser Permanente Best Practice Collaborative approach with group clinics and education on disease self-care in primary care settings. The Kaiser programmes are interdisciplinary and incorporate motivational interviewing to promote self-care. The benefit is a focus on active participation. But, as previously noted, demanding active, independent participation can be detrimental to some clients' health.

A third and newer model is that of high-risk care management developed by managed care insurers to control costs and to improve the care management of persons living with multiple chronic illnesses. The guided care nurse model represents this approach (Boyd et al., 2007). This model emphasizes coordination and nonduplication of services that are individualized to meet clients' unique needs. A specially educated nurse works in a primary care practice with two to five physicians and manages care for 50 to 60 older clients. An electronic health record is used to communicate among team members. The focus of guided care nursing interventions is on comprehensive assessment and monitoring of chronic conditions, coaching to aid in self-management of diseases, referral and coordination of services to secure needed resources and to facilitate transitions between healthcare settings, and provision of caregiver education and support. A key component of this model is that the client's highest priority needs for health must be addressed by the nurse. This is a multipronged approach with many client-centred aspects.

Other types of programmes are case management programmes led by social workers, state-funded programmes for low-income persons with chronic illnesses, and wellness management programmes in senior centres (Lynch et al., 2005). All these promote self-care in some fashion. However, a limitation is that most of these programmes have a very narrow focus. Therefore, the clients' holistic health needs are not always addressed.

More innovative, comprehensive programmes need to be developed in the future to help promote self-care in persons living with chronic illnesses. These could be located in housing units or community-based sites where persons with chronic illnesses congregate—for example, churches, shopping centres, and grocery stores. Future models should incorporate the recommended multipronged approaches and address needs related to multiple chronic illnesses. All models need to adopt a client-centred and holistic perspective so that interventions can be tailored to meet clients' unique needs, values, and lifestyles.

Evidence-Informed Practice Box

Purpose: Examined relationship between perceived autonomy, representing the potential for self-care action, and internal and external self-care resources from the perspective of the MRM self-care model.

Research design: Descriptive, correlational study

Sample: The study used a convenience sample of 120 older adults aged 60 to 101 years who resided in the community and who attended a senior centre. All could read and write English. Most were women, White, not currently married, and lived alone. More than 80% had Medicare insurance, with 79% also insured by another health insurance policy. More than 62% used two or more community care services, and on average they used 2.1 services; the most frequent services were meals, health screenings, housing, and information and referral.

Setting: Six senior centres in Manhattan, New York City

Findings: Participants demonstrated relatively high scores on perceived autonomy. They also scored highly on functional ability, indicating the group was independent. The internal self-care resources of White race and functional status were significantly correlated to perceived autonomy. Social support, overall and that from family, friends, and significant others, separately, and satisfaction with service utilization were the only external

(continues)

self-care resources significantly linked to perceived autonomy. Using a multiple linear regression model, perceived autonomy was predicted by race, service satisfaction, and social support.

Implications: In this relatively independent sample of older persons, functional status was linked to perceived autonomy. Thus, those who have declining functional abilities need to be given support to care for self. Furthermore, social support was also related to perceived autonomy, indicating self-care can be facilitated through social support. It is unclear why White race was related to self-care, represented by perceived autonomy. However, the sample was predominantly White. Further study is warranted. The finding regarding satisfaction with services and its linkage to perceived autonomy is important. This may reflect that these services were a good match and met the participants' unique needs. In practice, it is important to ask clients to evaluate service satisfaction as an indicator of meeting self-care needs.

Source: Matsui & Capezuti (2008).

OUTCOMES

Grey, Knafl, and McCorkle (2006) developed a framework for describing and organizing outcomes of self-management programmes. The categories of outcomes also apply to programmes other than ones that promote self-care. The categories are condition outcomes, individual outcomes, family outcomes, and environmental outcomes. Positive outcomes in each category would be optimal.

Condition Outcomes

These outcomes indicate the individual's adherence and responsiveness to treatment regimens. For example, in persons with diabetes, hypertension, and osteoarthritis, outcomes include reduced levels of hemoglobin A1c, decreased systolic blood pressure by 5 mm Hg and decreased diastolic by 4.3 mm Hg, and pain reduction, respectively (Chodosh et al., 2005). Following recommended screening procedures (Berg & Wadhwa, 2007) was also a condition outcome. Other outcomes might include morbidity, mortality, and improved or stable functional status (Burnette et al., 2004; Grey et al., 2006; Lynch et al., 2005).

Individual Outcomes

Any outcomes that reflect clients' perceptions regarding health status, quality of life, and well-being are included in this category. Connectedness to others, transcendence, a sense of well-being (Leenerts et al., 2002), life satisfaction (Borg et al., 2006), satisfaction with health care (Matsui & Capezuti, 2008), and reports of needs being met (Inglis et al., 2006) are examples. Quality of life and physical, mental, and spiritual health ratings (Boyd et al., 2007; Campbell & Aday, 2001), increased health-related knowledge, and a greater sense of being in control of one's situation or sense of autonomy are other individual outcomes (Campbell & Aday, 2001).

Family Outcomes

Outcomes that indicate an effect on the family of the person receiving the promotion intervention are included in this group. Depression in caregivers, improved family functioning, and degree of caregiver burden (Grey et al., 2006) are examples of family outcomes.

Environmental Outcomes

Outcomes that reflect the costs of health care or influence the healthcare system are considered environmental outcomes. For example, cost reductions, unplanned hospital admission rates, lengths of stay, and frequencies of healthcare utilization (Inglis et al., 2006) fall into this category. In addition, nonduplication of services (Boyd et al., 2007), decreased nursing home admissions, and use of ambulatory services may be included in this category (Berg & Wadhwa, 2007; Lynch et al., 2005).

SUMMARY

Healthcare professionals caring for persons with chronic illness need to be aware of their role in helping clients to achieve self-care of their condition. Despite the differing approaches to the concept of self-care addressed throughout this chapter, HCPs should continue to reflect upon their role to assess, advise, agree, assist, and arrange self-management plans for individuals living with chronic illness. Engagement within this process will help to improve client outcomes by providing concrete care plans, helping clients to prevent and to recognize acute exacerbations of their condition(s), and continuing to provide client education that is guided by the client's needs. Most importantly, the HCP should be available for support and education for the client and support their decision-making process throughout their illness trajectory.

STUDY QUESTIONS

1. Define self-care as it relates to persons living with one or more chronic illnesses.
2. Identify the relationship between self-care and health outcomes. Why is self-care a key concept to positive health outcomes?
3. How can nurses promote self-care in the clients for whom they care? Identify the key elements of a self-care supportive intervention.
4. Delineate at least one positive outcome for the individual client, family, and healthcare system as a result of the individual client demonstrating self-care in relation to his or her chronic illness.

INTERNET RESOURCES

Center for Self and Family Management of Vulnerable Populations, Yale University School of Nursing: nursing.yale.edu/Centers/ECSMI/

Communities Putting Prevention to Work: Chronic Disease Self-Management Programme: www.aoa.gov/AoARoot/PRESS_Room/News/2009/03_18_09.aspx

Expert Patients Programme Community Interest Company (EPP CIC) in the UK: www.selfcareconnect.co.uk/

Family Caregiver Alliance, Taking Care of YOU: Self-Care for Family Caregivers: www.caregiver.org/caregiver/jsp/content_node.jsp?nodeid=847

Guided Care: www.guidedcare.org/index.asp

(continues)

INTERNET RESOURCES (Cont.)

Health Literacy in Canada: A Healthy Understanding: www.ccl-cca.ca/ccl/Reports/Health Literacy.html

International Orem Society for Nursing Science and Scholarship: www.orem-society.com/

Living Well with a Chronic Condition: www.calgaryhealthregion.ca/cdm

Self-Management Science Center, University of Wisconsin–Milwaukee, College of Nursing: www4.uwm.edu/smsc/

The Society for the Advancement of Modeling and Role-Modeling: mrmnursingtheory.org/index.html

Stanford Self-Management Programmes: patient education.stanford.edu/programs/

Supporting Self Care in Primary Care—The Book. Chapter 14 has many suggestions for promoting self-care in clients (and self): www.self careconnect.co.uk/167

Understanding the Affordable Care Act: www.healthcare.gov/law/introduction/index.html

For a full suite of assignments and additional learning activities, use the access code located in the front of your book and visit this exclusive website: **http://go.jblearning.com/kramer-kile**. If you do not have an access code, you can obtain one at the site.

REFERENCES

Barlow, J. H., Sturt, J., & Hearnshaw, H. (2002). Self-management interventions for people with chronic conditions in primary care: Examples from arthritis, asthma and diabetes. *Health Education Journal, 61*(4), 365–378.

Beattie, B. L., Whitelaw, N., Mettler, M., & Turner, D. (2003). A vision for older adults and health promotion. *American Journal of Health Promotion, 18*(2), 200–204.

Berg, G. D., & Wadhwa, S. (2007). Health services outcomes for a diabetes disease management program for the elderly. *Disease Management, 10,* 226–234.

Bickerstaff, K. A., Grasser, C. M., & McCabe, B. (2003). How elderly nursing home residents transcend losses of later life. *Holistic Nursing Practice, 17*(3), 159–165.

Bliss, D. Z., Fischer, L. R., & Savik, K. (2005). Managing fecal incontinence: Self-care practices of older adults. *Journal of Gerontological Nursing, 31*(7), 35–44.

Borg, C., Hallberg, I., & Blomqvist, K. (2006). Life satisfaction among older people (65+) with reduced self-care capacity: The relationship to social, health and financial aspects [Electronic version]. *Journal of Clinical Nursing, 15*(5), 607–618. Retrieved from http://onlinelibrary.wiley.com/doi/10.1111/j.1365-2702.2006.01375.x/abstract

Boyd, C. M., Boult, C., Shadmi, E., Leff, B., Brager, R., Dunbar, L., Wolff, J. L., & Wegner, S. (2007). Guided care for multimorbid older adults. *The Gerontologist, 47,* 679–704.

Boyd, C. M., Reider, L., Frey, K., Scharfstein, D., Leff, B., Wolff, J., . . . Boult, C. (2010). The effects of guided care on the perceived quality of health care for multi-morbid older persons: 18-month outcomes from a cluster-randomized controlled trial. *Journal of General Internal Medicine, 25*(3), 235–242.

Britz, J., & Dunn, K. (2010). Self-care and quality of life among patients with heart failure. *Journal of the American Academy of Nurse Practitioners, 22*(9), 480–487.

Burnette, D., Mui, A. C., & Zodikoff, B. D. (2004). Gender, self-care and functional status among older persons with coronary heart disease: A national perspective. *Women & Health, 39*(1), 65–84.

Campbell, J., & Aday, R. H. (2001). Benefits of a nurse-managed wellness program: A senior center model. *Journal of Gerontological Nursing, 27*(3), 34–43.

Canadian Public Health Association. (2008). Health literacy in Canada: A healthy understanding. Canada: Author. Retrieved from http://www.ccl-cca.ca/ccl/Reports/HealthLiteracy.html

Chodosh, J., Morton, S. C., Mojica, W., Maglione, M., Suttorp, M. J., Hilton, L., . . . Shekelle, P. (2005). Meta-analysis: Chronic disease self-management programs for older adults. *Annals of Internal Medicine, 143,* 427–438.

Chriss, P. M., Sheposh, J., Carlson, B., & Riegel, B. (2004). Predictors of successful heart failure self-care maintenance in the first three months after hospitalization. *Heart & Lung, 33,* 345–353.

Coleman, E. A., Smith, J. D., Frank, J. C., Min, S-J., Parry, C., & Kramer, A. M. (2004). Preparing patients and caregivers to participate in care delivered across settings: The care transitions intervention. *Journal of the American Geriatrics Society, 52,* 1817–1825.

Cortes, T., Lee, A., Boal, J., Mion, L., & Butler, A. (2004). Using focus groups to identify asthma care and education issues for elderly urban-dwelling minority individuals. *Applied Nursing Research, 17*(3), 207–212.

DiMatteo, M. R., Lepper, H. S., & Croghan, T. W. (2000). Depression is a risk factor for noncompliance with medical treatment: Meta analysis of the effects of anxiety and depression on patient adherence. *Archives of Internal Medicine, 160*(14), 2101–2107.

Dyer, C. B., Goodwin, J. S., Pickens-Pace, S., Burnett, J., & Kelly, P. A. (2007). Self-neglect among the elderly: A model based on more than 500 patients seen by a geriatric medicine team. *American Journal of Public Health, 97,* 1671–1676.

Edwardson, S. R., & Dean, K. J. (1999) Appropriateness of self-care responses to symptoms among elders: Identifying pathways of influence. *Research in Nursing & Health, 22,* 329–339.

Erickson, H. C., Tomlin, E., & Swain, M. A. (1988). *Modeling and role-modeling: A theory and paradigm for nursing* (2nd ed.). Lexington, SC: Pine Press.

Erickson, H. L. (2006). *Modeling and role-modeling: A view from the client's world.* Cedar Park, TX: Unicorns Unlimited.

Grey, M., Knafl, K., & McCorkle, R. (2006). A framework for the study of self- and family management of chronic conditions. *Nursing Outlook, 54,* 278–286.

Haber, D. (2002). Health promotion and aging: Educational and clinical initiatives by the federal government. *Educational Gerontology, 28,* 253–262.

Handley, M., MacGregor, K., Schillinger, D., Sharifi, C., Wong, S., & Bodenheimer, T. (2006). Using action plans to help primary care patients adopt healthy behaviours: A descriptive study. *Journal of the American Board of Family Medicine, 19,* 224–231.

Hertz, J. E. (1996). Conceptualization of perceived enactment of autonomy in the elderly. *Issues in Mental Health Nursing, 17*(3), 261–273.

Hertz, J. E., & Baas, L. (2006). Self-care: Knowledge, resources, and actions. In H. L. Erickson (Ed.), *Modeling and role-modeling: A view from the client's world* (pp. 97–120). Cedar Park, TX: Unicorns Unlimited.

Hertz, J. E., & Rossetti, J. (2006, March). *Senior apartment residents' reported self-care activities.* Paper presented at the 2006 Midwest Nursing Research Society Conference, Milwaukee, WI.

Inglis, S. C., Pearson, S., Treen, S., Gallasch, T., Horowitz, J. D., & Stewart, S. (2006). Extending the horizon in chronic heart failure: Effects of multidisciplinary, home-based intervention relative to usual care. *Circulation, 114,* 2466–2473.

Leenerts, M. H., Teel, C. S., & Pendleton, M. K. (2002). Building a model of self-care for health promotion in aging. *Journal of Nursing Scholarship, 34*(4), 355–361.

Lorig, K. (2001). Arthritis self-management. In E. A. Swanson, T. Tripp-Reimer, & K. Buckwalter (Eds.), *Health promotion and disease prevention in the older adult: Interventions and recommendations* (pp. 56–80). New York, NY: Springer.

Lubben, J. E., & Damron-Rodriguez, J. A. (2003). An international approach to community health care for older adults. *Family and Community Health, 26*(4), 338–349.

Lynch, M., Estes, C. L., & Hernandez, M. (2005). Chronic care initiatives for the elderly: Can they bridge the gerontology-medicine gap? *Journal of Applied Gerontology, 24,* 108–124.

Maddox, M. (1999). Older women and the meaning of health. *Journal of Gerontological Nursing, 25*(12), 26–33.

Maslow, A. H. (1962). *Toward a psychology of being.* New York, NY: John Wiley & Sons.

Matsui, M., & Capezuti, E. (2008). Perceived autonomy and self-care resources among senior center users. *Geriatric Nursing, 29*(2), 141–147.

McDonald-Miszczak, L., & Wister, A. V. (2005). Predicting self-care behaviors among older adults coping with arthritis: A cross-sectional and 1-year longitudinal comparative analysis. *Journal of Ageing and Health, 17,* 836–857.

Mendias, E. P., & Paar, D. P. (2007). Perceptions of health and self-care learning needs of outpatients with HIV/AIDS. *Journal of Community Health Nursing, 24*(1), 49–64.

Musil, C. M., Morris, D. L., Haug, M. R., Warner, C. B., & Whelan, A. T. (2001). Recurrent symptoms:

Well-being and management. *Social Science & Medicine, 52,* 1729–1740.

Naik, A., Dyer, C., Kunik, M., & McCullough, L. (2009a). Patient autonomy for the management of chronic conditions: A two-component reconceptualization. *American Journal of Bioethics, 9*(2), 23–30.

Naik, A., Dyer, C., Kunik, M., & McCullough, L. (2009b). Response to commentaries on "Patient autonomy for the management of chronic conditions: A two-component re-conceptualization." *American Journal of Bioethics, 9*(2), W3–W5.

Naik, A., Teal, C., Pavlik, V., Dyer, C., & McCullough, L. (2008). Conceptual challenges and practical approaches to screening capacity for self-care and protection in vulnerable older adults. *Journal of the American Geriatrics Society, 56,* S266–S270.

Orem, D. (2001). *Nursing: Concepts of practice* (6th ed.). St. Louis, MO: Mosby.

Potempa, K., Butterworth, S., Flaherty-Robb, M., & Gaynor, W. (2010). The healthy ageing model: Health behaviour change for older adults. *Collegian, 17*(2), 51–55.

Registered Nurses' Association of Ontario. (2010). Strategies to support self-management in chronic conditions: Collaboration with clients. Toronto, ON: Author. Retrieved from http://www.rnao.org/Storage/72/6710_SMS_Brochure.pdf

Resnick, B. (2001). Promoting health in older adults: A four-year analysis. *Journal of the American Academy of Nurse Practitioners, 13*(1), 23–33.

Resnick, B. (2003). Health promotion practices of older adults: Model testing. *Public Health Nursing, 20*(1), 2–12.

Rogers, A., Kennedy, A., Nelson, E., & Robinson, A. (2005). Uncovering the limits of patient-centeredness: Implementing a self-management trial for chronic illness. *Qualitative Health Research, 15,* 224–239.

Ryan, P., & Sawin, K. (2009). The individual and family self-management theory: Background and perspectives on context, process, and outcomes. *Nursing Outlook, 57*(4), 217–225.

Scollan-Koliopoulos, M., & Walker, E. (2009). Multigenerational timeline and understanding of diabetes and self-care. *Research & Theory for Nursing Practice, 23*(1), 62–77.

Sharkey, J., Ory, M., & Browne, B. (2005). Determinants of self-management strategies to reduce out-of-pocket prescription medication expense in homebound older people [Electronic version]. *Journal of the American Geriatrics Society, 53*(4), 666–674. Retrieved from http://onlinelibrary.wiley.com/doi/10.1111/j.1532-5415.2005.53217.x/full

Singleton, J. K. (2000). Nurses' perspectives of encouraging clients' care-of-self in a short-term rehabilitation unit within a long-term care facility. *Rehabilitation Nursing, 25*(1), 23–35.

Sutherland, D., & Hayter, M. (2009). Structured review: Evaluating the effectiveness of nurse case managers in improving health outcomes in three major chronic diseases. *Journal of Clinical Nursing, 18*(21), 2978–2992.

Wang, H. H., Hsu, M. T., & Want, R. H. (2001). Using a focus group study to explore perceptions of health-promoting self-care in community-dwelling older adults. *Journal of Nursing Research, 9*(4), 95–104.

Washburn, S., Hornberger, C., Klutman, A., & Skinner, L. (2005, May). Nurses' knowledge of heart failure education topics as reported in a small Midwestern community hospital [Electronic version]. *Journal of Cardiovascular Nursing, 20*(3), 215–220. Retrieved from http://journals.lww.com/jcnjournal/Abstract/2005/05000/Nurses__Knowledge_of_Heart_Failure_Education.14.aspx

Yip, Y. B., Sit, J. W. H., & Wong, D. Y. S. (2004). A quasi-experimental study on improving arthritis self-management for residents of an aged people's home in Hong Kong. *Psychology, Health & Medicine, 9,* 235–246.

CHAPTER 13

Client and Family Education

Original chapter by Elaine T. Miller
Canadian content added by Joseph C. Osuji

INTRODUCTION

For most clients and their families a chronic illness is a life-changing event uniquely affecting them as they deal with the added demands and long-term nature of the particular disease. Perhaps more importantly, chronic illnesses neither always have a similar trajectory of presentation and management (e.g., asthma, heart disease, depression, cancer, stroke, arthritis, diabetes, and hypertension) nor discriminate according to age, race, gender, socioeconomic status, culture or ethnicity, or learning capability. Furthermore, the client's and family's response and resources to cope with chronic illnesses may vary tremendously, requiring healthcare professionals (HCPs) to be attuned to each client's and family's particular needs, expectations, resources, and personal goals.

Data from the Public Health Agency of Canada indicate that chronic illnesses cost Canadians at least 190 billion dollars annually, which is more than half of the Canadian annual healthcare spending budget (www.phac.gc.ca). In the global context more than 60% of all deaths are attributable to chronic diseases

(Strong, Mathers, Leeder, & Beaglehole, 2005; World Health Organization, 2005). The World Economic Forum projects that by 2030 the aggregate global cost of treating just five common chronic illnesses (cancer, diabetes, heart disease, mental disorders, and chronic respiratory diseases) will top 4 trillion dollars (see report at www.weforum.org/reports/global-economic-burden-non-communicable-diseases). The Chronic Disease Prevention Alliance of Canada also reports on the cost of chronic disease in Canada (www.gpiatlantic.org/pdf/health/chronic canada.pdf).

Most chronic diseases (e.g., pulmonary, hypertension, heart disease) could be prevented or better managed by adopting a more client-centred, multidisciplinary approach that fosters client and family involvement, client self-management, and continuous quality improvement (Partnership to Fight Chronic Disease, 2010). For example, Woodhouse, Peterson, Campbell, and Gathercoal (2010) found a significant reduction in the costly use of emergency department visits by high-user clients with chronic pain who received targeted educational/behavioural interventions to better manage their condition. Thus, the central aspects of the care-delivery process encompass maximizing client and family coping with chronic illness; improving their knowledge, attitudes, and behaviours; and using HCPs to provide a more unified approach and subsequent monitoring, management, and evaluation of care outcomes. Given that many clients and their families are likely to experience more than one chronic illness in a lifetime, it is critical for HCPs to be cognizant of the potential interplay of diverse chronic illnesses that may influence the client's and family's responses to further losses such as incontinence, fatigue, diminishing cognitive function, or mobility.

Educating clients and their families is critical to successful coping with chronic illnesses and overall long-term quality of life. The family also frequently serves as the client's primary support system, affecting the client's decision making about health, seeking health care, and adherence to recommended healthcare management (e.g., taking prescribed medication, following a diet, having a recommended procedure or test) (Falvo, 2011). Although commonalities often exist, each client and family situation has its distinctive characteristics that require HCPs to approach every situation carefully and systematically without making assumptions as to the client's and family's resources, capability to learn, and ability to achieve educational outcomes. Moreover, HCPs must continually assess the factors influencing the client's and family's educational needs, the teaching and learning approach, and evaluation of short- and long-term outcomes. Another central element in this educational process is identifying what clients and their families want to learn, their priorities in terms of their educational needs, and having mutual goal setting, so that clients, families, and HCPs are working together to achieve common goals.

Because numerous factors contribute to the success or failure of client and family education pertaining to chronic illness, this chapter presents an overview of the fundamental elements that should be considered and clarifies the state of evidence-informed knowledge pertaining to client and family education related to chronic illnesses. Even though much is known regarding client and family education, the literature and research do not suggest simple solutions or approaches that optimize this educational process in all situations. In addition, the nature of the chronic disease(s) and the specific attributes of the learner(s), such as age, gender, race/ethnicity, culture, socioeconomic status, motivation, self-efficacy, psychological conditions (depression, bipolar disorder), sensory deficits (low-level vision, hearing impairment, literacy, learning capability), and/or learning disabilities, significantly influence how the HCP approaches and evaluates the success of each client and family educational encounter.

The primary focus of this chapter is the adult learner. However, a basic distinction is described regarding key learning differences between adults and children. Finally, because this chapter only purports to present a broad overview of key issues affecting client and family educational processes regarding chronic illnesses, it is highly recommended that additional evidence-informed resources be obtained to more specifically target the chronic illness and client population of concern, recognizing that research and the associated findings continue to expand the science of what is known.

TEACHING–LEARNING PROCESS

The teaching–learning process is characterized by multifaceted, dynamic, and interactive exchanges that are fundamental to client–family education and nursing practice. Teaching involves a deliberative, intentional act of communicating information to individuals in response to their identified educational needs and with the objective of achieving a desired outcome (Bastable, 2006; Falvo, 2011). Learning, on the other hand, assists the individual to acquire new knowledge, skills, and/or attitudes that can be measured (Bastable, 2006). A review of the literature reveals more than 50 major teaching–learning theories that can shape an educational intervention (Learning Theories Knowledge Base, 2011).

Although many theories and frameworks are applicable to client and family education, behaviourist theory, social–cognitive learning theory, humanistic learning theory, and constructionist theory have been identified as particularly helpful in shaping educational interventions. Each offers a different orientation of what is most important and what should be the HCP's focus of attention when educating individuals with chronic illness and their families. In addition, each has a particular perspective in terms of how teaching and learning are defined, measured, and structured, as well as the phases of learning.

For example, the *behaviourist framework* states that learning is the result of connections between the stimuli in the environment and the individual's responses (Skinner, 1974). So, if an educator wants a client and/or family to learn new information or alter their attitudes and responses, such as the new need for a client to receive a subcutaneous insulin injection twice daily, the educator would alter the conditions in the environment (e.g., information available on the hospital educational cable system) and reinforce positive new behaviours when they occur (e.g., praise when the injection is given correctly).

On the other hand, *social–cognitive theory* includes role modelling as a central concept and offers a different approach to teaching clients and their families to perform the same task (Bandura, 1986). In the situation described earlier, using social–cognitive theory the nurse educator would demonstrate how to perform the insulin injection and then have the client, if capable, perform the insulin injection when next scheduled.

One of the best known humanistic frameworks is Maslow's hierarchy of needs. If this theory was applied to the preceding scenario, the educator would first need to fulfil lower level needs, such as physiological needs and safety, before teaching the client how to perform the insulin injection.

Finally, *constructionist learning theory* offers an additional alternative theoretical perspective to guide the HCP's educational encounter, asserting that learners are actively creating meaning as they learn. When viewed from this constructionist orientation, learning is perceived as contextual, requiring not only time, social contact, and motivation but also creating meanings that foster learning over time and its application (Hein, 1991). In the case of learning how to properly give an insulin injection, the constructionist theory provides a framework to connect the client's understanding/meaning of how the insulin injection should be correctly given, the client's motivation to learn this activity, the time required to correctly perform this task, and the contribution of the HCP who is teaching this skill.

In summary, theoretical frameworks offer alternative ways to approach a teaching–learning situation involving clients and their families. Because there are a myriad of theoretical frameworks, it is important that HCPs determine what is most relevant to their situations, examine available evidence-informed research pertaining to that framework (preferably evidence published in the last 5 years), and then translate that framework to their particular client–family interactions and systematically evaluate the efficacy of using that perspective to direct their educational interventions.

In conjunction with the numerous teaching–learning theories that guide the HCP's client–family educational encounters, it is valuable to contemplate several basic assumptions underpinning these interactions. According to Petty (2006), learning involves "an active process of making sense and creating a personal interpretation of what has been learned" (p. 8), rather than simply an exact interpretation of what has been taught. What occurs is more than just a storing of personal interpretations of facts and ideas, it is "also linking them in a way that relates ideas to other ideas, and to prior learning, and so creates meaning and understanding" (Petty, 2006, p. 8). When viewed from this perspective, learners construct meaning that is more easily applied to solve problems, make judgments, and assist clients and their families to perform the numerous tasks associated with living with one or more chronic illnesses. Evidence is steadily expanding to support the constructivism perspective and its positive outcomes (Muijs & Reynolds, 2005). In addition, results from multiple meta-analyses of educational research reinforce the pivotal influence that feedback and reinforcement exert on individual as well as group learning (Petty, 2006).

CASE STUDY

Mrs. McGill is a 63-year-old grandmother with a history of chronic obstructive pulmonary disease and clinically defined obesity (body mass index > 30) as well as two falls in the last 4 months resulting in bruises but no fractures. About 6 months ago she was also diagnosed with type 2 diabetes and is receiving medication, but getting her blood sugars under control and adhering to her diet restrictions have been somewhat of a challenge. Mrs. McGill lives with her husband of 34 years and is currently raising two grandsons, ages 6 and 10. Although she loved being a substitute English teacher in the high school where she taught, Mrs. McGill has been unable to do so since obtaining custody of her two grandsons 9 months ago. Her husband, who is a pharmacist, still works part-time and is very supportive of his wife. The couple lives with their grandsons in a comfortable duplex.

Discussion Questions

1. What appears to be the primary educational objectives for Mrs. McGill?
2. What additional assessment data would be helpful in identifying your educational objectives and structuring your related interventions?
3. What teaching method(s) are most appropriate and what is your rationale for this decision?
4. What websites or national practice guidelines may assist in helping to develop your teaching plan?
5. Briefly describe your teaching plan in terms of objective(s), content, timeline, and teaching strategies.

SIGNIFICANCE OF CLIENT AND FAMILY TEACHING TO PRACTICE AND HEALTHCARE COSTS _____

Practice standards/guidelines from the different nursing associations in Canada and across the globe consistently identify health teaching as a fundamental component of nursing practice. Even in the early writings of Florence Nightingale, teaching was recognized as a prominent nursing activity (Nightingale, 1860). In addition, all provincial nurse practice acts include teaching within the scope of nursing practice responsibilities and as essential to promoting optimal health and disease management of clients and their families.

The expectation is that clients and families assume an active role in this process and have responsibilities just as the educator does. They should indicate when they do not understand the information and must take responsibility for self-management of their needs when capable (e.g., medication, safety, nutrition, pain). Moreover, the educator is expected to consistently and comprehensively assess the client and family's learning needs and barriers affecting the educational outcomes. In addition, client educational activities must be coordinated, tailored according to the clients and families needs/abilities, and evaluated to determine if learning has occurred. It is imperative to draw the distinction between client education and self-management education. *Client education* typically addresses issues that reflect common problems related to a specific disease. This information may focus on disease-specific information or technical skills. The goal of this type of education is compliance and is based on the underlying theory that disease-specific knowledge creates behaviour change, which in turn produces better outcomes (Registered Nurses' Association of Ontario, 2010). The HCP delivers client education. On the other hand, *self-management education* encompasses issues identified by the client. This type of education is based on the theory that greater client confidence in making life-improving changes increases clinical outcomes. The overall goal is increased self-efficacy and improved clinical outcomes. The client takes a problem-solving approach to address his or her chronic condition. Educators may be nurses, HCPs, or other individuals who are living with the disease (Registered Nurses' Association of Ontario, 2010).

Education plays a pivotal role in a client's ability to self-manage a particular chronic illness. For instance, improved patient education correlates with increased quality of life and adherence to treatment in clients that underwent kidney transplant surgery (Curcani & Tan, 2011), in the prevention of stroke and heart diseases (Vecchione, 2011), and reduced coronary heart disease risk factors in Chinese patients after percutanous coronary intervention (Gao et al., 2011), as in many other chronic illnesses. With regard to heart disease and stroke, Gao and colleagues (2011) further emphasized that much of the burden associated with these two diseases can be eliminated by reduction of major risk factors such as high blood pressure, high cholesterol, tobacco use, limited physical activity, and poor nutrition. By targeting client and family education on those modifiable risk factors, the likelihood of heart disease and stroke can be significantly diminished and personal and financial costs reduced.

Basic Differences Between Child and Adult Learners

The term "pedagogy" is defined as the art and science of teaching children, whereas "andragogy" refers to adult learning (Bastable, 2006). When teaching children versus adults the key principles operating during the teachable moment are distinctly different, as indicated in **Table 13-1.**

Quality of Research and Evidence

When developing educational interventions for clients and their families, it is important to first determine the quality of the evidence forming the basis for the planned actions. Evidence-informed practice, formerly referred to as evidence-based practice, refers to a problem-solving approach used in practice that combines the following three components: the best available evidence, the HCP's clinical expertise, and the client's values and preferences (Melnyk & Fineout-Overholt, 2010).

The highest level of evidence is a well-conducted meta-analysis and systematic review of randomized controlled trials (Craig & Smyth, 2002; Melnyk & Fineout-Overholt, 2010). However, a review of the literature reveals a sizable portion of present knowledge directing our educational interventions is of a lower level of evidence, such as single randomized trials, nonrandomized studies, consensus opinion of experts, and case studies. Results of a systematic review of 139 educational randomized controlled trials involving more than 22,000 clients with diabetes, asthma, or congestive heart failure revealed that many of these randomized controlled trials draw inappropriate conclusions, with researchers frequently tending to overgeneralise their findings and include opinions not based on research evidence (Boren, Balas, & Mustafa, 2003). Therefore, educators need to carefully scrutinize the level of available evidence that underpins their practice,

Table 13-1 Comparison of Assumptions Pertaining to Teaching and Learning for Children and Adults

Pedagogy (Children)	Andragogy (Adults)
Rely on others to decide what is important to learn. Teacher is dominant. Learning is teacher led.	Decide for themselves what is important to learn (self-directive).
Expect what they learn will be helpful in the future.	Expect what they learn is immediately useful/applicable.
Have little or no experience on which to build knowledge/skill.	Have abundant experience.
Possess little ability to serve as a resource to teacher or classmates.	Possess great ability to serve as a resource to teacher and other learners (active student role).
Expect to be taught and take no responsibility.	Like to take control of the situation.
Not necessarily ready to learn.	Imply their motivation to learn, because they are present in the learning situation.
View learning as a process of acquiring information to be used at a later time.	View learning as a process of increasing competence to achieve a fuller life potential.

Sources: Bastable (2006), Conner (2005), Knowles (1998), and Mihall & Belletti (1999).

determine whether stated implications in research studies extend beyond the documented evidence, and recognize the tentative nature of our knowledge.

An excellent illustration of how knowledge evolves is demonstrated by the Internet and the increasing prevalence of online learning that has reshaped, in many instances, the education of clients, families, and HCPs worldwide. In a study investigating clients seeking trends for additional health information regarding their disease/health problem, Rahmqvist and Bara (2007) identified from a sample of 24,800 respondents that young and middle-aged clients primarily use the Internet to expand their knowledge. However, they stress the inherent quality issues associated with public access to a blend of poor- as well as high-quality, evidence-informed online health information. Their findings were reaffirmed by Gremeaux and Coudeyre (2010), who performed a systematic review of the Internet and therapeutic education of patients and found that HCPs must work to create quality sites that provide accurate evidence-informed data and best practices pertaining to chronic disease management for clients and their families.

Assessment of the Learner

A critical aspect of the client and family educational process is the assessment phase that shapes the other steps in the process, such as planning the educational event/program, its implementation, and evaluating outcomes. However, just as vital signs are obtained to determine the client's physiological state, so too must certain essential information be obtained in this initial assessment that will affect how the education is structured, delivered, and evaluated. Because it is assumed the client and family

dealing with the chronic illness are equal partners with the HCP, the following are critical questions to ask the client and family:

- What information do you want provided? Recognize that the client and family may identify different needs. If so, make sure each of their needs is addressed.
- Are there any new skills that you want to learn or ones you want to review?
- What are your specific educational goals? You may need to give an example (e.g., correctly identify signs/symptoms of hypoglycemic reactions; know what to do when an insulin reaction occurs and how to correctly give an insulin injection). The HCP must recognize that client and family goals can focus on knowledge, attitude (i.e., self-efficacy), and/or skill acquisition.
- Of the goals identified, what is most important? Once again, the client and family may differ markedly in specific goals and priorities. Listen carefully to both of them.
- What do you perceive as factors that affect your ability to achieve these educational goals? How will barriers be overcome?
- Do you feel confident using the information provided to you? If not, how may I assist you in increasing your confidence and ability to use this information?

When clients and family members are providing answers, the HCP must always be an astute listener, nonjudgmental, capable of developing individualized and attainable client and/or family goals, and reflect back to the client and family their understanding of what has been heard (Miller, 2003). While collecting the relevant client and family data the HCP needs to be organized, perform the assessment in a timely manner, and be aware of readability of assessment materials. In addition, the client with chronic illness often has associated limitations that affect the assessment (e.g., easily fatigued and diminished hearing and/or vision and/or comprehension).

Influences on Teaching and Learning

This section identifies a variety of factors that may influence the teaching–learning process; however, the list is not all inclusive because each individual with chronic illness is unique and teaching–learning may be influenced by other factors.

Family Structure and Function

Families can vary significantly in structure and function. The chronic illness of a family member can precipitate changes in the family structure and function, as do changes associated with marriage, raising children, or death of a family member. When a family member has a chronic illness, the family's response to this change and its capability to adapt and make decisions can influence their receptiveness to education. When the client and family experience high anxiety, it can markedly interfere with their ability to receive and comprehend information, maintain normal patterns of family functioning, and use appropriate coping skills. Because culture and lifestyle affect the development of family norms and beliefs, differences in these client/family and HCP factors can affect the dynamics of the educational process (Rankin, Stallings, & London, 2005). Once these beliefs and values are identified, they can be addressed through individualized teaching. It is imperative, therefore, that the family structure, function (i.e., roles, resources, strengths, and weaknesses), and norms be considered in the assessment and educational planning process.

For client education to be effective, the family should be included in client teaching (e.g., fall-reduction strategies, reporting concerns related to care and safety). Because the client's family may be large with varying functions, the HCP must determine the primary family member who should receive the relevant education. Just as in the case of the client, the HCP needs to assess the primary family caregiver's role, expectations, learning needs/goals, learning style, fears, concerns, cognitive and physical abilities, and present knowledge pertaining to the client's healthcare needs (Bastable, 2006). Moreover, the client and the family member may need to receive similar information, reinforcement, and feedback related to their knowledge and/or skill performance. In many instances the family member is the single most important factor in determining the success or failure of the teaching plan (Haggard, 1989).

Culture

When working with clients and their families, culture can dramatically affect how educational activities are structured, delivered, and evaluated. The client's and family's culture comprise "an integral part of each person's life and includes knowledge, beliefs, values, morals, customs, traditions, communication patterns, and habits acquired by members of a society" (Bastable, 2006, p. 455). When educating clients and families, an important initial step is becoming culturally sensitive. This refers to the process of becoming aware of one's own biases and prejudices about another culture or ethnic group. Cultural competence, a higher level, denotes educational interventions reflecting knowledge, understanding, respect, and acceptance of the client's and/or family's culture (Bastable, 2006).

For a successful educational encounter to occur, HCPs and clients and their families must bridge these cultural differences through the use of effective interpersonal communication. This establishment of common understanding between HCPs and clients and their families is facilitated by the HCP performing the following:

- Explore and respect the client's/family's beliefs, values, meaning of the chronic illness, preferences, and needs.
- Identify what will build rapport and trust. Potential sources of information to assist in this process are other colleagues, family members of the client, community groups, and reputable websites.
- Determine if there are any common views or interests.
- Identify own biases and assumptions.
- Maintain and convey an unconditional positive regard. Be an excellent listener, be open and nonjudgmental, and use consistent perception checks to assess comprehension of what has been communicated.
- Become knowledgeable of the culture and health disparities/discrimination of the particular client's/family's culture. Review some of the websites listed at the end of this chapter that provide a starting point for resources from reputable sources.
- Use interpreter services when needed.

Cultural differences make each client and family situation unique, but there are also essential considerations in communication, interactions, and the ultimate delivery of any educational activity. Culturally unsafe practices are defined as "any actions that diminish, demean or disempower

the cultural identity and well being of an individual" (Cooney, 1994, p. 7). Because culture has been linked to cancer-related beliefs and practices, Kreuter and associates (2003) examined the effects of culture on responses to cancer education materials and determined that responses to culturally tailored materials were no different from other materials, regardless of the women's cultural characteristics. In another study investigating factors predicting prostate cancer information seeking by 52 African American men, it was discovered that the men increased their awareness by obtaining accurate information regarding the disease, early detection and screening, and treatment. However, negative beliefs such as fear, distrust, and inconvenience of the symptoms and treatment were identified. It was further revealed that peers, siblings, and religious leaders had a significant influence on the study subjects' behaviours.

In an integrative review that focused on Hispanic adults and their beliefs about type 2 diabetes, Hatcher and Whittemore (2007) identified several valuable findings to consider when developing educational interventions for this population. After reviewing 15 research studies, they identified that generally Hispanic adults' understanding of the etiology of diabetes was an integration of biomedical causes (e.g., heredity) and traditional folk beliefs. With knowledge of the importance of heredity and folk beliefs in how Hispanics view diabetes, Hatcher and Whittemore (2007) recommended this as a starting point to clarify misconceptions and develop individualized plans of teaching and care. Results from this synthesis of the research literature highlight the necessity of obtaining specific knowledge of how race and culture can affect the structure, implementation, and evaluation of educational outcomes.

Healthcare practices and health-seeking behaviours are culturally bound (Peterson, Soncar, Sherman-Slate, & Luna, 2004; Shahid, Finn, Bessarab, & Thompson, 2009). Language and culture have been described as protective factors for health because they build resilience and serve as buffers to the negative effects of risks. When health educators use indigenous languages and culture to develop teaching materials, this increases the potential for positively impacting aboriginal peoples' health and wellness (McIvor, Napoleon, & Dickie, 2009). Butow, Tattersall, and Goldstein (1997) highlighted the sensitivities involved in communicating with cancer patients and their families in aboriginal communities. McIvor et al. (2009) concluded that "aboriginal cultures and languages contribute positively to build well being and therefore are positive factors against risks" (p. 19). Models of health education must therefore be culturally friendly to indigenous people to make a difference in their health behaviours.

Determination of the family's sense of burden, ability to cope, and the role of culture is another aspect of the client and family assessment that needs to be taken into consideration when planning individualized educational activities. In a study involving 138 family caregivers of clients with chronic obstructive pulmonary disease, Cain and Wicke (2000) discovered that African American caregivers experienced less burden than their White counterparts. Similar levels of burden occurred in men compared with women and spouse caregivers compared with nonspouse caregivers. In addition, younger caregivers indicated more burden than those aged 55 and older. Although these findings are not generalisable beyond this study, the researchers acknowledge the importance of educators being cognizant of contextual factors such as caregiver burden and age and how these factors may affect other activities such as client and family teaching. **Table 13-2** provides additional resources to facilitate cultural competence with diverse client and family populations.

Gender and Learning Styles

In addition to cultural background, gender and learning styles have a significant influence on the learner's willingness and ability to respond to and apply educational content. Numerous studies have identified gender differences in the structure of the brain and how it functions (Gur et al., 1999; Luders et al., 2008; Witelson, Beresh, & Kigar, 2006). **Table 13-3** provides an overview of basic gender differences that have been identified, but educators are strongly encouraged to individually determine the applicability of these differences to a particular client and family population (Connell & Guzelman, 2004; Gurian & Ballew, 2003; Sax, Bryant, & Harper, 2005).

With the increased usage of online courses and web-based educational materials, research reveals variations in learning styles of online students and students in face-to-face courses (Garland & Martin, 2005). Moreover, these researchers determined that gender is related to learning style and engagement. In their study involving seven online courses and 168 students (102 female and 66 male), there was a significant relationship with regard to male students who favoured an abstract conceptualization mode of learning and how many times they accessed the communication area of Blackboard, an online course management system. Female students, meanwhile, were more highly motivated to perform required class activities than male students. The researchers emphasized that

Table 13-2   Cultural Competence Resources for Client–Family Education
Center for Human Diversity. Provides consulting and training in cultural competence, diversity, and customer service: www.centerforhumandiversity.org
Canadian Public Health Association. Cultural competency: www.cpha.ca/en/activities/safe-schools/culture.aspx
Ontario Volunteer Centre Network. A guide for cultural competency: Application of the Canadian code: www.hhsc.ca/body.cfm?id=1782
Indigenous Cultural Competency Programme: www.culturalcompetency.ca/post-training/resources /federal-resources
National Center for Cultural Competence. Increase the capacity of health and mental health programs to design, implement, and evaluate culturally and linguistically competent service delivery systems (there is also a Spanish version): www11.georgetown.edu/research/gucchd/nccc/
Centre for Addiction and Mental Health. Culture counts: Resources-ethnocultural communities/cultural competence: www.camh.net/About_CAMH/Health_Promotion/Community_Health_Promotion/Culture_ Counts_Guide/culture_counts_ethno_resources.html
Network for Multicultural Health Research on Health and Healthcare: www.multiculturalhealthcare.net/
Hamilton Health Sciences. Building cultural competency in practice: www.hhsc.ca/body.cfm?id=1782
Cultural Human Resources Council: www.culturalhrc.ca/index-e.asp
Working together to end racial and ethnic disparities: One physician at a time. AMA toolkit designed to help physicians eliminate health care disparities: www.ama-assn.org/ama1/pub/upload/mm/433/health_disp_kit .pdf

faculty constructing online courses need to be aware of how discussions, chats, and groups are influenced by gender, while keeping in mind that postings may be intimidating to some female students. Garland and Martin (2005) further stressed the need for additional studies that investigate the relationship between online learning, learning style, and gender as well as the importance of considering gender equity in building and designing online courses and educational programs.

In another study involving an online health-education program, Women-to-Women, Cudney, Sullivan, Winters, Paul, and Orient (2005) were interested in determining issues and solutions in a sample of 50 middle-aged women with cancer, diabetes, multiple sclerosis, or rheumatoid arthritis who lived in rural communities. The problems identified included difficulties carrying out self-management programs, negative fears/feelings, poor communication with HCPs, and disturbed relationships with family and friends. Self-identified solutions pertained to problem-solving techniques that were tailored to their rural lifestyle. Although most women indicated their health promotion problems were not easily solvable, they continued to identify feasible ways to self-manage their chronic illnesses

Table 13-3 Comparison of Brain-Based Learning Differences According to Gender		
	Males	**Females**
Deductive and inductive reasoning	Are more inclined to use deductive thinking	Prefer inductive thinking
Abstract and concrete reasoning	Gravitate to abstract arguments	Perform better with concrete analysis
Language usage	Write, read, and speak but usually less than females; in a group of males one or two tend to dominate	Usually prefer writing, reading, and speaking more words than males
Logic and evidence	Tend to ask for more evidence to support a claim	Tend to be better listeners, more secure in conversation, and require less control of discussion compared with males
Symbolism usage	Respond to pictures with males; more dependent on pictures, diagrams, and graphs in their learning process	Respond to pictures, but not as dependent on pictures, diagrams, and graphs as males to learn

Sources: Connell & Guzelman (2004), Gurian & Ballew (2003), and Sax et al. (2005).

(e.g., small achievable goals, taking one day at a time, taking responsibility for being informed, improving communication with HCPs, being proactive in family relationships, being able to say "no"). Results from this study affirm the importance of performing research to expand the best available evidence to guide our practice.

Just as gender differences need to be assessed, many educators indicate that determination of the individual's learning style is equally important. The presumed method by which an individual learns best is defined as one's learning style. The difficulty is that there are more than 80 learning style models and limited scientific evidence to support any of them (Coffield, Moseley, Hall, & Ecclestone, 2004; Stahl, 2002). Despite the controversy over the presence and quality of the evidence, it is still worthwhile to ask clients and families what approach to learning they prefer (e.g., spoken word, reading, writing, doing, or interacting). With this

information the HCP can then more effectively plan the teaching interventions. Moreover, age, intelligence, motor skills, degree of impairment, anxiety, and past experiences can significantly affect an individual's ability to learn (Rankin et al., 2005). Along with the aforementioned factors, educational activities must be adapted to clients' and families' style of learning and preferences regarding what they need to learn.

Readiness to Learn, Self-Efficacy, and Readiness to Change

Once the learning needs of the client and family are identified, determination of their readiness to learn and self-efficacy are important next steps. Readiness to learn refers to the time when learners are receptive to learning, whereas self-efficacy indicates they have confidence in their capability of attaining a particular goal (Bastable, 2006). For learning to occur, clients and family members must be ready to learn and possess average to high self-efficacy.

Readiness to learn is manifested in a variety of areas such as physical readiness, emotional readiness, experiential readiness, and knowledge readiness. More specifically, physical readiness can be affected by the client's ability to perform the task, the task's complexity, environmental conditions that keep the client's attention and interest, the client's health status, and gender (Bastable, 2006). Research supports that women are more receptive to medical care and less likely to take risks associated with their health compared with men (Bertakis, Rahman, Helms, Callaham, & Robbins, 2000). Emotional readiness to learn, on the other hand, has been demonstrated to be affected by anxiety level, strength of one's support system, motivation, state of mind, and developmental stage (Bastable, 2006). Previous positive as well as negative learning experiences can dramatically affect experiential readiness of clients and family members. Therefore, HCPs planning an educational activity should identify any previous learning successes and failures and prior ways of coping with similar situations and understand the potential influence of culture and human motivation. Finally, readiness to learn new knowledge can be influenced by what the client or family member already knows, their cognitive ability, any learning disabilities, and general learning style (Bastable, 2006; Muijs & Reynolds, 2005; Rankin et al., 2005).

When assessing clients and family members for readiness to learn, self-efficacy must also be determined. In the research literature a strong sense of self-efficacy, confidence in one's ability to achieve a behaviour, has repeatedly been demonstrated to have significant positive influence on accomplishing a health-promoting behaviour

change in individuals with chronic illness (Coleman & Newton, 2005; Osborne, Wilson, Lorig, & McColl, 2007; Tung & Lee, 2006).

Readiness to change is another increasingly familiar term applied to chronic illness and reducing unhealthy behaviours. Although readiness to change has varied definitions, the best known emerges from the transtheoretical model of change (TTM), which involves intentional decision making and was developed to promote effective interventions to facilitate positive behavioural change. TTM is a model that reflects an integration of constructs from other theories and describes how individuals modify problem behaviours such as smoking, limited exercise, and overeating to acquire a more positive behaviour (Prochaska & DiClemente, 1983; Prochaska, DiClemente, & Norcross, 1992; Prochaska & Velicer, 1997). The central organizing construct is stages of change, but the model also includes other variables (e.g., self-efficacy, processes of change, decisional balance, and temptation). TTM focuses on stage-focused interventions pertaining to the individual's readiness to change an unhealthy behaviour (e.g., smoking, limited exercise). Within TTM, there are five stages of readiness to change (i.e., precontemplation, contemplation, preparation, action, and maintenance). Measurement instruments with demonstrated reliability and validity can be obtained at the Cancer Prevention Research Center website (2008).

Developmental Stage

Chronological age provides a basic indication of clients' and family members' projected physical, cognitive, and psychological state of development. When planning a teaching–learning activity for a client and family member, consideration of the clients' or family members' developmental stage is pivotal, along with past learning experiences, stress level, physical and emotional health, personal motivation, environmental conditions, and available support systems (Bastable, 2006).

Within the literature there are several prominent developmental theorists who have shaped how HCPs view life stages (Erikson, 1968; Piaget, 1951, 1976). In contrast with childhood, where learning is student centred, adult learning tends to be more problem centred, with the primary emphasis on how to apply new knowledge and skills to immediate problems (Bastable, 2006). Adults tend to be more resistant to change, which is why establishing mutual goals and an action plan with HCPs markedly improves the achievement of educational outcomes (Miller, 2003; Rankin et al., 2005).

Table 13-4 provides a brief overview of the developmental stages of adults, the major attributes of the learner, and the most applicable teaching strategies. A common misconception is that older adults cannot learn. Older adults who are provided information at a slower rate, taught relevant material, and provided with positive feedback are very capable of learning new knowledge and skills (Bastable, 2006; Mauk, 2010). Because depression, grief, and loneliness are not restricted to older adults, these factors can markedly affect any client's or family members' ability to concentrate on content being presented. HCPs, moreover, must be continually aware of other potential cognitive as well as physical limitations (i.e., pain, fatigue, diminished vision, reduced hearing) that can affect the ability of clients and family members to learn. **Table 13-5** provides a listing of recommended resources for HCPs to identify how to optimally structure and evaluate educational activities involving older adults.

Literacy

Low levels of health literacy are prevalent even in most Western countries (Begoray & Kwan, 2011), and this has been associated with negative health outcomes. The Canadian Council on Learning (2007) reported that the majority of adult Canadians (60%) do not have the necessary skills to manage their health adequately. Throughout the entire healthcare delivery process, low literacy levels can affect the ability of clients and family members to read and comprehend health information (e.g., discharge instructions, labels on prescription bottles), which serves as an important prerequisite to adherence and overall successful client outcomes (Bastable, 2006; Lasater & Mehler, 1998; Nielson-Bohlman, Panzer, & Kindig, 2004). A variety of measurement tools is available to HCPs to assess the readability of written educational materials as well as reading capability of clients and family members. **Table 13-6** provides a brief description of several tools that have proved useful.

SYSTEM FACTORS THAT INFLUENCE THE TEACHING AND LEARNING PROCESS

To ensure an optimal client, family, and HCP educational situation, certain elements need to be in place. The following system factors can significantly contribute to positive educational outcomes (Edwardson, 2007; Nobel, 2006; Rankin et al., 2005):

- Preparation of the HCP in terms of knowledge of the educational content and teaching capabilities
- Cultural competence and knowledge related to all other factors that help to personalize

Table 13-4   Linking Developmental Stage with Learner Characteristics and Teaching Strategies

Developmental Stage	Learner Characteristics	Recommended Teaching Strategies
Young adulthood (18–39.9 years)	Peak body function	Immediate application
	Self-directive	Active participation
	Independent in learning	Learning needs to be convenient, self-paced, and blend of visual and written
	Making decisions about career, education, social roles	Tend to like group interaction
	Competency-based learner	Organized materials and presentation
	If has a chronic illness, tends to want to learn as much as possible to remain independent and lead as normal a life as possible	Use past experiences as a resource for learning
		Provide practical answers to their problems
		Give opportunity for immediate application of teaching
		Seek credible/evidence-informed information
Middle age (40–64.9 years)	Well-developed sense of self	Maintain independence and perhaps reestablish what constitutes normal life patterns
	Usually at career peak	Assess prior positive and negative learning experiences
	Concerned about physical changes	Identify potential stressors
	Reexamines goals and values	Provide information that fits to life problems and/or concerns; use past experiences as a resource for learning
	Confident in abilities	
	Tends to want to reduce unsatisfying aspects in life	Provide practical answers to their problems
	May be experiencing midlife crises	Give opportunity for immediate application of teaching
Older adult (65 years and older)	Cognitive changes	Use concrete examples
	Decreased ability to think abstractly	Build on past experiences
		Make information relevant
	Reduced short-term memory	Allow time for processing and responses
	Increased reaction time	Use verbal interactions and coaching
	Focus on past life experiences	Encourage active involvement
	Motor and sensory losses	Keep explanations brief (20–40 min)
	Auditory and visual changes	Speak distinctly and slowly
	Hearing loss especially with high-pitched tones, consonants, and rapid speech	Minimize distractions while teaching
		Avoid shouting—if large group, microphone may be needed
	Decreased peripheral vision	Use large font in handouts
	Decreased risk taking	Avoid glares
		Provide a safe environment
		Keep teaching sessions short
		Provide rest periods
		Rooms where conducted should be neutral temperature (not too hot or cold)

Sources: Bastable (2006), Mauk (2006), and Rankin et al. (2005).

Table 13-5 Helpful Resources to Facilitate Teaching and Learning of Older Adults	
Organization	**Website**
Active Living Coalition for Older Adults	www.alcoa.ca
Association for Gerontology in Higher Education	www.aghe.org
The John A. Hartford Foundation Institute for Geriatric Nursing	www.hartfordign.org
Info for Seniors	www.seniorsinfo.ca
Canadian Association on Gerontology	www. cagacg.ca
National Council on Aging	www.ncoa.org
Osher Lifelong Learning Institute	www.olli.gmu.edu

the educational approach (i.e., age, developmental stage, and cognitive and physical status related to the chronic illness)

- Required resources for effective teaching (e.g., equipment/technology, materials—booklets, figures)
- Time limitations that permit updating teaching plans, evaluation tools, and developing/updating educational protocols
- Coordinating educational activities that are consistent with discharge plans and other important client and family information that needs to be communicated
- Succinct and timely documentation of what was taught, when, and the outcome, so others can build on and reinforce prior teaching
- If client and family education is not valued by the system and rewards are not given for educational excellence and positive outcomes
- If there is inadequate record-keeping and reimbursement policies that reimburse fully for direct, hands-on illness interventions, but poorly for client/family education and interventions via telephone and computer

The following strategies (Bastable, 2006; Falvo, 2011; Mayer & Vallaire, 2007; Petty, 2006) may serve as a starting point when assessing and educating clients and families with low literacy:

- Materials should not be above 5th-grade level and should be culturally appropriate.
- Keep sentences short and limited to 20 words or fewer if possible.
- Speak and write using short words with only one or two syllables whenever possible. Rely on common words that are easily recognized by most individuals.
- Put the most important information first and limit focus on what the client and family member need to know.
- Clearly and simply define technical words or ones that are unfamiliar (e.g., *fasting blood glucose, hypertension*) or replace with simpler words (*high blood pressure* for *hypertension*).
- Remember that those with low literacy skills may require more time to read and absorb the materials.

Table 13-6   Tools to Access Readability of Educational Materials and Individuals' Reading Comprehension

Measurement Tools to Assess Readability of Educational Materials	**Measurement Tools to Assess an Individual's Reading Comprehension**
Flesch formula	*Wide Range Achievement Test (WRAT)*
In use more than 70 years to assess news reports, adult educational materials, and government publications. Based on a count of two basic language components: average sentence length in words and average word length measured in syllables per word of selected samples of text (Flesch, 1948; Spadero, 1983). Helpful web sources to assist with these calculations are www.readabilityformulas.com /flesch-reading-ease-readability-formula.php and www.csun.edu/~vcecn006/read1.htm	WRAT is a word-recognition screening test that typically takes about 5 min to complete. It assesses the client's ability to recognize and pronounce a list of words out of context to determine reading skills. It has two levels of testing: Level 1 is for children 5–12 years; Level 2 is for individuals older than 12 years of age (Doak, Doak, & Root, 1996). Helpful web source is www4.parinc.com /Products/Product.aspx?ProductID=WRAT4
Fog formula	*Rapid Estimate of Adult Literacy in Medicine (REALM)*
Assesses the reading level of materials from 4th grade to college level. One of the easier tools to use with the calculation based on the average sentence length and percentage of multisyllabic words based on a sample of 100 words (Bastable, 2006; Spadero, 1983). Helpful web sources are www.readabilityformulas.com /gunning-fog-readability-formula.php and www.thelearningweb.net/fogindex.html	The REALM tests the client's ability to read medical and health-related vocabulary (advantage over the WRAT), takes less time, and has easy scoring (Duffy & Snyder, 1999). Although the test has validity, it offers less precision and reliability than other word tests (Hayes, 2000). Sixty-six medical and health-related words are placed in three columns ranging from short and easy to more difficult. Clients are to begin reading the words from the top and go down. The total number of correctly pronounced words is the raw score that is then converted to a grade range (Doak et al., 1996). Helpful web source is Faculty-Development/MediaLibraries /Faculty-Development/Media/PDF/The-REALM-Test- (Hazen-3-07-07).pdf
SMOG formula	*Test of Functional Health Literacy in Adults (TOFHL)*
This formula has been used primarily to evaluate the grade-level readability of patient educational materials and can measure reading level with as little content as 10 sentences. This formula determines readability from grades 4 to college level and is based on number of multisyllable words (3 or more) within a set number of sentences (McLaughlin, 1969). Helpful web source is www.readabilityformulas.com /smog-readability-formula.php	TOFHL is a newer measurement tool to assess clients' literacy skills and actually uses hospital materials (i.e., appointment slips, informed consent documents, and prescription labels). The test consists of two parts: reading comprehension and numeracy (Bastable, 2006). It has demonstrated validity and reliability, takes approximately 20 min to administer, and has an English and Spanish version (Quirk, 2000). Helpful web source is education.gsu.edu/csal/TOFHLA.htm

- Visual presentation (a picture is worth a thousand words) can be especially helpful to someone with low literacy skills.
- Avoid abbreviations.
- Use consistent words throughout the presentation (e.g., don't switch from "diet" to "menu" to "dietary prescription").
- Organize information into "chunks" that facilitate recall. Use numbers only when necessary and realize that statistics are usually confusing and meaningless for the low-literate client and family member.
- Keep the number of items in a list to no more than seven.
- Keep teaching sessions short and preferably no longer than 10 to 15 minutes.
- Use the teach-back method with clients to ensure they understand their care routine and warning signs if there is a problem (i.e., signs of a wound infection or urinary tract infection, signs of a stroke or heart attack—not myocardial infarction). Never ask, "Do you understand?" Ask the patient to explain the processes or state the signs of an infection, stroke, or heart attack. These perception checks are an important part of the teaching–learning process and enable the HCP to assess whether learning is occurring as planned. Plus, these perception checks allow the HCP to redirect his or her activities if the client and/or family educational outcomes are not being achieved as planned.
- Have your written materials reviewed by a literacy expert to determine the grade reading level. Also, ask the client and family member a question to determine their specific ability to read and comprehend what is described. In addition, do not assume that the teaching materials address all client and/or family concerns. Ask if there is something missing or whether they have questions about anything that is not included in the materials provided. Remember too that blending written materials combined with auditory interactions enhances learning and retention of information.
- Present information one step at a time to pace instruction and allow clients and family members to understand each step and ask questions before moving on to the next step.

In conjunction with the system challenges just identified, HCPs must also consider other diverse attributes (i.e., age, gender, culture, developmental stage, literacy, and functional status) that make each client and family educational encounter unique. In addition, what is the best available evidence that will help shape these interventions? Townsend, Bruce, Hooten, and Rome (2006) also assert that HCPs do not always recognize the tensions and ambiguities permeating clients' experiences, particularly those who have multiple chronic illnesses. Results of this research revealed that clients with chronic illness use multiple techniques to manage their symptoms and frequently felt pressure to manage "well" and have a "normal life" for both their families and HCPs.

Despite the limited strong evidence to support all aspects of HCPs' educational interventions, the research continues to expand as do the meta-analyses and systematic reviews that synthesize the evidence and identify additional areas to be explored. To more comprehensively document the specific contribution of nursing to the education and self-care of clients with chronic illness. Edwardson (2007) recommended two focus areas for research. The first is to measure the outcomes of client and family education and have this information included in both the clinical and administrative databases. Secondly, whenever possible, the client and family educational process and outcomes should be separated according to type of education, objectives, timing, dose (i.e., strategies, length), and so forth. In addition, systematic reviews and meta-analysis suggest that inpatient education followed by some form of post-discharge intervention may be the most promising approach to reduce hospitalizations (Gonseth, Castillion, Banegas, & Artalejo, 2004). However, for this care system to succeed, databases from ambulatory care, acute care, and after-care services need to be linked to monitor symptoms, monitor adherence to treatment prescription, and modify treatment plans as needed (Edwardson, 2007).

EDUCATIONAL INTERVENTIONS FOR THE CLIENT AND FAMILY _____

As indicated earlier, multiple factors should be carefully assessed and considered in the development of an educational plan for clients with chronic illness and their families. Because of the variance in how these elements manifest, the mutually established goals by the client, family, and HCP; associated interventions; and outcomes will need to be uniquely planned, implemented, and evaluated. In most instances nurses are the principal HCP who participates in this ongoing educational process and provides the continuity of care for clients with chronic illness and their families.

Development of the Teaching Plan

The teaching plan provides the overall blueprint or outline for instruction that clearly defines the relationship among the behavioural objectives, instructional content, teaching strategies, timeframe for teaching, and methods of evaluation (Bastable, 2006). All aspects work together to achieve a predetermined goal that should be mutually agreed on by the client and family and HCP. The domains of learning that are to be accomplished divide into one of three domains: cognitive (knowledge), psychomotor (physical activities), and affective (attitudes or emotions). When constructing teaching plans to address these learning domains for specific chronic illnesses, HCPs should also refer to published practice standards such as those from the Agency for Healthcare Research and Quality, specialty nursing groups, and the Heart and Stroke Foundation, which present evidence-informed guidelines. The specific teaching plan includes the following aspects: purpose of the teaching plan, goal(s), broad statement of what is to be achieved, objective(s) that need to be specific and measurable, content covered to achieve each objective, teaching strategies, time required, and evaluation methods to determine if the learning has occurred. Key aspects of the teaching plan are described, followed by a specific example.

Teaching Strategies

Knowing how to use varied teaching strategies to achieve educational objectives can make client and family education more interesting, challenging, and effective for HCPs and learners (Rankin et al., 2005). A general overview of common teaching strategies and their predominant characteristics is presented in **Table 13-7.** For the client with chronic illness, the research strongly supports that combining multiple teaching methods during several educational sessions consistently produces more positive client outcomes than single teaching methods and events (Bastable, 2006; Beranova & Sykes, 2007; Edwardson, 2007; Joanna Briggs Institute, 2006). However, the HCP must also remain

Table 13-7　General Overview of Common Teaching Strategies

Teaching Strategy	Learning Domain	Learner Role	Teacher Role	Strength	Weakness
Lecture	Cognitive	Passive	Presents information	Cost effective; targeted to larger groups	Not individualised
Group discussion	Cognitive; affective	Active, if learner participates	Directs and focuses discussion	Share emotions and ideas	Shy or dominant members affect participation; may lose focus
One-to-one teaching	Cognitive; affective; psychomotor	Active	Presents information and encourages individualised learning	Tailored to client's or family member's needs and goals	Great diversity; labour intensive; learner isolated
Demonstration	Cognitive	Passive	Modelling of skill or behaviour	Preview of skill or behaviour, can ask questions	Need individual or small group to visualize
Return demonstration	Psychomotor	Active	Individualised feedback to refine skill performance	Immediate feedback	Labour intensive; anxiety may affect actions
Gaming	Cognitive; affective	Active, if client–family participates	Oversees pacing; debriefs	Stimulates learners' enthusiasm and participation	May be too competitive; over-stimulating
Simulation	Cognitive; psychomotor	Active	Designs situation; facilitates learning; debriefs	Practice a reality situation in a safe setting	Labour intensive; equipment costs/access; scheduling issues
Online learning	Cognitive; affective	Passive, but can be active if participates in group discussions, problem solving, group projects	Usually designs program/ class; presents information; provides active learning exercises, discussions, case studies, and group projects	Learners usually at a distance; flexibility when access learning content and activities; learners need to be motivated; feedback provided is usually individualised and immediate	Need equipment to access; lack of personal contact; accessibility; all feedback may not be instantaneous
Computer-assisted instruction	Cognitive; affective	Active	Purchases or designs program; expected to provide feedback to student	Individualised instruction; learner controls pace of the learning; can program to receive feedback; valuable modality if hearing impaired, learning disability, or aphasic	Must have equipment and software

Sources: Bastable (2006), Miller (2010), and Wantland, Portillo, Holzemer, & Slaughter (2004).

cognizant of the system factors contributing to the success and/or failure of the teaching and learning process.

A pivotal aspect of any client and family teaching event is preparing measurable objectives that can be achieved in the timeframe specified. For example, the client with diabetes may need to learn the signs and symptoms of a hypoglycemic reaction. An appropriate measurable objective could be "Ms. Jones will state four signs/symptoms of a hypoglycemic reaction by the end of this 12-hour shift."

Increasingly, more clients with chronic illness and their family members are receiving education regarding disease management from web-based sources, with the young to middle aged being the biggest consumers (Beranova & Sykes, 2007; Lee, Yeh, Liu, & Chen, 2007). Research from a new survey published by the Pew Research Center's Internet and American Life Project and the California Healthcare Foundation found that 80% of Internet users look online for health information, making it the third most popular online pursuit after email and using a search engine (Fox, 2011). For clients with chronic illness, the use of the Internet provides a means to encourage behaviour change necessitating knowledge sharing, education, and greater understanding of their condition. Results of a meta-analysis comparing web-based and non–web-based education of chronically ill adults (mean age, 41.2 years) from 1996 to 2003 revealed substantial evidence that web-based interventions improved behavioural change outcomes (Wantland et al., 2004). The specific positive outcomes identified were increased knowledge of nutritional status, increased knowledge of asthma treatment, increased exercise time, slower health decline, and 18-month weight-loss maintenance. Web-based interventions that were relevant and individually tailored had more and longer website visits. Wantland and associates further discovered that sites with chat rooms increased social support scores of the users. They cautioned, however, that the long-term effects on individual persistence with the chosen therapies and the cost effectiveness of the web-based therapies and hardware and software development demand ongoing evaluation.

Learning Curve

Whenever a learner is acquiring knowledge, an attitudinal change, or motor skill, there is a learning curve (Bastable, 2006). Typically, individual learning curves are irregular, with fluctuations attributed to changes in the learner such as attention, energy, ability, or situational factors (Gage & Berliner, 1998). In the case of clients with chronic illness, learning to walk again after a stroke may take time and create frustration, as expectations do not match physical capability. Because learning may not always occur in a linear fashion, HCPs must recognize this and assist clients and their families when they experience anger, discouragement, or depression associated with achievement not progressing as anticipated. In addition, research supports that retention of learning is enhanced when there are opportunities to see, hear, observe demonstrations, discuss, and practice as well as teach others (Bastable, 2006; Muijs & Reynolds, 2005; Petty, 2006).

Evaluation

Evaluation of educational outcomes is a critical step in the teaching and learning process. It encompasses a systematic and continuous activity that involves collecting and using information to determine whether the educational objectives have been achieved. This outcome evaluation is labelled summative evaluation, but there can also be formative evaluation. Formative evaluation occurs during the actual teaching process when the implementation is still in process. Formative evaluation permits the HCP to adjust or change aspects of the implementation process that may improve the quality or delivery of the educational program or session. For instance, the HCP may decide to use a web-based program and face-to-face demonstration of a task to clients and their families. On the basis of immediate negative feedback received regarding a client's unfamiliarity with computers and reluctance to use such a program, the HCP may decide to replace the web-based education with a small group discussion involving the client and family.

When performing any type of evaluation, it is also important to identify what outcome is being measured, how and when the data will be collected, and then how data will be interpreted. For example, assume the HCP and client have established the following outcome objective: "Client will state three signs/symptoms of hypoglycemia by the end of a 12-hour shift." Determination of achievement for this objective is straightforward. Yet, sometimes barriers occur that hinder the evaluation process, such as lack of clarity regarding what is being evaluated, lack of ability to perform the evaluation, and, finally, fear of punishment or low self-esteem (Bastable, 2006). With regard to lack of ability, the HCP may not know how to construct a short test to determine if the client and family have a basic understanding of diabetes or feel comfortable orally quizzing them to assess their learning. In other situations clients may be too ill to learn the information, how to perform a new task, or respond as they anticipate the HCP wants them to.

In many settings practice guidelines or protocols identify how formative and summative evaluations are to be conducted and what information needs to be documented. Data from the evaluation process, especially as they apply to the teaching and learning process for the client and family, can be extremely valuable as the chronic illness progresses and additional knowledge, attitudinal, and psychomotor skills need to be developed.

Example of a Teaching Plan

This teaching plan shown in **Table 13-8** was developed in accordance with the following case situation. You have a newly diagnosed client with diabetes who is going to be discharged in the next 48 hours. The client is a 24-year-old White man who is single and lives alone. He is currently working as a cashier at a grocery store but wants to go to college. He also tells you that his parents live about 2 hours away and are concerned about him, but they work full-time and called once while he was in the hospital. Given that you are his primary care nurse, you need to make sure the four objectives presented in Table 13-8 are accomplished.

The specific approach to this client considers such elements as gender, culture, learning curve, importance of feedback, and reinforcement. Given the content and objectives of this specific teaching plan, it is recommended that *not all* of this teaching occur at the same time. The teaching plan pertaining to the first three objectives could be performed, and then teaching of the fourth objective could occur later in the day. During this second educational session, review the key points associated with the first teaching episode. Furthermore, make sure that each teaching session is not interrupted and that there is adequate time to permit questions from the client and family, who should also be present if at all possible.

Table 13-8   Sample Teaching Plan

Objectives	Content (Topics)	Time Frame	Teaching Strategy	Evaluation Method
The client will be able to	a. Definition of hypoglycemia compared with hyperglycemia	5 min	One-to-one teaching presentation.	Use several vignettes and then ask client to identify signs and symptoms of each from a list. Need 100% correct response.
1. Distinguish the signs and symptoms of hypoglycemia from hyperglycemia.	b. Signs of hypoglycemia c. Signs of hyperglycemia		Visual materials: poster listing signs and symptoms of hypoglycemia and hyperglycemia, booklet to keep.	
Cognitive domain of learning	d. Actions to take when each is present		If client has difficulty getting the content correct, repeat teaching as well as discuss other strategies that may facilitate retention of the information.	Ask immediate action when each is present. Must get all correct.
2. Demonstrate ability to correctly perform a finger stick and reading of glucose level.	a. Purpose of client glucose self-monitoring b. Key aspects in the correct performance of a finger stick and accurate reading of the results	20 min	One-to-one teaching presentation. Provide a demonstration of the correct technique. Then, have client perform the finger stick and interpretation of results. Nurse provides feedback, reinforcement of behaviours, and may have client do this again if needed. May have online or hospital TV channel available so that client can review this again.	Client correctly performs the finger stick and glucose interpretation. Have a video of incorrect performance of this skill or nurse incorrectly do and client identify incorrect elements performed.
Psychomotor domain of learning				
3. Verbalize confidence in performing key elements in glucose monitoring.	a. Importance of daily monitoring of blood glucose in the continued management of diabetes	2 min	One-to-one teaching and blend brief discussion, reinforcement, and feedback.	Have rate on a scale of 0 = no confidence to 10 = complete confidence in performing daily glucose monitoring.
Affective domain of learning	b. Accountability and self-monitoring associated with a chronic disease			

(continues)

Table 13-8 Sample Teaching Plan *(continued)*

Objectives	Content (Topics)	Time Frame	Teaching Strategy	Evaluation Method
4. State purpose, dose, time to take, and side effects of single medications prescribed at discharge. *Cognitive domain of learning* During the second interaction when this fourth objective is the focus, assess the client's retention of the correct information associated with objectives 1–3.	Medication prescribed—including purpose, dose, time to take, side effects, and other considerations	10 min	One-to-one teaching, poster, or other written materials to provide a blend of visual and auditory information is advisable. Determine if the client has any questions since receiving instruction pertaining to objectives 1–3.	Orally and/or on paper list the medication's purpose, dose, time to take, prominent side effects, and other considerations. Assess knowledge, actions, and attitudes pertaining to objectives 1–3 with the same evaluation standard as in the first encounter.

SUMMARY

Education serves as an essential vehicle to provide the client and family with the knowledge, skills, and confidence to address the many facets associated with living with a chronic illness. Although numerous factors contribute to the success or failure of this educational process, HCPs and nurses in particular play a fundamental role as part of their scope of practice and other national standards.

Research evidence continues to expand and guides the assessment of all learners, teaching plan development, and ultimate educational outcomes. Teaching and learning is a complex process and requires consideration of many elements such as family structure and function, culture, gender, learning styles, readiness to learn/change, self-efficacy, developmental stage, literacy, socioeconomic status, resources, and learning capability. In addition, as HCPs partner with clients and their families during this educational process, it is critical that the HCPs assess their educational objectives and redirect their actions when needed. Because well over 50% of the Canadian adult population has at least one chronic illness, the teaching and learning process is paramount to attaining greater quality of life and adapting to the frequently dynamic nature of most chronic diseases.

Another central ingredient that is sometimes overlooked is the mutual goal setting that occurs among the client, family, and HCP. Working together, clients are much more inclined to achieve the planned educational objectives whether targeted at knowledge, attitudes, and/or behaviours pertaining to the chronic health problem.

Evidence-Informed Practice Box

Purpose and background: Client education is an important intervention in the management of heart disease. This article is a systematic review of the literature that examined the educational interventions implemented for clients with heart failure that assessed their related outcomes.

Methods: Randomized control trials from 1998 to 2008 in CINAHL, MEDLINE, EMBASE, PsychINFO, and the Cochrane Library were reviewed with the search terms: *patient education, educational intervention, self-care* in combination with *heart failure*. Two reviewers independently examined 1,515 abstracts.

Results: A total of 2,686 patients in 19 studies met the inclusion criteria for this literature review. The initial intervention for all reported studies was typically a one-to-one educational intervention. Seven of these studies had a theoretical framework for their educational intervention. Of the studies reviewed, 15 revealed the educational intervention had a significant positive outcome on at least one of the desired outcomes.

Conclusions: Even though there were improvements in educational outcomes, the study samples varied considerably. As a result it was difficult in this systematic review to determine the most effective educational strategy because of the variance in delivery methods, duration of the interventions, and the outcomes evaluated. A client-centred approach to education based on an educational theory and evaluated consistently with that framework is recommended.

Source: Boyde, Turner, Thompson, & Stewart (2010).

STUDY QUESTIONS

1. What are the pros and cons of three teaching strategies that can be used to educate an individual with a chronic illness?
2. What is the difference between pedagogy and andragogy and what affect does it have on your approach to teaching?
3. What are major factors that should be considered when planning an educational session for a client with chronic illness?
4. How may the approach of an educational intervention differ if the client is a man compared with a woman?
5. How may cultural and ethnic/race differences specifically affect how you structure and evaluate the outcomes of a specific educational intervention?
6. How would you specifically assess the literacy of a client and his or her family?
7. What is the difference between a formative and summative evaluation?
8. What level of evidence provides the greatest confidence in the applicability of research findings to practice?

For a full suite of assignments and additional learning activities, use the access code located in the front of your book and visit this exclusive website: **http://go.jblearning.com/kramer-kile**. If you do not have an access code, you can obtain one at the site.

REFERENCES

Bandura, A. (1986). *Social foundations of thought and action: A social cognitive theory.* Englewood Cliffs, NJ: Prentice Hall.

Bastable, S. B. (2006). *Essentials of patient education.* Sudbury, MA: Jones & Bartlett.

Begoray, C. D., & Kwan, B. (2011). A Canadian exploratory study to define a measure of health literacy. *Health Promotion International, 27*(1), 23–32.

Beranova, E., & Sykes, C. (2007). A systematic review of computer based software for educating patients with coronary heart disease. *Patient Education and Counseling, 66*(1), 21–28.

Bertakis, K., Rahman, A., Helms, L. J., Callaham, E., & Robbins, J. (2000). Gender differences in the utilization of health care services. *Journal of Family Practice, 49*(2), 147–152.

Boren, S., Balas, E., & Mustafa, Z. (2003). Evidence-based patient education for chronic care. *Abstract Academy Health Meeting, 20*(788). Retrieved from http://gateway.nlm.nih.gov/MeetingAbstracts/102275756.html

Boyde, M., Turner, D., Thompson, D. R., & Stewart, S. (2010). Educational interventions for patients with heart failure: A systematic review of randomized controlled trials. *Journal of Cardiovascular Nursing, 26*(4), E27–E35.

Butow, P. N., Tattersall, M. H., & Goldstein, D. (1997). Communication with cancer patients in culturally diverse societies. *Annals of the New York Academy of Sciences, 806,* 317–329.

Cain, C. J., & Wicke, M. N. (2000). Caregiving attributes as correlates of burden in family caregivers coping with chronic obstructive pulmonary disease. *Journal of Family Nursing, 6*(1), 46–68.

Canadian Council on Learning. (2007) *Health literacy in Canada: Initial results from the international adult literacy and skills survey.* Retrieved from http://www.ccl-cca.ca/pdfs/HealthLiteracy/HealthLiteracyinCanada.pdf

Cancer Prevention Research Center. (2008). *Measures.* Retrieved from http://www.uri.edu/research/cprc/measures.htm

Coffield, F., Moseley, D., Hall, E., & Ecclestone, K. (2004). *Learning styles and pedagogy in post-16 learning: A systematic and critical review.* Retrieved from http://www.pedagogy.ir/images/pdf/learning-styles-pedagogy.pdf

Coleman, M., & Newton, K. (2005). Supporting self-management in patients with chronic illness. *American Family Physician, 72*(8), 1503–1510.

Connell, D., & Guzelman, B. (2004). *The new gender gap: Why are so many boys floundering while so many girls are soaring?* Retrieved from http://teacher.scholastic.com/products/instructor/Mar04_gendergap.htm#bio

Conner, M. L. (2005). Andragogy and pedagogy. *Ageless Learner, 1997–2004.* Retrieved from http://agelesslearner.com/intros/andragogy.html

Cooney, C. (1994). A comparative analysis of transcultural nursing and cultural safety. *Nursing Praxis in New Zealand, 9*(1), 6–11.

Craig, J. V., & Smyth, R. L. (2002). *The evidence-based practice manual for nurses.* New York, NY: Churchill Livingstone.

Cudney, S., Sullivan, T., Winters, C., Paul, L., & Orient, P. (2005). Chronically ill rural women: Self-identified management problems and solutions. *Chronic Illness, 1,* 49–60.

Curcani, M., & Tan, M. (2011). Effect of the education given to the patients undergone kidney transplantation in the life quality and compliance to treatment and anxiety levels and depression levels. *Health Medicine, 5*(4), 753–758.

Doak, C. C., Doak, L. G., & Root, J. H. (1996). *Teaching patients with low literacy skills* (2nd ed.). Philadelphia, PA: Lippincott.

Duffy, M. M., & Snyder, K. (1999). Can ED patients read your patient education materials? *Journal of Emergency Nursing, 25*(25), 294–297.

Edwardson, S. (2007). Patient education in heart failure. *Heart and Lung: Journal of Critical Care, 36(*4), 244–252.

Erikson, E. H. (1968). *Identity: Youth and crisis.* New York, NY: Norton.

Falvo, D. R. (2011). *Effective patient education: A guide to increased adherence* (2nd ed.). Sudbury, MA; Jones & Bartlett.

Flesch, R. (1948). A new readability yardstick. *Journal of Applied Psychology, 32*(3), 221–233.

Fox, S. (Pew Internet Project and California Healthcare Foundation). (2011). *Health topics.* Retrieved from http://www.pewinternet.org/Reports/2011/HealthTopics.aspx

Gage, N. L., & Berliner, D. C. (1998). *Educational psychology* (6th ed.). Boston, MA: Houghton Mifflin.

Gao, Y., Li, Y., Zheng, J., Wang, R., Meng, H., Zhang, L., Jin, Y., Wang, S., & Li, R. (2011). The effects of a comprehensive health education program in Chinese patients after percutanous coronary intervention. *Institute of Integrative Omics and Applied Biotechnology Journal, 2*(7), 23–30.

Garland, D., & Martin, B. (2005). Do gender and learning style play a role in how online courses should be designed? *Journal of Interactive Online Learning, 4*(2), 67–81.

Gonseth, J., Castillion, G. P., Banegas, J. R., & Artalejo, F. R. (2004). The effectiveness of disease management programmes in reducing hospital re-admission in older adults with heart failure: A systematic review and meta-analysis of published reports. *European Heart Journal, 25*(18), 1570–1590.

Gremeaux, V., & Coudeyre, E. (2010). The Internet and therapeutic education in patients: A systematic review of the literature. *Annals of Physical and Rehabilitation Medicine, 53*(10), 669–692.

Gur, R. C., Turetsky, B., Matsui, M., Yan, M., Bilker, W., Hughett, P., Gur, R. E. (1999). Sex differences in brain gray and white matter in healthy young adults: Correlations with cognitive performance. *Journal of Neuroscience, 19*(10), 4065–4075

Gurian, M., & Ballew, A. C. (2003). *The boys and girls learn differently: Action guide for teachers.* San Francisco, CA: Jossey-Bass.

Haggard, A. (1989). *Handbook of patient education.* Rockville, MD: Aspen.

Hatcher, E., & Whittemore, R. (2007). Hispanic adults' beliefs about type 2 diabetes: Clinical implications. *Journal of the American Academy of Nurse Practitioners, 19*(10), 536–545.

Hayes, K. S. (2000). Literacy for health information of adult patients and caregivers in a rural emergency department. *Clinical Excellence for Nurse Practitioners, 4*, 35–40.

Hein, G. E. (1991). *Constructivist learning theory. Institute of inquiry.* Retrieved from http://www.exploratorium.edu/ifi/resources/constructivistlearning.html

Joanna Briggs Institute. (2006). Educational interventions for mental health consumers receiving psychotropic medication. *Best Practice, 10*(4), 1–4.

Knowles, M. (1998). *The adult learner: The definitive classic in adult education and human resource development.* Houston, TX: Gulf Publishing.

Kreuter, M., Steger-May, K., Bobra, S., Booker, A., Holt, C., Lukwago, S., & Sugg Skinner, C. (2003). Sociocultural characteristics and responses to cancer education materials among African American women.

Cancer Control: Journal of the Moffitt Cancer Center, 10(5), 69–80.

Lasater, L., & Mehler, P. S. (1998). The literate patient: Screening and management. *Hospital Practice, 33*(4), 163–165, 169–170.

Learning Theories Knowledge Base. (2011). *Constructivism at learning-theories.com.* Retrieved from http://www.learning-theories/constructivism.com

Lee, T., Yeh, Y., Liu, C., & Chen, P. (2007). Development and evaluation of a patient-oriented education system for diabetes management. *International Journal of Medical Informatics, 76*, 655–663.

Luders, E., Narr, K., Bilder, R., Szeszko, P., Gurbani, M., Hamilton, A., . . . Gaser, C. (2008). Mapping the relationship between cortical convolution and intelligence: Effects of gender. *Cerebral Cortex, 18*(9), 2019–2026.

Mauk, K. L. (Ed.). (2010). *Gerontological nursing: Competencies for care* (2nd ed.). Sudbury, MA: Jones & Bartlett.

Mayer, G. G., & Vallaire, M. (2007). *Health literacy in primary care: A clinician's guide.* New York, NY: Springer.

McIvor, O., Napoleon, A., & Dickie, K. M. (2009). Language and culture as protective factors for at risk communities. *Journal of Aboriginal Health, 1*(5), 6–26.

McLaughlin, G. H. (1969). SMOG-grading: A new readability formula. *Journal of Reading, 12*, 639–646.

Melnyk, B. M., & Fineout-Overholt, E. (2010). *Evidence-based practice in nursing and healthcare* (2nd ed.). Philadelphia, PA: Lippincott.

Mihall, J., & Belletti, J. (1999). Adult learning styles and training methods. *FDIC ADR presentation handouts.* Retrieved from http://justice.gov/adr/workplace/pdf/learstyl.pdf

Miller, E. (2003). Readiness to change and brief educational interventions: Successful strategies to reduce stroke risk. *Journal of Neuroscience Nursing, 35*(4), 215–222.

Muijs, D., & Reynolds, D. (2005). *Effective teaching: Evidence and practice* (2nd ed.). Thousand Oaks, CA: Sage.

Nielson-Bohlman, L., Panzer, A. M., & Kindig, D. A. (2004). *Health literacy: A prescription to end confusion.* Washington, DC: National Academies Press.

Nightingale, F. (1860). *Notes on nursing: What it is and what it is not.* New York, NY: D. Appleton and Co.

Nobel, J. (2006). Bridging the knowledge–action gap in diabetes: Information technologies, physician incentives and consumer incentives converge. *Chronic Illness, 2*, 59–69.

Osborne, R., Wilson, T., Lorig, K., & McColl, G. (2007). Does self-management lead to sustainable health benefits in people with arthritis? A 2-year transition study with 452 Australians. *Journal of Rheumatology, 34*(5), 1112–1117.

Partnership to Fight Chronic Disease. (2010). *An unhealthy truth: Rising rates of chronic disease and the future of health care in America.* Retrieved from http://www.caaccess.org/pdf/6_unhealthy_truths .pdf

Peterson, S., Soncar, B., Sherman-Slate, E., & Luna, L. (2004). The social construction of beliefs about cancer: A conceptual discourse analysis of racial differences in the popular press. *Journal of Applied Behavioural Research, 9,* 201–229.

Petty, G. (2006). *Evidence based teaching: A practical approach.* United Kingdom: Nelson Thornes.

Piaget, J. (1951). *The origin of intelligence in children.* New York, NY: International Universities Press.

Piaget, J. (1976). *Behavior and evolution.* Richmond, CA: McCutchen Publishing.

Prochaska, J. O., & DiClemente, C. C. (1983). Stages and processes of self-change of smoking: Toward an integrative model of change. *Journal of Consulting and Clinical Psychology, 51,* 390–395.

Prochaska, J. O., DiClemente, C. C., & Norcross, J. C. (1992). In search of how people change: Applications to addictive behavior. *American Psychology, 47*(9), 1102–1114.

Prochaska, J. O., & Velicer, W. F. (1997). The Transtheoretical Model of health behavior change. *American Journal of Health Promotion, 12,* 38–48.

Quirk, P. A. (2000). Screening for literacy and readability: Implications for the advanced practice nurse. *Clinical Nurse Specialist, 14*(1), 26–32.

Rahmqvist, M., & Bara, A. (2007). Patients retrieving additional information via the Internet: A trend analysis in a Swedish population, 2000–2005. *Scandinavian Journal of Public Health, 35*(2), 533–539.

Rankin, S. H., Stallings, K. D., & London, F. (2005). *Patient education in health and illness* (5th ed.). Philadelphia, PA: Lippincott.

Registered Nurses' Association of Ontario. (2010). *Strategies to support self-management in chronic conditions: Collaboration with clients.* Toronto, ON: Author. Retrieved from http://www.rnao.org /Storage/72/6710_SMS_Brochure.pdf

Sax, L., Bryant, A., & Harper, C. (2005). The differential effects of student-faculty interaction on college outcomes for women and men. *Journal of College Student Development, 46*(6), 642–657.

Shahid, S., Finn, L., Bessarab, D., & Thompson, S. C. (2009). Understanding, beliefs and perspectives of aboriginal people in Western Australia about cancer and its impact on access to cancer services. *BMC Health Services Research, 9,* 132–140.

Skinner, B. F. (1974). *About behaviorism.* New York, NY: Merrill.

Spadero, D. C. (1983). Assessing readability of patient information materials. *Pediatric Nursing, 4,* 274–278.

Stahl, S. A. (2002). Different strokes for different folks? In L. Abbeduto (Ed.), *Taking sides: Clashing on controversial issues in educational psychology* (pp. 98–107). Guilford, CT: McGraw-Hill.

Strong, K., Mathers, C., Leeder, S., & Beaglehole, R. (2005). Preventing chronic diseases: How many lives can we save? *Lancet, 366*(9496), 1512–1514.

Townsend, C., Bruce, B., Hooten, M., & Rome, J. (2006). The role of mental health professionals in multidisciplinary pain rehabilitation programs. *Journal of Clinical Psychology, 62*(11), 1433–1443.

Tung, W. C., & Lee, I. F. (2006). Effects of an osteoporosis educational programme for men. *Journal of Advances in Nursing, 56*(1), 26–34.

Vecchione, M. (2011). Primary stroke prevention and community education. *Medicine and Health Rhode Island, 94*(12), 369–371.

Wantland, D. J., Portillo, C. J., Holzemer, W. L., & Slaughter, R. (2004). The effectiveness of web-based vs. non-web-based interventions: A meta-analysis of behavioral change outcomes. *Journal of Medical Internet Research, 6*(4), 40–71.

Witelson, S., Beresh, H., & Kigar, D. L. (2006). Intelligence and brain size in 100 postmortem brains: Sex lateralization and age factors. *Brain, 129*(2), 386–398.

Woodhouse, J., Peterson, M., Campbell, C., & Gathercoal, K. (2010). The efficacy of a brief behavioral intervention for managing high utilization of ED services by chronic pain patients. *Journal of Emergency Nurses, 36*(5), 399–403.

World Health Organization. (2005). *Preventing chronic diseases: A vital investment.* WHO global report. Geneva, Switzerland: Author.

CHAPTER 14

Chronic Illness and the Family

Christina H. West and Linda L. Binding

INTRODUCTION

When a person is diagnosed with a chronic illness, the entire family enters the unfamiliar, uncertain, and often unexplored world of illness. In this place of illness family life is interrupted, and families face the need to adapt to illness in ways that bring significant challenges and complexities to their lives. Chronic illness is experienced by individuals, but it is also important to remember that illness is experienced by the entire family. Each member of the family will be profoundly affected by their experience of living with illness. Family members' illness experiences can be filled with suffering, sadness, grief, and despair, but these altered lives are also filled with love, relational connection, and even joy. Chesla (2005) described the in-between space in which families find themselves when chronic illness occurs. She suggested that the chronically ill and their families "live with days of intense suffering . . . mixed with moments of delight and possibility. They live lives filled with both" (p. 373). Barnard (1995) articulated this as the existential paradox of chronic illness. Chesla (2005) further stated that "those with chronic illness simultaneously confront their limitations and losses at the same time that they lean toward possibility, hope, and new openings" (p. 373).

Within the field of chronic illness care many clinicians and researchers have focused predominantly on the individual's experience rather than the experience of the family (Charmaz, 2002; Chesla, 2005; Kleinman, 1988). Within such conceptualizations, the contextualized, particular, and relational nature of chronic illness has not been well attended. Our approach to this chapter is to explicitly assume that chronic illness is a relational, contextual, and systemic experience (Rolland, 1984, 1994, 2005, 2011; Wright & Bell, 2009; Wright & Leahey, 2005, 2009; Wright, Watson, & Bell, 1996). Illness is not only experienced in the lives of ill individuals but also in the lives of those who love, support, and care for the ill person. Our concern for addressing the family in chronic illness is not necessarily to ensure family members remain healthy and able to fulfil caregiving roles for the ill family member; alternatively, we emphasize the need to address the illness suffering experienced by the entire family, including all family members who are a part of that family system.

We begin this chapter by describing the complex interaction between the illness trajectory of chronic illness with individual and family life cycle development. This part of the discussion is guided by Rolland's (1984, 1994, 2005, 2011) family systems-illness model, which is "a normative, preventive framework for assessment and intervention with families that are facing chronic and life-threatening conditions" (Rolland, 2011, p. 348). Rolland's (1984, 1994) psychosocial typology for chronic illness is described, as well as specific applications for clinical practice. This discussion also includes a consideration of multigenerational perspectives. Our reflection of the complex interaction between chronic illness and family life cycle development is also informed by McGoldrick, Carter, and Garcia-Preto's (2011) stages of family life cycle development.

Next, we discuss chronic illness and the experience of family caregiving. Qualitative research findings that explored the family experience of caring for a child with a progressive, neurodegenerative illness at home (Rallison, 2009) were highlighted within the context of this discussion.

Finally, we have explored family systems intervention practices that may be helpful to clinicians working with families in the context of the chronic illness experience. The discussion of these relational intervention practices is guided by the Illness Beliefs Model (IBM) (Wright & Bell, 2009; Wright et al., 1996) and the Calgary Family Assessment and Intervention Models (Wright & Leahey, 2005, 2009). The specific family interventions explored are circular questioning practices, encouraging the sharing of illness narratives and commendation practices.

Stanley Hauerwas (1986) suggested that our human response to suffering often reflects an internal, individual process rather than a social one. He goes on to consider the role of those who care for those who suffer (p. 26):

> It is the burden of those who care for the suffering to know how to teach the suffering that they are not thereby excluded from the human community, in this sense our primary role is to bind the suffering and the non-suffering into the same community.

We need to remember that the suffering other is not only the ill person but also the family; family members who live with illness experience their own unique suffering, on both an individual and relational level. Chesla (2005) asked how we do this and how is it possible to bind those who suffer in illness and the nonsuffering in the same community? She turned to Arthur Kleinman (1988), who stated the act of binding those suffering with the nonsuffering might occur through the practice of listening deeply to illness narratives, the illness stories of those who are ill.

The chronically ill are not the only ones who need to have someone listen empathically to their illness stories. There is a pressing need for healthcare professionals to attend better to the illness suffering of the entire family, including the unique illness experiences of all family members.

UNDERSTANDING THE COMPLEX INTERACTION BETWEEN CHRONIC ILLNESS AND FAMILY LIFE CYCLE DEVELOPMENT

When working with clients and their family members in the context of chronic illness, it is important to understand that families grow and change over time. Family members will face developmental stages and tasks related to individual and family life cycle development as they concurrently face challenges across the changing phases of the chronic illness trajectory. The complexity of simultaneously attending to the needs of the individual client and family can be attributed in part to the ongoing interaction of challenges posed by individual, family, and chronic illness life cycle development (Rolland, 1988, 1994, 2005, 2011; McGoldrick, Carter, & Garcia-Preto, 2011). There is a need for ongoing adjustment, adaptation, and role changes as family members face the experiences of growth and crisis that are an inherent part of living in the presence of chronic illness. For the healthcare professional the challenge lies in the ability to think and practice relationally and to identify and explore the developmental and relational challenges that are occurring at multiple system levels simultaneously (Bell & Wright, 2011; Rolland, 1988, 1994, 2005, 2011).

Family life cycle stages, which include specific emotional, instrumental, and relational tasks, have been previously described (Carter & McGoldrick, 2005; McGoldrick et al., 2011; Wright & Leahey, 2009). They include "leaving home, emerging young adults, joining of families through marriage/union, families with young children, families with adolescents, launching children and moving on in midlife, families in late middle age, and families nearing the end of life" (McGoldrick et al., 2011, pp. 16–17). These life cycle stages may appear to provide a framework for "normative" family development, but there has been a growing acknowledgement of the individuality of each family in clinical practice and the highly contextual and variable nature of family life cycle development (McGoldrick et al., 2011; Wright & Leahey, 2009). Within their recent work on the expanded family life cycle, McGoldrick and colleagues (2011) articulated some significant family life cycle influences, including but not limited to family transitions related to divorce (Ahrons, 2011;

McGoldrick & Carter, 2011); single parenting (Anderson & Anderson, 2011); African American families living in poverty (Moore Hines, 2011); lesbian, gay, bisexual, and transgender individuals (Ashton, 2011); and the influence of migration on family life cycle development (Falicov, 2011). In a similar manner Wright and Leahey (2009) delineated the following family life cycle types: middle-class North American, divorce and postdivorce, remarried, professional and low-income, adoptive family, and lesbian, gay, bisexual, intersexed, transgendered, and twin-spirited family life cycles. Further information on these variations within family life cycle development theory can be found in McGoldrick et al. (2011) and Wright and Leahey (2009).

The family's ability to meet the challenges within each phase of the chronic illness trajectory is affected significantly by the tasks they face in individual and family life cycle development. This is particularly relevant when the family's experience with chronic illness is "out of sync" or "off-time" with expected lifespan development (Rolland, 2011, p. 361). The encounter of chronic or life-threatening illness, loss, and death are expected within the developmental stages of families in later life and/or families nearing the end of life (McGoldrick et al., 2011). When chronic illness occurs earlier in the lifespan its presence is considered "out of phase," leading to an increased risk for families to experience significant disruption and crisis within family life cycle development (Neugarten, 1976; Rolland, 2011) as well as family functioning. Dr. John S. Rolland, Clinical Professor of Psychiatry at the University of Chicago Pritzker School of Medicine, family therapist, and co-director/co-founder of the Chicago Centre for Family Health, developed an internationally recognized family systems-illness model for understanding and addressing the interface between chronic illness and the family (Rolland, 1988, 1994, 2011). The family systems-illness model is based on extensive clinical work and research with families facing serious physical disorders and loss, illness trajectories, and components of family function (**Figure 14-1**).

The model includes a focus on multigenerational issues related to the way families have historically organized themselves concerning experiences of illness, crisis, loss, and/or death. The exploration of core family beliefs that have guided the behaviour, organization, and meaning related to experiences of chronic illness are central in the process of assessment and clinical intervention with families (Rolland, 2005, 2011).

Chronic Illness: Psychosocial Typology

Within the family systems-illness model proposed by Rolland, there is a careful articulation of a psychosocial typology of chronic illness. Rather than a traditional focus on the biological and pathological disease process, Rolland (1984, 1988, 2005, 2011) outlines the specific psychosocial demands that family members face with the emergence of different types of chronic illness.

The onset of chronic illness may be acute or gradual. When chronic illness has an acute onset, such as severe myocardial infarction, the psychosocial demands of illness must be faced by family members in a short period of time, which requires a more intense and rapid organization of resources, management skills, and support networks to meet specific, time-sensitive challenges. In addition to multiple instrumental demands, family members must cope with addressing intense emotional responses and uncertainty. Managing the emotional responses and uncertainty will be faced in both acute and gradual onset chronic illness, but this is frequently intensified within the acute onset experience with illness (Rolland, 1984, 1994, 2011).

The course of chronic illness may be progressive, constant, or relapsing/episodic (Rolland,

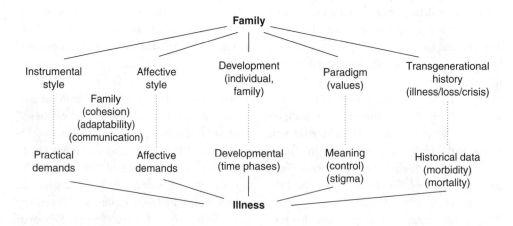

FIGURE 14-1 Interface of chronic illness and the family.
Source: Excerpted from: Rolland, J. S. (1988). Family Systems and Chronic Illness: A Typological Model, *Journal of Psychotherapy and the Family, 3*(3), 143-168. Reprinted with permission from Family Systems Medicine.

2011). When illness progresses gradually over an extended period, there is time for family members to adapt slowly, but there is limited reprieve from the ongoing presence of illness in family life and from its associated demands, caregiving tasks, and emotional influence on the family. Family members will face constant and ongoing role changes and adaptation. Family members need to take responsibility for new caregiving tasks and may be at increased risk for exhaustion as time progresses. When chronic illness is characterized by a constant course, an initial diagnostic phase is followed by a stable phase where there is a defined level or incapacitation (e.g., spinal cord injury) (Rolland, 2011). The family may face periodic recurrences, but there exists a "semipermanent change that is stable and predictable over a considerable time span" (Rolland, 2011, p. 351). Alternatively, when chronic illness has an episodic or relapsing course, family members face a movement back and forth between "stable low-symptom periods with periods of flare-up or exacerbation" (Rolland, 2011, p. 351). Although periods of stability may be characterized with low demands in relation to caregiving, there is often an increased level of uncertainty and unpredictability, as well as a need for the family to alternate between different forms of family organization and family roles on an ongoing basis (Rolland, 2011).

The chronic illness may be life-shortening, and the expectation or prediction related to the possibility of death is one of the crucial influences determining how profound the psychosocial impact will be on the client, as well as on family members (Clarke-Steffen, 1993a, 1993b, 1997; Cohen, 1993, 1995a, 1995b; Gagliardi, 1991; Gravelle, 1997; Powell-Cope, 1995; Rolland, 2011). Disability may include changes in cognition, sensation, movement, and physical disfigurement and can also include social

stigma (Rolland, 2011). The level, nature (progressive or stable), and timing of disability all impact the way family members experience stress and their ability to adapt over time (Rolland, 2011). As incapacitation occurs or develops progressively the family will face new or continuing responsibilities for caregiving. The level of uncertainty within illness, the nature of the treatment and its progression over time, the amount of hospitalization required, and the presence and intensity of pain and suffering, as well as other symptoms, will also have a profound impact on the family's experience with chronic illness (Rolland, 2011).

The Dynamic and Unfolding Nature of Chronic Illness: Family Impacts

Rolland (1994, 2005, 2011) previously challenged the assumption that chronic illnesses such as cancer or physical disability (i.e., spinal cord injury) are experienced by individuals and family members as constant states. He argued that chronic illness is a dynamic and unfolding experience that occurs over different time phases (crisis, chronic, terminal). Each time phase is thought to present unique developmental tasks and psychosocial challenges that call for "significantly different strengths, attitudes, or changes from a family" (Rolland, 2011, p. 352).

The crisis phase is defined as the time between the emergence of symptoms and when the initial adjustment to the diagnosis and treatment plan occurs. Rolland (1994, 2005, 2011) drew on the previous work of Rudolf Moos (1984) to describe both the instrumental or practical tasks encountered by family members in the crisis phase of chronic illness, as well as some of the more pressing general and existential tasks. Families often need to adapt to a complex medical regime and new relationships with various healthcare professionals, while simultaneously working to create meaning within chronic illness. They may experience intense and ongoing grief related to the loss of family normalcy as well as other illness-related losses (Moos, 1984; Rolland, 2011; West, 2011). During this time of crisis, there is a pressing need for family members to redefine relationships, roles, and responsibilities, which can lead to a marked reorganization of family life (McCubbin, Balling, Possin, Frierdich, & Bryne, 2002; Moos, 1984, Patterson, Holm, & Gurney, 2004; Rolland, 2011; West, 2011).

In contrast to the time of crisis, in the chronic time phase families face the ongoing, day-to-day, "long haul" (Rolland, 2011, p. 352) of living with illness in their midst. The day-to-day experience of living with illness may have more of a constant nature but can also be characterized by illness progression and episodic/relapse-related changes. The critical developmental task focuses on the "family's ability to maintain a semblance of a normal life with a chronic illness and heightened uncertainty" (Rolland, 2011, p. 352). Within a recent qualitative family intervention study West (2011) explored the illness suffering of family members living with childhood cancer. Within this research there was an analysis of both videotaped clinical work and research interviews with family members and nurse clinicians. In one of the clinical sessions a mother spoke about how the ongoing, never-ending nature of her suffering was more difficult to live with than actually having to face her child's death. This mother used a metaphor of being on the road to Disneyland to describe her family's life before illness.

When her child became ill, this mother faced many new obstacles and described her long, ongoing experience with illness as one of falling off the road and becoming stuck in the muck and mire. Within her words there is a glimpse into how the real-life challenges of ongoing chronic illness can profoundly challenge a family's ability to maintain the sense of normalcy that Rolland (2011) speaks of in relation to the chronic phase of illness. This is a critical area for exploration and intervention when working with clients and family members in the context of chronic illness. The following clinical excerpt is taken from a videotaped clinical intervention, which was based on the Illness Beliefs Model (Wright & Bell, 2009; Wright et al., 1996), a family systems nursing practice model for family level intervention. The therapeutic conversation between a nurse clinician and mother occurred at the Family Nursing Unit, University of Calgary:

> **Clinician:** And when we talk about suffering . . . we're talking about suffering on many levels. And I'm wondering if I could ask you a little bit about that. . . . What's been the most awful part, of all the experiences that you have gone through in the last few years?
>
> **Mother [crying as she speaks]:** It just seems never ending. . . . It just makes you tired. . . . and I think that's why I never feel like myself. . . . I'm perpetually in a state of flux, I don't feel like I have stable footing ever. I mean it was hard enough, I was really young when I had her. . . . I did the best that I could, and I raised her really well. . . . I got into university, and I was doing it all by myself, and I worked so hard, and I had a vision and determination. . . . And I've lost it . . . it's like I've lost me, because of what's happened. I can't seem to get back on the road. You're driving towards your goal . . . you're going to Disneyland, that's your main goal . . . so you have to work hard, and you have to earn money. . . . And then on the way, there are good things that happen. You take little mini-breaks, you enjoy your work, you get validation. . . . Yes, you have

fall backs, you get tired . . . but along the way, you're building and you're working towards that goal, of getting to Disneyland. On my way, I was doing it! I could see it happening. And, I was doing everything I could to be a good mother. . . . And then all of a sudden, "bang," she gets sick. And then it was like the stops on the way to Disneyland got bigger, and we didn't just stop, we were taking detours, backroads. The next thing you know there isn't a road to drive on anymore, to get where I want to go. It's like I'm stuck in the mire now . . . I'm in the muck. I'm stuck, I can't get out. And it's all I can do to walk around in the bush and gather enough berries . . . and I guess meet up with whoever I can meet up with in the woods, who can give me some validation and love.

In this therapeutic conversation the mother spoke of how long it had taken for her to move forward in life, given the intense grief she experienced over the symbolic loss of the daughter she had known before illness. This example shows the ongoing struggle families face within the chronic time phase as they try to move forward in life as individuals, and a family.

> **Mother:** Like it's taken a long time to move forward, I've been grieving the loss of my little girl for so long. . . . And that's why I'm so tired . . . because this never ends. It's always one thing after the next, and it's just . . . how much can one person take? It's exhausting. (Permission to use this excerpt of therapeutic conversation from the Family Nursing Unit, University of Calgary granted by Dr. Janice M. Bell.)

The Illness Beliefs Model (Wright et al., 1996; Wright & Bell, 2009) is another family systems–based assessment and intervention approach to clinical work with families who are suffering in the context of living with chronic and/or life-threatening illness. This model focuses on addressing the illness beliefs that lie at the heart of

a family's suffering. Clinicians consider how the illness beliefs of family members, the patient, and healthcare professionals intersect in a manner that can increase or alleviate a family's suffering as they live with illness. Within this Family Systems Nursing model, there is a careful, relationally based exploration and subsequent challenging of those illness beliefs that may be intensifying family challenges and suffering. The clinician purposely adopts a relational stance that is nonhierarchical, collaborative, and strengths-based (Tapp, 2000; Wright & Bell, 2009; Wright & Leahey, 2005, 2009; Wright et al., 1996) as they coevolve a therapeutic conversation with the patient and family members (Wright & Bell, 1996; Wright et al., 1996). The following are specific illness beliefs the clinician explores in this approach (Wright & Bell, 2009, p. 181):

- Beliefs about illness suffering
- Beliefs about diagnosis
- Beliefs about etiology
- Beliefs about prognosis
- Beliefs about healing and treatment
- Beliefs about illness mastery, control, and influence
- Beliefs about religion and spirituality
- Beliefs about the place of illness in the lives and relationships of family members

As the patient and family members enter the chronic time phase described by Rolland (1984, 1988, 1994, 2005, 2011), beliefs about mastery, control, and influence are often particularly important for clinicians to explore with the family. The ideas about exploring illness beliefs related to mastery, control, and influence described within the Illness Beliefs Model are credited to the field of narrative therapy, in particular the work and writing of Michael White (1988/1989, 2007; White & Epston, 1990). One of the approaches that Wright and Bell (2009) described for exploring illness beliefs is intentionally inviting clients and their family members into the role of expert, by asking about their illness experience and the influence they believe they have over illness. Wright and Bell (2009) included the following excerpt from a clinical therapeutic conversation shared by a nurse clinician, Mark (an adult living with multiple sclerosis [MS]), and his elderly parents, who were playing an active caregiving role in his life and illness. This excerpt illustrates how a clinician might work to explore beliefs about healing and treatment and, in particular, beliefs about mastery, control, and influence over illness (p. 204):

LMW: [Clinician]	Can I shift a bit and ask if there is anything else you want to ask me, Mark?
Mark:	No, I don't think so.
LMW:	Okay, is there anything else about experiencing MS that you think would . . . help me to understand better? Anything else you want to tell me about your experience that you think would . . .
Mark:	Well, it's just very frustrating to deal with.
LMW:	Yes. Do you feel like it rules your life at this point, or do you feel like you are able to rule MS sometimes?
Mark:	Well, a lot of things I don't do because of it.
LMW:	Yes. Are there any ways that you think you influence MS, that you have an influence over it?
Mark:	Yes.
LMW:	Yes? Terrific, can you tell me what those are? What ways do you think you influence the MS?
Mark:	Well, not really influence, things that I do in spite of it.

When the clinician asks whether Mark feels MS rules his life or whether he is able to rule MS sometimes, she is purposefully embedding her belief that it is possible for Mark to have increasing influence and control over his illness. In asking this question she is inviting him to look for and recognize the possibility of reclaiming a sense of normality in his life, as well as influence over MS. These questions could be asked of different family members, and the very act of having family members witnessing one another's responses may open up even more possibilities for the family, to claim influence over illness, as a family in relationship with a difficult illness experience, and with one another. We explore the use of circular questions within therapeutic conversations with families living with chronic illness later in this chapter (see Intervention with the Family in the Context of Chronic Illness).

Many clients and families living with chronic illness one day may face what Rolland (2011) identified as the terminal phase of illness. Within this time phase, death is expected at some time in the not too distant future. The uncertainty experienced within illness then shifts from whether the illness will shorten a family member's life to questions that focus on the length of time the family has left together and the quality of life that will be possible during the days, months, and even years left to live. During this time families continue to face the challenge of living well with chronic illness, but there is a new focus on creating memories as a family, saying good-bye, letting go, anticipatory grief, and preparing for death, in part through life and relationship review and legacy exploration (Rolland, 2011). The caregiving responsibilities held by family members often become intensified during this period, particularly when clients wish to remain at home until the time of death. The support of professional caregivers through home palliative care programs and caregiver respite programs, as well as the ongoing support from informal networks of care, becomes critical during this time of illness.

Application to Clinical Practice: Exploring the Interface of Illness, Individual, and Family Life Cycles

When meeting with the client and family in the context of chronic illness, it is important for clinicians to understand the reciprocal interaction between three developmental life cycles: those of the individual, family, and the chronic illness trajectory (Rolland, 2011). As mentioned earlier, each of these life cycles shares common themes related to developmental phases, tasks, and psychosocial challenges. Development in one life cycle (i.e., the chronic illness trajectory) will have an impact on the other life cycle experiences and development over time. Rolland (2011) argued that "illness is a significant marker event that can both colour the nature of a developmental period and be coloured by its timing in the individual and family life cycle" (p. 356).

The entrance of chronic illness into family life initiates an "inside-the family-focused process of socialization to illness" (Rolland, 2011, p. 357). The intense emotional experiences of chronic illness, as well as the emergence and progression of disability, lead to ongoing and potentially fluctuating demands that a family increase their flexibility, relational closeness, and cohesion. Families may need to pull together in a new and more intense manner than they have before in their efforts to support not only the ill family member but also one another (Rolland, 2011; Wright & Bell, 2009; Wright & Leahey, 2005, 2009; Wright et al., 1996). Of

critical importance is whether there is a close fit between the inward pull of the illness experience and what is occurring from a family and individual life cycle perspective.

Rolland (2011) offers two questions that are key to clinical assessment and intervention with the family in the context of chronic illness: "What is the fit between the psychosocial demands of a condition and family and individual life structures and developmental tasks at a particular point in the life cycle? Also, how will this fit change as the course of illness unfolds in relation to the family life cycle and the development of each member?" (p. 357).

Chronic Illness and Families with Young Children

When a young child is diagnosed with a chronic illness, developmentally the family is intensely focused on childrearing (Carter, McGoldrick, & Petko, 2011). Within this illness context significant emotional and practical challenges will emerge for parents, well siblings, and extended family members. For these families there is a natural focus inwards, as the couple works to make space for young children in the family system and faces the tasks of childrearing and household responsibilities while simultaneously working to create financial stability for the family. When a young child becomes ill the socialization process of the chronic illness can heighten the inward developmental focus that already exists within family life (Rolland, 2011). Family organization and structure, as well as family roles and relationships, must all change in an effort to meet illness-related tasks and responsibilities (Björk, Wiebe, & Hallström, 2009; Clarke-Steffen, 1990, 1993a, 1997; Kelly & Ganong, 2011; McCubbin, Balling, Possin, Frierdich, & Bryne, 2002; Moody, Meyer,

Mancuso, Charlson, & Robbins, 2006; Nicholas et al., 2009; Patterson, Holm, & Gurney, 2004; West, 2011; Woodgate, 2001, 2006).

When family resources and supports are stressed significantly and over a prolonged period of time, there may be significant limitations in the parents' ability to fully meet the child development needs of well siblings. Grandparents can similarly experience a "developmental detour" (Rolland, 2011, p. 358) as they commit to family life cycle alterations in their efforts to assist with the child care of well siblings or the ill child. What may occur is a split or separation within the family unit. The well siblings who are cared for at home by fathers, grandparents, extended family members, or family friends become one subgrouping within the family unit (father–well siblings), whereas the ill child and mother/parents who are together for most of the time in the hospital setting become another family subgroup. The parental–ill child relationship can become intensified throughout the treatment period, which is a family pattern that may continue within and beyond the chronic illness experience (Björk et al., 2005, 2009; Brody & Simmons, 2007; McCubbin et al., 2002; Nicholas et al., 2009; Patterson et al., 2004; West, 2011; Woodgate 2001, 2006; Young, Dixon-Woods, & Heney, 2002).

Parents often work very hard to protect the ill child and well siblings from illness-related distress, but these efforts can inadvertently leave children feeling left out, uncertain, and unsupported. The following excerpt from a recent research study that focused on the illness suffering of families living with childhood cancer reflected this experience (West, 2011, pp. 99, 100):

> **Father:** I think that's the first crack . . . as you . . . come out of the cancer problem. . . . Wow! Yeah, okay . . . we had all these people [well siblings] that, somehow . . . the curtain closed, and they were excluded.
>
> **Mother:** We were actually trying to protect them from some of the sorrow, some of the tragedy and pain and hardship that was going on there. . . .
>
> **Sister (Lizzie, 12 years old):** . . . it passes on to you . . . and even if you do protect us from it, it will still come back onto us.
>
> **Brother (Jason, 14 years old):** The problem is, that those two [parents], and Cameron [ill child], were experiencing it the most. . . . I was kind of kept in the dark. I really had no idea what was going on. And then, when cancer stopped, everyone changed. I changed, Rachael was changed, mom was changed, dad was changed. Lizzie was changed, everyone was changed, and we could never be the same people again, we could never be the same family again.

Within these words there is evidence of the disconnection that occurred between these parents and the well siblings during the course of childhood cancer treatment. Also evident is the grief experienced as family members witnessed the profound changes that occurred in each family member as well as in the entire family.

The event of chronic illness in a parent during this family life cycle stage also invites significant illness-related stress and strain into family life. Rolland (2011) compared this family experience with the entrance of a new family member into the family system, a family member "with special needs that will compete with those of the real children for potentially scarce family resources" (p. 358). The following case example illustrates the complexity that is involved when a parent becomes chronically ill during the "families with young children" (McGoldrick et al., 2011) life cycle stage.

CASE STUDY

John and his wife Sue asked to meet with members of the interdisciplinary healthcare team. John had a severe head injury at work in the construction industry 1 year ago and has been unable to work since that time. John is receiving workers' compensation, which supports the family's financial needs at this time. The family has struggled with John's physical and cognitive recovery. John has experienced severe headaches since his injury and is followed by a chronic pain specialist. Five months ago John developed a clinical depression, which is being treated by a psychiatrist. John had become increasingly distant in his marital relationship with Sue and, although he receives disability income, has expressed feelings of uselessness after his accident and anger at "the system" when he was still unable to return to work after 6 months. Sue, a stay-at-home mom, has been looking after their two children ages 6 and 8 years. Sue voiced her anger and disappointment with John as she believed he had withdrawn from his parenting responsibilities. Sue missed having her husband as a partner in parenting their children and said it was almost as if she was now a single parent, with three children in the home. John had grown up in a family in which physical strength and a strong work ethic were highly valued, and he had been financially independent since graduating from high school. When John was injured, Sue's mother had stayed with them to help look after the children, but she was unable to stay longer than a month. Sue had relied on friends and neighbours for as long as she could and now feels overwhelmed and exhausted. She stated that if she complained to John, he distanced himself even more.

Discussion Questions

1. What family life cycle task is most challenged by this illness experience? What family roles have changed because of the presence of illness in family life? What have been some of the relational/systemic impacts of the change in family roles?
2. What family relationship is experiencing the most difficulty? How might you approach clinical intervention with this family?
3. What strengths do you see in this family, based on your reading of the case study? Explain.
4. What gender influences do you see at play in this case study? What family and marital outcomes might you want to explore further?

Discussion first centred on the severity of John's depression symptoms and the ongoing care he was receiving from his psychiatrist. John expressed his worry that he was failing Sue as a husband because he was unable to work and fulfil the role of "provider" for the family. Sue missed John's partnership in parenting their children and believed his retreat from his parenting role had deeply affected her willingness to be intimate with him. John and Sue explored ways that John could still support his family, and he began to be more involved as a father. Over time, John was retrained and was able to take on a less demanding job that helped him feel he was a contributing member of the family. John continued to be followed by a psychiatrist for his depression, and the family continued to meet with the nurse and social worker to discuss the home situation.

Chronic Illness and Families Who Are Launching Children and Moving On in Mid-Life

When families are in a life cycle stage focused on launching children or have recently transitioned through that family milestone, the emergence of chronic illness can significantly affect the expected developmental path they had been on previously. Each family member, as well as the couple dyad, may have their autonomy and growing independence threatened by the intrusion of chronic illness. For example, when a young adult becomes ill, this may lead to a "heightened dependency and return to the family of origin for disease-related caretaking" (Rolland, 2011, p. 357). Whether these family patterns of interaction are temporary or become more permanent depends on both the severity of illness and family dynamics (Rolland, 2011).

The impact of individual development will also be significant. For example, adolescents are focused on identity formation and building stronger connections with their peers. The need to revert to a previously experienced dependent relationship with parents may seriously impede an adolescent's individual development, which would normally be focused on peer and intimate relationships as well as career planning (Garcia-Preto, 2011; Rolland, 2011). These relational patterns of interaction will also be influenced by the nature of the chronic illness trajectory. When disease is progressive in nature, "the continuous addition of new caregiving demands keeps a family's energy focused inward on the illness. In contrast, after a family develops functional adaptation, a constant-course disease . . . permits greater flexibility to enter or resume life cycle planning" (Rolland, 2011, p. 358).

CASE STUDY

Jane, aged 45, was diagnosed with MS 8 years previously at the age of 37, two years after the birth of her third child. The Andersons have three children, two daughters ages 17 and 19 and a son age 14. Initially, Jane was successfully treated with medication and had been able to continue working as a social worker except for periods of relapse. Recently, however, she recovered poorly from her last relapse and was now in a wheelchair and unable to return to work. Her husband, Jeff, is a lawyer who had been able to continue his practice due to short-term help when his wife had a relapse. Their oldest daughter, Rita, had completed her first year of university studies in another city and had a steady boyfriend. Their second daughter, Leanne, was looking forward to finishing her last year of high school and also entering university. Roy, their 14-year-old son, had done reasonably well in middle school but was recently increasingly truant at school and started wearing "gothic" clothing, including chains and other articles that were seen by the school as dangerous. Last week he was suspended from school. After Jane's serious relapse Rita immediately quit her summer job and returned home, which caused friction with her younger sister who had "taken over" her bedroom. Roy's behaviour shocked and frightened the rest of the family who had never considered such behaviour as fitting into their family.

CASE STUDY   (Continued)

WWW

Discussion Questions

1. In working with this family, what goals might you hope to work on collaboratively?
2. What family life cycle developmental tasks need to be addressed? What do you believe the family's priorities might be? If different from your own goals for the family, how would you approach that difference in clinical practice?
3. How has the transition in the trajectory of this chronic illness affected various individual life cycle stages of development? Identify the family life cycle stage, illness impacts, and potential areas for collaborative intervention. What family life cycle developmental tasks are challenged in this case study?
4. What beliefs and fears about illness might be contributing to the behaviours of various family members?

Clinical intervention with this family initially revolved around discussions about the worsening symptoms of Mrs. A's illness and what this change meant to each member of the family. These discussions helped to dispel some fears the three children had about the possibility of their mother's early death. After some discussion concerning family of origin issues, it was revealed that Jeff's mother had become severely withdrawn when he was 12 years old, after the death of his 4-year-old sister. His mother had understood this death as her fault, and as Jeff stated, "I didn't have a mother after that." Discussion then focused on ways in which Jeff could become more present to his own children, particularly his 14-year-old son, who had been distancing himself from the family and seeking company with counter-culture friends. Further discussion included ways in which the two daughters, who were feeling drawn back into the family, could resume their respective activities while still being emotionally involved with the family. After some of the priority family concerns had been addressed, marital issues were also addressed with Jeff and Jane.

Life-Transition Periods and Life Structure–Maintaining Periods

When chronic illness occurs it is important for clinicians to consider whether family members are in a time of life transition or a time of maintaining family life structure. The emergence of chronic illness often leads to a "loss of the family's pre-illness identity" (Rolland, 2011, p. 359), which requires a family to move into a significant period of transition, where they will face

changing family roles, responsibilities, and relationships. Rolland (2011) suggested that when family transition coincides with illness-related transitions, "issues related to previous, current, and anticipated loss will often be magnified" (p. 359). The family may face complex challenges related to the way illness becomes integrated into planning for an upcoming developmental phase in the family life cycle. At times, illness may be granted a more central place in family life than is warranted, or alternatively, it may be inadequately attended to, in transition planning (Rolland, 2011, p. 359).

The family's experience with illness may be very different when they are in a period of building and maintaining the family life structure. During these times family members have an expectation that life should be relatively stable. The family meets a challenge when chronic illness creates the need for adjustment and the move into an illness-related time of transition. "To successfully navigate this kind of crisis, family adaptability requires the ability to transform their entire life structure to a prolonged transitions state" (Rolland, 2011, p. 360). What is highlighted in this discussion is the value of approaching care of the chronically ill and their family members from a family systems perspective. From this perspective clinicians have an understanding of the complex and ongoing interaction between individual, family, and chronic illness life cycles. The focus is not only on the ill member but the entire family, which includes a careful consideration of each individual family member (Rolland, 2011, p. 360):

> Illness and disability in one family member can profoundly affect the developmental goals of another member. For instance, disability in an infant can be a serious roadblock to a mother's mastery of child-rearing, and a life-threatening illness in a married young adult can interfere with the well spouse's readiness to become a parent.

Each family member will have an individual experience with illness, which is affected significantly by the stage of individual and family life cycle development. When adopting a systems perspective, there is an understanding that these unique, changing experiences with illness will have an impact on other family members as the illness changes over time. It is important for clinicians to assist family members to find a balance between attending to the demands created by illness, without sacrificing "their own or the family's development as a system" (Rolland, 2011, p. 360). Conversations that focus on what control and influence illness has over family life can open up possibilities for a means to "strike a healthier balance with life plans as a way to minimize overall family strain and relationship skews between caregivers and the ill member" (Rolland, 2011, p. 360). Within this work it is important for clinicians to support family members in working through complex experiences of "guilt, overresponsibility, and hopelessness" (Rolland, 2011, p. 360). External resources such as community support, family support groups, and respite care may help family members find a better balance between pursuing individual and family goals, while simultaneously supporting and caring for an ill family member.

Multigenerational Perspectives: Implications for Practice

Healthcare professionals often focus exclusively on the family who is visible and present within healthcare interactions. It is important for the assessment of the family to move beyond this, with a purposeful effort to elicit multigenerational perspectives on illness. Attention to different generations within the family will assist the clinician in learning about core family illness beliefs (Wright & Bell, 2009) that have been passed on between family generations, as well as the family patterns developed in the past when illness, loss, and death have entered family life (Rolland, 2005, 2011). Rolland (2011) and other family systems clinicians (Wright & Bell, 2009; Wright & Leahey, 2005, 2009) advocated for the use of genograms and ecomaps in exploring the relational patterns that families have developed over time. Rolland (2011) suggested that a "chronic illness-orientated genogram focuses on how a family organized itself and adapted as an evolving system around previous illnesses and unexpected crises in the current and previous generations" (p. 362). Illness-related relationship changes, patterns of coping, and particular areas of vulnerability, strength, and competence need to be explored with family members within the family genogram discussion (McGoldrick, Gerson, & Petry, 2008; Rolland, 2011; Wright & Leahey, 2005, 2009).

A multigenerational assessment allows the clinician to explore the way families have organized themselves concerning illness in the past and their approach to the practical, emotional, relational, and spiritual tasks presented by past illnesses. "What did they learn from those experiences that influences how they think about the current illness? Whether they emerged with a strong sense of competence or failure is essential information" (Rolland, 2011, p. 326). More information on attending to multigenerational experiences with illness, loss, and crisis can be found in Rolland (2011) and McGoldrick et al. (2011).

CHRONIC ILLNESS AND FAMILY CAREGIVING: AN EXPERIENCE MARKED BY COMPLEXITY, UNCERTAINTY, AND ONGOING CHANGE

Within the chronic illness experience, those who are ill, as well as their family members, require holistic, comprehensive care that includes a focus on emotional, social, and spiritual care as well as on the physical aspects of illness. In this section, however, we focus specifically on the family caregiving experience. As part of this discussion we highlight findings from a qualitative, hermeneutic research study conducted by Lillian Rallison (2009) at the University of Calgary (Calgary, Alberta) entitled, "Living in the In-Between: A Hermeneutic Study of Families Caring for a Child with a Progressive Neurodegenerative Illness at Home." Within her writing Rallison used the metaphor of hands to explore the complex experience of family caregiving, such as "weary hands," "hands that keep everything moving smoothly," and "busy hands" (pp. 108–143).

Over the course of a chronic illness family members will be asked, and expected, to take responsibility for multiple medical caregiving tasks, activities of daily living, as well as the ongoing provision of emotional and spiritual care for their loved ones. Previously, we discussed how the nature and type of disability vary dramatically between types of chronic illness as well as across the changing trajectory of chronic illness (Rolland, 1984, 1994, 2005, 2011). This variability will create changing needs related to both physical caregiving and emotional and spiritual care.

As we enter this discussion about family caregiving, it is important to clarify that some individuals will require the level of care provided in institutional settings (acute and long-term care) and that not all families are willing or able to provide home-based care over the long term. The ability of the family to care for an ill family member will be affected by the severity of the chronic illness, the level and intensity of medical caregiving required over time, and individual and family life cycle challenges that are simultaneously occurring. There is a growing societal expectation that such ongoing, often specialized, care be provided in the home or through community-based care (McQuillan & Finally, 1996; Monterosso, Kristjanson, Aoun, & Phillips, 2007; Rallison, 2009; Romanow, 2002; Stein, 2001; Stevens, 2004). For example, in Canada one of the key recommendations put forward by the Romanow commission (2002), which focused on the future of health care in Canada, was to strengthen and expand home care, which promoted an increasing shift of care from institutional settings to the home environment.

The decision about where and how best to provide care for family members living with chronic illness is emotionally charged and multifaceted. Home-based care is financially cost effective for the healthcare system; however, the reliance on family members as care providers creates multiple stressors within the family system (Hunt, 2003; Rallison, 2009; Rolland 1984, 1994, 2005, 2011; Wright & Bell, 2009; Wright & Leahey, 2005, 2009). For these arrangements to work effectively family members, friends, and communities must play central roles in creating and implementing complex plans of care.

The following excerpt is from a mother caring for her 3-year-old daughter living with a progressive, neurodegenerative illness at home. This letter was written in an effort to advocate for increased funding support for the caregiving responsibilities this family faced in the home environment (Rallison, 2009). Within Rallison's (2009) discussion of the intensity of medical caregiving, the metaphor of "hands that keep everything running smoothly" (p. 103) was used. This mother's words give a glimpse into the complex and intensive medical care that can be required at home and also emphasize the extraordinary effort family members need to make to obtain adequate funding support (Rallison, 2009, p. 109):

Imagine trying to hold an oxygen mask on a seizing child who is turning blue, because she stops breathing for thirty seconds every ten minutes. Imagine again that you have to hold this child in the right position for her to breathe because without your support, she cannot hold up her own head, and can't swallow her saliva especially during seizures, so she gags and chokes on it and needs suctioning. This child heats up so fast that it is difficult to keep replacing the cool cloths to cool her, but you must keep going, because if her temperature doesn't come down . . . her seizure won't stop. You need to suction her saliva to stop her from choking at the same time. You need to also crush her pills, administer her medicine, wash her food bag, warm her feed, and push it through her g-tube because if her food is cold she gags. . . . While juggling this important and impossible set of life saving tasks, you need to be thinking hard about what has triggered the seizure, because if she has not had a bowel movement today then her seizures won't stop until you help her go. Or if she had a bath that was slightly too warm, that might have triggered her seizures. Oh and don't forget to time how long the seizure lasts and record the description.

Family Caregivers and Family Caregiving Systems

Today, the term "family caregiver" extends beyond the traditional family boundary. "Caregiver" is defined as anyone who provides assistance to another in need. The "informal caregiver" is anyone who provides care without pay and who usually has a relationship with the care recipient. "Family caregiver" is a term used interchangeably with informal caregiver and can include family, friends, neighbours, and community members. Motivations for caregiving, such as love, duty, or obligation (often based on ethnicity and culture), strongly influence a caregiver's willingness to accept a primary caregiving role (Geister, 2005). Additional reasons given by family caregivers for accepting their role are their expectations of themselves and others, religious or spiritual experiences, and role modelling (Piercy & Chapman, 2001).

Although it is ideal to have extended family members and friends involved in caregiving, as well as in the provision of emotional support for the family, there can be significant challenges and even hesitation from extended family members about their ongoing involvement over the course of a long-term, chronic illness. When this hesitation occurs family members may experience significant disappointment, anger, and sadness and associated impacts on family relationships. Even when extended family members and friends live close by, they may not always be willing to support family members in a significant manner. Rallison (2009) interpreted this as the "hesitant hands of extended family members and friends" (p. 112). Within that research one single mother who worked full-time and struggled to care for her teenage daughter over many years of progressive, chronic illness described her family's hesitation as follows (Rallison, 2009, pp. 112, 113):

> My mom and dad live next door . . . but my mom is not the kind of person who says "can I help you out?" Basically that's been very hard. . . . My sister has been very good . . . [she's] a nurse, who has been very committed and very caring. But I have not [had] one other family member who has even offered to take Shelley in all these years, and that hurts a lot . . . I just haven't had that kind of family support like some families do sometimes.

Early caregiving research identified a care recipient and a caregiver as separate entities: the caregiver had primary responsibility for the care and well-being of the care recipient. These studies often did not recognize that caregiving usually occurs within the context of larger, more complex family systems (Palmer & Glass, 2003; Rolland, 1994, 2005, 2011) or other social networks (Weitzner, Haley, & Chen, 2000). More recently caregiving research has placed more emphasis on the dynamics of the family relationships (Badr & Acitelli, 2005; Palmer & Glass, 2003; Rallison, 2009; Rolland, 1994, 2005, 2011; Sebern & Whitlatch, 2007). As expected, these studies indicated that the dynamics of the family or other close personal relationships that existed before the illness experience can profoundly impact caregiving relationships within the illness experience. The increasing number of stepfamilies and nontraditional family compositions also add significantly to the complexity of caregiving.

Today, people of both genders and of all ages, ethnicities, and economic classes occupy positions as caregivers with varying levels and types of responsibilities, especially in long-term care arrangements. Changes to the social structure of the family have resulted in more families where both parents work outside the home (Vanier Institute of the Family, 2010). This "sandwich generation" is not always available to provide full-time care for aging family members, which has created a new level of caregivers: children and adolescents. At times these young caregivers assist with or may even assume care of adults or children living with chronic illness in their homes (Hunt, Levine, & Naiditch, 2005; Lackey & Gates, 2001). Although this occurs in some families, parents have also reported trying to protect well siblings from the responsibility of physical caregiving and from emotional and spiritual distress (Rallison, 2009; West, 2011).

Family Caregiving Challenges: Letting Go and Embracing a Life Beyond Illness

Family caregivers face multiple problems, issues, and concerns throughout their caregiving experiences. Over the last 20 to 30 years there has been a blurring of the lines of responsibility for long-term caregiving, as families have been expected to take on more and more responsibilities for care in the home (McQuillan & Finally, 1996; Monterosso et al., 2007; Rallison, 2009; Romanow, 2002; Stein, 2001; Stevens, 2004). Increased technology, higher acuity, and competing demands on available caregivers have created an imbalance between the demand for family care and the ability of family caregivers to provide care. Family caregivers are being asked to provide highly technical treatments, administer complex medication regimens, provide labour-intensive hands-on care, and monitor the medical conditions of very ill family members.

One responsibility that has remained constant over time is the extensive decision-making demands placed on family caregivers. When the dependent family member cannot make decisions or has difficulty communicating choices, the responsibility for countless decisions associated with managing daily life falls to the caregiver. These decisions include the initiation, timing, and provision of assistance from informal and formal sources; integration of caregiving demands into work and family life; and planning for future long-term care needs (McAuley, Travis, & Safewright, 1997; Travis & Bethea, 2001).

Family Caregiver Strain or Burden

Caregiver strain and burden are multidimensional, closely related concepts that include both the subjective perceptions of caregivers, such as role overload, and objective factors, such as physical care needs of the care recipient. Caregiver strain is usually related to the stress, hardship, or conflicting feelings one has when performing the caregiving role (Hunt, 2003). For example, a caregiver may feel a high level of role strain when trying to decide between caring for an ailing parent and maintaining gainful employment. One area of caregiver research that has focused heavily on caregiver strain is dementia care.

Caregiving is more stressful and produces more emotional and physical strain when the caregiver is caring for a person with dementia or Alzheimer's disease (Ory, Hoffman, Yee, Tennstedt, & Schulz, 1999). Caregivers of persons with dementia are more likely than nondementia caregivers to say they suffer mental or physical problems as a result of caregiving (Ory et al., 1999). Caregivers also report higher levels of strain when they perceive the patient to be manipulative, unappreciative, or unreasonable (Nerenberg, 2002).

Caregiver burden is defined as "the oppressive or worrisome load borne by people providing direct care for the chronically ill" (Hunt, 2003, p. 28). Burden is relative to the level of the care recipient's disability, including behavioural and cognitive issues, the extent of care required, and the caregiver's level of worry or feelings of being overwhelmed (Nerenberg, 2002; Rallison, 2009). Financial strain also contributes to the level of caregiver burden (Evercare & National Alliance for Caregiving, 2007; Rallison, 2009). Caregiver burden has been associated with increased depressive symptoms in caregivers of patients with stroke (Chumbler, Rittman, Van Puymbroeck, Vogel, & Qin, 2004), coronary artery bypass (Halm & Bakas, 2007), and Alzheimer's disease (Mausbach et al., 2007), among others. Higher levels of depression have been found among dementia caregivers who cared for persons with moderate to severe functional impairment and greater amounts of behavioural disturbance (wandering and aggression) than among nondementia caregivers (Meshefedjian, McCusker, Bellavance, & Baumgarten, 1998). A study of caregivers and patients with dementia (n = 5,627) found 32% of caregivers were classified as clinically depressed on the basis of elevated scores on the Geriatric Depression Scale (Covinsky et al., 2003). When caregivers' appraisals of the burden of caregiving are high, there is greater likelihood of caregiver depression and depressive symptoms (Clyburn, Stones, Hadjistavropoulos, & Tuokko, 2000).

A gender component appears to be associated with caregiver strain. Within Canada the "5.5 million hours of unpaid informal caregiving for household members and individuals not residing with them" (Zukewich, 2003, p. 18) is more likely to be done by women. Female caregivers experience more psychiatric disorders than male caregivers (Yee & Schulz, 2000) and are much more likely than men to report being depressed or anxious and to experience lower levels of life satisfaction. The irony is that although they report more caregiver burden, role conflict, or strain, women are more likely than male caregivers to continue caregiving responsibilities over the long term. Women are less likely than men to obtain assistance from others with caregiving. Finally, women are less

likely than men to engage in preventative health behaviours, such as rest, exercise, and taking medications as prescribed while caregiving (Burton, Newsom, Schulz, Hirsch, & German, 1997). Providing female caregivers, as well as other family members, with the permission to rest, to seek out additional assistance, and to find a balance in caregiving is an important focus for family intervention in chronic illness (Wright & Leahey, 2009).

Caregivers for spouses have reported a higher incidence of depression and stress than those caring for a disabled parent (Gordon & Perrone, 2004). The caregiving roles and responsibilities may have a major impact on the relationship itself. It is important for healthcare professionals to realize that the relationship between the caregiver and the spouse receiving the care needs to be supported and nurtured in terms of love, affection, and intimacy (Gordon & Perrone, 2004). Children and adolescents who have functioned in the role of caregiver report difficulty watching their loved one progress with a chronic problem; they have memories of unpleasant smells and sights and also report feeling helpless because of their lack of knowledge and fear they will not be able to deal with a crisis (Lackey & Gates, 2001).

Financial Impact of Caregiving

An aspect of the chronic illness experience that may create significant strain for caregivers is the financial burden related to care needs in the home and community environment. There are different degrees of financial impact on families, depending on their particular caregiving situations and financial resources; however, the financial stresses that come with long-term chronic illness cannot be understated. The impact may range from minimal to considerable, depending on the extent to which other informal caregiving is available, what formal services are used, and how they are financed.

It is estimated that many informal caregivers in Canada are 45 years of age or older, representing approximately 2.7 million Canadians (Canadian Research Network for Care in the Community [CRNCC], 2011; Cranswick & Dosman, 2008). The growing population of seniors in Canada as well as changing family structures, including delayed age of marriage, declining fertility rates, increasing numbers of Canadian households headed by single parents, and people living alone, all lead to a national trend in which fewer family members are available to provide informal caregiving (Keefe, Legare, & Carriere, 2005). Increasing mobility of family and the growing geographical distances between family members are also contributing to the limitations and stresses inherent in the family caregiving experience (CRNCC, 2011). It has been estimated that informal caregivers provide approximately 80% of the care associated with chronic illness in Canada (Fast, Niehaus, Eales, & Keating, 2002), and the economic value of this care has been estimated to be equivalent to between 25 billion (Hollander, Liu, & Chappell, 2009) and 83.7 billion Canadian dollars (Zukewich, 2003).

The current public health system for in-home and community-based services within Canada is based on a shared-cost model. Family caregivers with significant financial resources can more easily afford to pay for home or community-based services out of pocket, before receiving reimbursement by the public system. Further, financial resources or the availability of private insurance through employment also allows some family members to augment the support they receive for in-home caregiving.

Hidden Costs of Family Caregiving

There are also hidden costs, economic and non-economic, related to the informal care of those who are ill, their caregivers, and other family members (CRNCC, 2011; Fast, Williamson, & Keating, 1999; Rallison, 2009). For example, caregivers may not be able to advance in their chosen careers due to the increased commitment of energy and time that would be required to fulfil those roles. Caregivers may also need to miss full and partial days of work due to the responsibilities of family caregiving (CRNCC, 2011). These economic impacts are thought to be particularly "devastating for women of the sandwich generation who generally earn less than their male counterparts, and look after children and aging parents" (CRNCC, 2011, p. 3). Additionally, one-third of caregivers report extra, ongoing financial expenses related to their caregiving responsibilities (Cranswick, 2003). Unfortunately, these costs are frequently ignored by policymakers focused primarily on containing costs of services. The emotional well-being of the care recipient, who struggles with conflicting issues of dependency and strain on the family, and the emotional well-being of the family caregiver, who struggles with loss of control and independence in his or her daily life, can become very tenuous in these situations (Pyke, 1999). The most dramatic economic costs to caregivers include giving up paid employment, lost income from unpaid leave or time off work, relinquishing career advancement opportunities, and the prospect of out-of-pocket expenses to support home care. Those in the lowest income categories have the highest economic burden. Employers need to consider flexible options to help the caregiver/employee meet the demands of multiple roles.

Family members who participated in Rallison's (2009) research study echoed the financial stress and burden previously documented in the literature. Hidden costs described by the families included the loss of income from one parent who needed to leave previous employment, adjustments to the family home and vehicle, cost sharing with government funding, and incidental costs such as parking, hotel, and food costs during medical visits/hospitalization (Rallison, 2009). Despite the publicly funded healthcare system in Canada, many of the illness costs that parents faced were not fully covered. A mother spoke of these costs as follows (Rallison, 2009, p. 118):

> I always had to advocate for the funds, but I also pay a lot out of my pocket as well. . . . And there is a high monetary cost with disability which is quite invisible, and yes, government funding pays for 75% of the bath chair, but my 25% is still 400 and some dollars. . . . It has been very, very difficult . . . like I realized that in 6 months last year, I paid . . . 3500 dollars myself in child care. These are the hidden costs that people don't recognize because any kind of support with families of children with disabilities is a cost sharing model, so you pay a certain percent and Shelley's care is expensive . . . well over $3000 a month, that the caregiver is getting. . . . So, financially, things are tough . . . and I don't spend. I don't have money to really take a holiday. I don't have money for anything.

Another significant finding within this research was that the funding each family had access to was highly variable and inconsistent. The family's ability to articulate their care and support needs through the writing of funding proposals and active lobbying was very influential in determining the level of funding support a family received (Rallison, 2009).

Moving from Physical, Mental, Emotional, and Spiritual Exhaustion to Letting Go

Family members face the risk of physical, mental, emotional, and spiritual exhaustion as they work day after day to care for and support their loved ones. Within the literature this experience of overwhelming exhaustion has been conceptualized by some as "burnout" (Nerenberg, 2002; Pines & Aronson, 1988). Parents caring for children with severe developmental disabilities or others caring for individuals with Alzheimer's disease are especially at risk for this experience of exhaustion. Very little research has been done on the exhaustion and burnout experienced by informal caregivers. One mother in Rallison's research described a time in her caregiving experience when she faced total exhaustion and came close to the point of total physical and emotional collapse (Rallison, 2009, pp. 118, 119):

> I remember one night when I really didn't have anybody to help me. . . . It was 4 in the morning, and Vince was working the night shift, and I really was by myself. Katie was having seizures . . . every 3 to 10 minutes, stopping breathing during those seizures, and gagging, and choking, and turning blue. I had to pee so bad. . . . So I raced to the bathroom . . . I sat down . . . and she woke up and had a seizure. . . . I just collapsed and went limp, and couldn't move, and I was crying . . . and thought to myself, "she is going to probably be dead" . . . luckily she

wasn't dead when I got back. . . . That was
what my life was. . . . It is hard to describe
how far past overwhelmed you can get before you finally actually do collapse.

For each of the families who participated in the
research conducted by Rallison (2009), an important shift happened in family life as the children continued to live with and progress in their
illness. Families became exhausted and overwhelmed with the care of their children at home,
but when they came to the point of breakdown or
complete collapse there was an eventual reaching out for help and request for support with
caregiving. At that point parents actively sought
out others, both informal and formal caregivers,
that allowed the families to weave "a creative
tapestry of shared care" (Rallison, 2009, p. 126).
The process of reaching out was not easy, and
the support of both informal and hired caregivers was very difficult to obtain. Further, their
ability to maintain ongoing support for their
child and family remained tenuous, uncertain,
and could "unravel" unexpectedly (Rallison,
2009, p. 130). The burden of finding support
and hired caregivers was laid completely on the
shoulders of family members. They had to find
the caregivers, hire them, pay them within a reimbursement program of shared care, and train
them for the care required.

For five of the six families participating in
this study there was a need to have "some form
of live-in caregiving to assist with the 24 hour
demands" (Rallison, 2009, p. 131). These parents gradually learned to let go of the full-time
care, only when they could trust the caregivers
who had been hired to care for their children.
This was a very difficult, emotionally painstak-
ing process for each parent, but once this support was in place the parents found new ways to

live and engage in their own lives, as well as in
the lives of their well children. When they became able to let go of the responsibility of caring for their children 24 hours a day and learned
to care for themselves in a different way, they
often believed they became better parents and
experienced an increased quality of life with
their children.

In such families the work to surrender the
guilt and continued efforts to claim more balance in individual lives also bring changes in
family relationships. For example, when this
mother claimed a new life of her own, there was
also a profound impact on her marital relationship (Rallison, 2009, p. 136):

We don't have to feel guilty about going
to a movie. We don't have to feel guilty
about sitting with each other and talking
for two hours. We don't have to feel like
we are neglecting Katie because we know
that someone is with her. . . . And time together is a lot less stressful. . . . It was a
very big change, and it was a wonderful
change, in that it introduces more possibilities for the future.

This mother also recognized that with the
changes she embraced in her life and in her relationship with the child's father, her child seemed
to be less stressed as well.

Family Caregiving: Experiences of Meaning and Growth

In the past, research on caregiver burden over-
shadowed experiences of meaning, strength, and
growth that are also an inherent part of caring
for and accompanying a family member through
the trajectory of chronic illness. As a result, less
is understood about how and why caregivers

commit to providing care even under difficult circumstances and in the context of their own suffering. Although not much has been published on satisfaction with caregiving, Kramer's (1997) review of research on positive aspects of caregiving noted that some caregivers experienced gain when assisting others. Gain was conceptualized as "the extent to which the caregiving role is appraised to enhance an individual's life space and be enriching" (p. 219).

Caregivers do report satisfaction with their role. Adults who functioned as caregivers during their childhood reported that their participation taught them responsibility, allowed them to be "part of the family," and provided opportunities to be "appreciated" and "useful" (Lackey & Gates, 2001). They also reported pride at learning skills at an early age (Lackey & Gates, 2001). Many couples believe that caring for their partner strengthened their relationship (Gordon & Perrone, 2004). Coherence and a sense of togetherness in caring for others was discovered by Pierce (2001) to be important for maintaining stability within the family. Through coherence, family caregivers felt connected, and this helped them survive in stressful times related to caring situations (Pierce, 2001).

Programs, Services, and Resources for Family Caregivers

Respite Programs and Services

Respite is temporary relief from caregiving responsibilities that provides intervals of rest and relief for the caregiver. Family members may provide respite for the primary caregiver by taking over some tasks; for example, children may assist their caregiving parents by shopping, cleaning, and fulfilling other household tasks. There are also formal sources of respite, such as adult day care, in-home and out-of-home respite support, and special weekend respite programs.

It is important for caregivers to recognize the warning signs that indicate they are becoming overwhelmed and are in need of increased support. For many caregivers the hardest step is acknowledging that help is needed; the next most difficult step is extending the effort to seek this help. Caregivers often feel guilty about seeking respite and delay using formal respite services until they are exhausted and debilitated. Ambivalence on the part of caregivers to make use of respite services is illustrated by a study of family caregivers' experiences with in-hospital respite care for family members with dementia (Gilmour, 2002). Caregivers' feelings varied from acceptance to qualified acceptance to marked ambivalence. Caregivers were torn between the need to have a break and the worry over the impact of the in-hospital respite care on their family member. It is important that healthcare professionals work closely with family members to decrease tensions and anxieties that relate to accessing respite care.

Caregivers need to see respite services as an expected and essential part of their formal support system, not as a sign of personal failure. Families need to understand that if they are to continue caregiving without becoming overwhelmed by the physical and social demands, it is important to build a strong support network using both informal and formal resources. For most families some form of respite care will be an important part of that support system.

When caregiving becomes too physically demanding or too emotionally exhausting, short-term institutional placement of a family member may be considered. Planned, short-term hospital admissions provide in-facility professional care while providing relief for the caregiver. These programs can prevent the threshold of family tolerance from being exceeded. To enhance family caregivers' comfort with this type of respite, it is important for healthcare professionals to put themselves in a secondary, supportive care provider role while simultaneously acknowledging the family as the authority on the care required (Gilmour, 2002). Family members are more fully able to relinquish care when they are confident their relative is receiving care comparable with what is provided at home and that the relative is not negatively affected by the hospital stay (Gilmour, 2002).

Home Care Programs

Home care has been expanded in recent years as a result of earlier hospital discharge, the increase in technically more complex therapies, and public policies that have encouraged the expansion of home care programs in Canada (Romanow, 2002). The home represents a different context for the provision of care than healthcare settings. Toth-Cohen and colleagues (2001) discussed four key factors that must be considered when providing care within the home setting: (1) understand the personal meaning of the home for the family, (2) view the caregiver as a "lay-practitioner," (3) identify the caregiver's beliefs and values, and (4) recognize the potential impact of the interventions on caregiver well-being.

Multiple benefits and challenges for the caregiver and the healthcare professional are present in home care (Toth-Cohen et al., 2001). Benefits for the caregiver include (1) saving time and mental and physical energy, (2) remaining in control and guiding interaction with the provider, (3) being more comfortable and at ease in one's surroundings, and (4) practicing newly learned skills in the context in which they will be used. Benefits for the healthcare professional include (1) gaining an in-depth understanding of the client, the caregiver, and the home context; (2) designing interventions tailored to specific home situations; (3) identifying safety issues of which caregivers may be unaware; and (4) observing caregiver and family interaction in the context in which it occurs.

INTERVENTION WITH THE FAMILY IN THE CONTEXT OF CHRONIC ILLNESS

Healthcare professionals are uniquely positioned to intervene with individuals and families who are living with chronic illness. In an effort to address the complex relational interactions that occur within families and between the family and illness, clinicians need to move beyond conversations that focus only on information about the disease and the provision of health-related education (Eggenberger, Meiers, Krumwiede, Bliesmer, & Earle, 2011; Wright & Bell, 2009). A family systems approach facilitates a more comprehensive focus on the family's patterns of interaction and the illness suffering of family members (Bell & Wright, 2011; Rolland, 2005, 2011; Wright & Bell, 2009; Wright & Leahey, 2005, 2009; Wright et al., 1996).

Within such an approach guidance is available to explore human suffering of families across the changing and uncertain trajectory of chronic illness. Family members are invited to share their stories of living with illness within a therapeutic conversation. The adoption of a specific relational stance is critical within this clinical practice. The clinician works to create a thoughtful and respectful collaboration with family members, which is nonhierarchical and marked by curiosity (Tapp, 2000; Wright &

Bell, 2009; Wright et al., 1996). Within the therapeutic conversation family relationships and illness suffering are explored. New interpretations of illness suffering and illness meaning, as well as alternative approaches to living in the presence of illness, are tentatively offered for the consideration of family members (Wright & Bell, 2009).

The intent of this discussion is to provide healthcare professionals with an introductory understanding of some family systems interventions that hold the possibility of lessening illness suffering when working with families in the context of chronic illness (Wright & Bell, 2009; Wright & Leahey, 2005, 2009). The intervention practices presented include the following: encouraging family members to share their illness narratives or stories of living with illness (Kleinman, 1988), the use of circular questioning practices (Tomm, 1987, 1988, 1989), and an explicit focus on family strengths through the practice of commendations (Houger Limacher, 2003, 2008; Houger Limacher & Wright, 2003, 2006).

Therapeutic Conversations

Within the relational intervention practices we describe, the clinician commits to engaging in purposeful, therapeutic conversations with family members. An important distinction between social and therapeutic conversations was articulated by Wright and Bell (2009, p. 32):

> Social conversations are those that occur as we move about in our daily life and interact with those we encounter. Therapeutic conversations are purposeful and time-limited. . . . Persons and clinicians engaged in therapeutic conversations come together for a particular purpose, generally because the clinician, a family member, or both,

have identified some emotional, spiritual, or physical suffering that needs to be alleviated, reduced, or softened.

Within a therapeutic conversation the clinician has the opportunity to promote family connection and communication and to strengthen the therapeutic relationship that is shared with family members. This very purposeful conversation provides an important opportunity for clinicians to explore with family members their experiences of illness suffering and to share stories of growth, courage, and love (Wright, 2005; Wright & Bell, 2009; Wright et al., 1996).

In a qualitative research study that focused on both the process and outcome of family systems intervention, Robinson (1994, 1998) found that one of the most helpful nursing interventions offered was bringing family members together to talk about their experiences of living with illness (Robinson & Wright, 1995). For many families the emotional intensity of the illness makes it very difficult for them to share their experiences with one another, without the support of a nurse or clinician (West, 2011). One mother who participated in a research study exploring the illness suffering of family members described the difference between sharing difficult conversations with her husband at home and participating in a therapeutic conversation guided by a clinician. Using a metaphor this mother described this difference as a fire burning out of control in a wild field versus a fire that burned safely within the physical boundary of a fire pit (West, 2011).

At the heart of the therapeutic conversation is the adoption of a particular relational stance (Tapp, 2000). A therapeutic conversation might be understood as a genuine conversation (Gadamer, 1989). Binding and Tapp (2008) further describe a genuine conversation as "a fundamental way of being with another . . . there is a quality of authenticity, unaffectedness, and sincerity which is brought to the discussion" (p. 122).

Encouraging the Sharing of Illness Narratives

An illness narrative is a person's own account of the human experience of living with an illness (Kleinman, 1988; Wright & Bell, 2009; Wright & Leahey, 2005, 2009; Wright et al., 1996). Kleinman (1988) articulated the term "illness narrative" and provided the following definition that can assist healthcare professionals to distinguish conversations that occur in the realm of illness rather than the realm of disease (p. 8):

> By invoking the term illness, I mean to conjure up the innately human experience of symptoms and suffering. Illness refers to how the sick person and the members of the family or wider social network perceive, live with, and respond to symptoms and disability.

The illness experience can be elicited from the family through collaborative family meetings in which family members are offered the opportunity to enter a therapeutic conversation and clinicians listen attentively to accept family members' experiences of fear, anger, and sadness, as well as those of hope and courage.

Often, families have not been asked for their unique understanding and experience of living with chronic illness or for their response to the events that have occurred after diagnosis (Wright & Leahey, 2009). In many instances family members have been unable to communicate their thoughts and feelings with the ill family member or other family members. The difficulties family members have in sharing their human experiences of living with illness can lead to feelings of isolation, relational disconnection, and undisclosed suffering (West, 2011). When a clinician is able to facilitate the creation of a therapeutic space in which family members share their illness narratives, a new experience of shared suffering can emerge, dispelling fear and apprehension concerning particular topics in family conversation (West, 2011). The clinician's willingness to explore painful and difficult topics with family members within the therapeutic conversation has been called "speaking the unspeakable" (Wright & Bell, 2009, p. 235). When a clinician "breaks the rules" and challenges the societal or family belief that sensitive topics such as death or anger cannot be raised in conversation, then a "family's belief about their inability to discuss sensitive issues is challenged, and new, facilitating beliefs may arise" (Wright & Bell, 2009, p. 236).

The illness narrative may differ widely between family members. In some cases of longstanding conflicts, family members may have struggled deeply with another family member's decision making over the course of an illness. In such instances the illness narrative between parents or spouses may diverge significantly. In other cases parents may find they have similar views but have not shared their difficulties with each other. In the latter case the telling of the narrative can be healing simply by expressing it to a third person in the company of a second family member. Many such expressions have their own benefit with little need for the clinician to intervene, except for short interjections of "listening noises," such as "yes, I can see that" or "it's so important for you to have shared that with your wife."

The meaning of the illness for each family member is another area that can be explored in the telling of the illness narrative. It can be helpful for a family to find meaning in illness that enhances their sense of mastery, competency, and strength. Family members also need to grieve for the loss of the life they knew before illness (Rolland, 2011). Fears of the future and the ability to adapt to the necessary changes caused by the illness can vary greatly from family member to family member (Rolland, 2011). The clinician's emotional presence and ability to receive and hold the illness narrative allows family members to witness one another's suffering in a manner that often has not been possible before. In this relational act of listening to, and witnessing of, another's illness narrative, family members sometimes come to new interpretations of their own suffering, as well as that of other family members (West, 2011). At other times the clinician may offer an interpretation that provides a new perspective on illness challenges (Wright & Bell, 2009).

The illness narrative that families present when asked is often surprising both in the extent of the difficulties families endure and in the strength and resilience that families possess. It can be a very moving experience for families to be given an opportunity to talk about their unique experiences with illness, particularly if their previous experience with healthcare professionals has been one of being questioned primarily about the medical diagnosis and treatment.

Illness Narratives: Challenges Faced by Healthcare Professionals

It can be very difficult for the clinician to avoid the temptation to "fix" a problem or defend the actions of other healthcare professionals when families share the distressing experiences they have had within the healthcare system. Often what family members need most is to be given an opportunity to share their difficult experiences and to have them acknowledged.

Exploring the illness narrative of family members can be challenging because of the tendency for each family member to see the narrative from their own point of view. This tendency can lead to conversations of blame and misinterpretation rather than ones of healing and restitution (Wright & Bell, 2009; Wright et al., 1996). It is helpful therefore for the clinician to ask questions in such a way that the problems are not viewed as residing within individual people but rather as occurring between people "in language and beliefs" (Wright & Bell, 2009, p. 46).

When listening to divergent narratives it is important to allow all members of the family to express their own experience and not to allow one member to take "air time" away from others. The clinician can play a pivotal role in facilitating this conversational process. After a short period of conversation a clinician may ask another member of the family, "What was this like for you? Did you experience it the same way, or was it different for you?" At other times the clinician may need to take a more purposeful stance, inviting one family member to join in silence as they listen to what another family member most wants to share about his or her experience with the illness.

This particular relational stance was described by the Milan family therapy team as neutrality (Selvini Palazzoli, Boscolo, Cecchin, & Prata, 1980). In adopting a stance of neutrality toward the family system, the clinician purposely works not to blame any one family member for the challenges the family is experiencing; the clinician does not take sides with one family member over another (Wright &

Bell, 2009). Miller (2002) described neutrality as an "evenly hovering attention" (p. 84), as well as an approach in which the clinician allows "the other 'to be' in his own right" (p. 84). In this way a different experience of family dialogue and communication becomes possible.

Circular Questioning Practices: Learning to Ask Relationally Focused Questions

The clinical practice of asking circular questions is a central intervention within the therapeutic conversation (Wright & Bell, 2009; Wright & Leahey, 2005, 2009; Wright et al., 1996). There are different types of questions that clinicians can ask, and each will have a different purpose and therapeutic intent. Questions can be asked to increase the clinician's understanding of the patient and the family situation or to increase or expand the understanding of family members' illness experiences. These circular questions have also been called "influencing questions" (Tomm, 1988, p. 1). It is in this sphere of influence that the use of circular and, in particular, reflective questions becomes more therapeutic. Some families living with chronic illness will manage the different phases and tasks within the trajectory of chronic illness with relative success. Other families, however, experience difficulty managing relational challenges that occur as illness evolves and interacts with individual and family developmental life cycles. These families may benefit significantly from circular questions within a therapeutic conversation.

Typically, we think of questions as having the primary purpose of eliciting factual information. The gathering of assessment data through the process of asking linear questions is one of the central activities of professionals within the healthcare field. Linear questions assist the clinician in defining illness challenges; they tend to focus on cause and content and hold an investigative character (Wright & Leahey, 2009). Circular questions, however, can have a deeper therapeutic effect than simply eliciting factual information. They can invite the recipient, as well as others who listen to the questions and responses, to ponder long after the question was posed.

Circular questions assist in the exploration of illness meaning, explanations family members have for illness, and the beliefs they hold about the relational patterns of interaction within their family. "With circular questions, a relationship between individuals, events, ideas, or beliefs is . . . sought . . . in a context of compassion and curiosity" (Wright & Leahey, 2009, p. 146). These questions may also invite family members into a reflection (Wright & Bell, 2009, p. 227). Maturana and Varela (1992) define the reflective experience as "the moment when we become aware of the part of ourselves which we cannot see in any other way" (p. 23). In asking circular questions we invite family members into a new view of themselves and of other family members.

These unique questions also offer clinicians an opportunity to share their beliefs with family members. For example, if a clinician were to ask the circular question, "When you think about the different ways your husband has supported you since you were diagnosed with cancer, what has been most meaningful for you?" she embeds the belief that the husband has shown support to his wife. In asking this question she also invites the wife into a reflection about how her husband has supported her and what has been most meaningful in that.

It is also important to highlight the importance of circularity (Selvini Palazzoli et al., 1980) in asking circular questions. It is not one question in isolation that will likely invite a family member into a new way of viewing an illness experience or family relationship but rather the careful and thoughtful "cycle of questions and answers between families and nurses" (Wright & Leahey, 2009, p. 147). A family member's response to one question will guide the clinician in the asking of the next question. "It is rarely one question alone . . . but the timing, spacing, placing, and sequencing of questions" (Wright & Bell, 2009, p. 228) that opens the possibility for a change in perspective. **Table 14-1** provides some descriptions and examples of different types of circular questions.

Commendation Practices: Focusing on Family Strengths in Therapeutic Conversations

When chronic illness enters a family's life, there is often a tendency for family members to focus on the difficulties and challenges that have become a part of their daily lives. The inherent strength and resilience that family members possess can become hidden or move outside of the family's view (Wright & Bell, 2009). Many people, both young and old, have not heard verbal confirmation of their value, strength, and resiliency. This is particularly true for family members who are living in the presence of chronic illness. Healthcare professionals can have a significant influence on the family's experience with illness by observing the strengths of family members and then articulating these observations in the course of a therapeutic conversation. The strengths of family members can be heard when clinicians invite the sharing of illness narratives (Wright & Bell, 2009). Further, the offering of a commendation can be an intervention on the clinician. Within commending practices, the clinician comes to see the family and the challenges they face very differently, as the clinician seeks evidence of strength, capability, and resiliency (Tapp, 2000).

Table 14-1	**Circular, Interventive Questions: Descriptions and Examples**	
Question Type	**Description**	**Example**
Difference questions	Explore "differences between people, relationships, time, ideas, or beliefs" (Wright & Leahey, 2009, p. 148)	What has been the greatest change in your relationship with your wife since you were diagnosed with prostate cancer?
Behavioural effect questions	Explore "the effect of one family member's behavior on another" (Wright & Leahey, 2009, p. 148)	When your wife started to cry in the family meeting, what did you find yourself thinking? Feeling?
Hypothetical/ future-orientated questions	Explore "family options and alternative actions or meanings in the future" (Wright & Leahey, 2009, p. 148)	If you were to look ahead 5 years from now, what do you believe you would be most proud of in the way your family has learned to live with this illness?
Triadic questions	Questions "posed to a third person about the relationship between two other people" (Wright & Leahey, 2005, p. 158)	When you are here at the hospital, what do you believe is the greatest challenge your husband faces at home in caring for your daughter?

Source: From Wright, L. M., & Leahey, M. L. (2009). *Nurses and Families: A Guide to Family Assessment and Intervention,* 5th edition, F.A. Davis Company, Philadelphia, PA. Used with permission.

A thoughtful commendation can have a great impact long after it has been offered to a family. Consider how family members might respond if a clinician were to share the following commendations: "I have noticed how carefully you listen to your husband when he speaks about his love for your son" or "I have noticed how you sit with your mother and hold her hand when she is in pain." Commendations need to be sincere and genuine, so it often takes some thought to choose the words that are offered to family members.

SUMMARY

In this chapter we explored the interaction between the stages of family life cycle development and the tasks and stages that occur across the trajectory of chronic illness. The psychosocial demands that unfold within family life in the context of chronic illness will vary with type of onset (acute or gradual), progression, and course of illness. The course may be progressive, constant, or relapsing and possibly life-threatening. Each of these will present unique and shifting challenges to the ill individual and to members of the family. Critical transition periods and a multigenerational perspective on chronic illness and the family life cycle were also considered within this discussion.

The developmental stages of the family as outlined by McGoldrick et al. (2011) and Rolland's (1994, 2005, 2011) theoretical and practice framework (family systems-illness model) for healthcare professionals who are working with families in the context of chronic illness informed our discussion. These frameworks highlight the complex developmental demands that families face and the way they interact with the multiple changes that are simultaneously imposed by the presence of chronic illness in

family life. The challenges that emerge can be particularly difficult when the normative changes within family life cycle development conflict with the demands of chronic illness. Two case studies were presented in an effort to highlight the complex practice issues healthcare professionals need to consider.

The family caregiving activities required during the course of chronic illness are multifaceted. Within this chapter we considered the increasing societal expectation in North America that much of the caregiving of the chronically ill be carried out by family members and other informal, unpaid caregivers. Experiences of meaning and growth and some of the intense challenges this has created for families were discussed, with a consideration of the increase in health-related technology, complex decision making, longer lifespans, and changes to the structure of the Canadian family. Within this discussion we also highlighted some qualitative, hermeneutic research on the family's experience of caring for a child with a progressive neurodegenerative illness at home (Rallison, 2009).

Family interventions that can be offered by healthcare professionals were presented in the final section of the chapter, with a specific focus on the importance of the clinician–family therapeutic relationship, encouraging the telling of the family's illness narratives, and exploring and challenging family members' illness beliefs. Circular questioning and the externalizing of internalized questions were also discussed, because these practices can assist clinicians to explore the illness narrative and illness beliefs within their therapeutic conversations with family members. Finally, commendations were discussed as a practice approach to facilitate an explicit focus on family strengths. The family interventions discussed are based on the Family Systems Nursing theoretical and practice frameworks provided in Wright and Leahey (2009) and Wright and Bell (2009).

It is important for clinicians to remember that many families living alongside chronic illness may feel isolated, alone, and discouraged. Many times the suffering experienced by family members is not acknowledged or attended to in practice. It is essential that professionals understand the reciprocal and systemic influence the illness has on family life and families have on the illness. The occurrence of chronic illness provides a unique challenge and opportunity for professionals to provide a new outlook, including an explicit focus on the strengths the family has shown throughout their particular journey. When new thoughts and interpretations are provided for family members, as well as shared among family members, new perspectives and strategies may be found for living better, or even living well, with chronic illness in the midst of family life.

ACKNOWLEDGEMENT

The authors of the previous American edition of the chapter Linda L. Pierce and Barbara J. Lutz are recognized for their work.

 For a full suite of assignments and additional learning activities, use the access code located in the front of your book and visit this exclusive website: **http://go.jblearning.com/kramer-kile**. If you do not have an access code, you can obtain one at the site.

REFERENCES

Ahrons, C. R. (2011). Divorce: An unscheduled family transition. In M. McGoldrick, B. Carter, & N. Garcia-Preto (Eds.), *The expanded family life cycle: Individual, family, and social perspectives* (pp. 295–306). Boston, MA: Allyn & Bacon.

Anderson, C. M., & Anderson, M. (2011). Single-parent families: Strengths, vulnerabilities, and interventions. In M. McGoldrick, B. Carter, & N. Garcia-Preto (Eds.), *The expanded family life cycle: Individual, family, and social perspectives* (pp. 307–316). Boston, MA: Allyn & Bacon.

Ashton, D. (2011). Lesbian, gay, bisexual, and transgender individuals and the family life cycle. In M. McGoldrick, B. Carter, & N. Garcia-Preto (Eds.), *The expanded family life cycle: Individual, family, and social perspectives* (pp. 115–132). Boston, MA: Allyn & Bacon.

Badr, H., & Acitelli, L. K. (2005). Dyadic adjustment in chronic illness: Does relationship talk matter? *Journal of Family Psychiatry, 19*(2), 465–469.

Barnard, D. (1995). Chronic illness and the dynamics of hoping. In S. K. Toombs, D. Barnard, & R. A. Carson (Eds.), *Chronic illness: From experience to policy* (pp. 38–57). Bloomington, IN: Indiana University Press.

Bell, J. M., & Wright, L. M. (2011). The illness beliefs model: Creating practice knowledge in family systems nursing for families experiencing illness. In E. K. Svavarsdottir & H. Jonsdottir (Eds.), *Family nursing in action* (pp. 15–51). Reykjavik, Iceland: University of Iceland Press.

Binding, L. L., & Tapp, D. M. (2008). Human understanding in dialogue: Gadamer's recovery of the genuine. *Nursing Philosophy, 9*(2), 121–130.

Björk, M., Wiebe, T., & Hallström, I. (2005). Striving to survive: Families' lived experiences when a child is diagnosed with cancer. *Journal of Pediatric Oncology Nursing, 22,* 265–275. doi:10.1177/1043454205279303

Björk, M., Wiebe, T., & Hallström, I. (2009). An everyday struggle—Swedish families' lived experiences during a child's cancer treatment. *Journal of Pediatric Nursing, 24*(5), 423–432. doi: 10.1016/j.pedn.2008.01.082

Brody, A. C., & Simmons, L. A. (2007). Family resiliency during childhood cancer: The father's perspective. *Journal of Pediatric Oncology Nursing, 24,* 152–165. doi: 10.1177/10434542 06298844

Burton, L. C., Newsom, J. T., Schulz, R., Hirsch, C. H., & German, P. S. (1997). Preventative health behaviors among spousal caregivers. *Preventative Medicine, 26,* 162–169.

Canadian Research Network for Care in the Community. (2011). In focus backgrounder: Informal caregiving. Retrieved from http://www.crncc.ca/knowledge /factsheets/pdf

Caputo, J. (2002). Good will and the hermeneutics of friendship: Gadamer and Derrida. *Philosophy &*

Social Criticism, 28, 512–522. doi: 10.1177/0191453 702028005663

Carter, B., & McGoldrick, M. (Eds.). (2005). *The expanded family life cycle: Individual, family, and social perspectives* (3rd ed.). Boston, MA: Allyn & Bacon.

Charmaz, K. (2002). Stories and silences: Disclosures and self in chronic illness. *Qualitative Inquiry, 8,* 302–328.

Chesla, C. A. (2005). Nursing science and chronic illness: Articulating suffering and possibility in family life. *Journal of Family Nursing, 11*(4), 371–387. doi: 10.1177/1074840705281781

Chumbler, N. R., Rittman, M., Van Puymbroeck, M., Vogel, W. B., & Qin, H. (2004). The sense of coherence, burden, and depressive symptoms in informal caregivers during the first month after stroke. *International Journal of Geriatric Psychiatry, 19*(10), 944–953.

Clarke-Steffen, L. (1990). The experience of families when a child is diagnosed with cancer. Unpublished doctoral dissertation. Portland, OR: Oregon Health & Science University.

Clarke-Steffen, L. (1993a). A model of the family transition to living with childhood cancer. *Cancer Practice, 1*(4), 285–292.

Clarke-Steffen, L. (1993b). Waiting and not knowing: The diagnosis of cancer in a child. *Journal of Pediatric Oncology Nursing, 10,* 146–153.

Clarke-Steffen, L. (1997). Reconstructing reality: Family strategies for managing childhood cancer. *Journal of Pediatric Nursing, 12*(5), 278–287.

Clyburn, L. D., Stones, M. J., Hadjistavropoulos, T., & Tuokko, H. (2000). Predicting caregiver burden and depression in Alzheimer's disease. *Journal of Gerontology, Social Sciences, 55B,* S2–S13.

Cohen, M. (1993). The unknown and the unknowable—Managing sustained uncertainty. *Western Journal of Nursing Research, 15,* 77–96.

Cohen, M. (1995a). The stages of the prediagnostic period in chronic, life-threatening childhood illness: A process analysis. *Research in Nursing and Health, 18,* 39–48.

Cohen, M. (1995b). The triggers of heightened parental uncertainty in chronic, life-threatening childhood illness. *Qualitative Health Research, 5,* 63–77.

Combrinck-Graham, L. (1985). A developmental model for family systems. *Family Process, 24,* 139–150.

Covinsky, K. E., Newcomer, R., Fox, P., Wood, J., Sands, L., Dane, K., & Yaffe, K. (2003). Patient and caregiver characteristics associated with depression in caregiving of patients with dementia. *Journal of General Internal Medicine, 18*(12), 1006–1014.

Cranswick, K. (2003). *General social survey cycle 16: Caring for an aging society.* Ottawa, ON: Statistics Canada. Retrieved from http://www.statcan.gc.ca

Cranswick, K., & Dosman, D. (2008). Eldercare: What we know today. *Canadian Social Trends, 86,* 48–56. Retrieved from http://www.statcan.gc.ca

Eggenberger, S. K., Meiers, S. J., Krumwiede, N., Bliesmer, M., & Earle, P. (2011). Reintegration within families in the context of chronic illness: A family health promoting process. *Journal of Nursing and Healthcare of Chronic Illness, 3,* 283–292.

Evercare & National Alliance for Caregiving. (2007). *Evercare study of family caregivers—What they spend, what they sacrifice.* Minnetonka, MN: Author. Retrieved from http://www.caregiving.org/data /EvercareNACCaregiverCostStudyFINAL20111907 .pdf

Falicov, C. J. (2011). Migration and the life cycle. In M. McGoldrick, B. Carter, & N. Garcia-Preto (Eds.), *The expanded family life cycle: Individual, family, and social perspectives* (pp. 336–347). Boston, MA: Allyn & Bacon.

Fast, J., Niehaus, L., Eales, J., & Keating, N. (2002). *A profile of Canadian chronic care providers: A report submitted to Human Resources and Development Canada.* Edmonton, AB: Department of Human Ecology, University of Alberta.

Fast, J. E., Williamson, D. L., & Keating, N. C. (1999). The hidden costs of informal elder care. *Journal of Family and Economic Issues, 20,* 301–326.

Gadamer, H. G. (989). *Truth and method.* New York, NY: Continuum.

Gagliardi, B. A. (1991). The family's experience of living with a child with Duchenne muscular dystrophy. *Applied Nursing Research, 4,* 159–164.

Garcia-Preto, N. (2011). Transformation of the family system during adolescence. In M. McGoldrick, B. Carter, & N. Garcia-Preto (Eds.), *The expanded family life cycle: Individual, family, and social perspectives* (pp. 232–246). Boston, MA: Allyn & Bacon.

Geister, C. (2005). The feeling of responsibility as core motivation for care giving—Why daughters care for their mothers. *Pflege, 18*(1), 5–14.

Gilmour, J. A. (2002). Disintegrated care: Family caregivers and in-hospital care. *Journal of Advanced Nursing, 39*(6), 546–553.

Gordon, P. A., & Perrone, K. M. (2004). When spouses become caregivers: Counseling implications for younger couples. *Journal of Rehabilitation, 70*(2), 27–32.

Gravelle, A. M. (1997). Caring for a child with a progressive illness during the complex chronic phase: Parents' experiences of facing adversity. *Journal of Advanced Nursing, 25,* 738–745.

Halm, M. A., & Bakas, T. (2007). Factors associated with depressive symptoms, outcomes, and perceived physical health after coronary bypass surgery. *Journal of Cardiovascular Nursing, 22*(6), 508–515.

Hauerwas, S. (1986). *Suffering presence.* Notre Dame, IN: Notre Dame University Press.

Hollander, M. J., Liu, G., & Chappell, N. L. (2009). Who cares and how much? The imputed economic contribution to the Canadian healthcare system of middle-aged and older unpaid caregivers providing care to the elderly. *Healthcare Quarterly, 12*(2), 42–49.

Houger Limacher, L. (2003). Commendations: The healing potential of one family systems nursing intervention. Unpublished doctoral dissertation. Alberta, Canada: University of Calgary.

Houger Limacher, L. (2008). Locating relationships at the heart of commending practices. *Journal of Systemic Therapies, 27*(4), 90–105.

Houger Limacher, L., & Wright, L. M. (2003). Commendations: Listening to the silent side of a family intervention. *Journal of Family Nursing, 9,* 130–135. doi: 10.1177/1074840703251968

Houger Limacher, L., & Wright, L. M. (2006). Exploring the therapeutic family intervention of commendations: Insights from research. *Journal of Family Nursing, 12,* 307–331. doi:10.1177/1074840706291696

Hunt, C. K. (2003). Concepts in caregiver research. *Journal of Nursing Scholarship, 35*(1), 27–32.

Hunt, G., Levine, C., & Naiditch, N. (2005). *Young caregivers in the U.S.* New York, NY: National Alliance for Caregiving and the United Hospital Fund.

Keefe, J., Legare, J., & Carriere, Y. (2005). *Developing new strategies to support future caregivers of the aged in Canada: Projections of need and their policy implications.* Social and Economic Dimensions of an Aging Population (SEDAP) Research Paper No. 140. Hamilton, Ontario. Retrieved from http://socserv .mcmaster.ca/sedap/p/sedap140.pdf

Kelly, K. P., & Ganong, L. H. (2011). "Shifting family boundaries" after the diagnosis of cancer in stepfamilies. *Journal of Family Nursing, 17*(1), 105–132. doi: 10.1177/1074840710397365

Kleinman, A. (1988). *The illness narratives.* New York, NY: Basic Books.

Kramer, B. (1997). Gain in the caregiving experience: Where are we? What next? *The Gerontologist, 37,* 218–232.

Lackey, N. R., & Gates, M. F. (2001). Adults' recollections of their experiences as young caregivers of family members with chronic physical illnesses. *Journal of Advanced Nursing, 34*(3), 320–328.

Maturana, H. R., & Varela, F. J. (1992). *The tree of knowledge: The biological roots of human understanding* (rev. ed., R. Paolucci, Trans.). Boston, MA: Shambhala.

Mausbach, B. T., Patterson, T. L., Von Känel, R., Mills, P. J., Dimsdale, J. E., Ancoli-Israel, S., Grant, I. (2007). The attenuating effect of personal mastery on the relations between stress and Alzheimer caregiver health: A five-year longitudinal analysis. *Aging & Mental Health, 11*(6), 637–644.

McAuley, W. J., Travis, S. S., & Safewright, M. P. (1997). Personal accounts of the nursing home search and selection process. *Qualitative Health Research, 7,* 236–254.

McCubbin, M., Balling, K., Possin, P., Frierdich, S., & Bryne, B. (2002). Family resiliency in childhood cancer. *Family Relations, 51,* 103–111.

McGoldrick, M., & Carter, B. (2011). Families transformed by the divorce cycle: Reconstituted, multinuclear, recoupled, and remarried families. In M. McGoldrick, B. Carter, & N. Garcia-Preto (Eds.), *The expanded family life cycle: Individual, family, and social perspectives* (pp. 317–335). Boston, MA: Allyn & Bacon.

McGoldrick, M., Carter, B., & Garcia-Preto, N. (Eds.). (2011). *The expanded family life cycle: Individual, family, and social perspectives* (4th ed.). Boston, MA: Allyn & Bacon.

McGoldrick, M., Carter, B., & Petkov, B. (2011). Becoming parents: The family with young children. In M. McGoldrick, B. Carter, & N. Garcia-Preto (Eds.), *The expanded family life cycle: Individual, family, and social perspectives* (pp. 211–231). Boston, MA: Allyn & Bacon.

McGoldrick, M., Gerson, R., & Petry, S. (2008). *Genograms: Assessment and intervention* (3rd ed.). New York, NY: W. W. Norton.

McQuillan, R., & Finally, L. (1996). Facilitating the care of terminally ill children. *Journal of Pain and Symptom Management, 12,* 320–324.

Meshefedjian, G., McCusker, J., Bellavance, F., & Baumgarten, M. (1998). Factors associated with symptoms of depression among informal caregivers of demented elders in the community. *The Gerontologist, 38,* 247–253.

Miller, M. E. (2002). Zen and psychotherapy: From neutrality, through relationship, to the emptying place. In P. Young-Eisendrath & S. Muramoto (Eds.), *Awakening and insight: Zen Buddhism and psychotherapy.* New York, NY: Taylor & Francis.

Monterosso, L., Kristjanson, L., Aoun, S., & Phillips, M. (2007). Supportive and palliative care needs of families of children with life-threatening illnesses in western Australia: Evidence to guide the development of a palliative care service. *Palliative Medicine, 21,* 689–696.

Moody, K., Meyer, M., Mancuso, C. A., Charlson, M., & Robbins, L. (2006). Exploring concerns of children with cancer. *Supportive Care in Cancer, 14,* 960–966. doi: 10/1007/s00520-006-0024-y

Moore Hines, P. (2011). The life cycle of African American families living in poverty. In M. McGoldrick, B. Carter, & N. Garcia-Preto (Eds.), *The expanded family life cycle: Individual, family, and social perspectives* (pp. 89–102). Boston, MA: Allyn & Bacon.

Nerenberg, L. (2002). *Preventing elder abuse by family caregivers.* Washington, DC: National Center of Elder Abuse.

Neugarten, B. (1976). Adaptation and the life cycle. *The Counseling Psychologist, 6*(1), 16–20.

Nicholas, D. B., Gearing, R. E., McNeill, T., Fung, K., Lucchetta, S., & Selkirk, E. K. (2009). Experiences and resistance strategies utilized by fathers of children with cancer. *Social Work in Health Care, 48,* 260–275. doi: 10.1080/0098138080259 1734

Ory, M. G., Hoffman, R. R. III, Yee, J. L., Tennstedt, S., & Schulz, R. (1999). Prevalence and impact of caregiving: A detailed comparison between dementia and nondementia caregivers. *The Gerontologist, 39*(2), 177–185.

Palmer, S., & Glass, T. A. (2003). Family function and stroke recovery: A review. *Rehabilitation Psychology, 48*(4), 255–265.

Patterson, J. M., Holm, K. E., & Gurney, J. G. (2004). The impact of childhood cancer on the family: A qualitative analysis of strains, resources, and coping behaviors. *Psycho-oncology, 13,* 390–407. doi: 10.1002/pon.761

Pierce, L. (2001). Coherence in the urban family caregiver role with African American stroke survivors. *Topics in Stroke Rehabilitation, 8*(3), 64–72.

Piercy, K. W., & Chapman, J. G. (2001). Adopting the caregiver role: A family legacy. *Family Relations, 50,* 386–393.

Pines, A. M., & Aronson, E. (1988). *Career burnout: Causes and cures.* New York, NY: The Free Press.

Powell-Cope, G. M. (1995). The experiences of gay couples affected by HIV infection. *Qualitative Health Research, 5*(1), 36–62.

Pyke, K. (1999). The micropolitics of care in relationships between aging parents and adult children: Individualism, collectivism, and power. *Journal of Marriage and the Family, 61,* 661–673.

Rallison, L. B. (2009). Living in the in-between: A hermeneutic study of families caring for a child with a progressive neurodegenerative illness at home. Unpublished doctoral dissertation. Alberta, Canada: University of Calgary.

Robinson, C. A. (1994). Women, families, chronic illness and nursing interventions: From burden to balance. Unpublished doctoral dissertation. Alberta, Canada: University of Calgary.

Robinson, C. A. (1998). Women, families, chronic illness, and nursing interventions: From burden to balance. *Journal of Family Nursing, 4*(3), 271–290.

Robinson, C. A., & Wright, L. M. (1995). Family nursing interventions: What families say makes a difference. *Journal of Family Nursing, 1*(3), 327–345.

Rolland, J. S. (1984). Toward a psychosocial typology of chronic and life-threatening illness. *Family Systems Medicine, 2*(3), 245–262. Retrieved from http://ovidsp .tx.ovid.com.ezproxylib.ucalgary.ca

Rolland, J. S. (1988). Toward a psychosocial typology of chronic and life-threatening illness. *Family Systems Medicine, 2*(3), 245–262.

Rolland, J. S. (1994). *Families, illness, and disability: An integrative treatment model.* New York, NY: Basic Books.

Rolland, J. S. (2005). Chronic illness and the family life cycle. In B. Carter & M. McGoldrick (Eds.), *The expanded family life cycle: Individual, family, and social perspectives* (3rd ed., pp. 492–511). Boston, MA: Pearson.

Rolland, J. S. (2011). Chronic illness and the life cycle. In M. McGoldrick, B. Carter, & N. Garcia-Preto (Eds.), *The expanded family life cycle: Individual, family, and social perspectives* (4th ed., pp. 348–367). Boston, MA: Pearson.

Romanow, R. J. (2002). *Building on values: The future of health care in Canada—Final report.* Ottawa, ON: Commission on the Future of Health Care in Canada.

Sebern, M. D., & Whitlatch, C. J. (2007). Dyadic relationship scale: A measure of the impact of the provision and receipt of family care. *The Gerontologist, 47*(6), 741–751.

Selvini Palazzoli, M., Boscolo, L., Cecchin, G., & Prata, G. (1980). Hypothesizing, circularity, neutrality: Three guidelines for the conductor of the session. *Family Process, 19,* 3–12. doi: 10.1111/j.1545–5300 .1980.00003.x

Stein, R. (2001). Home-based comprehensive care services for children with chronic conditions. *Children's Services: Social Policy, Research, and Practice, 4*(4), 189–201.

Stevens, M. (2004). Care of the dying child and adolescent: Family adjustment and support. In D. Doyle, G. Hanks, N. Cherney, & K. Calman (Eds.), *Oxford textbook of palliative medicine* (3rd ed., pp. 806–821). New York, NY: Oxford University Press.

Tapp, D. M. (2000). The ethics of relational stance in family nursing: Revisiting the view of "nurse as expert." *Journal of Family Nursing, 6*(69), 69–91. doi:10.1177/107484070000600105

Tomm, K. (1987). Interventive interviewing: Part II. Reflexive questioning as a means to enable self-healing. *Family Process, 26*(6), 167–183.

Tomm, K. (1988). Interventive interviewing: Part III. Intending to ask lineal, circular, strategic, or reflexive questions? *Family Process, 27*(1), 1–15.

Tomm, K. (1989). Externalizing the problem and internalizing personal agency. *Journal of Strategic and Systemic Therapies, 8*(1), 54–59.

Toth-Cohen, S., Gitlin, L. N., Corcoran, M. A., Eckhardt, S., Kearney, P. (2001). Providing services to family caregivers at home: Challenges and recommendations for health and human service professions. *Alzheimer's Care Quarterly, 2*(1), 23–32.

Travis, S. S., & Bethea, L. S. (2001). Medication administration by family members of elders in shared care arrangements. *Journal of Clinical Geropsychology, 7,* 231–243.

Vanier Institute of the Family. (2010). *Families count: Profiling Canada's families IV.* Retrieved from http ://www.vanierinstitute.ca

Weitzner, M. A., Haley, W. E., & Chen, H. (2000). The family caregiver of the older cancer patient. *Hematology and Oncology Clinics of North America, 14,* 269–281.

West, C. H. (2011). Addressing illness suffering in childhood cancer: Exploring the beliefs of family members in therapeutic nursing conversations. Unpublished doctoral dissertation. Alberta, Canada: University of Calgary.

White, M. (1988/1989). Externalizing of the problem and re-authoring of lives and relationships. *Dulwich Centre Newsletter,* 3–21.

White, M. (2007). *Maps of narrative practice.* New York, NY: W. W. Norton.

White, M., & Epston, D. (1990). *Narrative means to therapeutic ends.* New York, NY: W. W. Norton.

Woodgate, R. (2001). Symptom experiences in the illness trajectory of children with cancer and their families. Unpublished doctoral dissertation. Winnipeg, Manitoba, Canada: University of Manitoba.

Woodgate, R. L. (2006). Life is never the same: Childhood cancer narratives. *European Journal of Cancer Care, 15,* 8–18. doi: 10.1111/j.1365–2354.2005.00614.x

Wright, L. M. (2005). *Spirituality, suffering, and illness: Ideas for healing.* Philadelphia, PA: F. A. Davis.

Wright, L. M., & Bell, J. M. (2009). *Beliefs and illness: A model for health.* Calgary, Alberta, Canada: 4th Floor Press.

Wright, L. M., & Leahey, M. (2005). *Nurses and families: A guide to family assessment and intervention* (4th ed.). Philadelphia, PA: F. A. Davis.

Wright, L. M., & Leahey, M. (2009). *Nurses and families: A guide to family assessment and intervention* (5th ed.). Philadelphia, PA: F. A. Davis.

Wright, L. M., Watson, W. L., & Bell, J. M. (1996). *Beliefs: The heart of healing in families and illness.* New York, NY: Basic Books.

Yee, J. L., & Schulz, R. (2000). Gender differences in psychiatric morbidity among family caregivers: A review and analysis. *The Gerontologist, 40,* 147–164.

Young, B., Dixon-Woods, M., & Heney, D. (2002). Identity and role in parenting a child with cancer. *Pediatric Rehabilitation, 5,* 209–214. doi: 10.1080 /136384902100 046184

Zukewich, N. (2003). Unpaid informal caregiving. *Canadian Social Trends, 70,* 14–18. Retrieved from http://www.statcan.gc.ca

CHAPTER 15

Health Promotion

Original chapter by Alicia Huckstadt
Canadian content added by Joseph C. Osuji

INTRODUCTION

Health-promoting behaviours strongly influence whether one prematurely succumbs to disease or whether one postpones and possibly avoids many major diseases. Yet, health promotion is often viewed as insignificant as healthcare systems scramble to treat heart disease, cancer, and other diseases that are often in advanced stages. Historically, Canada has been in the forefront for innovations and research on health promotion and how health promotion can change the course of different diseases. The once believed single causation theory of morbidity has now been largely replaced by multifactorial causation theories and chronicity of conditions. Improved recognition and management of disease processes, better sanitation, immunizations, and other health measures have increased the longevity of Canadians. The life expectancy in the early 1920s was the late 50s; it has now increased to the upper 70s for men and early 80s for women (Statistics Canada, 2012). Diseases that once brought sudden death have been surpassed by chronic disease. Canadians are living longer but not necessarily healthier. The Public

Health Agency of Canada (2012a) projected that chronic diseases accounted for 66.9% of all deaths in Canada each year.

Societal influences and individual lifestyle choices have negatively influenced health. According to Health Canada (2012a), smoking remains the leading cause of preventable death in Canada. Smoking causes deaths from lung and other cancers, chronic lung disease, heart disease, and stroke. Exposure to second-hand smoke causes premature death and disease in others who do not smoke themselves. Other smokeless tobacco use also causes cancer and other conditions.

Following closely behind tobacco use as a major health risk is obesity. The prevalence of obesity among adults shows upward trends, and there have been increases in overweight children. According to the Heart and Stroke Foundation of Canada (2012), almost 60% of all Canadian adults, or 14.1 million Canadians, are overweight or obese according to clinical measures such as body mass index or waist-to-hip ratios. As researchers study the condition, long-term obesity has been associated with avoidable hospitalizations and substantial risk for health complications (Schafer & Ferraro, 2007). Obesity is associated with increased risk of diabetes, stroke, heart disease, some cancers, hypertension, osteoarthritis, gallbladder disease, and disability (Health Canada, 2012c). However, it is important to note that not all individuals who are clinically defined as overweight or obese will develop health issues, and it is important not to stigmatize people based on size.

Modifiable health-risk behaviours—smoking, poor diet, physical inactivity, and excessive alcohol consumption—are the major underlying causes of much of the illness, suffering, and early death related to chronic illness (Sweet & Fortier, 2010). These factors and the other modifiable behavioural risk factors listed previously are believed to be the genesis of heart disease, malignant neoplasm, cerebrovascular disease, diabetes mellitus, and other chronic diseases. The escalating healthcare costs, disease, and deaths associated with these factors make health promotion essential for all.

DEFINING HEALTH PROMOTION IN CHRONIC ILLNESS

Canada has been a world leader in health promotion (Barr et al., 2003). The World Health Organization (1986) definition of health promotion is "the process of enabling people to increase control over and to improve their health" (p. 1). Health promotion is a multidimensional concept and focuses on maintaining or improving the health of individuals, families, and communities. Minimizing preventable health risk factors such as tobacco use, inadequate diets, and physical inactivity would substantially decrease the development and severity of many chronic diseases and conditions (Cory et al., 2010).

Health promotion for individuals with chronic or disabling conditions is commonly defined as efforts to create healthy lifestyles and a healthy environment to prevent secondary conditions, such as teaching people how to address their healthcare needs and increasing opportunities to participate in usual life activities. These secondary conditions can be the medical, social, emotional, mental, family, or community problems that an individual with a chronic or disabling condition likely experiences. Healthy living refers to the "practices of population groups that are consistent with supporting, improving, maintaining and or enhancing health" (Public Health Agency of Canada [PHAC], 2012b). For individuals with chronic illness, this implies the capacity to make healthy choices such as healthy eating and engaging in physical activities.

Health-promoting activities can be implemented at the public level or the personal level and involve passive or active strategies (Greiner & Edelman, 2010). Passive strategies, such as those used in food industry sanitation, decrease infectious agents in foods and improve public health. National, provincial, and local public and private agencies are given the responsibility to provide passive strategies to promote health for their constituents. Active strategies, such as engaging in better personal nutrition or activity regimens, depend on the individual and/or family becoming involved (Edelman & Mandle, 2006). Although both strategies are essential, this chapter focuses primarily on active strategies for individuals with chronic illness and their families.

Health promotion applies to all individuals regardless of age or disability. The goal of health promotion is to increase the involved person's control over his or her health and to improve it.

Leddy (2006) added that health promotion is mobilizing strengths to enhance health, wellness, and well-being.

Health promotion in chronic illness involves individual behavioural change for positive lifestyle activities, accepting one's condition and making the necessary adjustments, decreasing the risk of secondary disabilities and preventing further disease, and striving for optimal health as well as systemic changes in the community and how health care is organized and delivered. Behavioural change becomes possible when environmental and political policies support the resources (Aro & Absetz, 2009). For instance, the Ottawa Charter for Health Promotion (World Health Organization, 1986) identified the prerequisites for health as peace, shelter, education, food, income, a stable ecosystem, sustainable resources, social justice, and equity. Health promotion action, according to the Charter, means building healthy public policies, creating supportive environments, strengthening community action, developing personal skills, and reorienting healthcare services.

Health promotion in chronic illness is important in maintaining and enhancing the function of the individual. It is also critical to prevent recurrence of some conditions. Often, families direct their energies toward the illness rather than health. The illness and its cascade of effects alter family dynamics, usual roles, and patterns of life (Heinzer, 1998). Managing medicines, conserving physical and mental energy, keeping appointments with healthcare professionals, adjusting finances, and learning new resources will likely require substantial effort. These new stressors often overtax the individual, and activities to maintain a healthy lifestyle are often ignored. Preventive health screening for other conditions may be forgotten by the client and

healthcare professional. Yet, health-promoting behaviours are crucial in the management of chronic conditions and are often the essential aspect in successful management. Individuals with chronic illness may develop comorbidities that could be avoided or minimized with early detection. Disease-specific preventive care needs and related physical, social, emotional, and spiritual well-being encompass health promotion for those with and without chronic illness. McWilliam, Stewart, Brown, Desai, and Coderre (1996) found in their phenomenological study exploring health and health promotion of 13 sample participants with chronic illness "a dynamically changing and evolving endeavor that encompassed four components: fighting and struggling, resigning oneself, creatively balancing resources, and accepting" (p. 5).

Undoubtedly, chronic illness presents numerous challenges to health promotion. The potential for these activities and overall health remains largely untapped in many individuals with chronic illness. Creating new ways of accomplishing health promotion often remains an unfilled goal for nurses and their clients with chronic illness. Efforts must go beyond the individual's chronic illness and limitations to include holistic health that focuses on personal goals, evidence-informed care tailored to the person, and a willingness to adjust the plan as needed. Determining individuals' perceptions of their condition, their aspirations, and their available resources and supporting their efforts to achieve health promotion is an ongoing process. Leddy (2006) emphasized that health promotion develops the individual strengths and environmental resources to find solutions rather than focusing solely on illness repair. Chronicity presents challenges to all those involved and can take precedence over other health considerations.

Nurses are ideally suited to promote the health of all individuals and their families. The holistic, caring perspective held by nurses provides opportunities to promote strengths at a time when others may perceive only threats to health. The consequences of failure to promote health are devastating. Additional morbidity, deaths, and financial strain for individuals, families, and society weigh heavy on the healthcare system. The rising healthcare costs and an aging population compound the problem.

ONLINE RESOURCES

The PHAC and Health Canada websites (www.phac.gc.ca and www.hc-sc.gc.ca) share the goal of helping people live longer and healthier lives; they feature health and safety topics on their home pages. These websites provide information on numerous diseases and conditions, case studies, government documents, action statements, emergency preparedness, environmental health, traveller's health, workplace safety, and other topics. One area, healthy living, is especially beneficial to consumers and healthcare providers for health in all life stages (further information is available at www.phac-aspc.gc.ca/hp-ps/hl-mvs/index-eng.php).

Specifically, the PHAC launched the Canadian best practices portal in November 2006 that is accessible to the general population (http://cbpp-pcpe.phac-aspc.gc.ca/about/portal-eng.html). This portal houses a compendium of community interventions related to chronic disease prevention, management and evidence-informed health promotion strategies that can be replicated elsewhere. Another website (http://centre4activeliving.ca/) provides a quick guide to healthy living, personal health tools, health news related to active living and

physical activities, and other information for healthcare providers/professionals who promote physical activity in their work life.

The Centre for Health Promotion, University of Ottawa (www.utoronto.ca/chp/) is a community–academic partnership committed to excellence in education, evaluation, and research. In a multidisciplinary, collaborative context it activates, develops, and evaluates innovative health promotion approaches in Canada and abroad. The Centre is an active, high quality, internationally recognized leader in health promotion and provides much valuable information on research and practice of health promotion. Finally, the Canadian Public Health Association presents an Action Statement for Health Promotion in Canada. This document can be accessed at www.cpha.ca/en/programs/policy/action.aspx.

CHALLENGES

These documents and other resources illustrate that health promotion and disease prevention are essential for all Canadians. The nation needs to continually work toward these goals; however, to do so requires changes in the healthcare system. Providing chronic health care once the disease has occurred is only a segment of the needed care. Many of the risks to health—obesity, diabetes, hypertension, heart disease, cancer, and other chronic conditions—often result from failure to engage in preventive care. More closely articulated preventive, public health, and policy programs are needed to promote a healthy life. Other factors, including genetics and environmental risks, contribute to chronic illness.

Health promotion can and should occur before the onset of chronic illness, and as early as possible. Health promotion ideally occurs throughout one's life and in concert with chronic conditions through the end of life. Health promotion is a lifetime activity and can include end-of-life planning for individuals and their significant others. Preparing for the physical and psychosocial changes that accompany death requires attention before crisis events. Preparation, dissemination, and discussion of advance directives with significant others can help set clear boundaries for honouring the wishes of clients (Rainer & McMurry, 2002).

BARRIERS

Reported barriers to health screening and other preventive care must be addressed. Unhealthy behaviours continue to increase in Canada, putting people more at risk for initial chronic illness and deterring health promotion practices among those with chronic illnesses. Cigarette smoking is the most important cause of premature death in Canada (Makromaski-Illing & Kaiserman, 1999) and accounts for 17% of all deaths (Rehm et al., 2002). According to data from the Canadian Tobacco Use Monitoring Survey 2002, the smoking rates in Canada have been on the decline for the past decade. Overweight, obesity, and physical inactivity are also considered risk factors for many chronic illnesses (Health Canada, 2002). The PHAC (2012b) reported that among Canadian adults, 50% of women and 44% of men are inactive and do not engage in up to 30 to 60 minutes of physical activities every day. Exercising regularly, eating a healthy diet, and not using tobacco can help people prevent and manage chronic diseases. However, many people in Canada and other countries do not have easy access to healthy foods and safe, convenient places to

exercise. These barriers have led to increasingly sedentary lifestyles for most Canadians.

Other barriers exist for health screening. Bryant, Fekete, and Major (2011) identified low level of understanding of screening as a wellness-related behaviour that was a common barrier to screening for colorectal cancer, whereas Brennenstuhl, Fuller-Thomson, and Popova (2009) implicated lower household income with lower odds of screening for colorectal cancer among Canadian women. Similarly, Lofters, Moineddin, Hwang, and Glazier (2011) studied the predictors of low cervical cancer screening among immigrant women in Ontario, Canada, and found that variables such as age, neighbourhood of residence, the influence of the primary care provider, and not having a female care provider were negatively associated with low levels of screening.

Little is known about how health screening and other preventive care affect outcomes. Norman et al. (2007) emphasized that we do not know what survivors of diseases like breast cancer must do to prevent recurrence. Data are needed on lifestyle change from prediagnosis to postdiagnosis, changes over time after diagnosis, and identification of potential lifestyle risk factors.

Health promotion has not been addressed well in the care of clients with numerous chronic health conditions. Capella-McDonnall (2007) reported that despite the recent focus on health promotion for persons with disabilities, adults who are visually impaired have not received adequate attention. Two conditions, overweight or obesity and physical inactivity, are problems for many persons with disabilities, including those who are visually impaired.

Problems with health literacy are commonplace in our society (Begoray & Kwan, 2011).

Health literacy is defined as the "ability to access, understand, evaluate and communicate information as a way to promote, maintain and improve health in a variety of settings across the life-course" (Rootman & Gordon-El-Bihbety, 2008, p. 11). It empowers people "to act appropriately in new and changing health-related circumstances through the use of advanced cognitive and social skills" (Speros, 2005, p. 633).

Poor health outcomes and less frequent use of preventive services are linked with low literacy. Individuals with low literacy are more likely to skip important preventive screening such as colonoscopy, Pap smears, and mammograms and are less likely to receive protective measures such as flu immunizations. Persons with low literacy are more likely to have chronic illness and are less able to manage it effectively. More preventable hospitalizations and use of emergency services are found among clients with chronic illness with limited literacy skills. People with limited literacy skills often lack knowledge about the nature and causes of disease and may not understand the relationship between lifestyle factors such as smoking, lack of exercise, and inadequate nutrition and poor health outcomes. Peerson and Saunders (2011) concluded that low levels of health literacy negatively impact self-management and disease prevention.

Other barriers to health screening and preventive care include associated costs, lack of knowledge/understanding, negative beliefs/attitudes, and lack of access, especially for those with limited geographical and/or functional ability. Other factors are addressed in the next section on Models, Theories, and Frameworks.

CASE STUDY `WWW`

Smith Jones is a 55-year-old man with hypertension, type 2 diabetes, and hyperlipidemia. Mr. Jones completed the 11th grade and worked as a mechanic until he could join the military. He served his country for 2 years and returned home. He lives at home with his wife of 35 years. Both he and his wife smoke, are overweight, and have sedentary jobs outside the home. Having raised three children, they now enjoy staying home and watching television together in the evenings. Neither has a physical exercise regimen even though both were told to increase exercise at their last medical appointment. Mr. Jones's last hemoglobin A1c was 8.1. He was scheduled for a colonoscopy but did not go for the appointment, stating he could not understand the informational brochure he was given. He reports he did receive a flu immunization this fall.

Discussion Questions

1. What are two health literacy implications in this case?
2. How would you tailor a health promotion program for Smith Jones and his family?
3. What theoretical framework would be useful for the health promotion program?

MODELS, THEORIES, AND FRAMEWORKS _____

An entire body of literature has evolved around the models and theories relating to health behaviour change. Considerable research has demonstrated success in changing behaviour with smoking cessation, alcohol abuse, and others using these theories. The most often used theories in 193 articles on health behaviour literature published in 10 leading public health, medicine, and psychology journals from 2000 to 2005 were the transtheoretical model, social cognitive theory, and health belief model (Painter, Borba, Hynes, Mays, & Glanz, 2008). In these articles most (68.1%) involved research that was informed by theory; others applied theory, tested theory, and sought to develop theory. The examples that follow are theories and models that may be useful in assessing change within chronic illness.

The *transtheoretical model* (TTM), by Prochaska, Redding, and Evers (2002), incorporates the processes and principles of change from several major theories in psychotherapy and human behaviour. The stages of change within the model are (1) precontemplation, which is no intention to change in the foreseeable future; (2) contemplation, the intention to change in the next 6 months; (3) preparation, the intention to take action within the next 30 days and some behavioural steps to change; (4) action, which is behaviour change for less than 6 months; and (5) maintenance, in which behaviour has changed for more than 6 months. These stages represent a temporal dimension to change and are helpful in identifying timing of change interventions. A last stage—termination, in which the individual who possesses total self-efficacy is no longer susceptible to temptation of unhealthy behaviour—is rarely used, because few individuals reach this level. In the TTM individuals weigh the pros and cons of changing (decisional balance) and determine their confidence (self-efficacy) that they can cope with high-risk situations without relapsing to unhealthy or high-risk behaviour specific to the situation.

The 10 processes of change of the TTM are activities that people use to progress through the stages of change: (1) consciousness raising (increasing awareness of the behaviour), (2) dramatic relief (experiencing increased emotions followed by reduced effect if appropriate action is taken), (3) self-reevaluation (assessing one's image with and without the unhealthy behaviour), (4) environmental reevaluation (assessing how one's social environment is affected by the unhealthy behaviour), (5) self-liberation (believing and committing to change), (6) helping relationships (building support for healthy behaviour change), (7) counterconditioning (learning that healthy behaviours can replace unhealthy behaviours), (8) contingency management (increasing reinforcement and probability that healthy behaviours will be repeated), (9) stimulus control (removing unhealthy behaviour cues and adding healthy behaviour cues), and (10) social liberation (increasing social opportunities to foster behaviour change) (Prochaska et al., 2002). The TTM has been used in numerous studies, including those involving smoking cessation, mammography screening, alcohol avoidance, and exercise and stress management. The TTM has been beneficial in tailoring interventions for the most appropriate stage of change.

The *theory of reasoned action* and the *theory of planned behaviour* offer another framework for examining factors that determine behavioural change. The framework focuses on motivational factors as determinants of the person's likelihood of performing a specific behaviour. The theory of reasoned action provides the rationale that the person's beliefs and values determine whether the person intends to change behaviour. The theory of planned behaviour adds that perceived behavioural control of facilitating or constraining conditions affect intention and behaviour. Beliefs affecting behaviour differ widely among persons, groups, and even specific behaviours of the same individual. The models help in understanding the likelihood of people performing a specific healthier behaviour and can provide a framework for interventions. These theories can be applied along with others to design and deliver behavioural change to improve research and practice (Montano & Kasprzyk, 2002).

The *health belief model* (HBM) is one of the most widely used conceptual frameworks to explain change in health behaviour and to provide a framework for interventions (Janz, Champion, & Strecher, 2002). The components of the HBM have been revised many times since the model's inception in the 1950s. Once a model to explain readiness to obtain chest x-ray screening for tuberculosis, the model has evolved beyond screening behaviours to include preventive actions, illness behaviours, and sick-role behaviour. The HBM now purports that individuals will take action to prevent, screen for, or control ill-health conditions if there is perceived susceptibility (persons regard themselves as susceptible to the condition), if there is perceived severity (persons believe it would have potentially serious consequences), if there are perceived benefits (persons believe a course of action available to them would be beneficial in reducing either their susceptibility to or the severity of the condition), and if the perceived barriers can be overcome (persons believe the anticipated barriers to [or costs of] taking the action are outweighed by its benefits) (Janz et

al., 2002). Determining strategies to activate persons' readiness to change (cues to action) can include providing information and awareness campaigns. Like the TTM, self-efficacy is an integral concept of the HBM. Researchers have tested interventions to increase positive change for each concept.

The *health promotion model* (HPM) integrates constructs from the expectancy-value theory and social cognitive theory and provides a nursing perspective to depict the multidimensional nature of persons pursuing health (Pender, Murdaugh, & Parsons, 2002). The HPM purports that behaviour change will occur if there is positive, personal value and a desired outcome. The HPM has been revised since its initial development in the early 1980s and is considered an approach-oriented or competence model. Pender et al. reported the HPM is different from the HBM in that it eliminates the negative source of motivation, fear or threat, from major motivating sources for health behaviour change. Pender et al. emphasized that elimination of the personal threat motivational factor provides applicability of the model across the lifespan. Self-efficacy is a major construct of HPM, and assumptions of the model require an active role of the person "in shaping and maintaining health behaviours and in modifying the environmental context for health behaviours" (Pender et al., 2002, p. 63). The HPM has been a framework for studies predicting its general health-promoting abilities and for specific health behaviours including hearing protection, exercise, and nutrition (Pender et al., 2002).

Theory and models are important in the understanding of health promotion and why people behave the way they do. Theory is also important in identifying variables that change these behaviours and help retain new behaviours. The importance of identifying mediating variables is often overlooked. Understanding relationships among variables could help refine health behaviour theories and design intervention studies.

In a recent study McQueen et al. (2010) examined the role of perceived susceptibility on colorectal cancer screening intention and behaviour. Perceived susceptibility is a psychosocial variable in several health promotion theories and is viewed as a motivating factor in behavioural change, but there is disagreement on how its mechanism affects behaviour. Results of this study showed perceived susceptibility was not limited to direct effects but was independent of perceived benefits, was mediated by the change in family influence, and moderated the change in perceived barriers and self-efficacy.

Ongoing work on theory and relationships between variables helps advance the understanding of health promotion and behavioural change. Some authors believe theory development has not kept pace with the evolution of health promotion practice (Crosby & Noar, 2010). Some of this disparity relates to the following problems: (1) theory is not grounded in practice, (2) theory is at the individual level and simplistic without attention to the contextual nature of human behaviour and environment, and (3) theory is inaccessible to practitioners who are facing increased demands to prevent disease and promote health (Crosby & Noar, 2010). Remedies that allow for the complexity of theory development for the future are daunting but something to which to aspire.

Health care frequently uses broad-stroke approaches to health promotion interventions in hopes that some health behaviours will change. Further development of theory will better frame questions surrounding health promotion. Caution should accompany new theory development as misleading data can exaggerate the theories' predictive accuracy (Weinstein, 2007). Often, studies in health promotion are based on correlational data with variables such as beliefs, attitudes, self-efficacy, intentions, diet, nutrition, preventive measures, and other human behaviours. Although these studies may provide descriptive information, correlations do not infer causation. Theory development needs to be carefully designed. Theory must be tested in practice-based contexts, allow cross-cultural transfer, be more inclusive of environmental changes, and effectively serve health promotion practice (DiClementi, Crosby, & Kegler, 2009).

INTERVENTIONS

Chronic diseases account for 66% of all deaths that occur in Canada each year (Public Health Agency of Canada, 2012a). These diseases also cause major limitations in daily living for those affected and their significant others. Although chronic diseases are among the most common and costly health problems, they are also among the most preventable. Adopting healthy behaviours such as eating nutritious foods, being physically active, and avoiding tobacco use can prevent or control the devastating effects of these diseases (PHAC, 2012c).

Nurses have been leaders in health promotion since the time of Florence Nightingale, whose pioneering work with the use of statistics demonstrated the positive effect of improved sanitation on the health of injured soldiers. Nurses have also led the healthcare profession in recognizing that health is a state of physical and mental wellness and that it is impossible to separate the former from the latter (Calloway, 2007).

Olshansky (2007), editor of the *Journal of Professional Nursing*, emphasized that nurses are the most appropriate health professionals to address health promotion. Nursing has role models within our profession, such as Nola Pender, who developed the HPM described previously. Nursing literature abounds with textbooks, articles, and other publications that include nursing's role in health promotion to individuals, families, communities, and populations. Yet, nurses cannot assume sameness for chronically ill persons, and nurses cannot assume resources are equally available to all. People with chronic illness may view health differently and have different goals defined within the limits of their illness.

Selected Examples of Health Promotion Interventions

A review of the literature provides examples of health promotion interventions for clients with chronic illness. The following discussion illustrates that much is yet to be examined. In an international study Huang, Chou, Lin, and Chao (2007) analyzed survey data including the health-promoting lifestyle profile and quality of life data of 129 outpatients from a medical centre who had systemic lupus erythematosus. These researchers found that a health-promoting lifestyle could not enhance the physical component summary of quality of life directly without an improvement in the fatigue disability, but a health-promoting lifestyle had a significant effect on the mental component summary of quality of life. This illustrates that although the physical aspects of the chronic condition may not improve without other physical changes, there can be improvements in psychological health.

Siarkowski (1999) emphasized the importance of including health promotion and illness management when working with insulin-dependent diabetes mellitus in children and their families. Siarkowski reviewed existing research and revealed factors that put children and their families at risk for poor adaptation. Health promotion is critical to minimize these risks.

Hope has been recommended as a health-promoting force. Hollis, Massey, and Jevne (2007) identified hope-enhancing strategies and sources to improve one's health. Blue (2007) studied 106 adults at risk for diabetes and found the theory of planned behaviour to be useful in explaining their healthy eating intentions and physical activity.

Health-promoting activities such as prevention of injuries may make the difference in whether one is able to live with chronic conditions. One example is preventing falls. Falls are one of the most common causes of injuries in older adults. These preventable accidents cause loss of independence, enormous financial costs, and possibly death. One evidence-informed program to prevent falls is exemplified in Ory and colleagues' (2010) analysis of community-dwelling older adults who participated in a matter of balance/volunteer lay leader model intended to reduce fear of falling and increase physical activity of participants.

Motivational Interviewing

Motivational interviewing incorporates behaviour change principles to promote healthy activities. Four guiding principles underscore motivational interviewing: (1) resist the righting reflex that helping professionals often have to set things right and assume patients are wrong, (2) understand and explore the patient's own motivation, (3) listen with empathy, and (4) empower the patient, encouraging hope and optimism (Rollnick, Miller, & Butler, 2008). Brodie and Inoue (2005) demonstrated the effectiveness of motivational interviewing over a traditional exercise program in increasing reported physical activity in older adults with chronic heart failure. Jackson, Asimakopoulou, and Scammell (2007) demonstrated in an experimental study of 34 clients with type 2 diabetes that motivational interviewing and behaviour change training significantly increased the participants' physical activity and stage of change.

Motivating Factors

Providing performance incentives, both financial and nonfinancial, have been explored in an effort to change behaviours in individuals and in communities. The following principles are helpful in guiding the development of any incentive design: (1) identify the desired outcome, (2) identify the behaviour change that leads to the desired outcome, (3) determine the potential effectiveness of the incentive in achieving the behaviour change, (4) link an incentive directly to the behaviour or outcome, (5) identify possible adverse effects of the incentive, and (6) evaluate changes in the behaviour or outcome in response to the incentive (Haverman, 2010). Researchers using a randomized study of 51 adults, all age 50, demonstrated that modest financial incentives were an effective approach for increasing physical activity among sedentary older adults (Finkelstein, Brown, Brown, & Buchner, 2008).

In a review of 26 studies (8 randomized controlled trials and 18 observational), use of pedometers significantly increased physical activity and significantly decreased body mass index and blood pressure (Bravata et al., 2007). The use of pedometers as a motivating factor with chronically ill persons capable of using a pedometer and the long-term effect of pedometers are yet to be investigated. Motivating factors have been identified in theories, models, and frameworks and positive motivators such as those in the HPM are congruent with nursing philosophical bases. Challenges for the future are to continue the testing and use of such frameworks in the health-promoting activities of persons and families with chronic illness.

Health Coaching

Health coaching is emerging as a new approach for preventing exacerbations of chronic illness and supporting lifestyle changes. This method partners health coaches with clients to enhance self-management strategies. "Coaching is a method of patient education that guides and prompts a patient to be an active participant in behaviour change" (Wilkie, Williams, Gravstad, & Mekwa, 1995, p. 9). Health coaching is one way of working with patients to ensure they understand, agree, and participate in the management of their chronic conditions (Bennett, Coleman, Parry, Bodenheimer, & Chen, 2010). According to Bennett et al., it is the process involved in assisting patients to gain knowledge, skills, tools, and confidence to be more active in their own care so that they can achieve their self-identified goals.

Registered nurses are well positioned to assume the role of a health coach for their clients living with chronic illness. The health coach roles as summarized by Bennett et al. (2010) include "providing self management support, bridging the gap between clinician and patient, helping patients navigate the health care system, offering emotional support and serving as a continuity figure" (p. 25).

The self-management of care model is used for lifestyle coaching programs based on collaborative goal setting and self-management health education (Rohrer, Naessens, Liesinger, & Litchy, 2010). A study examined the usefulness of self-rated health metrics in assessing telephonic coaching programs targeting weight, exercise, stress, and nutrition. Although these coaching programs showed positive improvements in all lifestyle interventions, the self-rated health metrics were correlated with improvements only in weight loss and exercise programs. Therefore, the coaching programs were successful, but self-ratings may not demonstrate the improvements in all areas (Rohrer et al., 2010).

Mass Media Campaigns

Beaudoin, Fernandez, Wall, and Farley (2007) used a mass media campaign of high-frequency paid television and radio advertising and bus and streetcar signage to promote walking and fruit/vegetable consumption in a low-income, predominantly African American urban population in New Orleans. Over 5 months of the campaign, these researchers found a significant increase in message recall measures and positive attitudes toward walking and toward fruit/vegetable consumption. It is unknown how many persons with chronic illness were included. It is likely many persons were at risk for future chronic illness. These efforts demonstrate population efforts to improve health that may be researched with chronic illness populations.

Snyder (2007) reviewed existing meta-analyses for effectiveness of health communication campaigns and found that the average

health campaign affects the intervention community by about five percentage points. Snyder concluded that successful campaigns likely to change nutrition behaviours need to include specific behavioural goals for the intervention, identification of the target population, communication activities and channels that will be used, provision of message content and presentation, and provision of techniques for feedback and evaluation.

Web-Based Programs

Verheijden, Jans, Hildebrandt, and Hopman-Rock (2007) found that web-based behavioural programs often reach those who need them the least. However, obese people were more likely to participate in follow-up than people of normal body weight. The researchers proposed that web-based programs are a nonstigmatising way of addressing the problem and suggested that weight management is better suited for this delivery method than many other health-related areas. Although this study was based in the Netherlands, it provides a source of potential research for other countries with similar health-promotion problems. Successful web-based interventions improve health knowledge and are effective in changing behaviours. These web-based interventions have been implemented primarily through interactive messaging and information dissemination but are wide open for expansion (Annang, Muilenburg, & Strasser, 2010).

Contracts

In a randomized, controlled trial of 77 children with persistent asthma, Burkhart, Rayens, Oakley, Abshire, and Zhang (2007) found the intervention group who received asthma education plus contingency management, including a contingency contract, tailoring, cueing, and reinforcement, significantly increased adherence to asthma self-management over the control group who received asthma education without the contingency management. However, in 30 trials involving 4,691 participants, Cochrane authors concluded that there is limited evidence that contracts can improve patients' adherence to health-promotion programs. Large, well-controlled studies are needed to recommend contracts in preventive health programs (Bosch-Capblanch, Abba, Prictor, & Garner, 2007). Contracts have been found useful in improving patient adherence in the management of diabetes mellitus (Delamater, 2006).

Health Literacy

Improving the use of health information is paramount in health promotion programs. The U.S. Department of Health and Human Services, Office of Disease Prevention and Health Promotion (2012) summarised the best practices for healthcare professionals to improve health literacy through providing effective communications and health services that are usable. **Table 15-1** outlines these practices.

Nath (2007) reviewed the literature between 1990 and mid-2006 for overcoming inadequate literacy in diabetes self-management and other chronic illnesses. The importance of culturally appropriate health literacy, improvement in self-efficacy, improved communication, and quality computer-assisted instruction were discussed as essential elements in tailoring health education. Nurses were recommended to address barriers related to inadequate literacy by (1) increasing sensitivity to the problem, (2) developing

literacy-assessment protocol, (3) creating and evaluating materials for target populations, (4) providing clear communication, (5) including health literacy in nursing curricula, (6) fostering decision making with patients, and (7) conducting research about literacy.

Additional Studies

Using telehealth to improve access, students in a community setting applied self-efficacy theory to help low-income older adults with chronic health problems to increase their practices of health promotion (Coyle, Duffy, & Martin, 2007). Although faculty and students favourably evaluated the activity, measurement of patient outcomes was not conducted. Like web-based programs, the effects of telehealth require further research.

Miller and Iris (2002) found that socialization and social support were central to the participation of older adults with chronic illness who participated in a wellness program. In this study participants recognized that chronic disease did not prohibit living a healthy lifestyle. The White Crane model of healthy lives for older adults used in this study contributed to understanding the way older adults view health for themselves. This model is also thought to be helpful in developing program evaluation measures.

A diet and exercise program to reduce cardiovascular disease risk was used with employees regardless of presence of chronic illness. There were significant differences between pre- and post-intervention for lipid profiles and weight. Self-reported levels of participation in the diet were significantly related to improvement in the low-density-lipoprotein levels (White & Jacques, 2007).

Table 15-1   Improving Health Literacy Interventions

When providing health information, is the information appropriate for the user?	Identify intended users of the information and services.
	Evaluate the users' knowledge before, during, and after the introduction of information and services.
	Acknowledge cultural differences and practice respect.
When providing health information, is the information easy to use?	Limit the number of messages. Keep it simple, and, in general, limit the information to no more than four main messages.
	Use plain language. Use familiar language and an active voice. Avoid jargon. See www.plainlanguage.gov for more information.
	Focus on the behaviour you want the person to change.
	Supplement instructions with visuals to help convey your message.
	Make written communication easy to read by using large font and headings and bullets to break up text; limit line length to between 40 and 50 characters.
	Improve Internet information by using uniform navigation, organizing information to minimize searching and scrolling, including interactive features. Apply user-centred design principles and conduct usability testing.
When providing health information, are you speaking clearly and listening carefully?	Ask open-ended questions.
	Use a medically trained interpreter for those who do not speak English or have limited ability to speak or understand English.
	Use words and examples that make the information relevant to the person's cultural norms and values.
	Check for understanding using a "teach-back" method to enhance communication.
Improve the use of health services.	Improve usability of health forms and instructions including plain language forms in multiple languages.
	Improve the accessibility of the physical environment including universal symbols, clear signage, and easy flow-through healthcare facilities.
	Establish a patient navigator program of individuals who can help patients access services and appropriate healthcare information.
Build knowledge to improve health decision making.	Improve access to accurate and appropriate health information.
	Increase self-efficacy and facilitate health decision making.
	Partner with educators to improve health curricula.
Advocate for health literacy in your organization.	Make the case for health literacy improvement.
	Identify how low health literacy affects programs.
	Incorporate health literacy into mission and planning.
	Establish accountability by including health literacy improvement in program evaluation.

The addition of health promotion to the usual care of frail older home-care clients was studied in Canada by Markle-Reid and coworkers (2006). These researchers found that proactively providing health promotion to older adults with chronic health needs enhanced quality of life but did not increase the overall costs of health care. Better mental health functioning, reduction in depression, and enhanced perceptions of social support were reported in the experimental group. The researchers concluded their finding underscored the need to provide health promotion for older clients receiving home care.

Age differences were found when researchers randomly assigned 111 young adults aged 18 to 36 and 104 older adults aged 62 to 86 to read health pamphlets with identical factual information for healthy eating but containing either emotional or nonemotional goals for the healthy behaviour. Basing their study on socioemotional selectivity theory and health promotion, the theory contends that as individuals get older, they perceive time as being increasingly limited, so emotionally meaningful goals with more immediate payoffs will be chosen over future-oriented goals. Older adults in this study evaluated health messages that contained emotional goals rather than the nonemotional, future-oriented or neutral goals more positively and the messages were better remembered and led to greater behavioural changes than in the younger adults. While cautioning generalization, these findings may suggest that health professionals should emphasize emotionally meaningful benefits when disseminating health messages to older adults (Zhang, Fung, & Ching, 2009). Similar results may be found in future studies of individuals with chronic illness, especially those perceiving time as being increasingly limited.

The adverse effects of obesity on chronic disease were supported when strong positive associations of age, gender, race/ethnicity, body mass index, and comorbidities were found with type 2 diabetes, hypertension, and hyperlipidemia (Crawford et al., 2010). The direct associations between body mass index and disease prevalence was consistent for both genders and across all racial/ethnic groups.

A shift from preventive home-care nursing functions to acute inpatient care functions has resulted in fragmented, expensive care for older adults with chronic illness rather than comprehensive and proactive care that is more likely to improve health outcomes. Providing the most appropriate services to older adults was the impetus for the following study. A two-armed, single-blind, randomized controlled trial of 288 older frail adults with chronic health needs, aged 75 and older, were evaluated in a Canadian study (Markle-Reid et al., 2006). The model of vulnerability by Rogers (1997) provided the theoretical basis for the study. Participants were randomly assigned to the usual home care or a "proactive" nursing health promotion intervention that included a health assessment combined with regular home visits or telephone contacts, health education about management of illness, coordination of community services, and use of empowerment strategies to enhance independence. Of the 288 patients randomly assigned at baseline, 242 completed the study (120 with the proactive nursing intervention, 122 in the control group). Results demonstrated that proactively providing the intervention group with nursing health promotion significantly resulted in better mental health functioning ($P = 0.009$), a reduction in depression ($P = 0.009$), and enhanced perceptions of social support ($P = 0.009$) while not increasing the overall costs of health care. Findings supported the need to provide nursing services for health promotion for older patients receiving home care. Implications from this study support the notion that health promotion efforts are productive in improving health outcomes and can be cost effective.

Many areas remain for further research to measure the effect of health-promoting frameworks and interventions with individuals and families with chronic illness. The earlier discussion provides a sampling of the current literature.

Guidelines

There are numerous easily accessible guidelines/schedules for health promotion, health screening, and preventive care at the PHAC website (www.phac.gc.ca) and other sources. Examples of guidelines are discussed here.

Immunizations are one of the most important discoveries in human history. Vaccines have helped save millions of lives worldwide and millions of dollars each year in unnecessary healthcare expenditures (Infectious Diseases Society of America, 2011). For example, the influenza vaccine alone can save thousands of lives by providing protection for persons with chronic illness. Immunized healthcare providers can decrease transmission of influenza to chronically ill persons. Recommended immunization schedules and information are easily obtained from the U.S. Centers for Disease Control and Prevention and the PHAC.

Several organizations provide guidelines that include health promotion for chronic conditions. Self-management education programs such as diabetes self-management education are outlined in the diabetes national standards (Kulkarni, 2006). Nurses are encouraged to use evidence-informed guidelines as they practice.

SUMMARY

The desired outcome for individuals with chronic illness and their families is to maintain and improve their overall health. Health-promotion activities should target the major causes of death—tobacco use, poor diet, physical inactivity, alcohol consumption, microbial agents, toxic agents, motor vehicle crashes, incidents involving firearms, risky sexual behaviours, and illicit use of drugs. These causes are responsible for the majority of deaths in Canada and most of the developed world. Measures are needed to research outcomes of health-promoting interventions across populations and disabilities. Further efforts to make activities accessible and studies to evaluate their effectiveness are encouraged. The challenge of the coming years will be to link existing and future research studies to practice.

Evidence-Informed Practice Box

Researchers in a recent study (Mayer et al., 2010) examined the healthcare costs and participation in a community-based health program for older adults. The program, called Enhance-Wellness, was designed to prevent disabilities and improve health and functioning. Earlier studies (Leveille et al., 1998; Phelan et al., 2002) demonstrated increased physical activity, improvements in health status, no decrease in functional status, and other positive health outcomes of the Enhance-Wellness program. Leveille and colleagues reported a multicomponent disability prevention and disease self-management program led by a geriatric nurse practitioner improved function and reduced inpatient utilization in chronically ill older adults. Phelan and colleagues demonstrated a health enhancement program reduced disability risk factors, improved health status, maintained functional status, and did not increase self-reported healthcare use. However, costs were not examined until the retrospective study by Mayer et al. (2010) in which program participants (n = 218) were matched for age and gender to nonprogram individuals (n = 654) and evaluated for 1 year after they began the program. Healthcare costs were $582 lower among the program participants than nonparticipants, but the differences were not significant. The preventive services score was significantly higher for participants, suggesting a stronger tendency of program participants to receive preventive services. Results of this study indicate that those participating in the health-promoting program did not cost more than nonparticipants. Future studies may show a significant decrease compared with nonparticipants, and studies that reveal combined positive health outcomes with reduced costs will undoubtedly add support to companies and communities to develop and maintain health promotion programs.

Numerous free resources are available through the federal government and other organizations. Many have been described throughout this chapter. Nurses are instrumental in promoting health. Stemming from our earliest work, nurses recognize the importance of health promotion. Like many other countries, health promotion and disease prevention is paramount in our costly, publicly funded healthcare systems. There are substantial but missed opportunities for promoting health and extending the lifespan that present an international challenge. Countries in Europe are struggling with strategies to improve the health of their aging populations and to control costs. Italy has one of the oldest populations in the world, with more than 20% of its population older than age 65 (Besdine & Wetle, 2010). Italy, like Canada, must be proactive in finding ways to minimize chronic illnesses and keep people healthy. Nurses and other health professionals must meet the challenge in designing and evaluating effective interventions that promote health and are accessible for all people.

STUDY QUESTIONS

WWW

1. Describe the importance of health promotion in chronic illness for all people.
2. Name the three major actual causes of death in Canada and compare this with other countries.
3. What is the goal of health promotion?
4. Identify a theory/model/framework useful in working with chronically ill individuals who need to change an unhealthy behaviour.
5. Discuss national documents that address health promotion and disease prevention.
6. What interventions can nurses use to promote health in persons with chronic illness?

REFERENCES

Annang, L., Muilenburg, J. L., & Strasser, S. M. (2010). Virtual worlds: Taking health promotion to new levels. *American Journal of Health Promotion, 24*(5), 344–346.

Aro, A. R., & Absetz, P. (2009). Guidance for professionals in health promotion: Keeping it simple—but not too simple. *Psychology and Health, 24*(2), 125–129.

Barr, V. J., Robinson, S., Marin-Link, B., Underhill, L., Dotts, A., Ravendale, D., & Salivaras, S. (2003). The expanded chronic care model: An integration of concepts and strategies from population health promotion and the chronic care model. *Hospital Quarterly, 7*(1), 73–82.

Beaudoin, C. E., Fernandez, C., Wall, J. L., & Farley, T. A. (2007). Promoting healthy eating and physical activity short-term effects of a mass media campaign. *American Journal of Preventive Medicine, 32*(3), 217–223.

Begoray, D. L., & Kwan, B. (2011). A Canadian exploratory study to define a measure of health literacy. *Health Promotion International, 27*(1), 23–32.

Bennett, H. D., Coleman, E. A., Parry, C., Bodenheimer, T., & Chen, E. H. (2010). Health coaching for patients with chronic illness: Does your practice "give patients a fish" or "teach patients to fish"? *Family Practice Management, 17*(5), 24–29.

Besdine, R. W., & Wetle, T. F. (2010). Improving health for elderly people: An international health promotion and disease prevention agenda. *Aging Clinical and Experimental Research, 22*, 219–230.

Blue, C. L. (2007). Does the theory of planned behavior identify diabetes-related cognitions for intention to be physically active and eat a healthy diet? *Public Health Nursing, 24*(2), 141–150.

Bosch-Capblanch, X., Abba, K., Prictor, M., & Garner, P. (2007). Contracts between patients and healthcare practitioners for improving patients' adherence to treatment, prevention and health promotion activities. *Cochrane Database of Systematic Reviews, 2*, 1–61.

Bravata, D. M., Smith-Spangler, C., Sundaram, V., Glenger, A. L., Lin, N., Lewis, R., . . . Sirard, J. C. (2007). Using pedometers to increase physical activity and improve health. *Journal of the American Medical Association, 298*, 2296–2304.

Brennenstuhl, S., Fuller-Thomson, E., & Popova, S. (2009). Prevalence and factors associated with colorectal cancer screening in Canadian women. *Journal of Women's Health, 19*(4), 775–784.

Brodie, D. A., & Inoue, A. (2005). Motivational interviewing to promote physical activity for people with chronic heart failure. *Journal of Advanced Nursing, 50*(5), 518–527.

Bryant, H. E., Fekete, S. V., & Major, D. H. (2011). Pan-Canadian initiatives in colorectal cancer screening: Adopting knowledge translation tools to accelerate uptake and impact. *Current Oncology, 18*(3), 111–118.

Burkhart, P. V., Rayens, M. K., Oakley, M. G., Abshire, D. A., & Zhang, M. (2007). Testing an intervention to promote children's adherence to asthma self-management. *Journal of Nursing Scholarship, 39*, 133–140.

Calloway, S. (2007). Mental health promotion: Is nursing dropping the ball? *Journal of Professional Nursing, 23*(2), 105–109.

Capella-McDonnall, M. (2007). The need for health promotion for adults who are visually impaired. *Journal of Visual Impairment & Blindness, 101*(3), 133–145.

Cory, S., Ussery-Hall, A., Griffin-Blake, S., Easton, A., Vigeant, J., Balluz, L., . . . Greenlund, K. (2010, September 24). Prevalence of selected risk behaviors and chronic diseases and conditions—Steps communities, United States, 2006–2007. *Morbidity and Mortality Weekly Report, 50*(SS-8), 1–9.

Coyle, M. K., Duffy, J. R., & Martin, E. M. (2007). Teaching/learning health promoting behaviors through telehealth. *Nursing Education Perspective, 28*(1), 18–23.

Crawford, A. G., Cote, C., Couto, J., Daskiran, M., Gunnarson, C., Haas, K., . . . Schuette, R. (2010). Prevalence of obesity, type II diabetes mellitus, hyperlipidemia, and hypertension in the United States: Findings from the GE Centricity electronic medical record database, *Population Health Management, 13*(3), 151–161.

Crosby, R., & Noar, S. M. (2010). Theory development in health promotion: Are we there yet? *Journal of Behavioral Medicine, 33*(4), 259–263.

Delamater, A. M. (2006). Improving patient adherence. *Clinical Diabetes, 24*(2), 71–77.

Department of Health and Human Services. (2012). *Quick guide to health literacy.* Retrieved from http://medicine.osu.edu/sitetool/sites/pdfs/ahecpublic/Quickguide.pdf

DiClemente, R. J., Crosby, R. A., & Kegler, M. C. (2009). Issues and challenges in applying theory in health promotion practice and research: Adaptation, translation, and global application. In R. J. DiClemente, R. A. Crosby, & M. C. Kegler (Eds.), *Emerging theories in health promotion practice and research* (2nd ed., pp. 551–568). San Francisco, CA: Jossey-Bass.

Edelman, C. L., & Mandle, C. L. (2006). *Health promotion throughout the lifespan* (6th ed.). St. Louis, MO: Mosby.

Finkelstein, E. A., Brown, D. S., Brown, D. R., & Buchner, D. M. (2008). A randomized study of financial incentives to increase physical activity among sedentary older adults. *Preventive Medicine, 47*(2), 182 187.

Greiner, P. A., & Edelman, C. L. (2010). In C. L. Edelman & C. L. Mandle (Eds.), *Health promotion throughout the lifespan* (7th ed., pp. 3–25). St. Louis, MO: Mosby.

Haverman, R. H. (2010). Principles to guide the development of population health incentives. *Preventing Chronic Disease Public Health Research, Practice, and Policy, 7*(5), 1–5. Retrieved from http://www.cdc.gov/pcd/issues/2010/sep/10_0044.htm

Health Canada. (2002). Smoking in Canada: An overview. Retrieved from http://publications.gc.ca/collections/Collection/H12-35-2002-1E.pdf

Health Canada. (2012a). Smoking and your body. Retrieved from http://www.hc-sc.gc.ca/hc-ps/tobac-tabac/body-corps/index-eng.php

Health Canada. (2012b). Obesity. Retrieved from http://www.hc-sc.gc.ca/hl-vs/alt_formats/pacrb-dgapcr/pdf/iyh-vsv/life-vie/obes-eng.pdf

Heart and Stroke Foundation of Canada. (2012). Statistics. Retrieved from http://www.heartandstroke.com/site/c.ikIQLcMWJtE/b.3483991/k.34A8/Statistics.htm

Heinzer, M. M. (1998). Health promotion during childhood chronic illness: A paradox facing society. *Holistic Nursing Practice, 12*(2), 8–17.

Hollis, V., Massey, K., & Jevne, R. (2007). An introduction to the intentional use of hope. *Journal of Allied Health, 36*(1), 52–56.

Huang, H. C., Chou, C. T., Lin, K. C., & Chao, Y. F. (2007). The relationships between disability level, health-promoting lifestyle, and quality of life in outpatients with systemic lupus erythematosus. *Journal of Nursing Research, 15*(1), 21–32.

Infectious Diseases Society of America. (2011). *Immunization/vaccination.* Retrieved from http://www.idsociety.org/Content.aspx?id=6346

Jackson, R., Asimakopoulou, K., & Scammell, A. (2007). Assessment of the transtheoretical model as used by dietitians in promoting physical activity in people with type 2 diabetes. *Journal of Human Nutrition and Diet, 20*, 27–36.

Janz, N. K., Champion, V. L., & Strecher, V. J. (2002). The health belief model. In K. Glanz, B. K. Rimer, & F. M. Lewis (Eds.), *Health behavior and health education theory, research, and practice* (3rd ed., pp. 45–66). San Francisco, CA: Jossey-Bass.

Kulkarni, K. D. (2006). Value of diabetes self-management education. *Clinical Diabetes, 24*(2), 54.

Leddy, S. K. (2006). *Health promotion: Mobilizing strengths to enhance health, wellness, and well-being.* Philadelphia, PA: F.A. Davis.

Leveille, S. G., Wagner, E. H., Davis, C., Grothaus, L., Wallace, J., LoGerfo, M., Kent, D. (1998). Preventing disability and managing chronic illness in frail older adults: A randomized trial of a community-based partnership with primary care. *Journal of the American Geriatrics Society, 46*(10), 1191–1198.

Lofters, A. K., Moineddin, R., Hwang, S. W., & Glazier, R. H. (2011). Predictors of low cervical cancer screening among immigrant women in Ontario, Canada. *BMC Womens Health, 11*(1), 20–30.

Makromaski-Illing, E. M., & Kaiserman, M. J. (1999). Mortality attributable to tobacco use in Canada and its regions, 1994–1996. *Chronic Disease Canada, 20*(3), 111–117.

Markle-Reid, M., Weir, R., Browne, G., Roberts, J., Gafni, A., & Henderson, S. (2006). Health promotion for frail older home care clients. *Journal of Advanced Nursing, 54*(3), 381–395.

Mayer, C., Williams, B., Wagner, E. H., LoGerfo, J. P., Cheadle, A., & Phelan, E. A. (2010). Health care costs and participation in a community-based health promotion program for older adults. *Preventing Chronic Disease Public Health Research, Practice, and Policy, 7*(2), 1–7.

McQueen, A., Vernon, S. W., Rothman, A. J., Norman, G. J., Myers, R. E., & Tilley, B. C. (2010). Examining the role of perceived susceptibility on colorectal cancer screening intention and behavior. *Annals of Behavioral Medicine, 40*, 205–217.

McWilliam, C. L., Stewart, M., Brown, J. B., Desai, K., & Coderre, P. (1996). Creating health with chronic illness. *Advances in Nursing Science, 18*(3), 1–15.

Miller, A., & Iris, M. (2002). Health promotion attitudes and strategies in older adults. *Health Education & Behavior, 29*(2), 249–267.

Montano, D. E., & Kasprzyk, D. (2002). The theory of reasoned action and the theory of planned behavior. In K. Glanz, B. K. Rimer, & F. M. Lewis (Eds.), *Health behavior and health education theory, research, and practice* (3rd ed., pp. 67–98). San Francisco, CA: Jossey-Bass.

Nath, C. (2007). Literacy and diabetes self-management. *American Journal of Nursing, 107*(6 Suppl.), 43–54.

Norman, S. A., Potashnik, S. L., Galantino, M. L., DeMichele, A. M., House, L., & Localio, A. R. (2007). Modifiable risk factors for breast cancer recurrence: What can we tell survivors? *Journal of Women's Health, 16*(2), 177–190.

Olshansky, E. (2007). Nurses and health promotion. *Journal of Professional Nursing, 23*(1), 1–2.

Ory, M. G., Smith, M. L., Wade, A., Mounce, C., Wilson, A., & Parrish, R. (2010). Implementing and disseminating an evidence-based program to prevent falls in older adults, Texas, 2007–2009. *Preventing Chronic Disease Public Health Research, Practice, and Policy, 7*(6), 1–6. Retrieved from http://www.cdc.gov/pcd/issues/2010/nov/09_0224.htm

Painter, J. E., Borba, C. P., Hynes, M., Mays, D., & Glanz, K. (2008). The use of theory in health behavior research from 2000 to 2005: A systematic review. *Annals of Behavioral Medicine, 35*, 358–362.

Peerson, A., & Saunders, M. (2011). Men's health literacy in Australia: In search of a gender lens. *International Journal of Men's Health, 10*(2), 111–135.

Pender, N. J., Murdaugh, C. L., & Parsons, M. A. (2002). *Health promotion in nursing practice* (4th ed.). Upper Saddle River, NJ: Prentice Hall.

Phelan, E. A., Williams, B., Leveille, S., Snyder, S., Wagner, E. H., & LoGerfo, J. P. (2002). Outcomes of a community-based dissemination of the health enhancement program. *Journal of the American Geriatrics Society, 50*(9), 1519–1524.

Prochaska, J. O., Redding, C. A., & Evers, K. E. (2002). The transtheoretical model and stages of change. In K. Glanz, B. K. Rimer, & F. M. Lewis (Eds.), *Health behavior and health education theory, research, and practice* (3rd ed., pp. 99–120). San Francisco, CA: Jossey-Bass.

Public Health Agency of Canada. (2012a). *Chronic diseases—most significant cause of death globally.* Retrieved from http://www.phac-aspc.gc.ca/media/nr-rp/2011/2011_0919-bg-di-eng.php

Public Health Agency of Canada. (2012b). Healthy living? Retrieved from http://www.phac-aspc.gc.ca/hp-ps/hl-mvs/index-eng.php

Public Health Agency of Canada. (2012c). Physical activity in Canada. Retrieved from http://www.phac-aspc.gc.ca/alw-vat/intro/canada-eng.php

Rainer, J. P., & McMurry, P. E. (2002). Caregiving at the end of life. *Journal of Clinical Psychology, 58*, 1421–1431.

Rehm, J., Baliunas, D., Brochu, S., Fischer, B., Gnam, W., Patra, J., . . . Taylor, B. (2002). *The cost of substance abuse in Canada 2002*. Ottawa, ON: Canadian Centre for Substance Abuse.

Rogers, A. C. (1997). Vulnerability, health and health costs. *Journal of Advanced Nursing, 26*, 65–72.

Rohrer, J. E., Naessens, J. M., Liesinger, J., & Litchy, W. (2010). Comparing diverse health promotion programs using overall self-rated health as a common metric. *Population Health Management, 13*(2), 91–95.

Rollnick, S., Miller, W. R., & Butler, C. C. (2008). *Motivational interviewing in health care: Helping patients change behavior*. New York, NY: Guilford Press.

Rootman, I., & Gordon-El-Bihbety, D. (2008). *A vision for a health literate Canada: Report of the expert panel on health literacy*. Ottawa, ON: Canadian Centre for Substance Abuse.

Schafer, M. H., & Ferraro, K. F. (2007). Long-term obesity and avoidable hospitalization among younger, middle-aged, and older adults. *Archives of Internal Medicine, 167*, 2220–2225.

Siarkowski, K. (1999). Children's adaptation to insulin dependent diabetes mellitus: A critical review of the literature. *Pediatric Nursing, 25*(6), 6–27.

Snyder, L. B. (2007). Health communication campaigns and their impact on behavior. *Journal of Nutrition Education and Behavior, 39*(2 Suppl.), S32–S40.

Speros, C. (2005). Health literacy: Concept analysis. *Journal of Advanced Nursing, 50*(6), 633–640.

Statistics Canada. (2012). Life expectancy at birth, by sex, by province. Retrieved from http://www.statcan.gc.ca/tables-tableaux/sum-som/l01/cst01/health26-eng.htm

Sweet, S. N., & Fortier, M. S. (2010). Improving physical activity and dietary behaviours with single or multiple health behaviour interventions? A synthesis of meta analysis and review. *International Journal of Environmental Research and Public Health, 7,* 1720–1743.

Verheijden, M. W., Jans, M. P., Hildebrandt, V. H., & Hopman-Rock, M. (2007). Rates and determinants of repeated participation in a web-based behavior change program for healthy body weight and healthy lifestyle. *Journal of Medical Internet Research, 9*(1), e1.

Weinstein, N. D. (2007). Misleading tests of health behavior theories. *Annals of Behavioral Medicine, 33*(1), 1–10.

White, K., & Jacques, P. H. (2007). Combined diet and exercise intervention in the workplace: Effect on cardiovascular disease risk factors. *Journal of the American Association of Occupational Health Nurses, 55*(3), 109–114.

Wilkie, D. J., Williams, A. R., Gravstad, P., & Mekwa, J. (1995). Coaching persons with lung cancer to report sensory pain: Literature review and pilot study findings. *Cancer Nursing, 18,* 7–15.

World Health Organization. (1986). Ottawa Charter for Health Promotion. First International Conference on Health Promotion, Ottawa, 21 November 1986. WHO/HPR/HEP/95.1. Retrieved from http://www.who.int/hpr/NPH/docs/ottawa_charter_hp.pdf

Zhang, X., Fung, H., & Ho-hong Ching, B. (2009). Age differences in goals: Implications for health promotion. *Aging & Mental Health, 13*(3), 336–348.

CHAPTER 16

Complementary and Alternative Therapies

Original chapter by Pamala D. Larsen
Canadian content added by Joyce M. Woods

INTRODUCTION

The use of complementary and alternative treatments has continued to increase in Canada (Anderson, 2009; Boon, Verhoef, Vanderheyden, & Westlake, 2006; Clarke, Romagnoli, Sargent, & Gudrun van Amerom, 2010; Ditte, Schulz, Ernst, & Schmid-Ott, 2011; Metcalfe, Williams, McChesney, Patten, & Jetté, 2010; Ramsay, 2009; Shahjahan, 2004; Williams, Kitchen, & Eby, 2011). What motivates an individual with chronic illness to try nontraditional therapies? If the traditional allopathic approach cannot provide a treatment that relieves suffering and improves quality of life, should healthcare providers help individuals with chronic illnesses find nonallopathic treatments that may help? What is the responsibility of the healthcare provider in providing this help? What is the role of government in balancing the safety of healthcare treatments with an individual's right to access alternative or complementary treatments? Addressing these questions in a scholarly, evidence-informed manner assists the healthcare professional in providing improved health care for clients with chronic illnesses.

DEFINITIONS

In North America we tend to think of complementary and alternative medicine (CAM) as something recently discovered. However, 80% of the world's population uses some form of CAM, and it has been used in societies such as Asia, Africa, India, and China for thousands of years. Most CAM practices have evolved with indigenous peoples and were introduced to North America and Europe through migration (Disease Control Priorities Project, 2007). Uncertainty exists about what to call these therapies and so there are many descriptors throughout the literature, such as complementary, alternative, integrative, nonscientific, unconventional, unorthodox, and marginal. The following definitions are presented to assist you in understanding their use.

CAM is used to describe diverse medical and healthcare systems, practices, and products not generally considered part of conventional (Western or allopathic) medicine (British Columbia Cancer Agency, 2007; National Centre for Complementary and Alternative Medicine [NCCAM], 2008a). However, over time some

CAM practices have been labelled as conventional medicine due to their acceptance in the Western world. Complementary medicine, now commonly called "integrative" medicine, refers to using alternative medicine combined with conventional treatment where there is evidence of safety and effectiveness (Cady, 2009). Alternative medicine refers to therapies used in place of conventional medical treatments (NCCAM, 2008).

Self-healing is the primary concept in CAM practices, emphasizing the natural ability of the body to heal itself. External sources are used to mobilize the health-promoting forces in the body (Micozzi, 2011). Some therapies labelled CAM within the Canadian context are considered conventional medicine in other cultures. What needs to be done to have CAM practices recognized and supported is addressed later in this chapter.

CAM is divided into types, as follows:

1. *Biologically based therapies:* Use things found in nature such as herbs, foods, special diets, and vitamins.
2. *Alternative medical systems:* Include homeopathic medicine, naturopathic medicine, traditional Chinese medicine, Ayurvedic medicine, and native medicine.
3. *Mind–body interventions:* Techniques designed to enhance the mind's capacity to affect body functions and symptoms. These include support groups, cognitive-behavioural therapy, hypnosis, meditation, prayer, mental healing and therapies that use creative outlets such as art, music, or dance that are least likely to interact adversely with conventional medicine, drugs, chemotherapy, and radiation therapy.
4. *Manipulative and body-based methods:* Based on manipulation and/or movement of one or more parts of the body (i.e., chiropractic or osteopathic manipulation, reflexology and massage).
5. *Energy:* Biofield therapies are used to create healing and wellness by affecting the energy fields believed to surround and/or penetrate the body. Examples of biofield therapies are Gigong, Reiki, and therapeutic massage, which all apply pressure or use placement of hands on the body (Cancer Center of Southeastern Ontario, 2012). Bioelectromagnetic-based therapies use electromagnetic fields such as pulsed fields, magnetic fields, or alternating-current or direct-current fields applied externally as treatment and for disease prevention and health promotion (Centre for Cooperative Medicine, 2011).

BENEFITS OF CAM

CAM practitioners are primary healthcare providers who offer a multitude of therapies that are safe, noninvasive, effective, and inexpensive compared with the ever-increasing cost of prescription drugs. The emphasis of these therapies is on prevention and wellness, not merely looking for preexisting conditions or treating symptoms. Other benefits include allaying the severe side effects of prescribed medication or treatments such as chemotherapy, providing support for improved healing, and providing the patient with the opportunity to be an active participant with a personal responsibility for meeting personal healthcare needs and practice choices. The practitioner is present for the patient and carefully listens while attending to the patient's emotional, spiritual, psychological, and physical needs. CAM practitioners help meet the growing shortage of healthcare providers, both in urban and rural areas (Alternative Medicine Examiners Council of Canada [AMECC], 2006).

USERS

The Fraser Institute Survey (2007), entitled "Complementary and Alternative Medicine in Canada: Trends in Use and Public Attitudes, 1997–2006," provides rich data on the use of CAM (**Table 16-1**). The 2006 survey, conducted to determine use, interviewed 2,000 Canadians from a randomly selected sample of adults 18 years of age and older. Seventy-four percent of Canadians used at least one alternative therapy sometime in their lives, and greater than one-half (54%) reported using at least one alternative therapy in the 12 months before the 2006 survey, which is an increase of 4% over the rate

Table 16-1   Use of Alternative Therapy for the 10 Most Frequently Reported Principal Medical Conditions, 2006

Rank	Condition	Percentage Reporting Condition	Percentage Using Alternative Therapy in Past 12 Months	Percentage Who Saw a Provider in the Past 12 Months	Three Most Commonly Used Alternative Therapies
1	Allergies	29%	62%	34%	Massage therapies, prayer, relaxation techniques
2	Back or neck problems	28%	71%	47%	Massage therapies, chiropractic care, prayer
3	Arthritis or rheumatism	21%	61%	31%	Prayer, massage therapies, chiropractic care
4	Difficulty with routine walking	17%	64%	39%	Prayer, massage therapies, chiropractic care
5	Frequent headaches	14%	70%	41%	Prayer, massage therapies, relaxation techniques
6	Lung problems	13%	63%	33%	Prayer, relaxation techniques, massage therapies
7	Digestive problems	11%	64%	39%	Prayer, massage therapies, relaxation techniques
8	Gynaecological problems	9%	66%	40%	Massage therapies, relaxation techniques, prayer
9	Anxiety attacks	9%	72%	45%	Relaxation techniques, prayer, massage therapies
10	Heart problems or chest pain	7%	60%	30%	Prayer, relaxation techniques, massage therapies

Source: Fraser Institute (2007). Reprinted with permission by The Fraser Institute.

of the 1997 survey. The 2006 survey increased the number of interviews from 1,500 to 2,000 for greater statistical accuracy when examining changes between 1997 and 2006. Respondents in both surveys were asked to indicate their usage from a list of 22 commonly used CAMs and therapies. The interviews were conducted at the same time of the year to minimize seasonal biases. The same questions were used for both surveys; however, split-sampling was used with questions related to beliefs and perception and healthcare policy option to reduce the questionnaire length to no more than 20 minutes to address a trend in lower survey responding. Further adjustments to the 2006 survey included weighing by age and gender to reflect actual proportions in the Canadian population and dropping questions related to support for a government-funded health savings account and demographic questions related to ethnicity and religious preference (Fraser Institute, 2007).

Similar patterns to 1997 were seen in the 2006 survey with the usage of an alternative therapy during a lifetime. Albertans (84%) had the highest rate of usage, followed closely by British Columbia (83%), whereas the lowest rates where experienced by Quebecers (67%) and Atlantic Canadians (63%). Use of alternative treatment is most common amongst 18- to 34-year-olds (58%), diminishing to 49% for seniors 65 years and older (Fraser Institute, 2007).

The same five alternative therapies headed the list, but there was a significant change in the order and the number of respondents using the top five alternative therapies from 1997 to 2006. Over a lifetime chiropractic care was the most common type of therapy used by Canadians (40%), up 4% over 1997. Massage usage was 35% in 2006, up 12% from 1997, followed by relaxation techniques (20%) and prayer (18%), both percentages slightly lower than in 1997.

However, in the 12 months before the 2006 survey, the responses to usage of alternative therapies for Canadians were as follows: massage (19%), prayer (16%), chiropractic care (15%), relaxation techniques (14%), and herbal therapies (10%). The main reason for using an alternative therapy in the 12 months before the survey was for health maintenance and vitality and illness prevention (Fraser Institute, 2007).

In the 2006 survey very little change was seen in the use of CAM in households with children under the age of 18 in the 12 months before the survey (15%, down from 17%). Most commonly used by children were chiropractic care (43%), herbal therapies (22%), and massage (21%). This differs from 1997 where chiropractic care was 39%, herbal therapies 29%, and homeopathy 21%. In 2006 herbal therapies, homeopathy, naturopathy, acupuncture, folk remedies, energy healing, spiritual healing by others, osteopathy, yoga, and high dose/megavitamins were more commonly used to treat an illness, whereas chiropractic care, massage, prayer, lifestyle diets, relaxation techniques, aromatherapy, imagery techniques, special diet programs, and self-help groups were used more often for maintaining wellness (Fraser Institute, 2007).

Individuals with chronic illnesses often feel frustrated with disease-focused, fragmented, time-limited traditional allopathic care. As a result they may turn to CAM practitioners, who may take more time to listen and evaluate not only their health problems but their entire lives. Specifically, these nontraditional healthcare services are noted for extensive clinical evaluations that focus on understanding individuals and their experiences in dealing with a chronic illness; continuity with care providers over time; active participation in care by clinicians, patients, and their family members; choice of individualized services; provision of hope; open communication and information sharing; and an emphasis on the meaning and spiritual components of dealing with chronic illnesses (Bezold, 2005; Oguamanam, 2006; Saydah & Eberhardt, 2006).

The most commonly reported health problems treated by CAM in the 2006 survey were allergies (29%), back and neck problems (28%), and arthritis and rheumatism (21%). Other conditions within the top 10 were difficulty with routine walking (17%), frequent headaches (14%), lung problems (13%), digestive problems (11%), gynecological problems (9%), anxiety attacks (9%), and heart problems or chest pain (7%). Data from the 2007 survey were consistent with the 1997 survey, demonstrating that CAM use was more prevalent among women; adults aged 18 to 34; those who were married, employed full-time, and with higher levels of education; and those with a family income of greater than $60,000 (Fraser Institute, 2007; Park, 2004).

Of the respondents, 53% (down from 54% in 1997) did not discuss their use of alternative therapies with their physician (Briggs, 2007; Fraser Institute, 2007). Clients may avoid telling their physician for fear of being scolded or dismissed or of the physician becoming angry and defensive, instead of exhibiting understanding behaviours. This lack of empathy may result in future reluctance to tell conventional practitioners about nonstandard treatments as well as loss of trust in allopathic providers (Fraser Institute, 2007; Oguamanam, 2006; Sleath, Callahan, DeVellis, & Sloane, 2005).

COSTS

In 2006 adults in Canada spent more than $5.6 billion out of pocket on visits to alternative medicine practitioners, compared with $2.8 billion in 1997. This was an average of $173, a sizable increase from $93 in 1997. Had this figure included herbs, vitamins, books, medical equipment, and special diet programs, it is estimated that the total out-of-pocket spending on alternative medicine in Canada would be $7.84 billion, another sizable increase over 1997 ($5.37 billion). Greater than 76% of Canadians have purchased natural health products such as vitamins and herbs, and approximately 70% of Canadians use these products at least once weekly (Fraser Institute, 2007; Laupacis & Born, 2011).

Canadians continue their usage of CAM at some point in their lives, despite the fact that alternative medicine and therapies are generally restricted by government health insurance plans or limited by private insurance plans, as is often seen for chiropractic and massage services. These costs are in addition to the $191.6 billion Canada was estimated to spend on health care in 2010, up from an estimated $182.1 billion in 2009 and $171.8 billion in 2008. Canada was in the top fifth, with spending similar to several other OECD countries, including the Netherlands (US$4,063), Austria (US$3,970), Germany (US$3,737), and France (US$3,696) (Canadian Institute for Health Information, 2010). These statistics support the need for CAM usage because the emphasis is on prevention and health promotion, which addresses the increasing incidence of chronic disease that absorbs a major portion of the healthcare spending budget.

REGULATION OF COMPLEMENTARY AND ALTERNATIVE PRACTITIONERS

No national policy, laws, regulations, or national programme exists in Canada for CAM because this power lies with the provinces and territories.

CAM practitioners seek licensure and regulation to ensure high standards of practice with qualified practitioners with a defined scope of practice. Licensure and regulation vary throughout Canada, with chiropractors being the only profession to have achieved this status in all provinces since 1992. For most CAM practitioners licensure has only occurred in certain provinces. For example, naturopaths are licensed in Alberta, British Columbia, Saskatchewan, Manitoba, Nova Scotia, and Ontario, and Quebec is actively lobbying for provincial regulation (Vogel, 2010). Massage therapy is licensed in British Columbia, Ontario, Newfoundland, and Labrador, with some transfer arrangements between provinces to use the titles of massage therapist, registered massage therapist, and massage therapy (Massage Therapy Association of Manitoba Inc., 2012; Why Massage Therapy.com, 2009). Traditional Chinese medicine is licensed in British Columbia and Ontario, but Alberta and Quebec have only licensed acupuncture. Aromatherapy is an unlicensed occupation, but practitioners who are members of the Canadian Federation of Aromatherapists may use the designation certified aromatherapy health profession, after successfully passing the Canadian Federation of Aromatherapists national exam, holding professional liability insurance, and having current cardiopulmonary resuscitation/first aid qualifications (Canadian Information Centre for International Credentials, 2011).

Government licensure often means a possibility of coverage of insured services. However, at times the government of Canada has stopped funding or "delisted" health services, but evidence also exists where services were reinstated after public protest. In 2009 the Alberta government "delisted" chiropractic services from its provincial health plan, becoming one of seven provinces, including Ontario and Quebec, that have dropped chiropractic from their health plans. These cuts ignore arguments that chiropractic services could relieve pressure on an increasingly strained medical system, which may save money over time, and are done solely as cost-cutting measures. Numerous responses submitted to Canadian newspaper websites reflecting widespread anger for cutting chiropractic services have been ignored, and chiropractic services have not been reinstated. Although the government stated "saving money" ($53 million) was the reason for the cuts, in the same budget funding for physician services was increased by 13.8%, or $365 million. This increase was to cover physical compensation following a new contract that awarded doctors a 15% fee increase over 3 years (Sinnema, 2009).

In 2009, the British Columbia Medical Association voiced concerns about proposed changes that would allow naturopaths to prescribe drugs, order lab tests, and use the title "doctor," stating the main concern was "safety and science" (Stueck, 2009). With the controversy that exists about CAM between professional groups, we can expect these concerns to continue.

Ontario is currently drafting standards of practice for homeopathy and traditional Chinese medicine, and province-appointed transitional councils for these CAM practices are establishing professional colleges, entry to practice requirements, standards of practice, and effective disciplinary systems. Homeopathy and traditional Chinese medicine are amongst the most used complementary and alternative practices, yet they remain almost entirely unregulated in Canada. Chinese medicine was first regulated in British Columbia, but Ontario is the only province to regulate homeopathy (Complementary and Alternative Medicine Law Blog, 2010).

Naturopathic medicine is regulated in British Columbia, Saskatchewan, Manitoba, Ontario, and Nova Scotia. Alberta was expected to follow with its own regulations in 2011. Only a few years ago naturopathic doctors in Ontario and British Columbia celebrated legislative gains that allowed them to prescribe drugs as well as natural products (Vogel, 2010).

Recognizing that 80% of the world's population depends on traditional medicines for primary health care, the World Health Organization (2008) and its Member States have cooperated to promote the use of traditional medicine for health care.

> "The collaboration aims to support and integrate traditional medicine into national health programs; encourage national policy and regulation for products, practices, and providers; increase access and preserve knowledge and resources; and upgrade skills and knowledge of traditional medicine providers to ensure patient safety and quality" (World Health Organization, 2008, p. 2).

In addition to being affiliated with a college that sets the standards for high quality service and addresses safety, ethical, and disciplinary issues, regulation also makes it possible for CAM practitioners to lobby for increased coverage by public and private health payers—a great economic benefit for both practitioner and consumer.

COMMON TREATMENT MODALITIES

CAM practices fall into broad categories, and Canada recognizes categories of CAM as grouped by NCCAM. These categories are natural products, mind–body medicine, manipulative and body-based practices, and other CAM practices (NCCAM, 2008).

Natural Products

In 2003 Canada's Natural Health Products Directorate indicated that 71% of Canadians used natural health products, which includes vitamins, minerals, herbs, homeopathic medicines, traditional Chinese medicines, probiotics, amino acids, and essential fatty acids. In 2004 Canadians spent an estimated $4.3 billion on natural health products that numbered between 40,000 and 50,000 products (Health Canada, 2004; Ramsay, 2009). In Canada, herbal medicines are sold in pharmacies as over-the-counter (OTC) medicines, in special outlets, in grocery stores and retail stores by licensed and unlicensed practitioners, and in multilevel marketing. All natural health products sold in Canada must have a product license, and a site license is required for all companies that manufacture, package, label, and import these products (Health Canada, 2005, 2011a).

A 2010 Ipsos-Reid survey showed that natural health product usage had risen to 73%, up from 71% in 2005 (Health Canada, 2011b, p. 6). The most notable rise was in the use of omega 3/essential fatty acids (18%, up from 3% in 2004) and herbal teas (11%, up from 0). A significant decrease was documented for the use of Echinacea (7%, down from 15%). The leading responses for using natural health products were health maintenance (85%), illness prevention and strengthening the immune system (79%), and general concern about personal health (76%). Seventy-one percent of Canadians surveyed believed natural health products are better for them than chemical products or drugs (Health Canada, 2011b).

The Natural Health Products Directorate was established in 1999 to develop a regulatory framework for natural health products marketed in Canada. The intent was to ensure that all Canadians could readily access safe, effective, and high quality products that allowed for freedom of choice and philosophical and cultural diversity (Natural Health Product Directorate, 2003). However, regulation of natural health products in Canada did not occur until 2003 under the Food and Drugs Act (Health Canada, 2010).

Since January 2004 natural health products have been regulated by the federal government and are defined as herbs, vitamins, minerals, essential fatty acids, and homeopathics used to prevent, diagnose, or treat disease; restore or correct function; or maintain or promote health. Natural health products must be safe for OTC use and therefore must have labels and package inserts that provide the information necessary for a consumer to safely and effectively use the product without consulting a healthcare provider and must be accessible without a prescription (Her Majesty the Queen, 2003; Moss, Boon, Ballantyne, & Kachan, 2006).

Greater than 10,000 herbal medicines have been registered under the current system. Although no national pharmacopoeia for natural health products exists, reference can be made to the following resources: *Compendium of Pharmaceuticals and Specialties, Canadian Drug Reference for Health Professionals, Compendium of Nonprescription Products, United States Pharmacopoeia, Herbal Medicines, Expanded Commission E Monographs, ESCOP Monographs, World Health Organization Monographs, Pharmacopoeia of the People's Republic of China, Physician's Desk Reference for Herbal Medicines, British Herbal Compendium,* and *British Herbal Pharmacopoeia* (World Health Organization, 2005).

The elderly are major consumers of prescription medicine, and concern has been expressed throughout the literature about rising costs, compliance, and appropriateness of use. Use of OTC products and natural health products by the elderly could be due to the increase in chronic disease with aging as well as efforts to counter undesirable effects of the aging process (Qato et al., 2008; Zarowitz, 2010a). However, the combination of an OTC dietary supplement and a prescribed medication could have serious side effects, particularly in the older adult. In a Mayo Clinic study of 1,795 adults averaging 55 years of age, 107 dietary supplement–drug interactions of significance were found. The five supplements accounting for 68% of the interactions were kava, garlic, biloba, St. John's wort, and valerian. The prescription medications most frequently implicated were warfarin, sedatives/ hypnotics, antidepressants, insulin, oral antidiabetic agents, hepatotoxic medications, oral contraceptives, and tramadol (Zarowitz, 2010b).

Mind–Body Medicine

Mind–body practices focus on interactions among the brain, mind, body, and behaviour. The intent is to use the mind to affect physical functioning and thus promote health. Main practices within this category include meditation, yoga, acupuncture, deep-breathing exercises, guided imagery, hypnotherapy, progressive relaxation, qigong, and tai chi (**Table 16-2**). Acupuncture is also a component of energy medicine, manipulative and body-based practices, and traditional Chinese medicine (NCCAM, 2008). Use of three of these practices—deep-breathing exercises, meditation, and yoga—increased significantly in the 2007 National Health Interview Survey compared with the 2002 National Health Interview Survey.

Acupuncture has been practiced in China and other Asian countries for thousands of

Table 16-2 Mind–Body Medicine		
Approach	**Therapeutic Method**	**Rationale**
Meditation	Refers to a group of techniques such as mantra meditation, relaxation response, mindfulness meditation, and Zen Buddhist meditation; elements include a quiet location, specific comfortable position, focus of attention, and an open attitude.	Practice is believed to result in a state of greater calmness and physical relaxation and psychological balance due to person learning to focus attention.
Yoga	Combines physical postures, breathing exercises, meditation, and the spirit.	Enhances stress-coping mechanism and mind–body awareness.
Acupuncture	Thin needles are inserted superficially on the skin in various patterns and left in place for 8–20 min.	Points along channels of energy are manipulated to restore balance; acupuncture is part of traditional Chinese medicine.

Sources: National Centre for Complementary and Alternative Medicine (2006a, 2007a, 2008c).

years, using scientific principles to treat illness by bringing the body into harmony, balance, and homeostasis. Acupuncture has been used in a wide variety of chronic conditions. A review of the Cochrane Database reveals three systematic reviews on acupuncture. Reviews include depression, chronic asthma, and stroke rehabilitation. The 2010 update of the original 2005 systematic review of acupuncture for depression now includes data from 30 studies. These 30 studies included 2,812 participants in the meta-analysis. Two clinical trials found acupuncture may have an additive benefit when combined with medication compared with medication alone. However, the authors concluded there was insufficient evidence to recommend the use of acupuncture for people with depression. Further, the results are limited by the high risk of bias in most trials meeting inclusion criteria (Smith, Hay, & Macpherson, 2010).

An updated review of a 2003 review of randomized clinical trials of acupuncture for chronic asthma included 12 studies with 350 participants meeting the inclusion criteria. Trial reporting was poor and trial quality inadequate. The authors found no change in the 2003 conclusion of insufficient evidence to make any recommendations of acupuncture in asthma treatment (McCarney, Brinkhaus, Lasserson, & Linde, 2009).

Five clinical trials of 368 participants met the inclusion criteria in a systematic review of acupuncture and stroke rehabilitation. These trials included both ischemic and hemorrhagic stroke in the subacute or chronic stage. There was no evidence of any effects of acupuncture on subacute or chronic stroke. This was an update to a 2006 Cochrane review (Wu et al., 2009).

In Canada acupuncture is currently regulated in British Columbia, Alberta, and Quebec and pending in Ontario. In nonregulated Canadian provinces anyone, regardless of their level of training, can practice traditional acupuncture. In these cases, and in all cases of nonregulated CAM practitioners, it is up to the consumer to become informed about the practitioner's level of training (Acupuncture Foundation of Canada Institute, 2012).

In some Canadian provinces healthcare practitioners are permitted to include acupuncture as part of their scopes of practice. For example, medical doctors and dentists can use acupuncture in all provinces and territories, although specific training may be required in some provinces. Physiotherapists can use acupuncture in all provinces except Quebec; however, some provinces have set standards of training. Chiropractors can use acupuncture in all provinces except British Columbia and Quebec. Alberta and Manitoba have set standards for use, and standards are pending in Ontario. Registered nurses can use acupuncture within the practice of nursing in some provinces, except Quebec. Naturopathic doctors can use acupuncture in their regulated provinces of British Columbia, Saskatchewan, Manitoba, and Ontario (Acupuncture Foundation of Canada Institute, 2012).

In the Fraser Institute survey of 2006, the top three health conditions treated with acupuncture were back and neck problems (30%), joint problems (11%), and any sprains or strains (10%). This was a change from 1997, where back and neck pain was 30%, frequent headaches 13%, and arthritis and rheumatism 8% (Fraser Institute, 2007). Acupuncture is widely accepted throughout the world. For example, in Germany 77% of pain clinics provide acupuncture (Disease Control Priorities Project, 2007).

Manipulative and Body-Based Practices

These practices focus on the structures and systems of the body and include the bones and joints, soft tissues, and circulatory and lymphatic systems. Spinal manipulation (chiropractic) and massage therapy are the primary practices within this area (NCCAM, 2008) (**Table 16-3**).

Massage therapy is based on the principle that body tissues function at optimal levels when arterial supply and venous and lymphatic drainage are unimpeded. It is designed to re-establish proper fluid dynamics through skin, muscles, and fascia and may include nerve pathways. Massage is generally applied in the direction of the heart to stimulate increased venous and lymphatic drainage, although different techniques may be applied depending on the objective. All techniques are of the passive variety (Coughlin & Delany, 2011).

A 2008 review of Cochrane Systematic Reviews revealed several reviews of massage therapy, all associated with a specific disorder. One condition typically associated with the use of massage therapy is low back pain. Massage in the Cochrane review was defined as soft tissue manipulation using hands or a mechanical device on any body part. Thirteen randomized trials with 1,596 participants were included in the review (Furlan, Imamura, Dryden, & Irvin, 2008). The authors concluded that massage might be beneficial for patients with subacute and chronic nonspecific low back pain, especially when combined with exercises and education.

The main emphasis of chiropractic care is on the spine and its effects on the central nervous system, the autonomic nervous system, and the peripheral nervous system. Chiropractors emphasize that adjusting the spinal joints and resolving subluxations assist in restoring normal nerve function and promote optimal health (Freeman, 2009). A Cochrane systematic review examined 12 studies involving 2,887 participants with low back pain who were using combined chiropractic interventions. It was

Table 16-3 Manipulative and Body-Based Practices

Approach	Therapeutic Method	Rationale
Massage	Encompasses many techniques. Therapists press, rub, and manipulate the muscles and other soft tissues of the body.	Numerous theories about how massage therapy may affect the body. One is the gate control theory that suggests massage helps to block pain signals to the brain. Other theories suggest that massage stimulates the release of certain chemicals in the body.
Reflexology	A practice in which pressure is applied to points on the foot and sometimes the hand with the intent to promote relaxation or healing in other parts of the body.	There are "reflex" areas on the feet and hands that correspond to specific organs (e.g., tips of the toes and the head).
Chiropractic medicine	Adjustments, high-velocity, and low-amplitude thrusts are made on the spinal column. Focuses on the relationship between body's structure, mainly the spine, and its functioning.	Rearranging displaced structures promotes healing, improves functioning, and decreases pain.

Source: NCCAM (2006b, 2006c, 2007b, 2010b).

concluded that combined chiropractic interventions slightly improved pain and disability in the short term and pain in the medium term for acute and subacute lower back pain. However, no current evidence suggests or negates that these interventions provide a clinically meaningful difference for pain or disability when compared with other interventions (Walker, French, Grant, & Green, 2010).

Other CAM Practices

This broad category includes Western and Eastern movement therapies such as Pilates, Rolfing, and the Feldenkrais method; traditional healers; manipulation of energy fields, such as magnet therapy; qigong; Reiki; healing touch; and whole medical systems such as Ayurvedic medicine, traditional Chinese medicine, homeopathy, and naturopathy (**Table 16-4**).

CHRONIC DISEASE AND CAM

Increasing numbers of individuals with chronic disease are using CAM. When traditional (i.e., Western) approaches to treating and managing chronic disease, whether benign or terminal, are ineffective, individuals and their families begin looking for alternatives. Here we focus on two conditions of morbidity and mortality in Canada: hypertension and cancer.

Hypertension

Among cardiovascular risk factors, hypertension is one of the most important. Studies have shown that only one-third of patients with hypertension achieve optimal control using drug therapy, which may be why many individuals with hypertension often seek alternative therapies. Studies have been conducted on a variety of CAM practices, but the best evidence exists for coenzyme Q10, qigong, slow breathing techniques, and meditation. Supplementation of vitamin D lowered blood pressure in two trials. Acupuncture reduced blood pressure in three trials, and melatonin was effective in two small trials. Caution must be taken when using drugs to treat disease, especially calcium-channel blockers or beta-blockers (Nahas, 2008).

Jain and Mills (2010) conducted a systematic review of biofield therapies (Reiki, therapeutic touch, and healing touch) on hypertension. There was little evidence that biofield therapies reduced systolic blood pressure and

Table 16-4   Other CAM Practices

Approach	Therapeutic Method	Rationale
Qigong	Self-initiated moving meditation consisting of movement, self-massage, meditation, and breathing. It is a combination of qi (life force, energy, creativity, consciousness, breath, function) and gong (cultivation or practice over time).	Qigong puts the body into the relaxation/regeneration state where the autonomic nervous system is predominately in the parasympathetic mode.
Traditional Chinese medicine	All aspects of the person are interconnected and interact with the environment. Acupuncture, herbs, and nutrition are used to promote health and internal and external balance.	Health and healing result from determining and resolving imbalances of energy flow in the body. Central to traditional Chinese medicine is yin-yang theory; qi, which circulates in the body through a system of pathways called meridians; the use of eight principles to analyze symptoms and categorize conditions; and five elements to explain how the body works (these elements correspond to organs and tissues in the body).
Homeopathic medicine	A whole medical system based on the principle of similars (or "like cures like"). Remedies are made from naturally occurring substances from plants, minerals, or animals. Common remedies include red onion, arnica, and stinging nettle plant.	This whole medical system seeks to stimulate the body's ability to heal itself by giving very small doses of highly diluted substances based on the principle of similars.
Reiki	Japanese technique for stress reduction and relaxation that promotes spiritual healing and self-improvement; administered through laying on of hands.	An unseen "life force energy" flows through us and is what causes us to be alive. If that energy is low, the likelihood of getting sick or feeling stress is high. Reiki is not taught in the traditional sense of the word but is transferred to a student during an "attunement" in a Reiki class given by a Reiki master.

Sources: International Center for Reiki Training. (1990–2011). *What is Reiki?* Retrieved from http://www.reiki.org/FAQ/WhatIs Reiki.html; NCCAM (2006d, 2009a, 2009b); and Qigong Institute (2004–2011).

conflicting evidence that biofield therapies reduced diastolic blood pressure when compared with no treatment.

In a study to assess the efficacy of acupuncture for treatment of essential hypertension, Kim and Zhu (2010) found no evidence to support the role of acupuncture in individuals with hypertension. Further, they noted a lack of rigorous trials and the need for better designed and powered studies to reach any conclusions.

One other well-designed randomized, controlled trial reported a positive result over the long term. Yin et al. (2007) reported significant declines in active acupuncture versus sham treatment after 8 weeks of twice-weekly treatments.

Acupuncture, as a part of traditional Chinese medicine, has been used to treat hypertension in China for greater than 2,500 years and is commonly used today to treat hypertension in China and the West. However, how this mechanism works is unclear. Yang and colleagues (2010) created an intervention protocol through the Cochrane Hypertension Group that was intended to quantify the blood pressure–lowering effects of acupuncture in adults with primary hypertension. Unique to this review was that studies included must have a control group of either placebo or sham acupuncture or no treatment.

Several CAM therapies are considered as part of an evidence-informed approach to the treatment of hypertension. However, further research based on cardiovascular outcomes is needed to prove potential benefits (Nahas, 2008).

Cancer

Up to 80% of Canadians with cancer use some type of CAM during their cancer experience; however, only 28% of cancer patients discuss their use of CAM practices with their oncology healthcare providers. A study on the frequent use of CAM by prostate cancer patients showed that 90% of the patients used CAM with the aim to improve quality of life (Ponholzer, Struhal, & Madersbacher, 2003). Of those who did discuss their CAM use, only 18% received the support they needed to make informed decisions.

The Complementary Medicine Education and Outcomes Program is a research program that studies the CAM needs of people living with cancer. They develop programs and resources to address the needs of the person with cancer, their support persons, and their healthcare providers by bringing the latest CAM research to conventional cancer care settings through education courses, lectures, published documents, and individualized information and decision support consultations. The Complementary Medicine Education and Outcomes Program is a joint venture with the University of British Columbia School of Nursing and the British Columbia Cancer Agency (2012).

Individuals with cancer use CAM for a variety of reasons, but according to the Canadian Cancer Society, "The purpose of a complementary therapy is not to treat the cancer itself. They help a person cope with cancer, its treatment or side effects, and to feel better. They take a holistic approach by focusing on the whole person" (Ovarian Cancer Canada, 2010). Most patients used CAM as a complementary practice to conventional therapies such as radiotherapy, chemotherapy, hormone therapy, and surgery (Adams & Jewell, 2007). Only 4% to 6% of Canadians with cancer leave conventional cancer care for alternative medicine (Ovarian Cancer Canada, 2010). Commonly used CAM practices included visualization, herbs, dietary treatment, meditation, spiritual healing, relaxation, homeopathy, hypnotherapy, and megavitamins (Adams & Jewell, 2007; Leis et al., 2003).

Reasons given for choosing CAM practices were dissatisfaction with conventional medicine; a "perceived" poor relationship, lack of interest, and disapproval of the therapies with some healthcare professionals; hope for a positive outcome; hope for control over treatment; and desperation on the part of patients to get cured (Bott, 2007). According to Robotin and Penman (2006), the gap in knowledge of healthcare professionals on CAM impacts decision making regarding the use of CAM. Most healthcare professionals admit they know very little about CAM cancer therapies, and most physicians obtain their information regarding CAM from patients. This lack of knowledge, communication, and relationship between patients and healthcare professionals decreases the likelihood of discussing potential benefits and risk of CAM therapies and could be a factor for the lack of approval and support for CAM use and the resulting negative attitudes and beliefs (Bott, 2007). Younger doctors were more likely to be in favour of CAM and also more likely to use CAM for themselves or a family member (Boon et al., 2000).

Jain and Mills (2010) conducted a systematic review of 66 clinical studies examining the use and effectiveness of biofield therapies (Reiki, therapeutic touch, and healing touch) in a variety of individuals with different chronic conditions. In their review they noted moderate evidence for positive effects on acute cancer pain; however, evidence was conflicting for longer term pain, cancer-related fatigue, quality of life, and physiological indicators of the relaxation response.

Complementary and alternative therapies are often used in symptom management in individuals with cancer. Boon, Olatunde, and Zick (2007) reported that 80% of their sample of 1,434 women with breast cancer used CAM for symptom management. To better understand this statistic, Wyatt, Skiorskii, Wills, and An (2010) used secondary data analysis in a sample of 222 stage I and stage II breast cancer patients to explore the association of CAM use, spending on CAM therapies, demographic variables, surgical treatment, and quality of life. Overall, 58.2% of the women used CAM, specifically the biologically based therapies; 77 women used vitamins; 25 used audiotapes; 18 used massage; 17 used spiritual healing; and some women used more than one CAM therapy. Alternative medical systems were used in 13 women. Individuals reporting lower quality of life are highly likely to use CAM therapies.

A 2008 review of 20 clinical trials found no convincing evidence that antioxidant supplements prevent gastrointestinal cancer but did find indications that some might actually increase overall mortality. The review looked at beta-carotene, selenium, and vitamins A, C, and E. Selenium alone demonstrated some preventive benefits. Research from the National Cancer Institute noted that higher intake of calcium may be associated with reduced risk of colorectal cancer but concluded that the available evidence does not support taking calcium supplements to prevent colorectal cancer.

A 2008 review of the research concluded that some botanicals used in Ayurvedic medicine and traditional Chinese medicine may have a role in cancer treatment. However, scientific evidence is limited because much of the research on botanicals and cancer treatment is in the early stages. It is unclear whether the use of vitamin and mineral supplements by patients with cancer is beneficial or harmful. There is a concern that some supplements might interfere with the cancer treatment.

A 2008 evidence-informed review of clinical options for managing nausea and vomiting in cancer patients noted that electroacupuncture was an option to be considered. A study of 380 patients with advanced cancer concluded that massage therapy may offer some limited relief for these patients. A 2008 review of botanical research concluded that some botanicals have shown promise in managing the side effects of cancer treatment. However, the reviewers did not find sufficient evidence to recommend any specific treatment (NCCAM, 2010).

Smith et al. (2010) conducted a study on the outcomes of therapeutic massage for 41 hospitalized cancer patients and reported a positive outcome for the study. They compared the outcomes of therapeutic massage on a group of patients and that of a nurse interaction on a control group. It was observed that pain, distress, anxiety, and sleep quality were worse in the control group and concluded that therapeutic massage helps to alleviate pain and distress and improves sleep patterns. Cassileth and Vickers (2004) conducted a much larger study of massage for cancer patients with a sample size of 1,290. The study setting was at a cancer centre, and most study subjects were inpatients (74%), with outpatients treated in their homes. Patients reported over 40% improvement in their pain and fatigue and over 50% in their anxiety levels.

Telephone interviews were conducted to ascertain CAM use among breast cancer (*BRCA*) mutation carriers enrolled in a high-risk breast and ovarian cancer screening study. Of the 164 *BRCA1* or *BRCA2* women in the analysis, 78% reported CAM use of prayer, lifestyle, and diet as the most commonly reported modalities. Using three or more CAM therapies was reported in 34% of the women. CAM use was associated with older age, higher education level, and higher levels of ovarian cancer worry (Mueller et al., 2008).

In a study funded by the National Cancer Institute, NCCAM, and the National Institute on Aging, researchers examined the interface between allopathic medical providers and CAM providers in a sample of older women with breast cancer. The qualitative study interviewed 44 women who were approximately 5 years post-diagnosis. For all but four women a diagnosis of breast cancer was not the catalyst for CAM use. The women highly valued their simultaneous relationships with both their CAM provider and their biomedical provider. Although the study focused on the interface of different practitioners, core results of the study reflected on broader beliefs of health, illness, and aging (Adler, Wrubel, Hughes, & Beinfield, 2009).

However, in cases where CAM has been used solely as an "alternative" to standard care, the outcome has been very poor. In a study on the outcomes of breast cancer patients who used alternative therapies as primary treatment, it was discovered that the sole use of CAM as primary treatment for breast cancer resulted in increased recurrence and death of patients (Chang, Glissmeyer, Tonnes, Hudson, & Johnson, 2006).

There are frequent studies in the literature on the use of CAM to prevent cancer, treat cancer, and control symptoms. In the October 2010 *NCCAM Clinical Digest,* the focus of the e-newsletter was "Cancer and CAM: What the Science Says." The following is a summary of the findings (NCCAM, 2010):

A 2007 review of clinical trials looking at the effectiveness of multivitamin/mineral supplements for cancer prevention found that few such trials have been conducted and that the results of most large-scale trials have been mixed. According to the National Cancer Institute, the following did not find sufficient evidence to recommend any specific treatment.

ISSUES

Issues concerning CAM therapies include research, dissemination of information, legislative matters, and quackery.

Research

Challenges in designing research studies to evaluate CAM practices include determining the appropriate therapy, amount to be administered, and population to receive the treatment. Criticisms of research on CAM treatments are that studies often do not use hypothesis testing, do not include large numbers of subjects, and do not randomly assign subjects to treatment and control groups, and often rely on subjective responses from clients rather than objective measures.

Adams and Jewell (2007) reviewed the many criticisms levelled against CAM. There tends to be agreement amongst researchers of insufficient research into CAM use by cancer patients and lack of "peer-reviewed" scientifically conducted research, in spite of the extensive use. Factors cited were lack of funding, insufficient patient numbers for a study, and more clinical trials including randomized control trials. Additional barriers to research on nontraditional treatments were lack of needed research skills among practitioners; lack of computers, libraries, and statistical support; problems obtaining suitable numbers of subjects; difficulties in comparing and interpreting research; and methodological issues such as individualized treatment and lack of control subjects for comparison. Allopathic and CAM require different types of evaluative research: Allopathic medicine demands scientific validation of the efficacy of a treatment on composite groups of patients using experimental and control groups, whereas CAM emphasises holistic, individualized treatment that is qualitative in nature (Boozang, 2003; Oguamanam, 2006). Most CAM modalities are based on beliefs, practices, and traditions of a culture; therefore, their potential benefits and effectiveness are based on experiences or testimonials of patients (Adams & Jewell, 2007).

Bausell (2009, p. 349) reviewed 45 CAM efficacy randomized controlled trials from four high-impact journals: *New England Journal of Medicine*, *Journal of the American Medicine Association*, *Annals of Internal Medicine,* and *Archives of Internal Medicine*. Bausell's review was based on three validity criteria: the existence of a placebo control, moderate attrition rates, and 50 or more participants in each group of the sample. Of the 26 trials meeting all three criteria, only 2 were judged to be supportive of the CAM therapy, whereas more than half (55.5%) of the 19 trials failing to meet one or more of the criteria reported positive results ($P < 0.001$). Of the two positive high validity trials, one was funded and authored by the herbal company marketing the product tested and one used a placebo control group of questionable credibility.

Several systematic reviews generated by the Cochrane Collaboration noted bias. Although many studies were examined in a systematic review, Cochrane authors often noted few randomized clinical trials that met study criteria. Walker and colleagues (2010), in their review of chiropractic and low back pain, noted that of the studies they reviewed, none looked at chiropractic interventions versus no treatment. Kim and Zhu (2010), in their review of acupuncture and hypertension, noted a lack of rigorous trials. Further, Jain and Mills (2010), in their systematic review, stated that the studies were of average quality and met minimum standards required for validity. Only 6 of 67 studies reviewed reported an effect size. Jain and Mills (2010) reported a lower overall study quality than previous authors.

The mission of the Canadian Interdisciplinary Network for Complementary and Alternative Medicine (IN-CAM) is to foster excellence in CAM research in Canada, which informs healthcare practitioners and healthcare consumers. Members of IN-CAM are eligible for CAM research funding and have membership in and are eligible for financial support to develop special interest groups related to CAM research. IN-CAM has created a database of outcome measures of relevance and importance to CAM research to assist in making practical information accessible (IN-CAM, 2012).

CAMline is an evidence-informed website on CAM for healthcare professionals and the public. The aim is to provide peer-reviewed, accessible, credible, practice and objective information on the safety and efficacy of CAM products, therapies, and practitioners, as well as a Canadian perspective on CAM (CAMline, 2012).

The CAM in Undergraduate Medical Education (UME) project was established in 2003 by a team of conventional and CAM educators as a Canadian medical education initiative. The project provides information on skills and attitudes and discusses CAM with patients in an informed and nonjudgmental manner. This project has developed a searchable digital resource repository of oriented teaching/learning resources, peer-reviewed curriculum guidelines, a set of CAM-related competencies for undergraduate medical education, and a guide to assist medical school educators teaching CAM in their schools. From 2001 to 2011 support from the CAM in UME was received from Lotte and John Hecht Memorial Foundation, Canadian Interdisciplinary Network for Complementary and Alternative Medicine Research, Sociobehavioural Cancer Research Network, Health Canada, Health Human Resources Strategies Division and Natural Health Products Directorate, and the Hospital for Sick Kids (IN-CAM, 2012).

The Canadian CAM Research Fund was established in 2009 as a partnership between IN-CAM and the Holistic Health Research Foundation of Canada to increase and enhance CAM research capacity in Canada. An annual competition is held to offer funding for research project proposals to encourage and support CAM research. Projects must have as a research priority one of the following: efficacy, effectiveness, and/or safety of CAM interventions (products, modalities, practices); evaluation of healthcare delivery models that incorporate CAM; development and evaluation/assessment of CAM specific policies in the context of healthcare delivery in Canada; or effectiveness and/or usefulness of knowledge translation activities related to CAM information dissemination to healthcare practitioners and the public (Natural Health Care Canada, 2011).

The Cancer and Complementary and Alternative Medicine Research Team, composed of 12 researchers and practitioners from across Canada, developed a coherent research program. The program includes the sociobehavioural aspects of CAM and cancer, CAM utilization in studies in ethnic cancer populations, exploration of appropriate methodologies to evaluate CAM interventions, testing CAM modalities, examination of evidence-informed decision making, and CAM information dissemination. The Cancer and Complementary and Alternative Medicine Research Team was established by the Sociobehavioural Cancer Research Network of the Centre for Behavioural Research and Program Evaluation funded by the National Cancer Institute of Canada with funds from the Canadian Cancer Society. In 2009, restructuring occurred, and it is now the Canadian Cancer Society Research Institute (2012). Examples of current research projects are as follows: a longitudinal and case-controlled study of women with breast cancer who decide to decline conventional cancer treatment and use CAM therapies (Canadian Breast Cancer Research Alliance funded: 2006–2010); Pathways: Understanding cancer patients' pathways of care: An international pilot study (Lotte and John Hecht Memorial Foundation, Norwegian Research Council: 2008–2010); Complementary Medicine Education and Outcomes Program; and the Lotte and John Hecht Memorial Foundation: 2008–2013 (IN-CAM, 2012).

The Canadian Institute of Natural and Integrative Medicine is a charitable organization that evaluates CAM through rigorous scientific research to help meet the demands of the public for more information about CAM and for access to these practices. The Canadian Institute of Natural and Integrative Medicine, in consort with the Faculties of Medicine and Nursing, the Calgary Health Region, and the Integrative Medicine Institute, is helping to facilitate the transformation of health care. Current projects funded through private donations and project grants include The LEAP Project—An Online Program for Young People Struggling with Depression (in collaboration with Alberta Health Services, the University of Calgary, and Mount Royal University); Nutritional Therapy & Asthma—New Research Project for Asthmatic Children (in collaboration with the Asthma Clinic at the Alberta Children's Hospital); Parent-delivered Massage—Randomized-Clinical Trial for Children (6–18 years old) diagnosed with cancer and their parents; and a Blood-Based Diagnostic Assay for Breast Cancer looking at early detection and response to treatment (Canadian Institute of Natural and Integrative Medicine, 2012).

Families frequently ask about the value of CAM therapies for asthma, particularly vitamin and mineral supplements. However, to date no studies have been done to decide if these supplements are effective, ineffective, or harmful.

Challenges continue for the Western biomedically dominated healthcare system and its practitioners as consumer enthusiasm for CAM continues. There is a growing need for evidence-informed research along with healthcare professionals who are able to talk in an informed and supportive manner, and this is hampered by the fact that CAM is not fully integrated or a research option in the Canadian healthcare system. Consistency with regulations, licensure, standards, and the development of a more comprehensive code of ethics to guide all disciplines toward the provision of safe and effective health services for Canadians would be beneficial. Today, one might ask the question, "Is CAM really alternative?" Surveys have indicated a readiness across the country for a concerted effort in providing information, support, and access to complementary and alternative health practices.

CASE STUDY

Mrs. Martin, a 70-year-old woman, developed rheumatoid arthritis when she was 18 years old. Her first symptoms were swelling in her left knee and ankle. She had just relocated from a rural community to an urban area, where she worked as a secretary full-time and attended college part-time. She was in a great deal of pain when she went to see a physician. The physician drained her knee, performed various diagnostic tests, and diagnosed her with rheumatoid arthritis. She was told to take 12 aspirin throughout the course of each day. No education regarding her illness, prognosis, or the potential side effects of her medication were provided. She was shy, deferred to authority figures, and was unprepared to advocate for herself.

She took a leave of absence from her job for a month, returned to the rural community in which she was raised, and rested. Her father had died when she was 4 years old. Her mother had an 8th-grade education. Her two older brothers and sisters lived nearby but were not actively involved in her life. After she had rested and began to feel a little better, she returned to her secretarial job and continued taking classes. Her left knee and both of her ankles remained swollen and painful, and the same symptoms developed in her fingers, wrists, and elbows. She had her knee drained and injected with steroid medication every other month; however, in a short time it would swell again. She felt fatigued and in pain.

Several years after her diagnosis, she married and had two children. During the course of her pregnancies her arthritis symptoms totally resolved. After each of her children was born her symptoms immediately came back. As the years went by she was followed closely by her primary care physician and saw a number of internists and rheumatologists. She took a variety of nonsteroidal anti-inflammatory agents.

Her joints were periodically drained and injected with a steroid. She tried gold shots without any relief. She went to physical therapists and was careful to eat a healthy and well-balanced diet. Over time her wrists, elbows, fingers, and feet developed joint deformities and contractures. Despite the deformities and pain she maintained an active lifestyle and balanced her household and maternal duties.

When she was 35, Mrs. Martin's symptoms became so severe she was unable to do any work and was bedridden for 6 months. Because of her severe pain she cried most of the time that she was awake. Her primary care doctor was empathetic but unable to help her. He referred her to a rheumatologist who failed to help relieve her suffering but told her, "You're doing fine for having a case of rheumatoid arthritis that is so aggressive."

Mr. Martin began to actively read about rheumatoid arthritis and search for ways to help relieve some of his wife's suffering. The couple tried a number of dietary programs without success. One day a friend mentioned to Mr. Martin that he knew of a woman with rheumatoid arthritis who had been in a wheelchair and was now walking. Mr. Martin tracked the woman down, and she told him about an alternative treatment for rheumatoid arthritis that seemed miraculous and had changed her life.

(continues)

CASE STUDY   (Continued)   `WWW`

Because this was an alternative treatment, it is not covered by the healthcare system and is only regulated in a few provinces in Canada. Against the advice of her rheumatologist, Mrs. Martin travelled to another province with her husband for therapy. Within 3 days Mrs. Martin's pain and swelling were reduced. She was walking, had resumed her household duties, and felt more energetic and in less pain than she had in her adult life. The contractures that had developed did not go away, so she began to use an alternative treatment weekly—massages to help with mobility, muscle relaxation, and pain minimization.

Over the years primary care physicians had not been willing to prescribe Mrs. Martin's alternative treatment, requiring her to travel yearly to another province to get her medication. However, they have been amazed at the change in her health status. Currently, although several newer allopathic treatments for rheumatoid arthritis are available, she does not see a rheumatologist. To determine if any of these allopathic treatments were appropriate for her, Mrs. Martin consulted with seven different rheumatologists. Each chastised her for her long-term use of an alternative, unproven therapy and was unwilling to discuss transitioning her to one of the newer allopathic treatments unless she completely stopped her existing medication (in order for them to do several months of workup). Consequently, because she is functioning well, considering the severity and length of time that she has had her disease, Mrs. Martin has opted to continue alternative treatment. She also has an array of vitamins, healthy nutrition, exercise, and rest. Mrs. Martin has been on this alternative regimen for 35 years. She adjusts her dosage daily in response to the presence of symptoms and continues to walk a half a mile each day, drive a car, do much of her own housework, and participate in social activities such as going to the opera.

Discussion Questions

1. What motivated Mrs. Martin to begin using alternative treatment for her rheumatoid arthritis?
2. What worked well for Mrs. Martin in the allopathic healthcare system, and what did not work well?
3. Healthcare professionals were absent from Mrs. Martin's care. What are some ways they could have—or should have—been involved in her care?
4. How will you help individuals who have chronic illnesses and choose to use alternative treatments to meet their healthcare needs?
5. What would you do if you or one of your family members developed a chronic illness that was continuing to cause worsening disability and suffering and allopathic healthcare providers were unable to offer effective treatment options?
6. What is the healthcare professional's role in advocating for expanded practice, changes in the healthcare system, and an open-minded approach with regard to alternative treatments for individuals with chronic illnesses?

This case study was developed by Dr. Lisa Onega.

Dissemination of Information

Journals developed for healthcare practitioners to address alternative, complementary, and integrative treatments include *Alternative Therapies in Health and Medicine, Complementary Therapies in Medicine, Evidence Based Complementary and Alternative Medicine, Journal of Alternative and Complementary Medicine, BMC Complementary and Alternative Medicine, Journal of Holistic Nursing,* and *Research in Complementary Medicine.*

Coelho, Pittler, and Ernst (2007), in an effort to categorize knowledge dissemination and compare it with previously published categorizations from 1995 and 2000, examined the 2005 contents of six major journals that publish research on alternative, complementary, and integrative treatments. Fewer articles than in previous years were about clinical trials (1995 had 28%, 2000 had 23%, and 2005 had 22%). Several additional journals were also reviewed, which had not previously been included in the 2000 and 1995 investigations. With these articles included (n = 363), only 19% of the manuscripts were classified as clinical trials. None of the journals published meta-analyses, and only 4% of the articles included a systematic review of the state of the science. The most common articles were about general alternative, complementary, and integrative topics (20%), phytomedicine (standardized herbal treatments) (14%), and homeopathy (11%). This survey of the literature indicated that although the number of individuals with chronic illnesses is increasing, the evidence-informed literature testing nonallopathic therapies to treat these individuals is decreasing. Clinicians who want to provide safe and effective options for their clients and families are in a quandary because they know that hope and options are essential both for treatment of disease and for healing the human spirit; however, they also know that scientific evaluation of treatment modalities is necessary.

Another study by Clarke and colleagues (2010) described the portrayal of CAM in mass print media magazines. The study was based on full-text articles in the English language using magazines with circulation rates of more than 1 million available in Canada and published in Canada or the United States during the years 1980 to 2005. *Maclean's* was included because it is the highest circulating national newsmagazine in Canada, even though its circulation is below 1 million. The Reader's Guide to Periodicals Index was used to locate CAM articles and the internal links mentioned. The articles located included the following CAM practices: acupuncture, chiropractics, naturopathy, holistic medicine, homeopathy, alternative medicine, and home remedies. A growth in the numbers of articles under the term CAM was noted over the years. In 1985, 9 articles were found; that number increased to 28 in 2004. Three themes emerged. The first theme was that medicalisation persists. This theme identified the following aspects: CAM is good but not good enough and therefore should be used as complementary in conjunction with conventional medicine, and CAM is potentially dangerous, lacking in evidence, used against the advice of conventional doctors, and should be used only after conventional medicine has been used and did not work. Theme 2 was related to individualism and consumerism and included holism and the uniqueness of the individual, the responsibility of the individual for health, and the fact that individuals as active consumers should have free choice. Theme 3 addressed costs and out-of-pocket expenses and lack of coverage by healthcare insurance programs. Profit motive was questioned both on medication and remedies and the huge profits earned by manufacturers of homeopathic remedies. Based on the significant amount of attention given to CAM by mass media, it should be considered as a contributor to CAM usage and understanding.

The Friends of Alternative & Complementary Therapies Society is a nonprofit, volunteer community organization that encompasses a broad range of physicians, nurses, CAM practitioners, academics, and consumer. The goal of the organization is to promote credible and practical health information about a variety of practices across cultures. This community is working to create an online repository of information about CAM therapies and practices (Friends of Alternative & Complementary Therapies Society, 2011).

Legislative Matters

Legal matters related to alternative and complementary therapies are discussed in the next two sections—paradigm issues and those specific to advanced practice nurses.

Paradigm Issues

Some critics of allopathic health care have argued that physicians, out of self-interest, have convinced legislators to restrict the scope of practice of CAM healthcare providers and limit choices for individuals with chronic illnesses. They believe because physicians work closely with hospitals, pharmaceutical companies, and reimbursers, they have persuaded these organizations to avoid partnering with nontraditional healthcare providers. Therefore, according to these critics, physicians, hospitals, pharmaceutical companies, and reimbursers have influenced policy and legislation to limit these practices and, when possible, to prosecute nonphysician

practitioners who offer competitive healthcare services (Boozang, 1998; Cuellar, Cahill, Ford, & Aycock, 2003).

Ultimately, a clash exists between proponents of the allopathic healthcare paradigm and proponents of the alternative and complementary healthcare paradigm. Advocates of the allopathic healthcare paradigm believe governmental regulation is based on scientific evidence, promotes safety, and ensures the treatment provided to persons with chronic illness is effective. Advocates of the nonallopathic healthcare paradigm believe individuals should have access to information and treatment, the freedom to evaluate benefits and risks, and ultimately decide for themselves their form of health care (Cuellar et al., 2003; Oguamanam, 2006).

Advanced Practice Nursing Issues

Advanced nursing practice is defined as "an umbrella term describing an advanced level of clinical nursing practice that maximizes the use of graduate educational preparation, in-depth knowledge and expertise, in meeting the health needs of individuals, families, groups, communities and populations" (Canadian Nurses Association, 2008). Canada recognizes two advanced nursing practice roles: the clinical specialist and the nurse practitioner. For the purposes of this chapter we reference the nurse practitioner. Nurse practitioners work within a holistic model of care, focusing on health management, health promotion, health protection, disease and injury prevention, and the determinants of health. They provide person-centred care, working with diverse client populations in a variety of practice settings. Nurse practitioners assess; counsel on both health and illness concerns; and advise on symptom management, self-care strategies, medication, and the benefits and potential risks of CAM, including the potential interactions between natural health products and OTC and/or prescribed medications. Actions associated with CAM require analyzing the effects of marketing strategies used to promote health products and CAM therapies (College of Registered Nurses of Nova Scotia, 2011, 2012).

Nurse practitioners providing care to individuals with chronic illnesses are often concerned about whether activities related to CAM treatment fall within acceptable legal parameters; they also worry about liability protection as it relates to nontraditional therapies (College of Registered Nurses of British Columbia, 2006; Cuellar et al., 2003). It is not uncommon for individuals suffering with chronic illness who believe they have exhausted allopathic options to ask a nurse practitioner to prescribe or administer nonallopathic treatments. Clinicians may feel persuaded by anecdotal evidence, compassion for clients and their families, and the belief the treatment is in their scope of practice; however, they may be concerned about how their provincial nursing regulators or their malpractice insurers would view their prescribing or administering of the requested treatment. Contacting the provincial nursing association and their practice insurer to obtain other perspectives may provide useful feedback about the desired treatment and assist the nurse practitioner in making wise decisions (Cuellar et al., 2003). Nurse practitioners should also be aware that provinces differ regarding licensure of nonallopathic practitioners.

STANDARDS FOR NURSING PRACTICE AND CAM

Registered nurses can be actively involved in the delivery of CAM or may assist clients to access and understand appropriate information to aid in decisions regarding treatment. The responsibility of the nurse in providing CAM therapies is based on the Code of Ethics and the Standards of Nursing Practice, and when a decision is made to participate in CAM healthcare practices, the primary duty of the nurse is to provide safe, competent, and ethical care. The standards for practice for CAM health care are as follows (College & Association of Registered Nurses of Alberta, 2011; College of Registered Nurses of British Columbia, 2012; College of Registered Nurses of Nova Scotia, 2005):

- Must have the necessary competence (knowledge, skill, judgment, and attitudes) to provide the therapy in a safe, competent, and ethical manner
- Must understand the purpose of the therapy, including indications, contraindications, risks, and expected outcomes and be prepared to provide care in the event of an expected or unexpected outcome of the therapy
- Must determine if the therapy is valid based on evidence-informed research, ascertain the therapy is not prohibited by law in Canada and/or the provincial jurisdiction, be certain there are policies in place in the practice setting to support CAM practices, and be authorized to perform the particular therapy by the agency
- Must have access to a pharmacist or other healthcare providers as necessary
- Must have the client complete an informed consent for the proposed therapy
- Must document all discussions, understandings, decisions, and consents
- Must practice within the legally authorized nursing scope of practice
- Must know the position of the provincial/territorial regulatory body on the provision of CAM and consult them as required.

CULTURAL CONSIDERATIONS AND CAM

Culture and ethnicity are key determinants of health. As a result these determinants may influence an individual's interaction with the healthcare system, healthcare providers, acceptance of and involvement in health promotion programs and services, lifestyle choices, and access to health information.

The Ontario Women's Health Council released a report in 2003 indicating that of 276 aboriginal women respondents, 72.1% consulted traditional healers and 42% sought out the services of medicine people. As well, about 34% of aboriginal peoples living in urban areas had access to traditional medicines. Inuit, Métis, and First Nations continue to consider traditional medicines and practices an important part of their lives.

Canada is diverse and complex in its cultural, geographical, and jurisdictional landscape. As a result some unique approaches to traditional knowledge, medicine, and public health have developed, based on indigenous culture, language, and knowledge. The Innulitsivik Health Centre in Puvirnituq, Nunavik, offers unique maternity services (pre- and postnatal care) provided by a team of both traditional Inuit midwives and Western medical practitioners, and protocols are set by an interdisciplinary council. The First Nations Health Program at the Whitehorse General Hospital integrates traditional knowledge and medicines in an inpatient setting to ensure quality and culturally sensitive holistic health care. Elders were part of all the development of the program and services. The Métis Addictions Council of Saskatchewan Inc. provides rehabilitation, education, and prevention services to all aboriginal peoples seeking support for drug and alcohol abuse in the province of Saskatchewan at Regina, Saskatoon, and Prince Albert. Their goal is lifelong recovery, restoring harmony through mental, spiritual, physical, and emotional care. Some centres provide cleansing ceremonies, healing rooms, traditional foods such as venison and moose meat, traditional medicines and natural herbs, and off-site practices such as sweat lodge ceremonies (National Aboriginal Health Organization, 2008).

Nursing education curricula are now available on cultural competency and cultural safety to create awareness and understanding of indigenous populations and their healthcare practices. Examples of health centres as mentioned previously are evidence that governments are recognizing true advancement of indigenous population health is possible if we recognize and work to eradicate structural inequalities (Stout & Downey, 2012).

QUACKERY

Although research verifying the effectiveness of most alternative, complementary, and integrative treatments is inadequate, practitioners have the responsibility to provide information regarding the known benefits and risks of the treatment (Chez & Jonas, 2005; Cuellar et al., 2003). When healthcare providers misrepresent treatments to consumers, they are committing fraud (Cuellar et al., 2003).

Quackery as treatment is defined as the promotion of unproven, disproved, and/or unsubstantiated methods that lack a scientifically plausible rationale (Barrett, 2009; Boozang, 1998). Boozang (1998) noted, however, that some nonallopathic treatments, although not yet adequately evaluated (unproven), may be helpful to clients. She emphasized the importance of heightened informed consent for any treatments outside of the accepted standard of care. Cuellar and colleagues (2003) stated that clinicians have a duty to present both traditional and nontraditional perspectives and assert that informed consent means providing information about allopathic and nonallopathic treatment options along with the associated benefits and risks.

PROFESSIONAL EDUCATION

CAM curricula have been developed within medical schools in the United States and United Kingdom over the past 10 years (Helms, 2006). A 1998 survey by Ruedy, Kaufman, and MacLeod (1999) reported that 81% of Canadian medical schools (13/16) were including CAM in their curricula; however, other evidence suggests that most of these schools are not providing CAM content in a formalized manner, and few have faculty-driven CAM initiatives or see CAM content as a priority (Verhoef, Brundin-Mather, Jones, Boon, & Epstein, 2004).

AMECC is the national accrediting agency for programs granting a doctoral degree in alternative medicine. It ensures high quality CAM education in Canada by offering a voluntary accreditation for 4-year graduate programs in CAM and certifies postdoctoral programs and physician residencies for alternative medicine family care and other specialties. Graduates of programs accredited by AMECC may apply for the complementary and alternative medicine physicians licensing examination administered by the Canadian Council of Examiners. By 2006, 28 CAM medical colleges in Canada were accredited by the AMECC (2006).

Approximately 180,000 medical doctors in the European Union have taken familiarization training and education in medical undergraduate programs in CAM modalities, some of which are optional and others mandatory. Most of the European Union Member States have universities that provide postgraduate courses in specific CAM therapies; other countries offer this education in private teaching centres (CAMDOC Alliance, 2010).

Nurses are at the forefront of healthcare delivery and need to have adequate knowledge about CAM to provide proper advice and have the skills to appropriately integrate CAM practices into holistic care (O'Regan, Wills, & O'Leary, 2010). Nursing schools have been slower to include classes in alternative and complementary treatments; however, this material is often integrated throughout graduate and undergraduate curricula. Few schools provide dedicated courses, although several schools have made a noteworthy commitment to nonallopathic theories. Mount Royal University in Calgary, Alberta, provides a senior option course in their undergraduate nursing program entitled "Integrative Healing Practices." This course provides information on traditional Chinese medicine, Ayurvedic medicine, native medicine, homeopathy, naturopathy, aromatherapy, orthomolecular therapies, nutritional therapies, herbal therapies, and healing modalities such as bodywork, mind–body practices, biological, spiritual, and energetic healing. The course examines what motivates individuals to try nontraditional therapies and asks whether healthcare providers have a responsibility to provide individuals with information related to complementary treatments (Woods, 2012). What is needed, however, is an enhanced education approach to expand the body of knowledge on CAM in nursing education and practice.

ETHICAL DECISION MAKING

Healthcare professionals working with individuals who have chronic illnesses may experience ethical decision-making challenges related to the use of nonallopathic treatment. The following case study provides an example. Thinking about one's values, beliefs, and rationale for decision making helps to prepare the advanced practice nurse for those unexpected and difficult challenges.

CASE STUDY

Dr. Thomas Smithton, a 58-year-old man, is a professor and owns a successful mathematical consulting business. Thomas has been happily married for 32 years to his wife, Patricia, who is a geologist. They have three children—Samuel, who is 30, married, has two children, and lives across the country; Jenna, who is 27, married, and lives in another province; and Ben, who is 25 and in graduate school in another province. Although their children are grown and do not live nearby, Thomas and Patricia maintain a close relationship with them.

Throughout his adult life Thomas has tried to maintain a healthy balance between work and family. He visits relatives once a year, has several good friends, and has many acquaintances. He eats healthy foods and exercises at a gym twice a week. He has never smoked cigarettes, used illegal drugs, or used alcohol excessively. He describes himself as a "high-energy person" and functions well on about 6 hours of sleep a night.

Thomas has been seeing Ms. Mason, a family nurse practitioner, for physical examinations and episodic visits for 15 years. He has excellent preventive health care and health habits. Thomas is known to Ms. Mason to always be on time for appointments, prepared, cooperative, and highly motivated. Ms. Mason considers him to be "the model patient, just an all around great guy." She provides care for the entire family and says "the whole family is special." She believes long-term relationships like these are what make being a nurse practitioner meaningful and rewarding.

About 2 years ago Thomas set up an appointment with Ms. Mason because he was feeling weak, had tripped over the carpet several times, and was dropping things. Ms. Mason did a neurological and muscle evaluation, laboratory work (including blood and urine studies with high-resolution serum protein electrophoresis, thyroid and parathyroid hormone levels, and 24-hour urine collection for heavy metals), and x-rays. She also referred him to a neurologist for further evaluation. The neurologist diagnosed him with amyotrophic lateral sclerosis (ALS), also known as Lou Gehrig's disease.

Thomas has been a model patient in living with his ALS; however, his illness has progressed. About a year and a half ago he took disability from his job at the university and several months later closed his consulting business. Patricia took family medical leave for 6 months to modify their house for a person with a disability, made sure business and legal

CASE STUDY (Continued)

matters such as power of attorney and advance directives were updated, and hired around-the-clock, live-in care. She has gone back to work out of financial necessity. Thomas's treatment team includes physical, occupational, and speech therapists; rehabilitation specialists; and two neurologists. He now uses a motorized wheelchair and is unable to feed himself or do any activities of daily living on his own.

Thomas's mind remains alert, and he and his wife have used the Internet to look for treatment options. They recognize that gold treatment is a long shot but have spoken to three individuals with ALS in different provinces who have experienced remission using gold treatment. These individuals have sent information regarding their dosage and where they obtained their medication. In addition, Thomas and Patricia have read information from homeopathic, alternative, and anecdotal sources that explain the rationale, procedures, dosing, and prescribing information for gold in ALS treatment. They have provided this information to their two neurologists, who have dismissed their requests to have this information reviewed.

Thomas and Patricia have a long-standing relationship with Ms. Mason; they trust her and know she cares about them as individuals, so they share the information they have gathered with her and ask her if she would be willing to order gold treatment for Thomas. They say they understand that she may feel uncomfortable with this request, but they ask her to put herself in their position, think about the evidence they have provided, and make a fair-minded decision. They also state they will be happy to sign any type of form stating they understand this is not the usual treatment but, under the circumstances, they want to take the risk because they believe the risk of trying this treatment outweighs the benefit of not trying the treatment.

Nurse practitioners in the province in which Ms. Mason works are independent. They are governed exclusively by the provincial nursing association. They do not practice under the supervision of physicians or as physician extenders. They are expected to abide by the regulations of the nursing association and provide care within their scope of practice. Ms. Mason contacts the provincial nursing association to obtain further clarification. The association representative says that if she is knowledgeable about a treatment and deems it to be appropriate, she should document her rationale and provide the treatment. Ms. Mason contacts her practice insurance company but is unable to speak with a lawyer. The service representative tells her careful documentation of care is necessary. She consults a trusted colleague and asks him about the case. He says there is "no way" he would ever prescribe a medication that was not approved by the U.S. Food and Drug Administration.

Ms. Mason cares about Thomas. She has worked with him for 15 years and knows he is a thorough, reliable, and careful person. She understands he is suffering from an incurable disease and that allopathic treatments offer no hope. She believes trust and offering hope are the most valuable interventions a nurse practitioner can provide to a person with a chronic illness.

(continues)

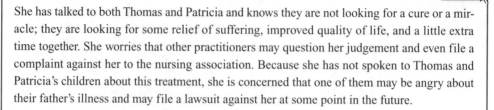

CASE STUDY   (Continued)

She has talked to both Thomas and Patricia and knows they are not looking for a cure or a miracle; they are looking for some relief of suffering, improved quality of life, and a little extra time together. She worries that other practitioners may question her judgement and even file a complaint against her to the nursing association. Because she has not spoken to Thomas and Patricia's children about this treatment, she is concerned that one of them may be angry about their father's illness and may file a lawsuit against her at some point in the future.

Discussion Questions

1. What should Ms. Mason do? What would you do?
2. How do ethical principles affect your decision?
3. How can you, as a practitioner, emotionally support the family even though you do not believe they should participate in the gold treatment?
4. How do your own values and beliefs influence your decisions in this situation?

This case study was developed by Dr. Lisa Onega.

INTERVENTIONS

Healthcare professionals considering the role of CAM treatment in the care of individuals with chronic illnesses need to be aware of their life experiences and feelings, promote wise decision making, deliver safe and effective care, and be informed about legal issues.

Self-Reflection

Healthcare professionals need to be aware of their own feelings about CAM treatments as they relate to chronic illness. Typically, most healthcare professionals are comfortable with complementary treatment; however, personal experience influences how they view alternative therapies that replace allopathic methods. Understanding one's own experiences and beliefs is essential to be present with individuals with chronic illnesses and understand their fears, concerns, motivations, and needs, without burdening them with personal biases that may inhibit them from making the wisest choices for their circumstances (Burman, 2003).

Decision Making

Healthcare professionals espouse individualized, holistic, and healing care; this requires considering the unique aspects, goals, and needs of each individual with a chronic illness. It is essential to partner with patients and view them as human beings, not cases with diseases (Burman, 2003; Chez & Jonas, 2005; Helms, 2006; Sleath et al., 2005; Wagner et al., 2005). Care should be accessible, affordable, compassionate, effective, efficient, evidence informed, patient focused, safe, and timely (Bezold, 2005; Chez & Jonas, 2005). To facilitate wise decision making on the part of the patient, the healthcare professional should address the following information with their patients (Cuellar, Rogers, & Hisghman, 2007):

- Find out all information about safety of the product.
- Look for warning signs; if it sounds too good to be true, it probably is.
- Be alert for new information; do your research on the CAM modality.
- Never try to diagnose or treat your own condition.
- Talk to your healthcare provider.
- Ask your healthcare provider for advice.
- Make a plan with your healthcare provider. How will the therapy fit into your medical treatment plan?
- Be open and honest.
- Ask your healthcare provider if he or she can refer you to someone knowledgeable about CAM.
- Share information you have about your therapy with your healthcare provider.
- Tell your healthcare provider about any CAM you are using and its benefits.
- Obtain licensing requirements for CAM practitioners in the province.
- Visit the CAM practitioner before your treatment and observe how the patients are treated.
- Consider the cost of the therapy and talk with your insurance company to find out whether services are covered.
- Ask the CAM provider important questions: Have you ever treated conditions like mine? Is the treatment effective? How long will it take for me to see results? Are you willing to work with my healthcare provider?

Legal Implications

Healthcare professionals wishing to incorporate alternative or complementary treatments into their activities should be certain that therapies comply with federal and provincial licensure and regulatory requirements. Close adherence to governmental requirements is challenging but necessary, because many of the individuals monitoring adherence to these requirements may have little understanding of nontraditional therapies (Burman, 2003; Cuellar et al., 2003; Helms, 2006).

Although individuals with chronic illnesses often use CAM treatments, healthcare professionals are challenged to maintain a balance between providing these therapies and protecting the public from potentially harmful interventions. Education about nonallopathic treatments can enable healthcare professionals to intelligently differentiate between clinical innovations that do not harm individuals and offer them hope and fraudulent or harmful treatments that rob individuals of dignity and economic resources (Burman, 2003; Cuellar et al., 2003, 2007; Sleath et al., 2005).

Healthcare professionals should share conceptual and evidence-informed information about CAM treatments with colleagues, legislators, and reimbursers. Regulatory reform to facilitate a flexible scope of practice with rigorous competency requirements will not only ensure public safety but will also enable clinicians to practice to their full scope of preparation, improve access to nontraditional therapies, and promote cost-effective treatment options. Provincial practice acts vary and therefore may or may not prohibit healthcare professionals from providing nonallopathic treatments. As knowledge increases, provincial practice competencies and standards need to be revised to incorporate healthcare professionals' rights to provide these services (Burman, 2003; Cuellar et al., 2003).

SUMMARY

Healthcare professionals caring for individuals with chronic illnesses need to balance an open-minded view of CAM treatments with a scientific, evidence-informed perspective. Healthcare professionals are in a unique position to bridge the gap between allopathic and nonallopathic health care by melding compassion, flexibility, and commitment to scientific and clinical excellence with common sense.

Individuals with chronic diseases may not have their needs met by the existing healthcare system, which is hampered by the dichotomous relationship between traditional and nontraditional schools of thought. The disciplinary perspective of healthcare professionals enables them to offer these individuals CAM options that address their specific circumstances.

ACKNOWLEDGMENT

Many thanks to Lisa Onega for her contribution to this chapter in the previous edition.

Evidence-Informed Practice Box

Researchers in the United Kingdom explored how 35 patients integrated CAM and orthodox medicine (OM) or traditional medicine in self-managing their chronic illness (Brien et al., 2011). Semistructured interviews were conducted with individuals who had a chronic benign condition for 12 months or longer and who were using CAM practices along with traditional medicine. Seven categories were developed from the interview data: (1) using CAM to maintain OM use, (2) using OM to support long-term CAM use, (3) using CAM to reduce OM, (4) using CAM to avoid OM, (5) using CAM to replace OM, (6) maximizing relief using both CAM and OM, and (7) returning to OM. These seven categories were neither mutually exclusive nor static. Changes in clients' behaviour occurred over time and were related to their treatment experiences, which either reinforced existing beliefs or inspired new beliefs. Clients used OM and CAM practices and integrated both approaches in managing their chronic illness. Given the nature of clients' decisions and beliefs changing over time, an ongoing discussion between CAM and OM practitioners is necessary.

Source: Brien et al. (2011).

STUDY QUESTIONS

www

1. Why do individuals with chronic illnesses use nontraditional treatments?
2. What are the four categories of alternative and complementary treatments outlined by the Centre for Cooperative Medicine?
3. How common is using nonallopathic therapy in Canada?

REFERENCES

Acupuncture Foundation of Canada Institute. (2012). Regulations in Canada. Retrieved from http://www.afcinstitute.com/AboutAcupuncture/RegulationinCanada/tabid/78/Default.aspx

Adams, M., & Jewell, P. (2007). The use of complementary and alternative medicine by cancer patients. *International Seminars in Surgical Oncology, 4,* 10. Retrieved from http://www.issoonline.com/content/4/1/10

Adler, S. R., Wrubel, J., Hughes, E., & Beinfield, H. (2009). Patients' interactions with physicians and complementary and alternative medicine practitioners: Older women with breast cancer and self-managed health care. *Integrative Cancer Therapy, 8*(1), 63–70.

Alternative Medicine Examiners Council of Canada. (2006). Complementary and alternative medicine. Retrieved from http://www.cpmdq.com/htm/govcandiencouncil.htm

Anderson, E. Z. (2009). Complementary therapies and older adults. *Topics in Geriatric Rehabilitation, 25*(4), 320–328.

Barrett, S. (2009). Quackery: How should it be defined? Retrieved from http://www.quackwatch.com/01QuackeryRelatedTopics/quackdef.html

Bausell, R. B. (2009). Are positive alternative medical therapy trials credible? Evidence from four high-impact medical journals. *Evaluation and the Health Professions, 32*(4), 349–369.

Bezold, C. (2005). The future of patient-centered care: Scenarios, visions, and audacious goals. *Journal of Alternative and Complementary Medicine, 11*(Suppl. 1), 77–84.

Boon, H., Stewart, M., Kennard, M. A., Gray, R., Sawka, C., Brown, J. B., . . . Haines-Kamka, T. (2000). Use of complementary/alternative medicine by breast cancer survivors in Ontario: Prevalence and perceptions. *American Society for Clinical Oncology, 18,* 2515–2521.

Boon, H. S., Olatunde, F., & Zick, S. M. (2007). Trends in complementary/alternative use by breast cancer survivors: Comparing survey data from 1998 and 2005. *BMC Women's Health, 30*(7), 4.

Boon, H. S., Verhoef, M. J., Vanderheyden, L. C., & Westlake, K. P. (2006). Complementary and alternative medicine: A rising healthcare issue. *Healthcare Policy, 1*(3), 19–30.

Boozang, K. M. (1998). Western medicine opens the door to alternative medicine. *American Journal of Law and Medicine, 24*(2–3), 185–212.

Boozang, K. M. (2003). National policy on CAM: The White House Commission report. *Journal of Law, Medicine and Ethics, 31*(2), 251–261.

Bott, J. (2007). An analysis of paper-based sources of information on complementary therapies. *Complementary Therapies in Clinical Practice, 13,* 53–62.

Brien, S. B., Bishop, F. L., Riggs, K., Stevenson, D., Freire, V., & Lewith, G. (2011). Integrated medicine in the management of chronic illness: A qualitative study. *British Journal of General Practice.* doi: 10.3399/bjgp11X556254

Briggs, J. (2007). Audio file about the 2007 National Health Interview survey CAM use data. Retrieved from http://nccam.nih.gov/news/multimedia/audio/nhisaudio.htm

British Columbia Cancer Agency. (2007). Complementary and unconventional therapies. Retrieved from http://www.bccancer.bc.ca/HPI/Unconventional Therapies/default.htm

British Columbia Cancer Agency. (2012). Complementary Medicine Education and Outcomes (CAMEO) program. Retrieved from http://www.bccancer.bc.ca/RES/ResearchPrograms/cameo/default.htm

Burman, M. E. (2003). Complementary and alternative medicine: Core competencies for family nurse practitioners. *Journal of Nursing Education, 42*(1), 28–34.

Cady, F (2009). Legal issues related to complementary and alternative medicine. *JONA's Healthcare Law, Ethics and Regulation, 11*(2), 46–51.

CAMDOC Alliance. (2010). The regulatory status of complementary and alternative medicine for medical doctors in Europe. Retrieved from http://www.camdoc.eu/Pdf/CAMDOCRegulatoryStatus8_10.pdf

CAMline. (2012). About CAMline. Retrieved from http://www.camline.ca/about/index.php

Canadian Cancer Society Research Institute. (2012). Current funding opportunities. Retrieved from http://www.cancer.ca/Research/Grants%20and%20Awards/Current%20funding%20opportunities.aspx?sc_lang=en

Canadian Information Centre for International Credentials. (2011). Information for foreign-trained practitioners of traditional Chinese medicine and acupuncture. Retrieved from http://www.cicic.ca/684/Acupuncturists_and_Practitioners_of_Traditional_Chinese_Medicine.canada?noc=3232.2

Canadian Institute for Health Information. (2010). Health care spending to reach $192 billion this year. Retrieved from http://www.cihi.ca/CIHI-ext-portal/internet/en/Document/spending+and+health+workforce/spending/RELEASE_28OCT10

Canadian Institute of Natural and Integrative Medicine. (2012). Closing the gap. Retrieved from http://www.cinim.org/index.php/main/page/about

Canadian Interdisciplinary Network for Complementary and Alternative Medicine. (2011). About us. Retrieved from http://www.incamresearch.ca/index.php?id=1,0,0,1,0,0&lng=en

Canadian Nurses Association. (2008). Advanced nursing practice: A national framework. Retrieved from http://www.srna.org/images/stories/pdfs/nurse_resources/2009_advanced_NP.pdf

Cancer Centre of Southeastern Ontario. (2012). Complementary therapies and alternate medicine. Retrieved from http://www.krcc.on.ca/patient_visitor/patient_visitor_CompTherap_AlternMed.asp

Cassileth, B. R., & Vickers, A. J. (2004). Massage therapy for symptoms control: Outcome study at a major cancer centre. *Journal of Pain and Symptoms Management, 28,* 244–249.

Centre for Cooperative Medicine. (2011). About biomagnetic therapy. Retrieved from http://www.cooperativemedicine.com/bioelectromagnetic-articles/about-bio-electromagnetic-therapy/

Chang, E. Y., Glissmeyer, R., Tonnes, S., Hudson, T., & Johnson, N. (2006). Outcomes of breast cancer in patients who use alternative therapies as primary treatment. *American Journal of Surgery, 192,* 471–473.

Chez, R. A., & Jones, W. B. (2005). Challenges and opportunities in achieving healing. *Journal of Alternative and Complementary Medicine, 11*(Suppl. 1), 3–6.

Clarke, J., Romagnoli, M. A., Sargent, C., & Gudrun van Amerom, B. A. (2010). The portrayal of complementary and alternative medicine in mass print magazines since 1980. *Journal of Alternative and Complementary Medicine, 16*(1), 125–130.

Coelho, H. F., Pittler, M. H., & Ernst, E. (2007). An investigation of the contents of complementary and alternative medicine journals. *Alternative Therapies in Health and Medicine, 13*(4), 40–44.

College & Association of Registered Nurses of Alberta. (2011). Complementary and/or alternative therapy and natural health products: Standards for registered nurses. Retrieved from http://www.nurses.ab.ca/Carna-Admin/Uploads/Complementary_Alternative_Therapy.pdf

College of Registered Nurses of British Columbia. (2006). Complementary and alternative health care: The role of the nurse. *Nursing-BC, 38*(3), 20–22.

College of Registered Nurses of British Columbia. (2012). Complementary and alternative health. Retrieved from https://www.crnbc.ca/Standards /ComplementaryAndAlternativeHealth/Pages/Default .aspx

College of Registered Nurses of Nova Scotia. (2005). Complementary and alternative therapies: A guide for registered nurses. Retrieved from http://www .crnns.ca/documents/Complementary%20and%20 Alternative%20Therapies%202005.pdf

College of Registered Nurses of Nova Scotia. (2011). Nurse practitioner competency framework. Retrieved from http://www.crnns.ca/documents/NS_NP_ Competency_Framework_Jun2011.pdf

College of Registered Nurses of Nova Scotia. (2012). Nurse practitioners standards of practice. Retrieved from http://www.crnns.ca/documents/NPStandards .pdf

Complementary and Alternative Medicine Law Blog. (2010). Complementary medicine regulations in Canada very mixed. Retrieved from http://www.cam lawblog.com/articles/health-trends/complementary- regulation-in-canada-very-mixed/

Coughlin, P., & Delany, J. (2011). Massage and touch therapies. In M. Micozzi (Ed.), *Fundamentals of complementary and alternative medicine* (4th ed., pp. 211–231). St. Louis, MO: Saunders Elsevier.

Cuellar, N. G., Cahill, B., Ford, J., & Aycock, T. (2003). The development of an educational workshop on complementary and alternative medicine: What every nurse should know. *Journal of Continuing Education in Nursing, 34*(3), 128–135.

Cuellar, N. G., Rogers, A. E., & Hisghman, V. (2007). Evidenced based research of complementary and al- ternative medicine (CAM) for sleep in the community dwelling older adult. *Geriatric Nursing, 28*(1), 46–52.

Disease Control Priorities Project. (2007). Complemen- tary and alternative medicine may reduce risk of some diseases. Retrieved from http://www.dcp2.org /file/93/DCPP-CAM.pdf

Ditte, D., Schultz, W., Ernst, G., & Schmid-Ott, G. (2011). Attitudes towards complementary and al- ternative medicine among medical and psychology students. *Psychology, Health & Medicine, 16*(2), 225–237.

Fraser Institute. (2007). Complementary and alterna- tive medicine in Canada: Trends in use and public attitudes, 1997–2006. Retrieved from http://www .fraserinstitute.org/uploadedFiles/fraser-ca/Content /research-news/research/publications/complementary- alternative-medicine-in-canada-2007.pdf

Freeman, L. (2009). Chiropractic. In L. Freeman (Ed.), *Mosby's complementary and alternative medicine: A research based approach* (3rd ed., pp. 283–309). St. Louis, MO: Mosby Elsevier.

Friends of Alternative & Complementary Therapies Society. (2011). News and events. Retrieved from http://www.thefacts.org/

Furlan, A. D., Imamura, M., Dryden, T., & Irvin, E. (2008). Massage for low back pain. *Cochrane Database of Systematic Reviews*, Issue 4. Art. No.: CD001929. doi: 10.1002/14651858. CD001929.pub2

Health Canada. (2004). Drugs and health products: General questions. Retrieved from http://www.hc-sc .gc.ca/dhp-mps/prodnatur/faq/question_general-eng .php

Health Canada. (2005). Baseline natural health products survey among consumers: Final report. Retrieved from http://www.hc-sc.gc.ca/dhp-mps/pubs/natur /eng_cons_survey-eng.php.

Health Canada. (2010). Natural health products. Retrieved from http://hc-sc.gc.ca/dhp-mps/compli- conform/info-prod/prodnatur/index-eng.php

Health Canada. (2011a). About natural health prod- uct regulation in Canada. Retrieved from http ://epe.lac-bac.gc.ca/100/200/301/pwgsc-tpsgc/por-ef /health/2011/135-09/report.pdf

Health Canada. (2011b). Natural health product track- ing survey—2010 final report. Ipsos Reid PRR 135-09, HCPOR-09-25. Retrieved from http://epe .lac-bac.gc.ca/100/200/301/pwgsc-tpsgc/por-ef /health/2011/135-09/report.pdf

Helms, J. E. (2006). Complementary and alternative ther- apies: A new frontier for nursing education. *Journal of Nursing Education, 45*(3), 117–123.

Her Majesty the Queen. (2003). Natural health prod- uct regulations. *Canada Gazette Part II, 137*(13), 1562–1607.

Jain, S., & Mills, P. J. (2010). Biofield therapies: Helpful or full of hype? A best evidence synthe- sis. *International Journal of Behavioural Medicine, 17*(1), 1–16.

Kim, L. W., & Zhu, J. (2010). Acupuncture for essential hypertension. *Alternative Therapies in Health and Medicine, 16*(2), 18–29.

Laupacis, A., & Born, K. (2011). Complementary & al- ternative medicine in practice and policy. Healthy debate, June 8, 2011. Retrieved from http://healthy

debate.ca/2011/06/topic/cost-of-care/caminpractice andpolicy

Leis, A., Verhoef, M. J., Deschamps, M., Doll, R, Tan, L., & Dewar, R. (2003). What determines use of complementary therapies by Canadian cancer patients. *Focus Alternative Complementary Therapy, 8,* 149.

Massage Therapy Association of Manitoba Inc. (2012). Registered massage therapists. Retrieved from http ://www.mtam.mb.ca/registered-massage-therapists .asp.

McCarney, R. W., Brinkhaus, B., Lasserson, T. J., & Linde, K. (2009). Acupuncture for chronic asthma. *Cochrane Database of Systematic Reviews*, 2003, Issue 3, Art. No.: CD000008. doi: 10.1002/14651858 .CD000008.pub2

Metcalfe, A., Williams, J., McChesney, J, Patten, S. C., & Jetté, N. (2010). Use of complementary and alternative medicine by those with a chronic disease and the general population—results of a national population based survey. *BMC Complementary & Alternative Medicine, 10*(58), 1–6.

Micozzi, M. (2011). Characteristics of complementary and alternative medicine. In M. Micozzi (Ed.), *Fundamentals of complementary and alternative medicine* (4th ed., pp. 1–8). St. Louis, MO: Saunders Elsevier.

Moss, K., Boon, H., Ballantyne, P., & Kachan, N. (2006). New Canadian natural health product regulations: A qualitative study of how CAM practitioners perceive they will be impacted. *BMC Complementary and Alternative Medicine, 6,* 18.

Mueller, C. M., Mai, P. L., Bucher, J., Peters, J. A., Loud, J. T., & Greene, M. H. (2008). Complementary and alternative medicine use among women at increased genetic risk of breast and ovarian cancer. *BMC Complementary and Alternative Medicine, 8*(17), 1–9. doi: 10.1186/1472-6882-8-17

Nahas, R. (2008). Complementary and alternative medicine approaches to blood pressure reduction: An evidence-based review. *Canadian Family Physician, 54*(11), 1529–1533.

National Aboriginal Health Organization. (2008). An overview of traditional knowledge and medicine and public health in Canada. Retrieved from http://www .naho.ca/documents/naho/publications/tkOverview PublicHealth.pdf

National Centre for Complementary and Alternative Medicine. (2008). CAM basics: What is comple-

mentary and alternative medicine? Retrieved from http://nccam.nih.gov/health/whatiscam/#types

National Centre for Complementary and Alternate Medicine. (2010, October). Cancer and CAM: What the science says. *NCCAM Clinical Digest.* Retrieved from http://www.nccam.nih.gov/health/providers /digest/cancer_science.htm

Natural Health Care Canada. (2011). The Canadian CAM Research Fund. Retrieved from http://reflexology .naturalhealthcare.ca/news.phtml?read=1606

Natural Health Product Directorate. (2003, November). *Overview of the natural health product regulations guidance document.* Ottawa, ON: Natural Health Product Directorate.

Oguamanam, C. (2006). Biomedical orthodoxy and complementary and alternative medicine: Ethical challenges of integrating medical cultures. *Journal of Alternative and Complementary Medicine, 12*(5), 577–581.

Ontario Women's Health Council. (2003). CIHR priority announcement—research personnel awards. Retrieved from http://www.cihr.ca/e/33786.html

O'Regan, P., Wills, T., & O'Leary, A. (2010). Complementary therapies: A challenge for nursing practice. *Nursing Standards, 24*(21), 35.

Ovarian Cancer Canada. (2010). Exploring complementary medicine (CAM). Retrieved from http ://ovariancanada.org/News---Events/Research- News-%281%29/CAMEO

Park, J. (2004). Use of alternative health care. *Health Reports, 16*(2), 39–42.

Ponholzer, A., Struhal, G., & Madersbacher, S. (2003). Frequent use of complementary medicine by prostate cancer patients. *European Urology, 43,* 604–608.

Qato, D. M., Alexander, G. C., Conti, R. M., Johnson, M., Schumm, P., Lindau, S. T. (2008). Use of prescription and over-the-counter medications and dietary supplements among older adults in the United States. *Journal of the American Medical Association, 300,* 286–778.

Qigong Institute. (2004–2011). What is Qigong? Retrieved from http://www.qigonginstitute.org/html /qigonghealth.php#AboutQigong

Ramsay, C. (2009). Unnatural regulation: Complementary and alternative medicine policy in Canada. Retrieved from http://www.fraserinstitute.org/research-news /display.aspx?id=13571

Robotin, M., & Penman, A. G. (2006). Integrating complementary therapies into mainstream cancer care:

Which way forward? *Medical Journal of Australia, 185,* 377–379.

Ruedy, J., Kaufman, D. M., & MacLeod, H. (1999). Alternative and complementary medicine in Canadian medical schools: A survey. *Canadian Medical Association Journal, 160,* 816–817.

Saydah, S. H., & Eberhardt, M. S. (2006). Use of complementary and alternative medicine among adults with chronic diseases: United States 2002. *Journal of Alternative and Complementary Medicine, 12*(8), 805–812.

Shahjahan, R. (2004). Standards of education, regulation, and market control: Perspectives on complementary and alternative medicine in Ontario, Canada. *Journal of Alternative and Complementary Medicine, 10*(2), 409–412.

Sinnema, J. (2009, April 8). Chiropractic cut from coverage. *The Edmonton Journal.* Retrieved from http://www.edmontonjournal.com/Health/Chiropractic+from+coverage/1476082/story.html

Sleath, B., Callahan, L., DeVellis, R. F., & Sloane, P. D. (2005). Patients' perceptions of primary care physicians' participatory decision-making style and communication about complementary and alternative medicine for arthritis. *Journal of Alternative and Complementary Medicine, 11*(3), 449–453.

Smith, C. A., Hay, P. P., & Macpherson, H. (2010). Acupuncture for depression. *Cochrane Database of Systematic Reviews,* Art. No.: CD004046.

Stout, M., & Downey, B. (2012). Nursing, indigenous peoples and cultural safety: Now what? Retrieved from http://www.contemporarynurse.com/archives/vol/22/issue/2/article/749/nursing-ind

Stueck, W. (2009, January 28). BCMA chief expresses worry over expanded role for naturopaths. *Globe and Mail.*

Verhoef, M., Brundin-Mather, R., Jones, A., Boon, H., & Epstein, M. (2004). Complementary and alternative medicine in undergraduate medical education: Associate deans' perspective. *Canadian Family Physician, 50,* 168–173.

Vogel, L. (2010). "Hodge-podge" regulation of alternative medicine in Canada. *Canadian Medical Association Journal, 182*(12).

Wagner, E. H., Bennett, S. M., Austin, B. T., Greene, S. M., Schaefer, J. K., & Vonkorff, M. (2005). Finding common ground: Patient-centeredness and evidence-based chronic illness care. *Journal of Alternative and Complementary Medicine, 11*(Suppl. 1), 7–15.

Walker, B. F., French, S. D., Grant, W., & Green S. (2010). Combined chiropractic interventions for low back pain. *Cochrane Database of Systematic Reviews 2010,* Issue 4. Art No.: CD005427. doi: 10.1002/14651858.CD005427.pub2

Why Massage Therapy.com. (2009). Massage therapy in Canada. Retrieved from http://whymassagetherapy.com/massage-therapy-canada.php

Williams, A. M., Kitchen, P., & Eby, J. (2011). Alternative health care consultations in Ontario, Canada: A geographic and sociodemographic analysis. *BMC Complementary and Alternative Medicine, 11,* 47.

Woods, J. (2012). *Integrated healing practices.* Calgary, AB: Mount Royal University, School of Nursing.

World Health Organization. (2005). National policy on traditional medicine and regulation of herbal medicines—report of a WHO Global Survey. Retrieved from http://apps.who.int/medicinedocs/en/d/Js7916e/9.2.html

World Health Organization. (2008). Traditional medicine. Fact sheet no. 134. Retrieved from http://www.who.int/mediacentre/factsheets/fs134/en/

Wu, H. M., Tang, J., Lih, X. P., Lau, J., Leung, P. C., Woo, J., & Li, Y. (2009). Acupuncture for stroke rehabilitation. *Cochrane Database of Systematic Reviews,* Issue 3, Art. No.: CD004131. doi: 10.1002/14651858.CD004131.pub2

Wyatt, G., Sikorskii, A., Wills, C. E., & An, H. S. (2010). Complementary and alternative medicine use, spending, and quality of life in early stage breast cancer. *Nursing Research, 59*(1), 58–65.

Yang, J., Feng, Y., Ying, L., Liu, G. J., Chen J., Ren, Y. L., & Liang, F. R. (2010). Acupuncture for hypertension (protocol). *Cochrane Database of Systematic Reviews,* Issue 11. Art. No.: CD008821. doi: 10.1002/14651858.CD00821

Yin, C., Seo, B., Park, H. J., Cho, M., Jung, W., Choue, R., . . . Koh, H. (2007). Acupuncture, a promising adjunctive therapy for essential hypertension: A double-blind, randomized, controlled trail. *Neurological Research, 29,* (Suppl. 1), S98–S103.

Zarowitz, B. (2010a). Complementary and alternative medicine. *Geriatric Nursing, 31*(2), 123–125.

Zarowitz, B. (2010b). Complementary and alternative medicine: Dietary supplement interactions with medication. *Geriatric Nursing, 31*(3), 206–211.

CHAPTER 17

Home Health Care

Original chapter by Cynthia S. Jacelon
Canadian content added by Joyce K. Engel

INTRODUCTION

Home health care in Canadian society has tradi-tionally been defined as care that is delivered at home. Although still primarily directed toward care in the home, home health care involves care of individual clients, in partnership with clients and families, and can also include direct care within shelters, group residences, schools, and the street (Stanhope, Lancaster, Jessup-Falcioni, & Viverais-Dresler, 2010). It includes "an array of services for people of all ages, provided in the home and community setting that encom-passes health promotion and teaching, curative intervention, end-of-life care, rehabilitation, support and maintenance, social adaptation and integration" (Canadian Home Care Association, 2011, p. 2). The following are goals of home health nursing (Health Canada, 1999):

- Assist individuals to maintain or improve health status and quality of life
- Assist individuals to remain as independent as possible

- Support families and family caregivers who are coping with the care needs of fam-ily members
- Help individuals to either stay at home or to remain at home with the support of treat-ments and care that they need

Care is provided by home care or home health nurses and homemakers as well as by physio-therapists, occupational therapists, speech ther-apists, and other healthcare providers. Home health nurses provide both direct care, which re-fers to physical care and face-to-face interaction (Stanhope et al., 2010), and indirect care, which involves activities such as case management, ad-vocacy, and consultation with other care provid-ers. Through case management, the delivery of home health care is coordinated with the efforts of clients, friends, and community to enable the frail elderly and others with a variety of acute, chronic, palliative, and rehabilitative needs to live independently and with dignity within the community. The focus of this chapter is on the roles of nurses and other skilled healthcare providers in the home.

Under the Canada Health Act home health care is not an insured service but is considered an extended health service that is subjected to reporting conditions, which has led to considerable diversity in the provinces and territories in how home health care is defined and delivered (Health Canada, 1999; Petrucka,, 2010). Currently, nine provinces have specific legislation related to home health care, and the remaining provinces and territories have orders-in-council that guide the delivery of home health care services (Canadian Home Care Association, 2011).

Home health care is the most rapidly expanding health service in Canada (Canadian Home Care Association, 2008a) and is considered an integral component of a gradual shift from acute, episodic care that is primarily institutionally based to community-based care. Currently, it is estimated that approximately 1 million clients across Canada receive publicly funded home care and approximately 500,000 are accessing home care (Canadian Health Care Association, 2009) that is provided by municipalities, not-for-profit organizations, and private providers and compensated by private insurance and through private funds. This number is expected to grow with an aging population, the increasing prevalence of chronic disorders, greater demands on the healthcare system, and the increasing expectation of Canadians that they will be able to choose their setting for care when health challenges occur (Canadian Home Care Association, 2012). Accessibility of home care enables Canadians to choose the setting in which their healthcare needs can be met and independence can be supported and is well positioned to play a key role in management strategies for

chronic disorders that emphasize choice and self-care (Canadian Home Care Association, 2012).

Home health nurses use holistic strategies to work with clients, families, and informal caregivers to manage disease or disability, and because home health is often intermittent, a primary aim of home health care is that of facilitating self-care. They practice in a highly autonomous and independent manner that nonetheless involves working with multiple stakeholders (Community Health Nurses of Canada, 2010) to provide care that includes intrathecal analgesia through computerized pumps, initiation and monitoring of intravenous solutions and medications, chemotherapy, drawing of blood, and management of Peripherally Inserted Central Catheter (PICC) lines (Underwood & Henteleff, 2010) and other nursing activities that would have occurred only within institutional settings a couple of decades ago. The autonomy and relative isolation of home health nurses in home and other settings demands a high level of professionalism, competence, and ethical practice. The specialty of home health nurses differs from other nursing specialties in that it is highly autonomous and the duration and frequency of care depends on the care delivery model and the holistic needs of the client, family, and caregivers.

HISTORY OF HOME CARE

In Canada, nursing began in the home, and only in the last century has it shifted from community to acute care and institutional care. Home health nursing has a long and respected history in Canada with its earliest roots in the delivery of health care in homes by members of religious orders in the early 17th century and later by women of the households who provided care for the mother during confinement and for those who were ill. These caregivers laid the foundations for home health care that has been formalized into public and private care of clients across the lifespan. Although it is predicted that most nurses will be practising in the community by 2020 (Villeneuve & MacDonald, 2006), the shift toward home health care has been slower than what many healthcare advocates may have envisioned.

The first formal district nursing association was formed in England by William Rathbone, a wealthy British businessman and philanthropist. The district nursing services, in which a nurse was assigned to a district in town, combined therapeutic nursing care and education for healthful living practices. Working with Florence Nightingale, he advocated for nursing throughout England in the mid-1880s (Stanhope & Lancaster, 2010) and founded a visiting nurses training school to ensure nurses had the necessary knowledge and skills to work successfully in a nursing setting (Hitchcock, Schubert, & Thomas, 2003).

By the late 19th century, doctors, nurses, and hospitals were desperately needed to meet the needs of isolated areas and of a growing population. Multiple stories of hardship and illness that were affecting women and children, which were influenced by these conditions, prompted Lady Aberdeen, the wife of the governor-general, to found the Victorian Order of Nurses (VON), the first formal organization of home nursing services, in 1897. Through Lady Aberdeen's efforts, Charlotte Macleod, who had studied with Florence Nightingale, was persuaded to come to Ottawa, where she helped set up the VON and became the first chief superintendent.

The early VON focused on maternity care as well as public health and the prevention and care of tuberculosis. The VON has continued to be an integral part of social and healthcare history in Canada and has been the origin of visiting nursing and coordinated home care programs in Canada. Today, this charitable organization has more than 75 different programs and services that are staffed by 4,500 healthcare workers and over 9,000 volunteers who provide services such as foot care clinics, respite care, and home-based palliative care (VON, 2009). These services contribute significantly to the mix of publicly and privately funded home health services that are offered in Canada.

Florence Nightingale's vision of trained nurses indirectly influenced community nursing in Canada and also found its way into the preparation of nurses. The first nursing school was established in St. Catharines, Ontario, in 1874 (Ross-Kerr, 2010). At the beginning of the 20th century trained nurses from these diploma programs worked in private duty, where they often lived and worked in the homes of their clients, thus primarily contributing toward meeting the healthcare needs of the affluent urban community that could afford their services. The contributions of the visiting nurse, however, were evident in other areas of practice. From 1911 to 1918 the Metropolitan Life Insurance Company proved contributions of visiting nurses decreased the mortality rates for infants, and by the end of World War I visiting nurses provided care wherever the client was situated and took care of several clients, instead a single client or family, as had been the practice of private-duty nurses. By 1920 the VON and Metropolitan Life Insurance nurses were well-established visiting nurse services for the sick and for maternity care, and the Red Cross had established nursing outposts for the provision of care to aboriginal people and new settlers in remote, isolated, and sparsely settled areas (Stanhope et al., 2010).

The United States also made strides in community and home health nursing at the end of the 19th and into the 20th century. The first visiting nurse associations to provide care in the needy person's home were established in Buffalo, New York (1985), Philadelphia, Pennsylvania (1986), and Boston, Massachusetts (1986). Charitable activities, supported by wealthy people, funded both settlement houses and the early visiting nursing associations. Together with Mary Brewster, Lillian Wald revolutionized the concept of public health and community nursing (Hitchcock et al., 2003). Lillian Wald is credited with developing the title of public health nurse, and with that the title of nursing care was broadened to encompass the health of individuals and the health, social, and economic needs of the community as a whole. In 1893 Wald and Brewster cofounded the first organized public health agency, New York City's Henry Street Settlement. The settlement hours provided a unique combination of social work, nursing, and social activism (Schoen & Koenig, 1997). The focus was public education to improve maternal and child health, communicable disease control, nutrition, and mental health. Lillian Wald, together with her friend, Lee Frankl, was instrumental in persuading the Metropolitan Life Insurance Company to use visiting nurses for home care on a fee-for-service basis and to establish an effective cost accounting system for visiting nurses, who assessed illness, taught health practices, and collected data from the Metropolitan Life policyholders (Stanhope et al., 2010).

By the 1930s private-duty nurses who had been the mainstay of home health services at the beginning of the century were largely unemployed. The VON focused on home nursing care, and outpost and district nurses continued to provide care for individuals and families in rural and remote locations (Stanhope et al., 2010). Public and community health services had been left largely to provincial jurisdictions, and although funding of these services had been largely through charitable organizations at the beginning of the 20th century, they were overwhelmed by the magnitude of healthcare problems and the challenges of communicable disease prevention and control. The funding solution of choice was transfer of the voluntary services to civic and municipal governments, which worked reasonably well in major urban centres such as Toronto but worked unreliably in rural areas, necessitating support by groups such as the United Farm Women for public health and community programs (Malowany, 2009).

The Weir Report (1932) discussed the challenges of public health nursing such as poor compensation and other issues such as transportation to rural and remote areas of Canada, physician resistance, and the lack of advanced skills and knowledge for nurses in public health, which were working as school nurses, industrial nurses, visiting and district nurses, and VON nurses. The report lamented that graduates from nursing programs were strongly focused on institutional care rather than on public health nursing, which was seen as being detrimental to recruitment of nurses into public health nursing during a time of projected shortages (Stanhope et al., 2010).

By the 1950s and 1960s the roles of the visiting nurse and public health nurse began to become more differentiated. The role of the public health nurse included regular visits to clients in the home, school, and community to provide immunization, prenatal clinics, and hospital liaison for discharged clients, with health promotion and disease prevention being the particular foci in the broader community rather than direct, bedside nursing care. Direct nursing care was provided by the VON, which provided these services in the home (Stanhope et al., 2010). Although their areas of concentration differed, both groups functioned independently in the delivery of nursing care outside of an institutional setting and shared the common goal of promoting, maintaining, and restoring health in the community (Hitchcock et al., 2003) (**Table 17-1**).

The collective successes achieved by visiting nurses, public health nurses, and public

Table 17-1   Similarities and Differences Between the Community Health Specialties of Public Health Nursing and Home Health Nursing

Variable	Similarities	
Setting	Nursing care is provided to clients in their residences or in a community environment.	
Independent nature of practice	Nurses practice independently outside of institutions.	
Control and environment	Client is an active participant in care decisions.	
	Control is shifted to the client.	
	Environment empowers the client.	
Family-centred care	The family is considered as a unit of care.	
	Family members contribute significantly to client care.	
Broad goals	Public health and home health services strive to promote, maintain, and restore health in the community.	
Differences	**Public Health Nursing**	**Home Health Nursing**
Focus of intervention	Population	Individual/family
Caseload acquisition	Case finding in community at large	Self, family or physician referral
Interventions	Continuous	Episodic
Orientation	Wellness	Wellness and illness
	Primary prevention	Primary prevention
		Secondary prevention
		Tertiary prevention
		Rehabilitation
Entry into services	Risk potential	Medical or social diagnosis or social diagnosis
	Social diagnosis	

Sources: Health Canada (1999) and Hitchcock et al. (2003).

health services created a shift in the focus of health care as a whole in the first half of the 20th century. Successes in teaching hygiene and decreases in immigration reduced the threat of communicable disease. Success in the community combined with advances in technology and hospital care began to result in changes to the population that home health nursing would ultimately serve. By the 1970s public health in Canada began to focus on reducing mortality and morbidity from chronic illnesses. Hospitals were beginning to realize that although they were the providers of acute care, they were also becoming the providers of care for individuals with long-term chronic disorders as survival from these disorders increased. The healthcare system began to look for ways to reduce increasing costs incurred by caring for persons with chronic illnesses and to accommodate the preferences of clients and early discharge from hospitals (Shah, 2003).

By the 1980s less funding support was being directed toward health promotion and disease prevention and more support was being given to acute care. With healthcare costs rising even more rapidly, alternatives to hospital care were considered. The first publicly funded home care program was initiated in Ontario in 1970, and by 1988 all provinces and territories had publicly funded short-term (acute) and long-term (chronic) home care programs. A federally funded program such as the Veterans Independence Program was implemented for aging war veterans that combined home care and community-based institutional care. Other federal initiatives included the implementation of home care programs for First Nations and Inuit peoples in 1999 and for the Royal Canadian Mounted Police in response to demands for in-home care. Currently, federal initiatives in home care in 606 First Nations reserves and

communities and in 53 Inuit communities has resulted in a wide variety of programs that include assessment and early intervention with leg ulcers, reduction in falls among older adults, smoking cessation programs, and integration of medical and social home care services (Canadian Home Care Association, 2010). Restructuring of home care in the provinces and territories has resulted in significant reorganization of healthcare delivery across Canadian health care into models such as regional health care that emphasize service planning and coordination (Canadian Home Care Association, 2011).

Home care has experienced enormous growth since its inception in the 1970s. Approximately 1 million clients receive publicly funded home care services annually, a number that has doubled over the past 15 years. In addition to those who receive public home care services, it is estimated that another 500,000 clients access services that are funded through private insurance or out-of-pocket funding. The greatest users of home care services are the oldest adults, with 42% of adults 85 years and older receiving home care (Canadian Home Care Association, 2011). The use of home care services is likely to increase with the aging of the Canadian population, changing policy and practices to emphasize healthcare services that are near home, acknowledging the importance of client choice to age in place or at home, increasing movement toward community care as a strategy to manage wait times in acute care, and managing chronic illness through approaches that include proactive home care programming (Canadian Home Care Association, 2011; Health Canada, 2011; Statistics Canada, 2010).

Home health nursing has become firmly established in the fabric of the Canadian healthcare system. Its potential to sustain the healthcare system was demonstrated in research in

2001 that found home care for older adults is less costly than institutional care (Hollander, 2001), and its value has been acknowledged in the Romanow Report (Romanow, 2002). Although home health care nursing has become more focused on secondary and tertiary prevention than public health nursing, each retains a focus on the primary preventive care of aggregates, so that both home health nursing and public health nursing are included as specialties under the descriptor of community health nursing (Stanhope et al., 2010) rather than being considered separate entities as is the situation in the United States.

ORGANIZATION AND FUNDING OF HOME HEALTH CARE IN CANADA

The organization of the healthcare system in Canada is determined, in large part, by the Constitution Act of 1867, which sets out the roles and responsibilities of the federal, provincial, and territorial governments in relation to health and social services. The division of responsibilities that was established through the Constitution Act provides provinces and territories with considerable control over the delivery of health programs within their individual jurisdictions. Under the Constitution Act, the provinces and territories have most of the responsibility to deliver health and social services, including the responsibility for establishing, maintaining, and administering hospitals and asylums. The federal government retains responsibility and control over health services and decisions for First Nations peoples living on reserves, Inuit, serving members of the Royal Canadian Mounted Police and Canadian forces, eligible veterans, inmates in federal penitentiaries, and refugee claimants (Health Canada,

1999, 2011). The federal government is also responsible for health protection and regulation (e.g., regulation of pharmaceuticals), disease surveillance, setting and administering national principles for health care, and providing financial support to the provinces and territories for health care. The level of responsibility and decision making that was given to provincial and territorial governments through the Constitution Act for the delivery of health care means there is considerable diversity in publicly funded healthcare programming and home care services among provinces and territories.

Before the Second World War health care in Canada was largely privately delivered and funded. In 1947 Saskatchewan began the movement toward a publicly funded, universal healthcare system in Canada by introducing a province-wide, universal hospital care plan. This was followed in 1962 in Saskatchewan by the introduction of a provincial medical insurance plan that provided medical (physician) care to all residents. By 1966 all provinces and territories provided publicly funded inpatient hospital and diagnostic services and universal physician services insurance plans, which solidified hospital, diagnostic, and physician services as essential or medically necessary services that were covered under the Canada Health Act (Health Canada, 2011) and ensured that all Canadians had access to hospital and medical care, regardless of the ability to pay (Petrucka, 2010).

Under the federal Canada Health Act, which was passed in 1984, the principles that had been included in earlier hospital and medical insurance acts of portability, accessibility, universality, comprehensiveness, and public administration were consolidated. The Canada Health Act also discouraged extra billing (fees above and beyond that paid for the service by the provincial or territorial plan) and user fees

(fees that are paid for an insured health service that is not payable by the plan), thus preserving the idea that all Canadians should have access to essential services, regardless of their income. The Act also established criteria for health insurance plans that had to be met by the provinces and territories in order for them to receive full federal case transfers for health. These criteria include reasonable access to medically necessary or essential hospital and doctors' services and ensuring that user fees and extra billing are not barriers to receiving care. It was left with the provinces and territories, however, in consultation with physician colleges and groups to determine which services would be considered medically necessary for the purposes of the provincial and territorial public health insurance plans. If a service is deemed medically necessary, then the full cost of the service must be covered in order for the province or territory to be in compliance with the Canada Health Act (Health Canada, 1999, 2011).

Funding for public health services in Canada is recovered through general revenue that comes from taxation and health premiums. Provincial and territorial governments receive assistance to fund medically necessary services through block federal cash and tax transfers. The block cash funding arrangement was established in 1977 under the Federal-Provincial Fiscal Arrangements and Established Programs Act and enabled the provinces and territories to invest the block fund or sum of money according to their priorities. Agreements between the federal and provincial and territorial governments in 2000 and 2003 resulted in increases to federal cash transfers for health expenditures and, under the Accord on Health Care Renewal in 2003, committed the governments to work toward initiatives to support long-term sustainability

and access. These initiatives included targeted reforms in primary health care, information technology (e.g., electronic records), enhanced access to diagnostic services and medical equipment, and enhanced accountability in health care. Further agreements on reforms and increased funding were reached by the governments in A 10-Year Plan to Strengthen Health Care in 2004, in which there was commitment to management of wait times, aboriginal health, primary health care, and a national pharmaceutical strategy, as well as reporting on these reforms (Canada Health, 2011).

When Canadians require health care they frequently turn first to primary care services, which, as the name suggests, is the first point of contact within the health system. Primary care services are increasingly comprehensive and include first contact health services (e.g., treatment of chronic illnesses, including mental health disorders, palliative care, rehabilitative services, and health promotion). Primary care also includes coordination of client care to facilitate continuity of services and movement through the health system when specialized care is required such as diagnostic services or care by allied health professionals (healthcare providers other than physicians or nurses) (Health Canada, 2011).

Secondary care services include those provided in hospitals, long-term and chronic care facilities, or the community. Referrals to home, community, and institutional care services can be made by clients themselves or their family, doctors, hospitals, and community agencies. The assessment of client needs is made by healthcare providers, and then services are coordinated with the goals of providing continuity in care by formal and informal caregivers (including family and volunteers). Palliative care falls under the umbrella of secondary services and may be delivered at home, in the community, or in hospitals and long-term care facilities (Health Canada, 2011).

One of the most serious limitations in the Canada Health Act is that it covers only medically necessary (hospital and physician) services, and secondary services, such as home care, are not provided for under the Act (Canadian Home Care Association, 2011; Health Canada, 2011; Stadnyk, 2002). However, nine provinces currently have legislation and policies related to public home care, and the remaining province and the territories have orders-in-council that direct the provision of public home health services and have increasingly relied on home health services as an important component of the health care system (Canadian Home Care Association, 2011). The control of provinces and territories over home health care has meant they have had the freedom to develop their own systems of care and funding for home health care programs, which largely observe the principles of Canadian medicare that are outlined in the Canada Health Act, although these principles are not mandated for home health care, because it not an insured service under the Act. This means, however, that there is considerable variation in eligibility for home care services, what home health services are publicly funded, residency requirements, service delivery, wait times, and access across Canada. Although provincial and territorial governments have some obligation to provide home healthcare services through public funds, there are no national standards, which means that home care can be driven by political decisions (Canadian Healthcare Association, 2009) and that care providers and clients must be alert to the nuances of home health care in the province or territory in which they reside.

APPROACHES TO HOME HEALTH SERVICES IN CANADA

Despite wide variations in mandates and principles for home healthcare services across Canada, there are consistent themes across the provinces and territories. In general, home care in Canada is defined as a variety of coordinated health and social services that "enable clients, incapacitated in whole or in part, to live at home, often with the effect of preventing, delaying, or substituting for long-term care or acute care alternatives. . . . it may address needs specifically associated with a medical diagnosis . . . and/or may compensate for functional deficits in the activities of daily living" (Health Canada, 1999, p. 6). These services include health promotion and teaching, curative intervention, support and maintenance, social adaptation, rehabilitation, and end-of-life care (Canadian Healthcare Association, 2009). Home care services, which are provided to individuals of all ages, are designed to complement and supplement the efforts of individuals to care for themselves (Canadian Home Care Association, 2011). It encompasses many different players including family caregivers, health professionals, employers, government departments and agencies, not-for-profit and for-profit organizations, and communities (Canadian Healthcare Association, 2009).

The purpose of home care programs is to provide the following (Canadian Healthcare Association, 2009; Health Canada, 1999):

- A substitution for acute and long-term care services for individuals who would need to enter or remain in hospitals and long-term facilities
- A maintenance and preventative function so that individuals with health and/or functional

deficits can remain at home, thereby retaining their independence and preventing health and functional breakdowns

- A preventative function for the system, which invests in client service and monitoring for an initial increase in short-term costs but lower long-term costs

The freedom of provinces and territories to choose funding and service delivery options for home health care has resulted in four basic models of home health service delivery across Canada (Canadian Healthcare Association, 2009; Health Canada, 1999):

- Assessment, case management and coordination, and discharge planning are provided by public employees (in Ontario, these are community care access centres), whereas all other services, such professional services (e.g., nursing and occupational therapy) and home support services, are contracted out to private providers. This model is used in Ontario.
- All professional services (including nursing care and other therapies, case management and coordination) are delivered by public (government) employees with home support (e.g., housework, meals, personal care) delivered by private agencies. This model is currently in place in British Columbia, New Brunswick, and Newfoundland and Labrador.
- Professional (e.g., nursing care) and home support services (e.g., housework, meals, shopping, personal care) are largely delivered by public employees. In this model, which is used in Manitoba, Saskatchewan, Nunavit, the Northwest Territories, Quebec, and Prince Edward Island, public employees also manage the services. There is little

or no involvement of intermediate agencies. Public and private providers provide professional home care services (e.g., nursing, physiotherapy, respirology and oxygen therapy) and home support services are contracted out. Public employees provide the overall coordination and administration of services. This model is used in Alberta and Nova Scotia.

CHALLENGES FOR HOME HEALTH CARE IN CANADA

An Aging Population

Projections by Statistics Canada (2010) indicate that the Canadian population will age rapidly until 2036, by which time all members of the Baby Boomer generation will have reached 65 years of age. The number of adults 65 years or older (or seniors) will reach between 23% and 25% in 2036 and will reach 24% to 28% in 2061. By 2036 the number of seniors will be nearly double that of the number of seniors in Canada in 2009 (Statistics Canada, 2010), with very old adults (80 years and older) representing the fastest growing segment of the Canadian population.

Surveys, such as the Health Care in Canada Survey, which has been administered annually since 1998 to the public and to members of selected health professionals, suggest that 89% of Canadians see at-home services as a desirable alternative to institutional care (Health Care in Canada Survey, 2000) and that a significant number of those surveyed (79%) support the increased development of community and home programs and services (Health Care in Canada Survey, 2007). Satisfaction levels have been found to be highest among seniors who are receiving home care, followed by supportive housing and those in facility care (MacAdam, Hollander, Miller, Chappell, & Pedlar, 2009). These findings suggest that home care is important to Canadians, even though many seniors who are living at home and using a combination of formal and informal caregiving and of private and publicly funded services report unmet needs (Canadian Home Care Association, 2011).

With aging, there is an associated acceleration of chronic illness, and chronic illness is the most important determinant in whether or not seniors use medically necessary services. Chronic diseases are now the major worldwide cause of death and disability (Canadian Home Care Association, 2011) and are expected to increase as the population ages. It is important, however, to remember that although older adults are the greatest users of long-term and chronic care services, a situation that will intensify with the aging of the population, children and younger adults also use home care services, which has resulted in the average age decreasing for those receiving healthcare services (Canadian Healthcare Association, 2009). Rising expectations, an aging population, and the increased prevalence of chronic disorders mean that in-home health and social services and governments may continue to be challenged to at least maintain, if not increase, the level of home health services, especially as it emerges as a vital component of the Canadian healthcare system (Canadian Healthcare Association, 2009).

Funding

Although spending on home care grew at an annual growth rate of 9.2% in the decade from 1994–1995 to 2003–2004, home care accounted for just 4.2% of total government health expenditures in 2003–2004 (Canadian Healthcare Association, 2009). A report from Ontario suggests that funding has not kept pace with demands for home care, which means that home care has shifted to providing fewer personal support services and professional interventions to an increasing number of individuals in Ontario (Ontario Home Care Association, 2010). This report highlights the magnitude of the contributions of informal caregivers such as friends and family members by suggesting that costs to the Ontario healthcare system would increase by $9.5 billion if these informal caregivers were reimbursed as employees (Ontario Home Care Association, 2010). In addition to the contribution that informal caregivers make to home care, it is estimated that 2% to 5% of Canadians paid privately for home care services, either through private insurance or out of pocket (Canadian Healthcare Association, 2009). These findings support recommendations from various sectors for expanded investment in home care to facilitate avoidance of hospital and long-term institutional care, quality of life, and overburdening informal caregivers, but also research to support the best mix of approaches, as well as standardized assessment and data that enable sharing across jurisdictions and determination of best practices (Canadian Healthcare Association, 2009; Health Canada, 1999; Ontario Home Care Association, 2010).

Access to Home Health Care

Despite gains in the delivery of home healthcare services, available funds are frequently targeted toward specific populations (Canadian Healthcare Association, 2009). Populations such as those suffering from mental illness, those who are dying, and those in aboriginal communities could be better served if home care could play a larger part in care. Home care for those who experience mental illness is effective in avoiding hospitalization and readmissions; barriers such as higher compensation to psychiatrists for inpatient care than for office visits and a lack of experienced mental health workers for specialized at-home care stand in the way of this larger role for home care. Despite the Romanow Report and the 2003 and 2004 First Ministers accords that made commitments to hospice palliative care, 70% to 75% of deaths still occur in hospitals, despite the preference of most individuals to die at home (Canadian Hospice Palliative Care Association, 2011). Individuals in aboriginal communities experience gaps in evening and weekend care, which means the care of young clients with lower care needs defaults to continuing care. Gaps in home care services for those who are mentally ill, dying, or aboriginal present unique challenges for Canada's healthcare system and for innovations in care delivery and technological solutions, such as telehealth.

Integration of Home Health Care with the Healthcare System

The full potential of home care can be realized in an integrated system, where home care is seen as a vital component in a continuum of care that includes long-term home care and support services, facility-based care, and supportive care and in which informal caregivers are supported financially through initiatives such as extending the current compassionate care benefit for informal caregivers of patients at the end of life from 8 to 26 weeks and providing tax relief. Electronic health records, telehealth, effective

case management (which is common activity for nurses in home health care), and a focus on bringing care to patients, rather than patients to care, are components of a transformed system in which there is a strong focus on effective communication among providers and systems and on outcomes of care. Initiatives such as alignment of home care personnel with primary care teams, establishment of interprofessional teams in primary care that enable patients to receive multiple services at one location, and collaborative partnerships between family physicians and home care case managers are additional strategies that are achieving increased integration between home care and primary care in provinces such as British Columbia, Alberta, Manitoba, and Ontario and that hold promise for seamlessness in home care and other areas of the healthcare system (Canadian Home Care Association, 2008b).

THEORETICAL FRAMEWORKS FOR MANAGEMENT OF CHRONIC ILLNESS IN HOME CARE

Home care nurses provide intermittent care and rely heavily on clients' ability to self-manage their health problems. As such, the nurse is in a unique position to apply frameworks for practice that help the nurse work with clients to promote independence. Midrange theories, applied in home care settings to help promote client's self-management of chronic health problems, conceptualize nursing care as based in relationships and coaching, and provide guidelines for collaborative decision making, are presented here. Also included are models for community-based care of clients with chronic illness and hospice care.

Self-Management and Family Management of Chronic Conditions

The framework for self- and family management of chronic conditions is designed to provide a structure for understanding factors influencing the ability of individuals and their families to manage chronic illness (Grey, Knafl, & McCorkle, 2006; Tanner, 2004) (**Figure 17-1**). The components of the framework are self-management, risk and protective factors including condition factors, individual factors, psychosocial characteristics, family factors, and the environment.

Self- and family management of chronic illness is defined as the decisions and activities individuals make on a daily basis to manage

their chronic health problems (Grey et al., 2006; Improving Chronic Illness Care, 2007; Ryan & Sawin, 2009). For some individuals, particularly those who are older or have cognitive deficits, engaging in self-management will be an ongoing challenge (Tanner, 2004). The nurse is challenged to help the client manage at the level of his or her ability (Jacelon, Furman, Rea, Macdonald, & Donoghue, 2011). The concept of self-management extends the responsibility of individuals with chronic illness beyond compliance and adherence to managing an ongoing condition within the context of their daily lives. In home care it is imperative that the nurse consider both the client's ability to self-manage and the family's ability to support the individual's self-management (Grey et al., 2006).

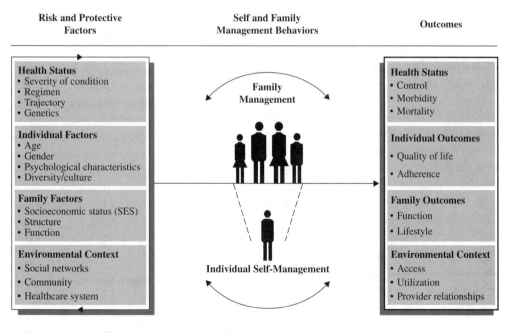

FIGURE 17-1   Self-management and family management framework.
Source: Grey, M., Knafl, K., & McCorkle, R. (2006). A framework for the study of self- and family management of chronic conditions. *Nursing Outlook, 54,* 278–286. Reprinted with permission by: Elsevier Inc.

The ability of individuals and families to manage chronic illness depends on the severity of the condition, the treatment regimen, the course of the disease, individual and family characteristics, and the environment in which individuals will manage their disease (Grey et al., 2006). The severity of the illness from the perspective of the individual with the chronic illness may not be the same as the nurse's perception. The meaning of the condition and the implications for management may be affected by the meaning of the illness to the individual and family. The etiology of the condition (e.g., a lifestyle disease such as emphysema as a result of smoking or a genetically determined disease) will affect the ability for self-management. The implications for the family in these situations may cause guilt or concern for the susceptibility of other family members. The treatment regimen for a chronic illness may be complex, requiring significant lifestyle adjustment. Individual factors such as the person's age, psychosocial situation, functional ability, self-perceived ability to manage the illness, education, and socioeconomic status all contribute to the individual's ability for self-management. Careful assessment by the nurse is imperative in providing care. Once an assessment is complete, the home care nurse is in a position to coach the individual or family in management of the illness.

In the model of self-management and family management, outcomes can include improved condition symptoms and improved individual and family outcomes such as better disease management, improved quality of life, or improved self-efficacy (Grey et al., 2006). The main goal of the model is to help the individual improve his or her health, using the broadest definition of health possible. The home care nurse supports the self-care and family's self-management, teaches them the skills needed to improve health, and coaches the individual and family on incorporating those activities into their daily lives.

Coaching as a Technique to Enhance Self-Management and Family Management

The home care nurse is in an excellent position to coach the client and family in the management of the chronic illness. Coaching, or motivational interviewing, is a strategy in which the nurse uses a combination of providing education, collaborative decision making, and empowerment to help clients manage their health needs (Butterworth, Linden, & McClay, 2007; Huffman, 2007, 2009). Health coaching has its roots in substance abuse counselling and has been found to be a relatively short-term, successful strategy. Health coaching is a client-centred approach to care with the focus on the issues and barriers to self-management.

To use health coaching, the home health nurse begins by asking the client what he or she is most concerned about. In this way the nurse can capitalize on the client's interest in resolving or managing a particular problem. The next step is to validate the client's feelings about his or her capacity to manage the problem. After this the nurse might help the client develop solutions to the problem by asking about what strategies the client has tried in the past and what strategies he or she might like to try (Huffman, 2007).

Relationship-Based Care

In this model relationship is the basis of nursing practice (Doane, 2002). Individuals are "viewed as contextual beings who exist in relation with other people and with social, cultural, political, and historical processes" (Doane & Varcoe, 2007, p. 198). Every day nurses engage in relationships with clients, other nurses, and healthcare professionals. This network of relationships forms a web of mutual dependencies (Doane & Varcoe, 2007). Relationship-based care is a model of human relating that reflects this web of interactions within the context of humanistic values (Hartrick, 1997). In the past models of nursing care have been based on behavioural models in which the nurse learns a set of communication skills and applies those skills when interacting with clients. This model is unique in that it is based on the recognition of the relational nature and complexity of human experience (Hartrick, 1997). Rather than enhancing communication between nurse and client, applying communication techniques may impede communication because the nurse may be focused on performing these techniques and unable to be "in-caring-human-relation" (Hartrick, 1997, p. 525). According to this model, "health and healing are promoted through the development of an increasing openness to learning and growth, an increasing capacity to tolerate ambiguity and uncertainty, and an increasing experience of empowerment and choice" (Hartrick, 1997, p. 525). For clients with chronic illness, this model of human relation may provide a means for the client, family, and nurse to grow in relationships with each other as well as in the relationship with the chronic illness.

Relationship-based care is not founded on problem identification and resolution but on responding to the client in a manner that acknowledges and supports the significance of the chronic illness as the client experiences it. Nursing action is based on five capacities: (1) initiative, authenticity, and responsiveness; (2) mutuality and synchrony; (3) honouring complexity and ambiguity; (4) intentionality in relating; and (5) re-imaging (Hartrick, 1997).

Initiative, authenticity, and responsiveness address the nurse's active concern for others

(Hartrick, 1997). Within this model these concepts are intertwined. The nurse takes the initiative to engage in relationship with the client. She or he is authentic, responding to the client and the situation in a way that is consistent with his or her personality and showing emotions as they arise. Finally, the nurse is responsive to the feelings, needs, and goals of the client. The nurse is mindful of her or his presence with the client and is attentive to the client with conscious listening.

The concepts of mutuality and synchrony explain the nature of relationships. Mutuality refers to the commonalities experienced by people in relationships. A mutual relationship is a negotiated, collaborative process where client and nurse both participate, make choices, and act (Doane & Varcoe, 2007). These commonalities include shared visions and goals, while acknowledging differences in perspectives. Synchrony describes the rhythms naturally occurring in the relationship, including synchrony between internal and external patterns and periods of silence (Hartrick, 1997).

The nurse honours complexity and ambiguity by acknowledging the complexity of human experience. The nurse, in relation with the client, seeks to uncover the numerous and possibly conflicting elements of the experience. Through this process of discovery the nurse and client begin to mutually make connections between seemingly disparate actions, feelings, and events. Through this process the client and nurse are able to appreciate the relevance of the experience and make choices regarding the management of the disease process (Hartrick, 1997).

Intentionality involves the nurse exploring his or her values and then maintaining consistency between personal values and values in use during professional practice. Each nursing moment is shaped by the actions and intentions of the nurse, the actions and responses of others, and the contexts within which those interactions occur (Doane & Varcoe, 2007). The intent of relational practice is to help clients understand the meaning of their health and healing experiences and to discover choice and power within the experiences (Hartrick, 1997). Reimaging is the process of questioning the usual ways of being in the world. Through this process the nurse can help clients transform their health and healing experiences and enhance their relational capacity (Hartrick, 1997).

The nurse who engages in relational nursing practice makes a conscious commitment to act using the values and goals of the nursing profession to attend to each client's unique context and situation, helping that person grow in health. Difficulty and suffering can provide a vehicle for meaningful relationships, which is the basis for ethical decision making. In these situations responsive nursing care creates the space for mutual experience and for nurse and client to develop clarity and courage to act in health-promoting ways (Doane & Varcoe, 2007).

In more recent work, Weydt (2010) identified other characteristics necessary for effective relationship-based care: clinical proficiency, interdisciplinary communication and teamwork, and continuity of nurse–patient–family relationships. In home care where a primary nursing care model is common, building relationships with clients to improve their self-management of chronic disease can help clients maximize their quality of life.

Chronic Care Model of Disease Management

Individuals with chronic disease require a new strategy for health management. The chronic care model (CCM) (**Figure 17-2**) was developed to change the way health care was delivered to individuals with chronic illness (Improving Chronic Illness Care, 2007) and is currently being trialled or being considered in a number of provinces, including British Columbia, Alberta, and Ontario. The model is designed to support the person with the chronic illness to self-manage his or her health using appropriate community and healthcare system resources. The home health nurse is in an excellent position to assist the client in managing his or her own health and chronic illness within the chronic care model.

Traditionally, the healthcare system in Canada has focused on providing acute care for acute illness in an episodic manner. Individuals with chronic illness require a proactive approach, combining self-management with effective use of community resources and the healthcare system (Improving Chronic Illness Care, 2007). Care is based on evidence-informed protocols that are then tailored to the needs of the individual client. Common areas of difficulty for self-management include managing multiple medications, recognizing early warning signs of condition changes, coordinating and appearing for multiple physicians' appointments, understanding the plan of treatment, and coordinating support services (Meckes, 2005).

According to the CCM, healthcare systems need to retool to provide planned visits focused on maintaining wellness. In this model clients are recognized as having the central role in managing their health. It is the role of healthcare providers to support clients' ability to self-manage their health (Improving Chronic Illness Care, 2007). The nurse can also affect the client's understanding of the disease process and choices for management. By being in the client's home, the home care nurse has a unique

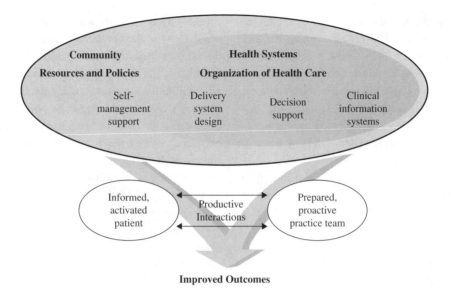

FIGURE 17-2 The chronic care model.
Source: Wagner, E. H. (1998). Chronic disease management: What will it take to improve care for chronic illness? *Effective Clinical Practice, 1,* 2–4.

perspective on the client's culture and the meaning of the illness in his or her life.

Recently, the CCM has been adapted to reflect care delivered by nurses in postacute care settings such as home care (Jacelon et al., 2011). In this version of the model the nurse and client are at the centre of the model. The nurse and client form a team where the nurse coaches and advises the client in effective self-management techniques. The home healthcare nurse may act as a case manager, helping the client navigate complicated interactions with several medical care professionals and guiding the client to seek medical care for condition changes in a timely manner. In addition, the nurse can encourage clients to engage with community organizations to help support their self-management strategies; these community agencies might include

food programs and disease-focused organizations (e.g., the Alzheimer's Association).

Philosophy of Hospice Care

The focus of hospice is the belief that each person has the right to die pain-free and with dignity, surrounded by those with whom the person is close, and that family members and informal caregivers will receive the necessary support to allow people to do so (National Hospice and Palliative Care Organization, 2007). Hospice care is a constellation of services with the goal of providing comfort and symptom management at the end of life (Stuart, 2003). To be eligible for hospice care physicians must determine that the patient has fewer than 6 months to live and the patient must be aware of the prognosis and willing to forgo treatment that may extend life. Hospice care can be offered in a specialized facility or in the individual's home. Recently, hospice services have begun to be offered in nursing homes and in some acute care facilities (Candy, Holman, Leurent, Davis, & Jones, 2011). Home healthcare agencies may offer hospice services in addition to their regular home care services.

Approximately 50% of the funding for hospice palliative care in Canada comes from private donors, and families bear up to 25% of home-based hospice palliative care services. The lack of sufficient, secure funding limits both scope and access to hospice palliative care, especially in rural, remote areas. Some, but not all, provinces and territories designate under provincial health plans and include hospice under home care or other health services budgets. Lack of public funding for home care and palliative hospice care increases the need for family caregivers, who must take on additional responsibilities such as spiritual care, personal care, administration of medications, and coordination of care (Canadian Hospice Palliative Care Association, 2011). Beginning in 2004 the Canadian Nurses Association offers a hospice palliative care certification to Canadian nurses.

considered a community nursing specialty, as is parish nursing and public health nursing. Even though the various specialties practice in different settings and with different client care units, all community health nurses are expected to meet the five standards of practice (**Table 17-2**) (Stanhope et al., 2010). When home health nurse competencies were developed and subsequently adopted in 2010, the community health nursing standards were used as an organizing framework for the competencies (**Table 17-3**) (Community Health Nurses of Canada, 2010).

As the need for home care services increases, it is anticipated that the shortage of nurses in home care may be more acute than in other areas of the healthcare system because of the unique characteristics required to be a successful home care nurse (Ellenbecker, 2004). Home care nurses are generalists who must possess unique skills, including "flexibility, creativity, and innovative approaches to situations and problems in the context of individual and environmental differences and widely varying resource availability" (American Nurses Association, 2008, p. 7). Home health nursing activities involve "teaching, curative interventions, end-of-life care, rehabilitation, support and maintenance, social adaptation and

HOME HEALTH NURSING

The Canadian Community Health Nursing Standards were initially adopted in 2003 and then edited in 2008. These standards form the basis of community health nursing practice in Canada and have been adopted by the Community Health Nurses of Canada. After 2 years of nursing practice, these standards become the basic expectations for nurses working in community health. Home health nursing is

Table 17-2 Canadian Community Health Nursing Standards of Practice
1. Promoting health
2. Building individual and community capacity
3. Building relationships
4. Facilitating access and equity
5. Demonstrating professional responsibility and accountability

Source: Adapted from Community Health Nurses Association of Canada (2008).

integration, and support for the family caregiver" (Canadian Home Care Association, 2008a, p. 2). Home health nurses "provide or manage the care of patients with a broad array of diagnoses across the lifespan and the health-illness continuum" (Community Health Nurses of Canada, 2010, p. 7). The practice of home health nurses is autonomous and independent but recognizes that the home health nurse is a guest in the patient's home. This unique position as a guest in the patient's home provides the home health nurse with the opportunity to observe the patient within the environment of family and home life, an environment that is usually reserved for family and friends (Stanhope et al., 2010). Within this environment the patient may feel more empowered to express concerns and ask questions

and to integrate the challenges of illness and aging with life and relationship patterns that are familiar. The intermittent nature of contact with the patient means that an objective of the home health nurse is assisting the patient and family to recognize their capacity for self-care or managing their own health needs. This implies that the home care nurse must see the patient and family as active and full partners in identifying needs, resources, and strengths that are implicated in managing their health needs.

Home Healthcare Team

The home healthcare team consists of the client, physicians, nurses, physical therapists, occupational therapists, speech therapists, medical social workers, home health aides, and informal caregivers. Each member of the team possesses a special skill set that collectively supports a comprehensive approach to assist the client in meeting his or her care needs.

Effective home care depends on groups of independent practitioners forming teams to provide services for clients. These practitioners have different skill sets and are not always from the same agency. The multiple practitioners on the home healthcare team have the knowledge and skills to identify clients' needs and address those needs through management of complex plans of care (Marelli, 1998). Each practitioner must have a strong grasp of the rules and regulations that govern home health care, the ability to pay attention to detail, well-developed interpersonal skills, strong clinical skills, a working knowledge of the changing economics of health care, and the ability to effectively prioritize and time manage challenging tasks and responsibilities.

Four models of team functioning are medical, multidisciplinary, interdisciplinary, and transdisciplinary (Mauk, 2007). In a medical

---

Table 17-3 Canadian Home Health Nursing Competencies

1. Elements of home health nursing
   a. Assessment, monitoring, and clinical decision making
   b. Care planning and care coordination
   c. Health maintenance, restoration, and palliation
   d. Teaching and education
   e. Communication
   f. Relationships
   g. Access and equity
   h. Building capacity
2. Foundations of home health nursing
   a. Health promotion
   b. Illness prevention and health protection
3. Quality and professional accountability
   a. Quality care
   b. Professional responsibility

Source: Community Health Nurses of Canada (2010).

model team the physician leader directs all functions of the team. Team members do not meet together but communicate through the physician. This team configuration is most common in acute care settings where the physician is in daily contact with the client. This model is not desirable in a home care situation because the client may not be in contact with the physician, the care providers are in the client's home, and independent decision making is a hallmark of this type of care.

The second type of team is the multidisciplinary team. In this model professionals work in parallel. Each provider develops goals for his or her interaction with the client, and coordination occurs at the supervisory level. The individuals who are providing care rarely communicate directly with each other. This model of care is common in long-term care settings in which a rigid bureaucratic structure exists. Multidisciplinary models also occur in home care settings. However, the nature of home care is that practitioners work independently and may interact with other professionals on the team only sporadically (Gantert & McWilliams, 2004).

Transdisciplinary teams are found in rehabilitation settings where team members and the client are in proximity daily. In this model the client and primary care provider work as a team with the counsel of all other team members (Mauk, 2007). Individual team members perform the interventions required for the client while the provider is with the client. Although this model is effective in rehabilitation settings, the nature of home care does not lend itself to this type of team function. The billing constraints in home care require that professionals perform the interventions within their scope of practice and do not reimburse for care outside

of that scope. This model works best in a capitated payment system, where the agency receives a predetermined amount of money for care regardless of who is providing the care.

The team configuration most effective in the home setting is the interdisciplinary team model. In an interdisciplinary team, professionals working with a client communicate directly with the client and each other. In this model the client is an integral part of the team, and professionals collaborate with the client to establish goals for care (Mauk, 2007). Effective interdisciplinary team collaboration has been associated with benefits for both practitioner and client. These include increased provider autonomy and job satisfaction and improved client outcomes and cost containment (Gantert & McWilliams, 2004).

Gantert and McWilliams (2004) identified three dimensions of interaction among interdisciplinary team members: networking, navigating, and aligning. Each dimension occurs along a continuum. The less interactive end of the continuum is representative of a multidisciplinary team, whereas the more interactive end is representative of a more interdisciplinary model. For networking, the continuum ran from isolation to connectedness. As communication among team members increased, so did feelings of connectedness among team members. Navigating had to do with how the team members trusted each other. The more contact team members had with each other, the more trust they exhibited with each other. Finally, the dimension of aligning described the strategies used to determine roles within the team. Team function ranges from the traditional organization hierarchy to a more fluid organization, where team members function autonomously and collaboratively (Gantert & McWilliams, 2004).

Coordination of Care

Care coordination is defined as services provided to individuals with chronic illness who are at risk for adverse outcomes and expensive care that remedy shortcomings in current health care by (Mathematica Policy Research, 2000)

- Identifying medical, functional, social, and emotional needs that increase risk of adverse outcomes and expensive care
- Addressing those needs through self-care education and optimization of medical treatment
- Monitoring progress and identifying problems early

Home care nurses and agencies are in an excellent position to incorporate the role of care coordinator into the role of the nurse because these high-risk individuals are often being treated by home care nurses. Nurses have a well-established relationship with physicians and the local healthcare system and are in an excellent position to incorporate technology into the plan of care through the use of telehealth strategies to augment care (Meckes, 2005).

Three major care coordination issues have been identified (Feldman, 2004). The first is coordination between the hospital and the home care agency at discharge from the hospital or at admission to the hospital from the home care agency. Transitions from one service to another are fraught with opportunities for miscommunication. The second issue for care coordination is strengthening the effectiveness and communication among the members of the interdisciplinary team (Feldman, 2004). The third issue is to improve the effectiveness of interaction between the formal and informal caregivers and to foster self-management (Feldman, 2004). This issue is described in more detail in the following section.

Formal and Informal Caregivers

In 2007, 2.7 Canadians 45 years and older provided care to an older adult with chronic health concerns (Cranswick & Dosman, 2008), and studies consistently suggest that between 70% and 80% of the care given to older individuals and those with chronic illness in the community is provided by family and friends (Keefe, 2011). Of those 45 years and older, 57% are women and 43% are men. Less than 1 in 10 are spouses, with a high number of informal caregivers being adult children (Cranswick & Dosman, 2008) who have other caregiving and work-related responsibilities. Ten percent of female caregivers are over the age of 75 years and 8% are men, which means these caregivers often have health concerns and disabilities and are in need of care themselves (Keating, Fast, Frederick, Cranswick, & Perrier, 1999; Rajonich, Keefe, & Fast, 2005). This caregiving includes a number of caregiving behaviours, many of which are also performed by professional and home support caregivers in formal home health services (**Table 17-4**).

Assessing the ability of unpaid caregivers to support the individual with chronic illness is critical to developing an effective plan of care. Tanner (2004) developed a 13-item scale, the Tanner Family Support Scale, to be used with individuals with chronic health problems to determine the availability of family support. The individual agrees or disagrees with such statements as, "My family members do as much as they can to help me with my health problems when I need help" (Tanner, 2004, p. 314).

Often, the home healthcare nurse and the recipient of care rely heavily on the informal caregiver. Collaboration and decision making often involve a triad rather than the usual nurse–client dyad (Dalton, 2003). However, the nurse must carefully negotiate the relationship to make sure the recipient of care is not silenced (Dalton, 2003). Dalton (2005) identified three types of decisions commonly made about nursing care: program decisions (goals and content

Table 17-4   Informal Caregiver Behaviours
Instrumental activities of daily living
Transportation
Grocery shopping
Housework
Managing finances
Preparing meals
Activities of daily living
Getting in and out of bed or chair
Dressing
Bathing or showering
Toileting
Eating
Incontinence
Helping with medications
Management of care
Finding services
Arranging for delivery of formal and informal services
Coordination of services
Social and emotional support
Provision of emotional support
Arranging for/enabling participation in social activities

Source: Armstrong & Kits (2001).

of care), operational control decisions (how the plan is implemented), and agenda decisions (timing and frequency of nursing visits and care delivery). Coalitions formed between two of the three parts of the triad can affect all care decisions. Home care nurses should collaborate with both the client receiving care and informal caregivers to optimize the benefit of the available professional care. Leff (2004) found that clients demonstrated higher satisfaction with care when they were included in decision making regarding goals, the plan, who (which disciplines and personnel) will provide care, how often and what time of day visits would occur, the activities occurring during the visit, how care is provided, and who will communicate with the physician.

Telehealth in Canada is growing rapidly and is facilitating home health care in many remote and rural areas in Canada, where there continues to be limited access to services because of geography, distance, and availability of services and providers. A study funded by Health Canada, provincial and territorial ministries of health, and Canada Health Infoway (the government-funded organization that partners with provinces and territories) found in 2010 more than 5,700 telehealth systems in approximately 1,175 communities across Canada (Gartner Incorporated, 2011), which represents an increase of 35% in telehealth usage over a 5-year period. Although the organization of telehealth services varies by province and territory, all provinces and territories currently have some form of telehealth delivery, which may follow a centralized model of services (such as in Ontario and Manitoba) or a decentralized delivery of services.

Many telehealth services involve emergency and specialist consultation, which enables clients in their communities to be assessed and treated from a distance without leaving their home communities. This aspect of telehealth is estimated to save elderly or ill Canadians living in remote and rural communities approximately $70 million in personal travel costs and the healthcare system in Canada approximately $55 million in travel and care costs (Gartner Incorporated, 2011). In addition to cost savings and increased accessibility of services, telehealth in Canada was found to improve timeliness in care, enhance care practices, provide support and education for health professionals in outlying areas, reduce unnecessary emergency room visits and hospitalizations, and increase the capacity of clients to manage their own care (Gartner Incorporated, 2011). In addition to these advantages, the wait times for specialized care such as wound care, crisis care, and endocrinology were found to be reduced.

Telehealth services that are specific to home health care are available in British Columbia, Ontario, Quebec, New Brunswick, Nova Scotia, and the Yukon. At present, it is estimated that approximately 2,500 clients are receiving home health services through home telehealth (Gartner Incorporated, 2011). These services enable home care nurses in Quebec, for example, to consult with wound specialists through telehealth about complex wound care concerns. Home care nurses in the East Kootney region of British Columbia are able to monitor the progress of clients who have been discharged from hospital and who have been diagnosed with congestive heart failure. These clients, who are given a monitor for at-home usage for 3 months after hospital discharge, are taught to use the system with the aid of text and voice prompts and to transmit their vital signs, oxygen saturation levels, and weight through encrypted information to home care nurses in centres such as Cranbrook

and Kimberly. The home care nurses examine the data and determine the next step, such as a home visit to the client or a client appointment with the physician. This approach has been found to enable faster detection of problems, facilitate the client's self-management of the disorder, increase the client's self-confidence, increase the confidence of health providers in the accuracy of results (as compared with self-reported results), and decrease the need for face-to-face visits. Other home telehealth programs provide for clients with chronic conditions such as chronic obstructive pulmonary disease, diabetes, and hypertension (Canada Health Infoway, 2011; Gartner Incorporated, 2011).

At present, home monitoring and care through telehealth is on par with Europe but lags behind the U.S. Department of Veteran Affairs, which has been using this technology for a number of years. With the exception of New Brunswick, pilots in home health monitoring have been successful but not self-sustaining, which remains a challenge for the full implementation of telehealth and telehomecare in Canada. In addition to funding and self-sustainability, other challenges to integrating telehealth in mainstream health care in Canada are as follows (Canada Health Infoway, 2011; Gartner Incorporated, 2011):

- Clinician reimbursement, which is seen to be critical to adoption of telehealth technologies and care
- Identification, measurement, and articulation of benefits, which affects adoption and support of telehealth delivery of healthcare services
- Licensing, which affects the ability of providers to provide care to clients in other provincial and territorial jurisdictions

- Technology implementation, such as integrating telehealth devices, solutions, and data with electronic health records, as successfully implemented in jurisdictions outside of Canada
- Governance, which refers to the organization, leadership, and resource allocation structures and processes for telehealth services (At present, provinces and territories are using both centralized and decentralized models of governance.)
- Professional development, which includes orientation and discussion of new roles and the possibilities inherent in working in the multidisciplinary teams that telehealth facilitates
- Maintenance and updating of care processes, such as data sharing and privacy and consent tools

The American Telemedicine Association has developed a training program for accreditation, and in 2006 Accreditation Canada enhanced its accreditation program to also include telehealth standards. Generic guidelines for telehealth programs, which include home telehealth guidelines and telemonitoring, involve determining client-inclusion criteria, explaining the program and obtaining client consent, protection of an individual's health information, home assessment for appropriateness of the plan, client/caregiver education, and a plan for performance improvement that includes the client (Britton, 2003).

The area of telehomecare is seen as an area of rapid growth in telehealth, with a potential to yield significant cost savings (approximately $540 million annually in inpatient costs and $23 million annually in emergency department visits) and to contribute positively to the care of clients with chronic disorders in their own homes and communities in terms of quality of life and self-management.

Clinical Care Classification System

The clinical care classification system was developed in 1991 by Saba as a way of predicting resource needs and measuring the outcomes of home care (Saba, 2002). Since then the system has gained credibility through independent research and use in clinical and educational settings (**Table 17-5**). The most recent update was in 2004 (Saba, 2004).

Table 17-5   The Clinical Care Classification System: 21 Care Components by Four Clinical Patterns

Health behavioural components
    Medication
    Safety
    Health behaviour

Functional components
    Activity
    Fluid volume
    Nutritional
    Self-care
    Sensory

Physiological components
    Cardiac
    Respiratory
    Metabolic
    Physical regulation
    Skin integrity
    Tissue perfusion
    Bowel elimination
    Urinary elimination
    Life cycle

Psychological Components
    Cognitive
    Coping
    Role relationship
    Self-concept

Source: Saba (2004). Clinical care classification (CCC) system. Retrieved from www.sabacare.com/. Used with permission.

The classification system consists of two standardized, interrelated terminologies: one for nursing diagnosis and another for nursing interventions. The two terminologies are classified by 21 care components and organized into four health patterns: behavioural, functional, physiological, and psychological, representing a comprehensive framework incorporated into an existing home healthcare record and linked to reimbursement software (Saba, 2002; more information on the clinical care classification system can be obtained at www.sabacare.com).

The home health industry is challenged to skillfully manage the risk, cost, resources, and outcomes of client care. All agency staff require a thorough education to be familiar with the rules and regulations for agency operations and how each staff member's skills and talents will be used to achieve agency goals. Clinicians need continuing education focused on maximizing the value of provided care. Accurate, thorough client assessments and rapid submission of these data are critical for the agency to obtain timely reimbursement.

OUTCOMES

The desired outcomes for home health care in the management of the client with chronic illness seem initially to be quite apparent. The positive effects of the health care delivered in the home to the client, as well as the positive effects of the caregiver support mechanisms that keep the client at home and do not necessitate institutionalization, are clearly important outcomes. However, establishing outcome criteria that are stable and dependable to measure outcome attainment is essential to know if positive effects are occurring to the advantage of the client and caregiver or simply because there is no alternative to providing care.

Maurer and Smith (2005) established nine possible outcome measures for evaluating the outcome attainment judged by changes in the population, the healthcare system within the community, or the environment: (1) knowledge; (2) behaviours and skills; (3) attitudes; (4) emotional well-being; (5) health status (epidemiology); (6) presence of healthcare system services and components; (7) satisfaction or acceptance regarding the program interventions; (8) presence of policy allowing, mandating, and funding; and (9) altered relationship with the physical environment.

Evaluating the outcomes of care rendered by any of the disciplines participating in home health care for the first five measures is inclusive in the care itself. The professionals and paraprofessionals who work within the home care team function within and by delivering care using these first five principles, thereby making their use as measurement variables relatively easy and functional. The last four outcome measures, however, have been a continuous struggle for home health care throughout the 20th and now the 21st centuries. These four measures are unpredictably influenced by the ups and downs of financial support, government regulations, management control in home health itself, and in the institutional care that passes clients on to in-home care.

Home health nurses can promote clients' self-management of their chronic diseases. The nurse can be effective in helping clients and their informal caregivers to maximize the support available to them. Using strategies such as coaching and telemedicine can help clients improve their self-care abilities. Resources such as protocols, care maps, and clinical pathways will become more useful, along with the incentive to explore advanced technologies such as point-of-service computers and telemedicine devices.

CASE STUDY

Ms. Lavoie is a 77-year-old woman with a diagnosis of congestive heart failure (CHF). She lives alone on the first floor of a two-family home in an urban neighbourhood. She has lived in the same house for 57 years. Over that time the neighbourhood has declined around her. Now there are many boarded-up houses on her street. Ms. Lavoie was admitted to the hospital after an exacerbation of her cardiac symptoms. While in the hospital the physician evaluated and adjusted her cardiac medications. It was determined that one of the contributing factors to the exacerbation of symptoms was Ms. Lavoie's diet. When interviewed at admission, it was clear that Ms. Lavoie had a poor understanding of her diet prescription.

After 5 days in the hospital, Ms. Lavoie was discharged from the hospital with orders for home care. Nurse Jones visited Ms. Lavoie for her intake interview within the regulated 48 hours after discharge from the hospital. At the first visit Nurse Jones completed the admission assessment including self-management and risk and protective factors including condition factors, individual factors, psychosocial characteristics, family factors, and information about the neighbourhood (environment). She collected the OASIS data and began teaching Ms. Lavoie about her new medications. Nurse Jones created a chart written in large print with the name of each medication, the purpose of each, and when Ms. Lavoie should take the medication. Nurse Jones developed a 60-day plan of care for Ms. Lavoie that included the number of visits, medications, diet education, treatments, and client-focused goals. The plan included skilled nursing services for teaching Ms. Lavoie about her medications, diet, and management of CHF and monitoring disease process; physical therapy to increase her daily activity, balance, and safety in the home; a nurse's aide three times weekly for help with activities of daily living; and a homemaker for assistance with instrumental activities of daily living. The nurse included telehealth services for close daily monitoring of Ms. Lavoie's CHF. The plan of care was subsequently signed by the physician.

Over the course of the first week of services the nurse visited twice more to coach Ms. Lavoie on using the telehealth equipment for daily weight and blood pressure monitoring, self-medication management, and diet. The nurse and physical therapist coordinated their visits so that they visited together on day 3 after discharge and thereafter visited on alternate days to maximize the presence of health professionals in the home. In collaboration with Ms. Lavoie, Nurse Jones organized the care schedule so that during the first 2 weeks after discharge from the hospital, someone on the healthcare team (registered nurse, physical therapist, certified nursing assistant, homemaker) visited Ms. Lavoie each day. By the end of the first 2 weeks Ms. Lavoie was stronger, was using the telehealth equipment to send her blood pressure information and weight to the home care office daily, and was making better diet choices. Nurse

CASE STUDY   (Continued)   www

Jones determined that she could decrease her visits to weekly as did the physical therapist. Nurse Jones continued to monitor Ms. Lavoie using the telehealth system.

At the beginning of week 4, using the telehealth data, Nurse Jones noted a sharp increase in Ms. Lavoie's weight and blood pressure. Nurse Jones telephoned Ms. Lavoie and made an appointment for a visit. During the visit Ms. Lavoie and Nurse Jones reviewed Ms. Lavoie's activities for the last 3 days. Ms. Lavoie reported that she had been feeling so much better that she had cooked one of her favourite meals, which may have been too salty. Nurse Jones reviewed the recipe with Ms. Lavoie and coached her on how to adjust the recipe so there was less sodium and how to divide the recipe into single servings and freeze them so Ms. Lavoie did not eat the entire casserole of eight servings every day until it was gone. In addition, Nurse Jones had Ms. Lavoie create a log where she could write down her weight and blood pressure every day so that she could use the information to self-manage her health.

Over the next week Ms. Lavoie's blood pressure and weight decreased, returning to baseline. The physical therapist determined that Ms. Lavoie had met her mobility goals. The plan was modified to discharge physical therapy and add walking to the certified nurse assistant activities. At week 6 the nurse helped Ms. Lavoie to transition from monitoring her blood pressure and weight on the telehealth equipment to using her own equipment, continuing to write down the results daily and looking for trends. Also during her visit at week 6 Nurse Jones discussed community resources that Ms. Lavoie might use to reduce her isolation and increase her activity outside the home.

Ms. Lavoie was discharged from home care services 7 weeks after discharge from the hospital. She was competently self-managing her CHF. Ms. Lavoie was consistently taking her medication according to the prescription, she could manage her diet to control her sodium and fluid intake, and she had increased her daily activity to include a trip (using public transportation for individuals with disabilities that would pick her up at her house) to the mall to take a short walk. Nurse Jones had developed a relationship with Ms. Lavoie in which they worked together to improve. Nurse Jones used coaching as a primary teaching strategy.

Discussion Questions

1. Describe the theoretical framework that Nurse Jones used to provide care to Ms. Lavoie.
2. What effect did telehealth have on Ms. Lavoie's outcomes?
3. Discuss the "team" concept used in Ms. Lavoie's care.
4. Describe the different patient education teaching strategies used in providing care to Ms. Lavoie.

Evidence-Informed Practice Box

A collaborative research study involving McMaster University researchers, community care access centre practitioners, and home support provider agencies (VON, Para-Med Home Health Care, Canadian Red Cross) examined the baseline characteristics and changes in health status and cost of use of health services associated with publicly funded services.

This study used data from a randomized controlled trial that examined the effects and costs of nursing health promotion intervention for older home care clients receiving home support services. Participants in the trial were 288 frail elderly people, 75 years and older, who were newly eligible for home support services (personal hygiene, routine activities of daily living, provision of prescribed supplies and goods). Subjects for the present study were 144 frail elderly people who were randomized into the usual home care (control) arm of the randomized controlled trial and divided into three groups, based on average weekly number of home support services used over a 6-month period. The sample was divided into three groups based on average use of home support services over 6 months: 0 hours/week, <1 hour/week, and >1 hour/week. Data related to cognitive status, functional health status, presence of depression, perceived social support, and coping style were collected, using validated questionnaires by individuals who were blinded to the study purpose at baseline and 6 months. Data regarding use of home support services were collected directly from computerized

records at a community care access centre, which account for number of home support hours used on a monthly basis. Data were analyzed using SPSS 15.0 for Windows and a number of statistical measures. The three groups were compared based on their characteristics at baseline (whether they used 0 hours of home support services/week, <1 hour of home support services/week, or >1 hour of home support services/week).

Findings from the study suggested the frail elderly who used the most home support services (>1 hour/week) were more likely to be depressed, have less effective coping styles, and to have moderate to severe cognitive impairment than the elderly in the other two groups, who used either no home support services or <1 hour a week. Cognitive impairment was found to contribute most to variation in and increased use of home support services.

Further findings from the study suggest that participants who used home support services for more than 1 hour a week had fewer days in hospital (5.3 days) than those who used services less than 1 hour a week (7.9 days in hospital), suggesting that the use of home support services is effective in reducing the need for hospitalization for the frail elderly. Notably, the cost for occupational health services was increased for the elderly who used the most hours of support services per week. These increases in occupational therapy costs were offset by lower costs for acute hospital and emergency room services, physiotherapy, and nursing, although this was not statistically significant.

The findings of this study suggest that the provision of even minimal home support services is effective in reducing hospital admissions and expensive hospital associated costs for frail elderly who have increased healthcare needs, although no increase in quality of life or functioning was observed. It further provides support for findings from other studies that suggest older adults with chronic and continuing care needs need home support services more than they do medical services.

Source: Markle-Reid et al. (2008).

HOME CARE SATISFACTION MEASURES

In health care objective measures of client satisfaction with care are often used as an indicator of positive outcomes. However, in home care it has been more difficult to measure client satisfaction with care (Geron et al., 2000). Although some scales of client satisfaction have been adapted from acute care, few measures have been developed specifically for home care. The Home Care Satisfaction Measure (HCSM) is a 60-item instrument measuring overall satisfaction with home care and satisfaction with five common services (Geron et al., 2000). The HCSM is designed to measure satisfaction with homemaker and home health aide services, case management, home-delivered meal service, and grocery service. The instrument is designed so that each service can be measured separately or the scores summed for an overall measure of satisfaction. The HCSM can be completed in person or by telephone. The HCSM evaluates client satisfaction with aspects of home care that are not usually covered by Medicare and private insurance.

SUMMARY

Positive client outcomes require that home care agencies become aware of the roles that clients, family, and caregivers play before the client is admitted for service. Home care providers, clients, families, and caregivers must enter into partnerships to provide the care needed for the client. Informal care providers need to know the significance of their roles in the plan of care, and nurses must enlist these informal caregivers to continue to provide care. In turn, the client's family must understand what can be expected from agency services.

Several forces are coming to bear on the need for home care services. As the population ages and individuals survive longer, chronic illness is increasing, and there is a social movement to decrease institutionalization in nursing homes in favour of keeping clients in their own communities. The home care industry is in an excellent position to create partnerships with clients and families to help clients stay in their own environments and manage their chronic illness.

STUDY QUESTIONS   WWW

1. What skills does a nurse need to be an effective home care nurse?
2. How can the interdisciplinary team maintain effective communication in the home?
3. Discuss how nurses might use home care outcome measures to improve the healthcare delivery system.
4. Describe how home care nurses differ in practice from public health nurses.

(continues)

STUDY QUESTIONS (Cont.)

5. Discuss the definition of "homebound" and how being homebound might affect an individual's ability to go to church regularly and how it might affect the provision of health care.

6. Describe the self- and family management of chronic illness model. How might you apply the model to an individual with type 1 diabetes?

7. Discuss how the home care nurse might use the CCM to provide care to a client with chronic illness.

8. How does including telehealth in the list of interventions affect the delivery of home care?

9. Discuss strategies the home care nurse might use to help a client and his or her family manage the disease process.

INTERNET RESOURCES

Canadian Home Care Association:
    www.cdnhomecare.ca
Canadian Hospice Palliative Care Association:
    www.chpca.net
Community Health Nurses of Canada:
    www.chnc.ca
Home Care Healthcare Nurses Association:
    www.hhna.org
National Association for Home Care and Hospice:
    www.nahc.org
Victorian Order of Nurses:
    www.von.ca

For a full suite of assignments and additional learning activities, use the access code located in the front of your book and visit this exclusive website: **http://go.jblearning.com/kramer-kile**. If you do not have an access code, you can obtain one at the site.

REFERENCES

American Nurses Association. (2008). *Home health nursing: Scope and standards of practice*. Silver Springs, MD: Author.

Armstrong, P., & Kits, O. (2001). *One hundred years of caregiving*. Ottawa, ON: Law Commission of Canada.

Britton, B. (2003). First home telehealth clinical guidelines. *Home Healthcare Nurse, 21*(1), 703–706.

Butterworth, S. W., Linden, A., & McClay, W. (2007). Health coaching as an intervention in health management programs. *Disease Management of Health Outcomes, 15*(5), 299–307.

Canada Health Infoway. (2011). Annual report 2010–2011: Towards critical mass: Moving from availability to adoption. Retrieved from http://www2.infoway-inforoute.ca/Documents/ar/AnnualReport_2010-2011_en.pdf

Canadian Healthcare Association. (2009). *Home care in Canada: From the margins to the mainstream: Policy brief*. Ottawa, ON: Canadian Healthcare Association.

Canadian Home Care Association. (2008a). Home care: Meeting the needs of an aging population. Retrieved from http://www.hc-sc.gc.ca/hcs-sss/alt_formats/hph-dgps/pdf/pubs/2005-cas-mgmt-gest/2005-cas-mgmt-gest-eng.pdf

Canadian Home Care Association. (2008b). Integration of care: Exploring the potential of the alignment of home care with other health sectors. Retrieved from http://www.cdnhomecare.ca/mediaphp?mid=185

Canadian Home Care Association. (2010). Mind, body, spirit: Promising practices in First Nations and Inuit home and community care. Retrieved from http://www.cdnhomecare.ca/content.php?doc=44

Canadian Home Care Association. (2011). Access to quality health care: The home care contribution. Retrieved from http://www.cdnhomecare.ca/media.php?mid=2844

Canadian Home Care Association. (2012). Home care 2020: A vision of health, independence, and dignity. Retrieved from http://www.cdnhomecare.ca/media.php?mid=2335

Canadian Hospice Palliative Care Association. (2011). Fact sheet: Hospice palliative care in Canada. Retrieved from http://www.chpca.net/media/7622/Fact_sheet_HPC_in_Canada_August_2011_FINAL.pdf

Candy, B., Holman, A., Leurent, B., Davis, S., & Jones, L. (2011). Hospice care delivered at home, in nursing homes and in dedicated hospice facilities: A systematic review of quantitative and qualitative evidence. *International Journal of Nursing Studies, 48*, 121–133.

Community Health Nurses of Canada. (2010). *Home health nursing competencies, version 1.0*. Toronto, ON: Author.

Cranswick, K., & Dosman, D. (2008). *Eldercare: What we know today. Canadian social trends.* Ottawa, ON: Statistics Canada.

Dalton, J. (2003). Development and testing of the theory of collaborative decision-making in nursing practice for triads. *Journal of Advanced Nursing, 50*(1), 22–33.

Dalton, J. (2005). Client-caregiver-nurse coalition formation in decision-making situations during home visits. *Journal of Advanced Nursing, 52*(3), 291–299.

Doane, G. (2002). Beyond behavioral skills to human-involved processes: Relational nursing practice and interpretive pedagogy. *Journal of Nursing Education, 41*(9), 400–404.

Doane, G., & Varcoe, C. (2007). Relational practice and nursing obligations. *Advances in Nursing Science, 30*(3), 192–205.

Ellenbecker, C. (2004). A theoretical model of job retention for home health care nurses. *Journal of Advanced Nursing, 47*(3), 303–310.

Feldman, P. (2004). Penny Feldman on home healthcare quality and research. *Journal for Healthcare Quality, 26*(3), 31–37.

Gantert, T., & McWilliams, C. (2004). Interdisciplinary team processes within an in-home service delivery organization. *Home Health Services Quarterly, 23*(3), 1–17.

Gartner Incorporated. (2011). Telehealth benefits and adoption: Connecting people and providers across Canada. Retrieved from http://www2.infoway_inforoute.ca/Documents/telehealth_report_2010_en.pdf

Geron, S., Smith, K., Tennstedt, S., Jette, A., Chassler, D., & Kastern, L. (2000). The home care satisfaction measure: A client-centered approach to assessing the satisfaction of frail older adults with home care services. *Journal of Gerontology: Social Sciences, 55*(5), S259–S270.

Grey, M., Knafl, K., & McCorkle, R. (2006). A framework for the study of self- and family management of chronic conditions. *Nursing Outlook, 54*, 278–286.

Hartrick, G. (1997). Relationship capacity: The foundation for interpersonal nursing practice. *Journal of Advanced Nursing, 26*, 523–528.

Health Canada. (1999). Provincial and territorial home care programs: A synthesis for Canada. Retrieved from http://www.hc-sc.gc.ca/hcs-sss/pubs/home-domicile/1999-pt-synthes/index-eng.php

Health Canada. (2011). Canada's health care system. Retrieved from http://www.hc-sc.gc.ca/hcs-sss/pubs/system-regime/2011-hcs-sss/index-eng.php

Health Care in Canada Survey. (2000). Health Care in Canada Survey 2000. Retrieved from http://www.hcic-sssc.ca/english/files/CurrentContent/2000/2000.hcic.pdf

Health Care in Canada Survey. (2007). Health Care in Canada Survey 2007. Retrieved from http://www.hcic-sssc.ca/english/files/CurrentContent/2007/2007.hcic.pdf

Hitchcock, J., Schubert, P., & Thomas, S. (Eds.) (2003). *Community health nursing: Caring in action* (2nd ed.). Albany, NY: Delmar.

Hollander, J. (2001). Final report of the study on the comparative cost analysis of home care and residential care services: University of Victoria, Centre on Aging. Retrieved from http://www.homecarestudy.com/reports/full-text/substudy-01-final_report.pdf

Huffman, M. (2007). Health coaching: A new and exciting technique to enhance patient self-management and improve outcomes. *Home Healthcare Nurse, 25*(4), 271–274.

Huffman, M. (2009). Health coaching: A fresh, new approach to improve quality outcomes and compliance for patients with chronic conditions. *Home Healthcare Nurse, 27*(8), 491–496.

Improving Chronic Illness Care. (2007). The chronic care model. Retrieved from http://www.improvingchroniccare.org/index.php?p=The_Chronic_Care_Model&s=2

Jacelon, C. S., Furman, E., Rea, A., Macdonald, B., & Donoghue, L. C. (2011). Creating a professional practice model for post acute care: Adapting the chronic care model for long-term care. *Journal of Gerontological Nursing, 37*(3), 53–60.

Keating, N., Fast, J., Frederick, J., Cranswick, F., & Perrier, C. (1999). *Eldercare in Canada: Context, content and consequences.* Ottawa, ON: Statistics Canada.

Keefe, J. (2011). Supporting caregivers and caregiving in an aging Canada. Retrieved from http://www.cdn homecare.ca/media.php?mid=2799

Leff, E. (2004). Involving patients in care decisions improves satisfaction: An outcomes based quality improvement project. *Home Healthcare Nurse, 22*(5), 297–301.

MacAdam, M., Hollander, J., Miller, J., Chappell, N., & Pedlar, D. (2009). Increasing value for money in the Canadian healthcare system: New findings and the case for integrated care for seniors. *Healthcare Quarterly, 12*(1), 38–47.

Malowany, M. (2009). Public health nursing in early 20th century. *Canadian Journal of Public Health, 100*(4), 249–252.

Marelli, T. (1998). *Handbook of home health standards and documentation guidelines for reimbursement.* St. Louis, MO: Mosby.

Markle-Reid, M., Browne, J., Weir, R., Gafni, A., Roberts, J., & Henderson, S. (2008). Seniors at risk: The association between the six-month use of publicly funded home support services and quality of life and use of health services in older people. *Canadian Journal on Aging, 27*, 207–224.

Mathematica Policy Research. (2000). Best practices in coordinated care: Prepared for health care financing administration. Retrieved from http://www .mathematica-mpr.com/pdfs/bestsum.pdf

Mauk, K. (2007). *The specialty practice of rehabilitation: A core curriculum.* Glenview, IL: Association of Rehabilitation Nurses.

Maurer, F., & Smith, C. (2005). *Community public health nursing practice.* St. Louis, MO: Elsevier Saunders.

Meckes, C. (2005). Opportunities in care coordination. *Home Healthcare Nurse, 23*(10), 663–669.

National Hospice and Palliative Care Organization. (2007). Caring connections. Retrieved from http://www .caringinfo.org/LivingWithAnIllness/Hospice.htm

Ontario Home Care Association. (2010). Home care in 2010—essential for an aging population. Retrieved from http://www.homecareontario.ca/public/docs /publications

Petrucka, P. (2010). The Canadian health care system. In P. A. Potter, A. G. Perry, J. C. Ross-Kerr, & M. J. Wood (Eds.), *Canadian Fundamentals of Nursing* (pp. 14–27). Toronto, ON: Elsevier.

Rajonich, R. J., Keefe, J., & Fast, J. (2005). Supporting caregivers of dependent adults in the 21st century: CPRN background paper. Retrieved from http://www .cewh-cesf.ca/pdf/acewh/SupportingCaregivers.pdf

Romanow, R. (2002). Building on values: The future of health care in Canada. Retrieved from http://www .hc-sc.gc.ca/english/pdf/romanow/pdfs/hcc_final_ report.pdf

Ross-Kerr, J. C. (2010). The Canadian health care system. In P. A. Potter, A. G. Perry, J. C. Ross-Kerr, & M. J. Wood (Eds.), *Canadian Fundamentals of Nursing* (pp. 28–40). Toronto, ON: Elsevier.

Ryan, P., & Sawin, K. J. (2009). The individual and family self-management theory: Background and perspectives on context, process, and outcomes. *Nursing Outlook, 57*(4), 217–225.

Saba, V. K. (2002). Home health care classification system: An overview. *Online Journal of Issues in Nursing, 7*(3). Retrieved from http://www.nursing-world.org/MainMenuCategories/ANAMarketplace /ANAPeriodicals/OJIN/TableofContents/Volume 72002/No3Sept2002/ArticlesPreviousTopic/HHCC AnOverview.html

Saba, V. K. (2004). CCC system, version 2.0. Retrieved from http://www.sabacare.com/Framework

Schoen, M., & Koenig, R. (1997). Home health care nursing: Past and present. *MedSurg Nursing, 6*(4), 230–234.

Shah, C. P. (2003). *Public health and preventive medicine in Canada.* Toronto, ON: Saunders.

Stadnyk, R. (2002). The status of Canadian nursing home care: Universality, accessibility, and comprehensiveness. A paper prepared for the Atlantic Centre of Excellence for Women's Health. Retrieved from http://www.acewh.dal.ca/eng/reports

Stanhope, M., & Lancaster, J. (2010). *Foundations of nursing in the community: Community-oriented practice* (3rd ed.). St. Louis, MO: Mosby.

Stanhope, M., Lancaster, J., Jessup-Falcioni, H., & Viverais-Dresler, G. A. (2010). *Community health nursing in Canada* (3rd ed.). Toronto, ON: Elsevier Canada.

Statistics Canada. (2010). Population projections for Canada, provinces, and territories. Retrieved from http://www.statcan.gc.ca/pub/91-520-x2010001-eng .htm

Stuart, B. (2003). Transition management: A new paradigm for home care of the chronically ill near the end of life. *Home Health Care Management & Practice, 15*(2), 126–135.

Tanner, E. (2004). Chronic illness demands for self-management in older adults. *Geriatric Nursing, 25*(5), 313–317.

Underwood, J., & Henteleff, A. (2010). Development of home health nursing competencies: Report submitted to the Community Health Nurses of Canada. Retrieved from http://www.chnc.ca/documents /DevelopmentofHomeHealthNursingCompetencies inCanada.pdf

Victorian Order of Nurses. (2009). History: A century of caring. Retrieved from http://www.von.ca/en/about .history.aspx

Villeneuve, M., & MacDonald, J. (2006). Toward 2020: Visions for nursing. Retrieved from http://www.cna-aiic.ca/CNA/documents/pdf/publications/Toward-2020-e.pdf

Weir, G. M. (1932). *Survey of nursing education in Canada.* Toronto, ON: University of Toronto.

Weydt, A. (2010). Mary's story, relationship-based care delivery. *Nursing Administration Quarterly, 34*(2), 141–146.

CHAPTER 18

Long-Term Care

Original chapter by Susan J. Barnes and Kristen L. Mauk
Canadian content added by Dawn Prentice

INTRODUCTION

Long-term care (LTC) is an umbrella term that refers to a range of services that address the health, personal care, psychoemotional, and social needs of persons with some degree of difficulty in caring for themselves. Although family members may assist those persons with age-related functional decline or with disabilities, LTC is often needed as time progresses to bridge the gap in care. The ideal LTC services promote independence of the person for as long as possible and allow him or her to remain at home as appropriate. LTC may be required because of disability associated with birth defects, injury, or the aging process. The concept of LTC may best be visualized on a continuum. Between the two ends of the spectrum—independence with minimal assistance at home versus skilled care in the nursing home—are many alternatives and options.

Care needs may be minimal or extensive (**Figure 18-1**). LTC services are offered in a variety of settings, which is discussed in greater detail later. There is a growing trend in community-based services. Often, persons visualize a nursing home setting when they think of LTC, but this setting is used by only a small portion of the population at any given time.

Nurses are in an excellent position to design and implement innovative, cost-effective, and visionary care modalities to provide high-quality LTC services for patients while preserving their dignity and personhood. Because of the holistic perspective that nurses have of the patient, family, and community, they are in an excellent position to act as change agents in the process of healthcare reform.

According to the 2001 Census 7% of seniors over the age of 65 years lived in dwellings such as nursing homes and hospitals (Turcotte & Schellenberg, 2007). Furthermore, living in an institution is age related and increases with age from 2% for older adults (seniors) 65 to 74 years of age to 32% for those aged 85 years and over (Turcotte & Schellenberg, 2007). In 2007, 2.7 million Canadians 45 years of age and over served as unpaid caregivers for seniors (Statistics Canada, 2008). The cost of providing health care to persons older than age 65 is three to five times greater than for younger persons. The changing demographics of the baby boomer generation entering the older age group will have a significant impact on the whole of society (Lomastro, 2006). In 2010 approximately 4.8 million Canadians were 65 years or older. By 2036 this number is expected to reach 10.4 million (Statistics Canada, 2010).

For many persons increased age is accompanied by one or more chronic illnesses.

In 2009, 89% of Canadian seniors had at least one chronic illness, with arthritis and rheumatism reported to account for 44% (Public Health Agency of Canada, 2009, as cited in The Chief Public Health Officer's Report on the State of Public Health in Canada, 2010). Moreover, one in four Canadians between the ages of 65 and 79 experienced four chronic illnesses in 2009.

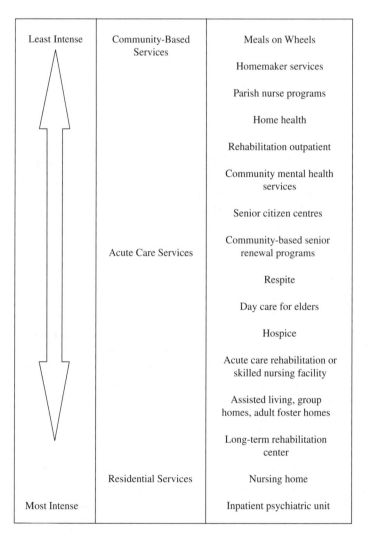

Least Intense	Community-Based Services	Meals on Wheels
		Homemaker services
		Parish nurse programs
		Home health
		Rehabilitation outpatient
		Community mental health services
		Senior citizen centres
	Acute Care Services	Community-based senior renewal programs
		Respite
		Day care for elders
		Hospice
		Acute care rehabilitation or skilled nursing facility
		Assisted living, group homes, adult foster homes
		Long-term rehabilitation center
	Residential Services	Nursing home
Most Intense		Inpatient psychiatric unit

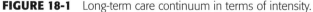

FIGURE 18-1   Long-term care continuum in terms of intensity.

These diseases included angina, asthma, arthritis or rheumatism, osteoporosis, high blood pressure, bronchitis, emphysema, chronic obstructive pulmonary disease, diabetes, heart disease, cancer, effects of a stroke, Crohn's disease, colitis, Alzheimer's disease, Parkinson's disease, cataracts, glaucoma, thyroid condition, mood disorder, and anxiety disorder (Statistics Canada, 2009).

Although perception of health declines as seniors age, in 2009 50% of seniors up to age 85 said they were in good health (Statistics Canada, 2011a). As the incidence of chronic disease grows, deficits in a person's ability to perform self-care often follow, which can eventually lead to the need for LTC services. According to a document from the American Association of Retired Persons (Houser, Fox-Grage, & Gibson, 2009), indicators of the need for LTC services include advanced age, living alone, poverty, less education, not owning a home, and not having a vehicle for transportation.

HISTORICAL PERSPECTIVES

Caring for a client with complex health needs over a long period continues to be a challenge for the healthcare system. Throughout history consideration given to the quality of care for older adults or other vulnerable populations is seen as a reflection of societal values (Koop & Schaeffer, 1976). In societies with more fluid resources, vulnerable populations such as the frail elderly or individuals with chronic illness are better cared for because of the availability of assistance with health care (Kalisch & Kalisch, 2004). History has demonstrated that in societies under strain caused by famine, war, or social upheaval, the vulnerable may not be able to

survive because of malnutrition, lack of health care, and the lack of ability of the family unit to provide support.

Before the 20th century older adults in the United States were usually cared for within extended family units (DeSpelder & Strickland, 2011). This finding is similar in Canada. Those without family to care for them might have gone to a facility supported by a religious organization or by charitable citizens, such as a poorhouse or almshouse. Changes in medical care altered hospital stays and allowed LTC to evolve, with group rest homes and private charitable homes providing care for chronically ill, dependent persons. Because life expectancies continued to increase, the demand for LTC increased. The Canada Health Act (1985) specifies that Canadian citizens are entitled to financial coverage for physician and medically necessary services. However, LTC including nursing home care is considered an "extended service" and not an insured service and therefore not funded under the Canada Health Act. Because LTC is governed by each provincial and territorial legislative body across the country, it is up to the provinces to determine how much of the long-term costs are publicly funded (Fernandes & Spencer, 2010). Thus, different provinces and territories offer a range of different types of services and for a variety of costs. Generally, the resident covers the accommodation costs.

As Western culture has evolved the family structure has been modified by the increasing number of women who work outside the home and are unavailable to care for aging parents (Gaugler & Teaster, 2006; Wagner, 2006). Current cultural values have made it less common for extended families to live together. However, Latino and Asian cultures often include extended families, with several generations living in the same household or nearby, which makes it possible for family members to look after the interests of vulnerable elder members and limits the need for formal LTC services (Leininger, 2002). In many cultures the concept of the "double caregiver" adds enormous stress to women who work and provide care for a family and ailing parents (Remennick, 2001). However, current North American values emphasize single-family dwellings, dual-income families, and transient lifestyles, which have led to families no longer residing in the same area, often geographically separated by great distance. This culturally driven environment has created a high demand for services from an already inefficient LTC system.

CONTINUUM OF CARE

Community-Based LTC

The premise of community-based LTC is to provide seamless, comprehensive programs to facilitate aging in place (Willging, 2006). However, much work needs to be done to operationalise the seamless aspect of transitions. A variety of services is available within the LTC continuum.

Current trends advocate using a case management approach to coordinate services and to ensure that individuals receive services in an efficient, timely fashion. Case management promotes aging in place with chronic illness, trying to keep a person in the home setting for a long as possible. The LTC system may be confusing to clients and families, but case managers can help to arrange and coordinate services such as Meals on Wheels, medical care, personal support workers, allied health care professional services, and companion services.

Respite care for family members who care for loved ones with chronic illness and disability is also a community-based service.

In Canada no one integrated system for the elderly exists, although all jurisdictions are moving forward with this agenda given the aging population and the incidence of chronic illness. Some provinces such as Ontario have implemented an aging at home strategy that focuses on providing enhanced home care services and community services to keep seniors at home as long as possible with support. The province of Quebec offers the Program of Research to Integrate the Services of Maintenance of Autonomy for clients 65 years and older who require the support of two or more social or health services to remain living in the community at home (MacAdam, 2009).

In the United States the Program of All-Inclusive Care for the Elderly (PACE) is another community-based alternative that promotes aging in place (Boult & Wieland, 2010). This program is an evidence-informed model of care whose services are often covered by Medicare and Medicaid. The National PACE Association (2011) stated that the average user is 80 years old, and preliminary studies suggest that involvement in a PACE program may slow functional decline for older adults. The PACE model combines dollars from different funding streams to deliver a comprehensive set of services focused on the health and well-being of the individual (National PACE Association, 2011). The number of states with participating organizations has increased to 30 in the last few years (the list of states with programs is found on the PACE website at http://www.npaonline.org). Continuing evaluation of this program in terms of cost to benefit to the funding agencies may make it available on a wider scale.

Residential LTC Settings

Residential LTC facilities are formal, organized agencies that provide care for persons unable to live alone because of physical or other problems but who do not require hospitalization. Persons living in residential care are not called patients but residents, because the LTC setting is their home. The most common types of residential LTC facilities are assisted-living centres/retirement homes and nursing homes. Many retirement communities combine independent living facilities and assisted living facilities, although these represent two different levels of care. Those living independently in a retirement community may do so because of declining health caused by chronic illness, safety factors, frailty, and the need for socialization. The decision to move from one's own home to a community living situation is difficult and often involves the advice of family members who are concerned about the older adult's ability to live alone safely. LTC residents are a vulnerable population who tend to have more chronic illnesses and may require advocacy from health or social professionals.

Persons in *assisted living* or *retirement homes* require some type of help with activities of daily living but require considerably much less care than those living in a nursing home. Data from the 2011 Canada Mortgage and Housing Corporation survey showed that 8.6% of Canadians (195,262) aged 75 years and older resided in assisted living facilities. Assisted living facilities provide autonomy for older adults, allowing them to live in a safe, home-like environment adapted for those with physical challenges. Assisted living provides personal space in the form of apartments or suites, meals through community dining, and transportation and social activities. A variety of amenities and services is available to the seniors. Some of the more popular services include 24-hour-call bell service, nursing services on site, transportation, exercise facilities, and movie theatres (Canada Mortgage and Housing Corporation, 2011). Required services can be purchased out of pocket, and rates vary depending on the level of services required and the type of accommodation desired. Assisted living centres may be found as freestanding facilities, as part of retirement communities, or attached to nursing homes to allow for smoother transition of care for those expected to need skilled nursing in the future.

CASE STUDY

www

Mrs. Saltano is an 89-year-old widow who lived alone for 2 years after her husband of 51 years died of colorectal cancer. For most of their lives Mr. and Mrs. Saltano lived in the same neighbourhood and in the same house where they raised their five children. Mrs. Saltano planned to stay in the family home after her husband's death, but she experienced bouts of loneliness and social isolation, despite being an active member of her local church before and after his death. She began to experience the effects of chronic illnesses, including having a bilateral knee replacement because of pain and decreased mobility from arthritis and taking more medications

(continues)

CASE STUDY   (Continued)

to control her high blood pressure and lower her cholesterol. With advancing age Mrs. Saltano also developed diabetes and some mild memory loss that her children found concerning. After one visit with the family at Christmas Mrs. Saltano's eldest daughter suggested that her mother explore the possibility of going to a retirement community designed for older adults.

Mrs. Saltano was absolutely opposed to leaving the home she had shared with her husband and where they had raised their family. She did not want to be in an "institution," as she called it, but she admitted to difficulty driving as a result of failing vision and said she did not feel safe living alone. Mrs. Saltano did consent to visit a nearby retirement community with two of her adult children and found that some old friends of hers who were also widowed were living there. Her friends seemed happy and active. The apartment she would have gave her privacy (and had its own kitchenette, refrigerator, and large bathroom) but also allowed the staff to check on her. Meals were served in a nice dining room with linen tablecloths and a formal menu, and a library, big screen TV, pool table, and exercise room were available. A beauty shop was on the premises, and transportation to doctors' offices and shopping was available for a nominal charge. Mrs. Saltano slowly warmed to the idea of moving to the continuous care retirement community, and so the arrangements were made. The quality of Mrs. Saltano's life improved significantly through socialization and activities in this new environment. Her adjustment to a change in living situation was facilitated by the attitudes of her children, the staff, and other residents.

Discussion Questions

1. What factors prompted Mrs. Saltano's children to encourage her to consider another living arrangement?
2. Was moving to a continuous care retirement community a prudent choice for Mrs. Saltano? Why or why not?
3. What problems and issues with adaptation to her new home is Mrs. Saltano likely to face?
4. What interventions might be helpful to assist with her adjustment?

Nursing homes, homes for the aged, and *special care homes* refer to facilities that provide skilled nursing services, personal care, and services such as meals, laundry, and housekeeping on a 24-hour basis. Nursing homes are LTC facilities for individuals with chronic illness, who are medically frail, or who are disabled. A number of facilities may include access to rehabilitation professionals or services for individuals who need assistance in reestablishing self-care abilities. Generally, the resident pays a copayment for this service, although some government subsidies may be available for those who qualify.

According to 2009–2010 data there were 2,136 LTC facilities for the aged in Canada, caring for 159,751 residents 65 years of age and older (Statistics Canada, 2011b). Of these, approximately 50% are for-profit and the rest are nonprofit facilities operated by municipal or provincial bodies or organizations having a religious affiliation.

Standards of Nursing Homes

There is a continued concern by those employed in LTC settings that facility structure and staffing are often based on minimal standards that contain costs instead of considering first what is desirable or needed for the client. However, as the baby boomer generation ages it is expected that its interest in this issue will influence the creation of higher standards, and quality of care may improve in LTC facilities.

Much of the care provided in the traditional nursing home setting is considered custodial care. Rehabilitative services are provided for those who have the capacity to regain function. Because the institutionalized individual may require a great deal of help with the physical aspects of care, such as bathing, dressing, eating, and space maintenance, the cognitive needs (emotional, psychological, and spiritual) may be considered less important. Activity programs are sometimes geared only toward one segment of the facility population. Care in LTC settings should include not only appropriate physical care but also appropriate social and cognitive stimulation.

LTC RECIPIENTS: A VULNERABLE POPULATION _____

Vulnerable individuals are those who are at increased risk for loss of autonomy, loss of self-will, injustice, loss of privacy, and increased risk for abuse. A vulnerable adult is defined as an individual who is either being mistreated or is in danger of mistreatment and who because of age and/or disability is unable to protect him- or herself (Teaster, 2002). A vulnerable individual can be described as one who has been judged by someone to be a nonperson. Examples of vulnerable persons in LTC may include those with physical, mental, or emotional problems; the elderly; those with dementia; and those who have been in prison. In a culture that values youth, energy, strength, and the ability to work, many devalue elders or those with chronic illness. Laws and practices differ between states in the areas of abuse, neglect, and protective services. Ultimately, it is the care providers and administrators in LTC who are responsible for maintaining an environment that supports the unique personhood of the client and protects the vulnerable.

Many individuals requiring LTC have already lost some autonomy and self-will because of illnesses that affect the individual's ability to make decisions or carry out intentional behaviour. Vulnerability is of special concern in these individuals. Decisions must be made for them regarding many aspects of life, such as eating, bathing, medication administration, socialization, and exercising religious practices. Some persons may benefit from the services of a guardian (discussed in the Substitute Decision-Making/Guardianship section).

Abuse in the home or in a residential facility is an extreme threat to the autonomy of the client. If the nurse providing care is the first to observe signs and symptoms of mistreatment, reporting these observations to management at the care facility is necessary. In the home the home healthcare nurse may be in a position to discover abuse and act as the primary advocate to prevent further abuse. The nurse may work with various agencies to ensure appropriate intervention is made. Because elder mistreatment is often subtle, the nurse must be persistent in reporting signs until action is taken. If abuse or neglect of the community-based client is profound, a move to residential care may be indicated.

PROBLEMS AND ISSUES IN LTC

There are a number of issues in LTC, ranging from overall system breakdown to individual treatment issues for clients in the system. The issues mentioned in this chapter are not an exhaustive list but can be considered an introduction to current problems.

Provision of Care

Along the continuum of LTC, problems in the provision of care include organization of services and access to care, gaps in public policy, funding, staffing, and standards of care. Specific issues vary within individual provinces or communities. It is imperative that the professional nurse involved in LTC is cognizant of the issues that affect delivery and quality of LTC services. Being a political activist to further the issues of the recipients of LTC is also important.

Gaps in Public Policy

In Canada the responsibility for paying for LTC services is usually shared between the provincial/territorial governments and the individual who needs those services. In an LTC facility the resident generally pays for accommodation costs. The amount of copayment varies across the country but generally is based on an assessment of the individual's income and means to pay (Canadian Healthcare Association, 2009). Additionally, some jurisdictions cover all drug and supply costs for residents in LTC facilities; however, in others the resident may need

to contribute out of pocket to cover these costs (Canadian Healthcare Association, 2009).

Partially because of the funding sources and partially because of the method of development of services, gaps exist in LTC services. Much policy work needs to be done related to transitions that individuals experience moving from one type of service to another because no overall umbrella of comprehensive care exists. The current healthcare reform effort is at least partially aimed at making transitions more seamless.

Funding

Gaps in service and public policy are both related to funding issues. In 2009, $17 billion of funding was spent on other institutional care, including facilities for the elderly (Canadian Institute of Health Information, 2009). Although these persons do not generally report difficulty obtaining medical care, 58% of those who need LTC report their needs as being unmet. This problem has led to additional consequences such as falls (Komisar, Feder, & Kasper, 2005). Private and nonprofit organizations also provide services for those in need of LTC. However, beyond the nursing home setting, piecing together a comprehensive LTC program for a frail elder with comorbidities who wishes to remain in the community is challenging. There are eligibility requirements for certain benefits, such as extended home care, as well as time limitations.

One view is that society has an obligation to provide for those in need, particularly the elderly, because of the labour and service they have provided (Tobin & Salisbury, 1999). Another view is that society is obligated to provide care for frail and chronically ill elders because of the sanctity of all human life and not simply because of work undertaken during the adult life. Philosophical origins play an important part not only in the establishment and continuation of programs but also in setting standards for ongoing programs.

Alternative financing for LTC needs to be explored. Although both PACE and social managed care plans offer alternatives to nursing homes and promote aging in place, it is evident that their scope and availability are significantly limited. In Arkansas, research revealed a need to expand health services because of unmet needs, suggesting policy recommendations to improve access to community-based care (Stewart, Felix, Dockter, Perry, & Morgan, 2006). In addition, a few strategies to fund LTC costs have arisen from the financial sector: reverse mortgages and life settlement. Both concepts focus on helping individuals liquidate assets (for example, a home or life insurance policy) to provide cash to privately pay to enter or remain in a facility (Feaster, 2006). Individuals considering this option should consult with a financial adviser.

Staffing and Quality of Care

Staffing in LTC facilities is mostly composed of unregulated healthcare providers commonly known as personal support workers. These individuals provide personal care for the residents such as assistance with eating, bathing, grooming, toileting, and ambulating. These unregulated healthcare providers are generally supervised by registered nursing staff or registered practical nurses (Canadian Healthcare Association, 2009).

One main issue associated with quality of care is the staffing in LTC facilities. Currently, there is no mandated minimum level of staffing. McGregor and Ronald (2011) purported that minimum staffing levels should be adopted in Canadian LTC facilities with a budget that can

only be used to provide direct nursing services. Furthermore, they suggested that information for staffing levels of LTC facilities and inspection reports should be easily accessible to the general public.

Given the acuity of the residents in LTC facilities today, there is a need for ongoing education to support the caregivers' abilities to meet the care demands of their residents. Currently, no standardized curriculum for personal support workers exists in Canada, leading to inconsistencies in the level of basic training required to work in the LTC homes. One recommendation is for the development of a consistent personal support workers curriculum for across Canada (Canadian Healthcare Association, 2009). Because most staff working in these facilities may be minimally trained personnel, client safety is a legitimate concern.

Staffing in nursing homes is also a continuing issue. There is conclusive evidence that a positive relationship exists between nursing staffing and quality of nursing home care. Fewer registered nurse and nursing assistant hours are associated with quality-of-care deficiencies (Arling, Kane, Mueller, Bershadsky, & Degenholtz, 2007; Harrington, Zimmerman, Karon, Robinson, & Beutel, 2000). The turnover rate for nursing assistants can be as high as 40% to 100% in some facilities. High turnover rates have been associated with poor quality care (Castle, Engberg, & Men, 2007). Recruitment and retention of qualified nursing assistants is an ongoing problem. Creating an environment that promotes teamwork, addresses care-related stressors, promotes positive communication, reduces paperwork inefficiencies and staffing shortages, and has high organizational morale has been shown to increase job satisfaction and commitment to the organization, but there are many other factors to consider in the complex process of staff turnover in these settings (American Association of Colleges of Nursing, 2011; Arling et al., 2007; Cherry, Ashcraft, & Owen, 2007; Donoghue & Castle, 2006; Sikorska-Simmons, 2006).

To complicate this situation, there is a projected shortage of healthcare professionals. In 2006 the average age of registered nurses in Canada was 45 years (Registered Nurses' Association of Ontario, 2009). The Canadian Nurses Association (2009) estimates that by 2022 there will be a shortage of at least 60,000 full-time equivalent registered nurses based on past healthcare trends, the retirement of nurses in the current workforce, and the aging nursing faculty.

Standards

The provinces and territories are responsible for the regulation and monitoring of LTC facilities. There is no mandated requirement across Canada for LTC facilities to participate in an external accreditation review. However, many LTC facilities do have an external review of their services conducted for quality assurance purposes. Once example is Accreditation Canada, a nonprofit organization that provides healthcare organizations such as LTC facilities with a peer review of the quality of services based on a set of standards of excellence. Their Qmentum Program has standards for LTC that focuses on quality improvement and patient safety (Accreditation Canada, n.d.). CARF Canada is another example of an accreditation body that provides an external review by an expert panel of practitioners for LTC homes and home care in Canada (CARF Canada, 2012).

Standards address issues such as nursing care hours per client, nursing assessments, care plans, accidents, fall prevention, prevention of pressure sores, use of physical restraints, nutrition, use of certain medications, and housekeeping services. In addition, facilities are to provide care for residents in a manner that maintains dignity and respect by providing grooming, appropriate dress, and promotion of independence in dining; allowing private space and property; and interacting respectfully. For example, nursing staff must not perform any invasive assessment or task in a public area but should take the resident to his or her room for procedures such as listening to lung sounds or checking a glucometer reading.

Harrington, Carrillo, Blank, and O'Brian (2010) pointed out that quality of care provided in nursing homes has long been a matter of great concern to consumers, professionals, and policymakers. If the regulation and inspection process is ignored, LTC residents may suffer. Some provinces such as Ontario have posted deficiency reports on the provincial website. The registered nurse is at times required to act as an advocate for the residents and to ensure compliance with minimal standards.

ETHICAL ISSUES IN LTC

Individuals who are chronically ill or frail are a vulnerable population often at the mercy of the caregivers in the LTC system. Healthcare professionals in LTC should have a solid understanding of the ethics involved in this type of care. Principles upon which decisions should be made include autonomy, nonmaleficence, beneficence, and justice (Beauchamp & Childress, 2009; Jonsen, 2007). The manner in which these principles are executed in the professional nurse–client relationship can make a visible difference in the quality of life of the

LTC resident. Some of the more common ethical issues are discussed herein.

Client Autonomy Versus Dependence

One principle of critical importance in LTC is autonomy. Healthcare professionals and caregivers should observe the particularly essential rule of bioethics: respect the autonomy of persons (Jonsen, 2007). Autonomy is sometimes misapplied or ignored (Kane, Freeman, Caplan, Aroskar, & Urv-Wong, 1990). It is possible for an individual to gradually lose increments of his or her autonomy because of limitations imposed by sensory deprivation, immobility, weakness, and cognitive impairment (Mezey, Mitty, & Ramsey, 1997). Research suggests that even frail elderly individuals who are homebound have a greater sense of personal control than those in nursing homes (Crain, 2001), making those living in facilities at greater risk for loss of decision making and independence. Loss of autonomy and development of excess disability are a problem for many LTC clients.

Excess Disability

Disability in excess of what is attributable to a chronic condition is often an unwanted consequence of care (Slaughter, Eliasziw, Morgan, & Drummond, 2009). It suggests a dependence of a resident on a caregiver to perform a task the client has the ability to perform. This phenomenon is a significant problem in the LTC setting. Depression, learned helplessness, and changes in sensorium contribute to increased dependence on caregivers. Caregivers may be unintentional contributors to excess disability. Providing unnecessary assistance or an inappropriate type of assistance can contribute to residents' dependency. "Factors influencing excess disability include: a desire of the caregiver to be helpful; lack of knowledge and skill of the caregiver; and lack of time and staff" (Remsburg & Carson, 2006, p. 584). An example of excess disability is dressing assistance provided to nursing home residents. Aides often do the dressing activities for residents to save time instead of allowing the residents to perform the activity at their own pace (Beck et al., 1997). This action moves the resident toward unnecessary and unwanted dependence.

Custodial Care

Using basic ethical principles, an issue arises whether providing minimal physical care for those with chronic illness is acceptable versus providing more comprehensive care extending beyond custodial physical care. This is particularly challenging in a residential LTC environment. As a result of regulation, funding, and staffing patterns for residential facilities the goal inadvertently becomes custodial care.

Physical issues of the resident are important, but those issues should not be the only focus. Mental health needs should also be considered in the chronically ill and elderly populations. With limited attention to these needs, the client is at risk of suffering boredom, anxiety, and, consequently, depression. In a 2004 study of LTC home residents from five provinces 44% of the residents experienced depression or some signs and symptoms of depression (Canadian Institute for Health Information, 2010).

Appropriate referral is a responsibility of the nurse who detects symptoms of emotional difficulties. Signs of depression include feeling nervous, empty, guilty, tired, restless, irritable, and unloved, and that life is not worth living.

Physical symptoms associated with mental health problems include eating more or less than normal, sleep disturbances, headaches, stomachaches, and an increase in chronic pain (Varcarolis & Halter, 2010). The risk of depression in the elderly increases with the presence of chronic illness and a loss of physical function (National Institute of Mental Health, 2010). If symptoms of depression are present in an LTC client, services are available to provide assistance.

End-of-Life Decision Making

Difficult and complex decisions at end of life are an inherent component of LTC. Many older adults lack the resources, or lack knowledge of the available resources, that could help with decision making at end of life. Although most older adults are approached about completing written documents to outline treatment preferences, many choose not to do so. Making one's wishes known in the event of terminal illness or incapacity is one approach to preserving autonomy for the older adult. Family issues may impact the elder's willingness to do this.

In the provinces and territories in Canada, an older person can make his or her wishes known by completing an advance directive for care, although the exact terminology may vary from one jurisdiction to another (Dunbrack, 2006). Basically, the individual can make his or her wishes for the following care decisions known:

- Who should make healthcare decisions for the person if he or she cannot
- The kind of medical treatment the person wants and does not want
- How comfortable the person wishes to be made

- How the person wants others to treat him or her
- What the person wants loved ones to know

Cultural and religious beliefs play an important part in end-of-life decision making. Some religions dictate that everything should be done to preserve life, whereas others support allowing natural death. For example, African Americans are generally opposed to placing a loved one in a nursing home, preferring family members to die at home. Healthcare professionals should familiarize themselves with the major traditions and practices of their clients so that culturally appropriate care can be provided.

In a study of older community-dwelling adults (with a mean of 80.7 years of age), a durable power of attorney for health care had been completed by 60.8% of respondents before death. However, a startling finding of this research was that persons with lower levels of cognitive functioning were less likely to have completed an advance directive than those older adults with higher cognitive functioning (McGuire, Rao, Anderson, & Ford, 2007). This research underscores the need for healthcare professionals to address advance directives with persons while they are capable of expressing their end-of-life wishes.

Abuse and Neglect of Vulnerable Adults

It is estimated that between 4% and 10% of Canadian seniors experience some type of abuse (Government of Canada, 2007). Police records show that in 2009 nearly 7,900 seniors were victims of violent crime. Of those, approximately one-third were committed by one of the victim's family members (Statistics Canada, 2011c). However, the actual incidence is hard to estimate because the data presented may underestimate the true extent of violence against seniors as many cases are not reported to the police (Statistics Canada, 2011b). It is believed that cases of abuse, neglect, or exploitation are grossly underreported because of fear, intimidation, lack of sound research, or other factors. Nursing home residents are particularly vulnerable to being victims of abuse (Lindbloom, Brandt, Hough, & Meadows, 2007).

Abuse can be categorized as domestic or institutional. Within these categories physical, sexual, and emotional/psychological abuse may occur as well as neglect, self-neglect, abandonment, and financial exploitation (National Center for Elder Abuse, 2011). Because of longer life expectancies for those with chronic illness, it is very likely that the incidence of abuse will increase (Teaster, 2002). The individual with chronic illness, if cognitively competent, may be hesitant to discuss the mistreatment because he or she fears the loss of the relationship or other reprisal by the perpetrator. If the individual is not capable of expressing information regarding the abuse, identification may be by forensic evidence. Physical abuse is the actual assault of an individual, and evidence exists with the presence of unexplained bruises, fractures, cuts, or burns in various stages of healing. Sexual abuse also falls within this category. The victim of such treatment is in danger and requires immediate advocacy. Physical abuse often escalates from neglect or other forms of abuse. Perpetrators often share similar characteristics such as lack of social support, history of being an abuse victim, and mental or emotional problems.

Neglect is defined as the lack of provision of basic necessities, such as food, water, and medical care. Neglect may be evidenced by poor hygiene, malnutrition or dehydration, pressure ulcers, and reports of being left in an unsafe condition or being left without resources to obtain necessary medications. Neglect can take place because of wilful intention or because home management has become overwhelming to the client's aging spouse or family. This type of abuse may be seen more frequently in homes where the caregiver lacks the knowledge or resources to provide care. Neglect can include self-neglect, which is defined as an individual losing the will or the ability to properly care for him- or herself. Abandonment is the extreme form of neglect.

The third type of elder abuse, exploitation, is defined as the use of an elder's resources without knowledge or consent for the gain of another. Signs of elder exploitation include the disappearance of monetary resources or the "taking over" of personal belongings without permission or consent (Fulmer, 1999). Financial abuse in the form of fraud or deception may also be considered exploitation and may come through family members who borrow money with no intention to repay it or from mail fraud schemes that attempt to cheat persons out of money by promising prizes and rewards.

In Canada the Criminal Code has laws that address elder abuse and neglect. In addition, the provinces and territories have structures in place that deal with protection of adults, human rights, and regulation of LTC facilities (Government of Canada, 2007). Currently, in Canada there is no mandatory reporting of elder abuse. Two provinces, Nova Scotia and Newfoundland, have some reporting requirements in their adult protection legislation (Canadian Network for the Prevention of Elder Abuse, 2011). Other provinces, for example Alberta and Manitoba, have specific reporting requirements for people in care homes, and Ontario has legislation in the Nursing Home Act that stipulates an individual who suspects a nursing resident is suffering from any type of harm or neglect is required to report his or her concerns to the administrator of the nursing home (Canadian Network for the Prevention of Elder Abuse, 2011).

INTERVENTIONS

Theoretical Frameworks for Practice

Using a theoretical framework to plan and implement nursing care in an LTC setting helps the nurse to avoid doing things simply "because they have always been done that way." Nurses draw from the sciences and use physiological theory, pharmacological theory, and theories of communication, change, caring, grief and bereavement, and ethics. A theoretical framework explains or guides one's practice. Mid-range theories are those defined as specific to particular caregiving situations and that have measurable outcomes. Theoretical frameworks give direction in the choice of interventions so that nursing care is tailored to each client.

Several middle-range frameworks are appropriate for LTC. The needs-driven dementia-compromised behavior model can assist the care professional in understanding how to better interact with dementia clients (Algase et al., 1996). This model hypothesizes that problematic behaviours in dementia clients are a result of needs that, when identified, can be addressed by the care provider, thereby avoiding a crisis. Such frameworks are helpful in assisting the care provider in solving problems encountered in the clinical area when dealing with LTC clients (Mitty & Flores, 2007a; Peterson & Bredow, 2004).

Any number of other mid-range theories may help enlighten the nurse's perspective on the LTC client and guide the planning of care. Examples include Kolcaba's (2003) theory of comfort, which can help nurses understand the importance of comfort and the need for relief of problematic symptoms and achievement of ease in the patient's daily life; the theory of unpleasant symptoms (Gift, 2004; originally developed by Lenz, Suppe, Gift, Pugh, & Milligan in 1995) also gives insight into a paradigm of understanding the challenges faced by those with chronic illness. Eakes (2004), building on previous researchers' work in the theory of chronic sorrow, discusses clients facing the loss of interpersonal relationships as well as physical functioning. These theories and others are available to the healthcare provider working in LTC.

Admission and Assessment in the LTC Setting

Admission to a nursing home can be very distressing to anyone. From the individual's perspective the move to a nursing home or even assisted living away from his or her personal home may symbolize the reality of the loss of health, autonomy, personal relationships, economic power, productivity, and independence. Adjustment to such facilities may evoke a mix of emotions. The stress of going into a facility in which one is surrounded by strangers can be difficult. In addition, the individual must adjust to schedules determined by others, instead of following routines established throughout a lifetime. In many nursing homes eating and bathing schedules are relatively fixed. Although not ideal, the resident is often the one who must change expectations to make allowance for the workload of the nursing home staff.

The decision to move to a nursing home is usually made after much consideration by the client and family. The transition may be made more smoothly when the client retains as much participation in the process as possible. The client should be encouraged to have input into choosing the facility and in planning the move. Retention of personal items gives the individual a better sense of self in the new facility. Admission to a nursing home may be one of the most traumatic life transitions. The nurse needs to assist in making the adjustment of the client to the facility as smooth as possible. The client experiencing psychological and emotional difficulty during the admission and transition into any LTC facility needs support from the attending nursing staff. The use of therapeutic communication techniques by the staff in addition to spending adequate time with a transitioning resident can make a difference in the level of anxiety and stress experienced. If indicated, the nurse should initiate a referral for the resident to be seen by mental health services. These services are generally an underused resource for elders.

Accessing community-based LTC services may seem a natural and necessary transition for an elder needing help with either rehabilitation or assistance with other aspects of care. For others, accessing services may create significant emotional turmoil. Once a frail elder can no longer stay in the community environment, the individual and family may decide that a move to another environment that provides needed services is necessary. For those who can afford assisted living, this option may be less emotionally traumatic. Individuals believe they have retained a great deal of autonomy while paying for the services they can no longer perform, such as food preparation, laundry, housekeeping, and medication management.

An accurate assessment of the client is the critical beginning for the client's experience in the LTC system. During the admission process to an LTC facility the care provider will complete a battery of paperwork that documents the client's condition and reason for admission. In residential nursing homes this assessment is important because it provides the basis upon which the care plan is developed and helps set the course for interventions designed to promote the highest level of functioning possible. It is imperative that the admission process not be limited to completing paperwork but includes gaining insight into the client to provide individualized care.

The Resident Assessment Instrument (RAI 2.0) is one example of the InterRAI instruments used in eight provinces and jurisdictions in Canada. Collectively, these instruments provide a standardized method of collecting patient data for the purposes of development of care planning that is specific to the individual's needs and can be used to track changes in clinical status (Hirdes, Mitchell, Maxwell, & White, 2011). In addition, the information collected is stored in a national databank that can be used for benchmarking outcomes across Canada. The RAI 2.0 used in nursing homes measures such items as functional levels, cognition levels, pain levels, behavioural changes, and levels of social engagement (Hirdes et al., 2011). Assessment is typically conducted within 14 days of admission and then quarterly for the remainder of the resident's stay. This information also helps in tracking the improvement or decline of a resident over time and whether or not quality indicators for care are being met. In the initial or follow-up assessment the assessment protocol summarizes vulnerable aspects of the client's life that may require special care planning, interventions, and reporting of progress or problems in the resident's chart.

Other assessment tools are available and can provide more specific or multidimensional information. Tools can help the nurse determine functioning in cognitive, communication, behavioural, and social support domains. Other instruments measure vision, personality, depression, affect, comorbidity, and quality of life (Teresi & Evans, 1997). Examples of individual tools that are readily available in the literature include the Katz index of activities of daily living (Katz, Downs, Cash, & Grotz, 1970), Older American resources and services (Fillenbaum, 1988), the Beck depression rating scale (Beck, Rush, Shaw, & Emery, 1979), and the Arthritis Impact Measurement Scales (Meenan, 1985).

A helpful website with a list of more than 30 assessment tools that can be downloaded for immediate use is http://hartfording.org/Practice/ConsultGeriRN/. For each assessment tool in the *Try This* series from the American Association of Colleges of Nursing/Hartford Foundation, explanation of the tool by an expert, validity and reliability information, the tool itself, and how to use it are succinctly provided.

Preservation of Autonomy of the Person

Healthcare professionals dealing with clients in LTC should carefully consider their own position as a moral force. Making decisions with a moral component is a part of everyday practice for most nurses. Understanding the concepts that provide the moral foundation for human existence is important. Those concepts typically include the following: autonomy, nonmaleficence, beneficence, justice, and professional–patient relationships (Beauchamp & Childress,

2009). Autonomy is in the forefront in LTC, and the concept is rooted in the idea of self-rule and independent decision making.

Autonomy

The role of the nurse in providing LTC along the continuum of care is to preserve the autonomy of the client. At the same time the client must be protected from harm. Balancing these issues is not always easy. The care provider should not assume because an individual has lost some physical autonomy, such as requiring personal assistance with daily hygiene, that the individual has given up his or her autonomy or is incapable of making his or her own decisions. Promotion of autonomy is accomplished by allowing the individual to make as many decisions as possible. In decisions that can impact health or health care, the nurse must provide the appropriate information to enable the client to make an informed decision. To more fully understand the concept of autonomy, the caregiver is encouraged to think about autonomy from the client's perspective when making caregiving decisions.

Individual decision making is a complex and multifaceted issue. Loss of decision-making capacity in one area does not indicate loss of all decision-making capacity. Decision-making capacity may fluctuate through the course of an illness, and determining the best approach to preserving safety and autonomy concurrently is important in order to incorporate client preferences. An example is a client's bathing twice a week as opposed to more frequent bathing. In that case the nurse might alter other interactions, such as frequency of spot baths or application of lotion to ensure skin integrity, while respecting the autonomy of the client.

Substitute Decision-Maker/Guardianship

Canadian laws are based on the assumption that one is "mentally capable" of making decisions about property, planning documents, and health care including admission to LTC facilities (Law Commission of Ontario, 2009). It is helpful for an individual to identify a substitute decision-maker in advance in the event that the individual is unable to make informed decisions for him- or herself because of a cognitive or other health problem. The substitute decision-maker may be a family member, a friend, or other, and the responsibility is to ensure safety and quality care for the person and to make decisions in the person's best interest. In complex cases involving large estates, difficult family relationships, or where there is no other substitute decision-maker, the court may choose to appoint a guardian who will assist in making legal decisions for the incompetent person. The appointment of a guardian by the court usually follows the legal determination of incapacity. The person who has been declared to be an incapacitated person is then no longer able to make any type of contractual decision independently. The guardian of the person is responsible for getting to know the person sufficiently to be able to make decisions in his or her best interest, to provide documentation to the court as needed on the status of the person, and may be responsible for a variety of tasks ranging from healthcare advocacy to managing finances to ensuring that daily care needs are being met. Different jurisdictions have varying rules, and guardians may be paid a small fee for their services.

In cases where the person has been legally deemed unable to make his or her own decisions, the designated substitute decision-maker or guardian must be informed of all important aspects of the person's life and is responsible for making decisions that are in the person's best interest, that is, on his or her behalf or at his or her behest. When a person has lost some degree of autonomy, the nurse must also act in a judicious way that protects the individual from harm or exploitation.

It is also possible for someone who has legally lost autonomy (been declared incompetent) to continue to participate in the decision-making process. For example, a person with early stage dementia may have a substitute decision-maker or guardian who is ultimately responsible for decision making in the person's best interest. However, as much as the person is able, the substitute decision-maker or guardian should involve the person in the decision-making process, seeking input and finding out the wishes of the person before taking any action. This kind of consideration can contribute significantly to quality of life for the LTC resident.

Decision making or autonomy can be viewed on a continuum. An example of this might be when a person with advanced dementia decides to walk the halls. Autonomous decision making in a small way is appropriate as long as other principles, such as the client's safety and the safety of others, are considered. It is the nurse's responsibility to recognize an individual's capacity for autonomy and preserve that capacity as much as possible (Casada da Rocha, 2009). Sometimes, the nurse must compromise what he or she perceives to be the best treatment. To preserve the autonomy of persons as long as possible, the substitute decision-maker or guardian should encourage as much participation as possible in decision making, while keeping in mind the goal of safety and quality care for the incapacitated person.

Enablement

The enablement process is defined as a professional intervention aiming to recognize, support, and emphasize the patient's capacity to have control over his or her health and life (Hudson, St. Cyr Tribble, Bravo, & Poitras, 2011). Enablement may even be appropriate for those with cognitive impairment (Dawson, Wells, & Kline, 1993). This perspective focuses on how the disease affects the client's ability to carry out day-to-day activities. The purpose of this intervention is to determine the client's existing abilities and to enhance those abilities. Three areas of human behaviour considered by this approach are self-care, social interaction, and interpretive abilities.

In the area of self-care, when the client is having difficulty achieving purposeful behaviours, certain nursing interventions can assist the caregiver in enhancing the client's abilities. These include object cueing, touch, direct physical assistance, and verbal prompting (Dawson et al., 1993). When a client with dementia loses many of the skills required for daily activity, there is the possibility of retention of some significant skill or pleasure, such as a music-related activity or game playing. The nurse should help preserve those abilities as much as possible by providing opportunities for their expression. Having a time to play cards or a music hour is often very meaningful to residents in LTC.

Advocacy: Role of the Ombudsman

Given that the responsibility for health care including LTC falls under the jurisdiction of the provinces and territories, the reporting of issues and complaints process varies across the country. In most provinces except for Ontario and New Brunswick (Ontario Ombudsman, 2012) the Ombudsman office is also able to investigate complaints about nursing home and LTC facilities. Ontario has a provincial hotline in place for individuals who wish to register a complaint about an issue in an LTC facility.

Nursing Care

Nursing care is the primary service provided by residential LTC facilities. The further one progresses along the LTC continuum, the more intense are the nursing care needs. Nursing care in LTC settings is much more complex than it has been in the past and requires greater knowledge and expertise on the part of the nursing staff to manage comorbidities and provide high-quality care to all residents.

Care that nurses provide in LTC facilities should be holistic and multidimensional. Approximately 40% of patients in LTC settings were 85 years of age and older in 2009–2010 (Statistics Canada, 2011b). Because most persons in LTC settings are older, nurses would benefit from education in gerontology. Yet the gerontological content in many Canadian nursing programs does not adequately prepare nurses to care for the complex needs of this population (Baumbusch & Andrusyszen, 2002; McCleary, McGilton, Boscart, & Oudshoorn, 2009). In the United States the American Association of Colleges of Nursing, with funding from the Hartford Foundation, has released a set of standards outlining geriatric content for inclusion in the baccalaureate educational process for nurses; each program should periodically review and update the curriculum to stay current and prepare expert nurses for practice (Thornlow, Latimer, Kingsborough, & Arietti, 2006).

Pain Management

It is important for the nurse in LTC to adequately assess pain and to provide adequate treatment of that pain (Fink & Gates, 2010). Of particular importance is assessing clients' suffering from the pain associated with arthritis, osteoporosis, or neuralgia. A great deal of information is available on appropriate pain management strategies, and the nurse dealing with such clients should access this body of literature. When implementing pain management strategies in the LTC setting, follow-up is critical. Pain relief varies for many reasons, and pain might not be relieved by a method that had previously been successful for the client. When pain is chronic and affects the ability of the client to function, current treatment strategies include routine regular administration of medication to manage the pain. Breakthrough pain, or pain experienced intermittently when a client is on routine pain medication, is then treated with "as-needed" medication. Addiction is not generally considered to be a major problem for elders suffering from chronic pain, but tolerance can become problematic.

For individuals unable to verbally express pain, its presence is noted in other ways. Evidence of pain may include facial expression (grimacing), groaning, body position, bracing, guarding, and rubbing of the painful body part. Alternative methods of dealing with pain should be considered. Massage, heat, cold, and support mechanisms such as knee or back braces may be helpful. The quality of life of the LTC client can be greatly affected by pain. With current advances in pharmacology and treatment most pain can be managed effectively.

End-of-life care requires an intense management of comfort levels. If the individual is suffering intractable pain, use of palliative sedation may be necessary. Guidelines for such aggressive symptom management must be accessed through a process of evidence-informed practice to ensure the most appropriate approach is used (Melnyk & Fineout-Overholt, 2010).

Disease Prevention and Health Promotion

Although it may be impossible to prevent some of the chronic diseases seen in the LTC population, others are certainly preventable. An important preventive health measure is the provision of flu and pneumonia vaccines to LTC residents. A vaccination program in residential facilities is essential and usually mandated by public health guidelines; in such settings infections such as influenza can spread rapidly and cause death among the frail elderly. These types of infections may affect a number of residents at one time and place a difficult burden on staff to deal with a number of acutely ill clients. Admission of clients to acute care settings in such circumstances is not unreasonable to ensure that all clients receive adequate nursing care during an outbreak of illness.

The National Strategy for Investing in Healthy Aging for Seniors focused on five areas that are considered to promote healthy aging in older adults: social connectedness, physical activity, healthy eating, falls prevention, and tobacco control (Healthy Aging and Wellness Working Group of the Federal/Provincial/Territorial [F/P/T] Committee of Officials [Seniors], 2006). One study of assisted living residents found that "social support is a key variable in bolstering residents' psychological well-being" (Cummings, 2002, p. 300). Thus, health promotion, even for those with existing chronic illness, emphasizes the same important strategies that healthcare professionals should encourage in LTC residents.

Cognitive Impairment

Individuals in LTC may suffer cognitive impairment from a variety of pathological processes. These processes may be either acute or chronic. Individuals with cognitive impairment caused by irreversible causes such as closed head injuries, stroke, or dementia from a number of pathological processes such as Alzheimer's disease, multi-infarct dementia, or Lewy body disease often need special assistance to manage activities of daily living. Individuals in LTC who have cognitive impairment caused by an acute condition (delirium) need to receive immediate intervention to reverse the cause of the impairment before permanent disability or death results.

The first and foremost consideration in dealing with cognitively impaired individuals is to determine whether the cognitive impairment is caused by delirium or dementia. Even an individual who has a diagnosis of dementia may experience a sudden change in cognition with an acute cause. Appropriate assessment of the condition can prevent unnecessary suffering or death.

Delirium is an acute condition brought on by one or more conditions that have altered brain functioning. The chief symptoms include sudden disturbance in consciousness and/or cognition. The underlying condition can be a single factor or a combination of conditions, which include but are not limited to fever, infection, allergic reaction, malnutrition, vitamin deficiency, drug toxicity (over the counter or prescription), drug interactions, food supplement toxicity, hyper- or hypoglycaemia, and hypoxia (Tullman, Mion,

Fletcher, & Foreman, 2008). The underlying condition can be life threatening and must be corrected or the incident may result in death. If the nurse providing care in the LTC setting determines that a client is suffering from delirium, it may be necessary to arrange transportation to an acute care facility where appropriate emergent care can be provided. In addition to these physiological processes, cognitive impairment can be brought about by psychosocial factors such as depression, change in health brought on by aging or disease, or change in location such as a move from a long-time home to live with another family member or a move to an institutionalized setting. The nurse assessing the patient should consider these possibilities to provide appropriate interventions.

Because of the physiological changes that occur with aging, the signs of delirium in a frail elder may develop over a period of days as a subclinical condition worsens to a crisis point. In addition, in a patient who has a complicated medication regimen, symptoms of increased confusion may initially be mild. The astute nurse will make the appropriate observations to detect delirium even when the symptoms are subtle. In a client population with fluctuating cognition, such as at many residential facilities, detection of delirium becomes more challenging.

Dementia differs from delirium in that the condition is chronic and the underlying pathological process is progressive and irreversible. An estimated 500,000 Canadians suffer from Alzheimer's disease or a related dementia (Alzheimer Society of Canada, 2010). In addition, it is estimated that between 40% and 80% of those living in nursing homes have a cognitive impairment (Centers for Disease Control and Prevention, 2009). Dementia is defined as the development of multiple cognitive deficits manifested by memory impairment and other problems, such as aphasia (inability to speak), apraxia (loss of ability to use familiar objects or carry out purposeful movements not caused by loss of sensory ability), and agnosia (loss of ability to determine the significance of sensory input, such as recognition of a familiar face or voice) (American Psychiatric Association, 2000). Primary dementias have no cure, and although a large investment is being made in drugs that could affect the progression of disease, outcomes of pharmacological interventions have shown varying levels of success.

Approximately 55% of dementia care is delivered in the home by a family caregiver with some type of community support (Alzheimer Society of Canada, 2010). In the community LTC setting the role of the nurse is to support the family caregiver with problem solving or identifying resources such as respite care, adult day care, or the local chapter of the Alzheimer Society. The nurse may play a key role in the decision making that takes place when caregiving for a demented loved one is negatively affecting the health of the spousal caregiver (Maas et al., 2004). When caregiving becomes overwhelming at home, the decision to place the individual with dementia in a residential facility is appropriate.

Periodic evaluation of individuals with chronic cognitive changes is necessary so that decline can be detected and care strategies adjusted. Many nurses working in the LTC setting rely on intuitive detection of cognitive changes, but this method can be improved by the inclusion of an objective measure of cognition such as the mini mental status exam (Folstein, Folstein, & McHugh, 1975) or the dementia rating scale (Alexopoulos & Mattis, 1991). Use of one or more of these instruments can provide data to track changes in cognitive functioning.

Nursing interventions that deal with dementia generally address one or more of three symptom domains: cognitive, functional, and/or behavioural. All clients with dementia demonstrate functional difficulties, whereas only some demonstrate behavioural problems. Dealing with individuals suffering from permanent cognitive impairment takes patience and understanding. It is important that the caregiver not lose sight of the client's perspective. It is more important to validate the client's personhood rather than to insist that he or she achieve "reality orientation." The client may find comfort in some behaviour, such as carrying a doll, and this behaviour, although not grounded in immediate reality, is grounded in the reality of a universal human behaviour regarding caring for others, specifically infants. An evidence-informed practice approach should be used in structuring care and the environment in LTC facilities responsible for patients with dementia. This ensures the patient benefits from the latest research findings regarding best practice in dementia care.

The nurse needs to work closely with the activity director to meet the needs of the clients and to find appropriate and enjoyable activities for those with dementia. The activity director is responsible for providing activities for residents; individuals at different stages of dementia enjoy different types of activities. Those with mild dementia may still enjoy activities requiring personal interaction and following rules such as games or group singing. Those with more advanced dementia may enjoy more isolated activities such as the opportunity to fold laundry or a task related to food preparation.

Many nursing homes and even some assisted-living centres have special care units for dementia clients. The environment in such settings allows for safe wandering. Ideally, the staff has received training specific to caring for clients with dementia. The units are generally set up with consideration given to lighting, colour, noise levels, congregate areas, and room setups. Such considerations are used to make the environment more pleasant for the residents. Again, an evidence-informed practice approach will ensure that the latest research findings are incorporated into the caring regimen.

CASE STUDY   `www`

Mr. Havlin is a 92-year-old man who resides in an Alzheimer's special care unit that is part of a nursing home. Mr. Havlin's prior occupation was as a union labourer, where he worked with his hands to help build bridges and roads. Before being diagnosed with dementia he lived at home with his wife, who died recently. The couple had no children and no other close relatives living in the area. Mr. Havlin's neighbours became concerned when he did not answer the door, had fallen several times at home, and appeared confused when they visited. Eventually, a community social worker became involved in his care, and a guardian was appointed for Mr. Havlin because of lack of available family members willing to assume this job.

Mr. Havlin spends much of his time wandering the halls on the Alzheimer's unit and sometimes displays combative, aggressive behaviour. The nursing staff members try to get Mr. Havlin more involved in group activities such as playing games and doing art projects, but his behaviour becomes agitated at these attempts.

Discussion Questions

1. Is it necessary for Mr. Havlin to be involved in group activities such as games and music therapy? What are the benefits or drawbacks to insisting on his involvement in these types of activities?
2. Is Mr. Havlin's wandering a common problem for persons with dementia? How is this best handled by the nursing staff?
3. Describe what types of therapeutic activities might be most appropriate for Mr. Havlin, considering his occupation and history.

Risk Reduction and Safety

One of the most important functions of the nurse in an LTC setting is to reduce risk and ensure client safety. In a community setting part of the home assessment includes a thorough examination of the environment to detect possible hazards and correct them. The most obvious hazards include throw rugs, electrical cords strung across traffic areas, stairs (especially those without handrails), loose tiles in the shower, slick flooring, small pets, and similar environmental conditions. In residential settings the nurse has similar responsibilities to ensure client safety. Facilities should provide a safe environment with adaptations for those with chronic health problems that would place them at higher risk for injuries or falls.

Safe patient handling has become an important issue in best nursing practice. Organized safety programs have been linked to positive outcomes for both patients and staff (Nelson, 2006; Nelson, Collins, Siddharthan, Matz, & Waters, 2008). Researchers found that implementing a safe patient-handling program in an LTC through the Veterans Administration system resulted in better quality of patient care for residents. Safe-handling programs included four key interventions: appropriate patient-handling equipment and devices, assessment protocols, safe lifting policies, and patient lift teams. Key areas of change for residents after implementation of the program were improved physical functioning, decreased sedentary states of residents, less deterioration in activities of daily living, decreased fall rate, and increased wakeful states in the mornings (Nelson et al., 2008).

Another important safety consideration is the use of restraints. Falls are a significant problem in LTC, and of persons who fall, 20% to 30% suffer significant injuries such as hip fractures (Cowley, Deibold, Gross, & Hardin-Fanning, 2006). Originally, restraints were thought to prevent injury to clients and were applied to ensure patient safety through limiting movement. Research has demonstrated, however, that restraints do the opposite and are likely to cause injury (Lekan-Rutledge, 1997). The Registered Nurses' Association of Ontario developed clinical practice guidelines that outline a list of alternatives to restraint use that is available for downloading (Registered Nurses'

Association of Ontario, 2012). The provinces are responsible for regulating restraint use in LTC facilities.

Exercise has emerged as the "most effective factor in reducing the risk of falls and injuries from falls" (Mitty & Flores, 2007b, p. 349). All LTC facilities should have an exercise plan and program available to residents. The ideal environment for LTC residents is restraint free, with environmental and staffing accommodations made to meet the needs of each resident and promote optimum physical functioning through exercise, adequate nutrition, and safety.

PALLIATIVE AND HOSPICE CARE

The World Health Organization defined palliative care as follows (2008, paragraph 1):

> An approach that improves the quality of life of patients and their families facing the problem associated with life-threatening illness, through the prevention and relief of suffering by means of early identification and impeccable assessment and treatment of pain and other problems, physical, psychosocial and spiritual.

The goal of this care is not curative but centres around comfort. It is both a philosophy of care as well as a treatment system, and not necessarily just for those considered terminally ill. In palliation, physiological needs are met and aggressive measures are taken for pain relief. A holistic view of the client should be maintained, and the personhood of the client is of primary consideration in this type of nursing care. Palliative care may be used in conjunction with life-prolonging care.

For adults, the World Health Organization described the goals of palliative care as follows (2008, paragraph 2):

- Provides relief from pain and other distressing symptoms
- Affirms life and regards dying as a normal process
- Intends neither to hasten nor postpone death
- Integrates the psychological and spiritual aspects of patient care
- Offers a support system to help patients live as actively as possible until death
- Offers a support system to help the family cope during the patient's illness and in their own bereavement
- Uses a team approach to address the needs of patients and their families, including bereavement counselling, if indicated
- Will enhance quality of life and may also positively influence the course of illness
- Is applicable early in the course of illness, in conjunction with other therapies that are intended to prolong life, such as chemotherapy or radiation therapy, and includes those investigations needed to better understand and manage distressing clinical complications

A person with chronic illness may benefit from palliative care services and yet not qualify for hospice. Palliative care services may be delivered in the hospital, at home by home care staff, in an LTC facility, or sometimes in a hospice that is a residential stand-alone building. Regardless of where palliative care is rendered, usually a team of trained professionals addresses the needs of the patient and the entire family. Depending on the jurisdiction many provincial plans will cover some of the costs

associated with palliative care, but in LTC facilities the residents are usually required to pay for some of these services. In the terminal phase of life appropriate care includes pain relief, comfort, and emotional and spiritual support for the client and family (Tarzian, 2000). The client and family can be referred for grief counselling related to the experience of incurable illness (Ferrell & Coyle, 2010). Death is a natural part of life, and the nurse should be prepared to facilitate the client's end-of-life transition and provide support to the family survivors (DeSpelder & Strickland, 2011).

RESEARCH IN LTC

The science of caring for those who have chronic illness is changing rapidly. Andersen and Horvath (2004) reported that 85% of seniors and 45% of the working adult population have at least one chronic illness. This growing burden of care for long-term health problems accounts for 78% of the nation's healthcare spending. Research often begins with clinical observations of problems or recurring events that require solutions. A number of Canadian nurse researchers have focused research programs on dealing with chronic illness and issues related to care of the elderly (e.g., Wendy Duggleby, Sandra Hirst, and Katherine McGilton). Nurses in a clinical role should take the opportunity to define a problem and propose a solution. A novice researcher may partner with a more experienced researcher to develop an idea into a researchable question. Local chapters of Sigma Theta Tau, the Honor Society of Nursing, are available to provide assistance.

As the body of literature grows, more opportunity for implementation of evidence-informed practice and translational research exists. The Registered Nurses' Association of Ontario has several evidence-informed practice guidelines on a variety of subjects pertinent to the elderly, including pain management and end-of-life care. These guidelines can be found at www .rnao.org/Page.asp?PageID=1212&SiteNodeID =155&BL_ExpandID=.

SUMMARY

Simple medical models are rarely sufficient to address desired outcomes for those with complicated chronic medical conditions (Mold, 1995). It is not sufficient to consider the quality of life based on absence of sickness, but one must consider the overall well-being of the client. Outcomes will vary along the LTC continuum. For community-based clients the overall outcome may be to remain in their homes as long as possible. Interventions to support that outcome may include client and family teaching on medication management, safety issues, or wound care. Rehabilitation may be a desired outcome for a community-based client after hospitalization.

For the resident in an LTC facility outcomes are different and may include a reduction in the exacerbations of a chronic illness such as congestive heart failure. A client in the rehabilitative area of the facility may determine living independently again to be an outcome. Outcomes for others may be to function at the highest potential within the limitations imposed by the chronic illness. A decrease in pain and/ or nausea might be an appropriate outcome for an individual in palliative care. Living each day with optimal quality of life is an outcome for most clients in LTC. Nurses can empower even frail older persons to obtain better outcomes by good listening skills, working with them to identify the meaning of frailty to each person, and identifying positive coping and self-care solutions (Hage & Lorensen, 2005).

Evidence-Informed Practice Box

The purpose of this study was: "(1) to explore barriers to pain management and those associated with implementing a pain management program in long-term care (LTC); and (2) to develop an interprofessional approach to improve pain management in LTC" (Kaasalainen et al., 2010, p. 503). Using a case study method seven focus groups were conducted at two LTC facilities with licensed nurses, unregulated health providers, and physicians. An additional 10 interviews were conducted with other health professionals, residents, and administration. Participants also completed a short survey about barriers to pain management in LTC. The findings indicated that barriers were present at the resident, staff, and organizational levels. The resident's inability or reluctance to report pain, inadequate time for the staff to assess residents' pain, and the need to implement education about pain management and best practices for all staff were identified. The authors concluded that a multilevel approach must be taken to ensure effective pain management in this population.

Source: Kaasalainen et al. (2010).

STUDY QUESTIONS

1. There are a number of issues in LTC today. What are the most essential issues for the provincial/territorial governments to address first?
2. Discuss the ethical principle of autonomy when constructing an appropriate plan of care for an LTC recipient.
3. Discuss the principle of autonomy in relation to the community-dwelling client versus the person in a residential facility.
4. Analyze nursing interventions that would most likely support the goals of an ideal LTC system.
5. How is LTC defined?
6. Describe the major settings in which LTC is provided, giving a specific example of each in your local community.
7. What are some of the precipitating factors for an individual to access the LTC system?
8. What are the major problems facing both caregivers and clients in today's LTC continuum?
9. What individuals are considered vulnerable populations?

INTERNET RESOURCES

Canadian Gerontological Nursing Association: www.cgna.net/
Canadian Hospice Palliative Care Association: www.chpca.net/Home
Canadian Patient Safety Institute: www.patientsafetyinstitute.ca/English/Pages/default.aspx

INTERNET RESOURCES (Cont.)

Geriatric Nursing Education Project: www.aacn.nche.edu/gnec.htm
Hartford Institute for Geriatric Nursing: hartfordign.org/
National Initiative for the Care of the Elderly: www.nicenet.ca/

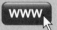

For a full suite of assignments and additional learning activities, use the access code located in the front of your book and visit this exclusive website: **http://go.jblearning.com/kramer-kile**. If you do not have an access code, you can obtain one at the site.

REFERENCES

Accreditation Canada. (n.d.). Long term care. Retrieved from http://www.accreditation.ca/our-clients/long-term-care/

Alexopoulos, G. S., & Mattis, S. (1991). Diagnosing cognitive dysfunction in the elderly: Primary screening tests. *Geriatrics, 46*(12), 33–38, 43.

Algase, D., Beck, C., Kolanowski, A., Whall, A., Berent, S., Richards, K., & Beattie, E. (1996). Need-driven dementia-compromised behavior: An alternative view of disruptive behavior. *American Journal of Alzheimer's Disease, 11*(6), 10–19.

Alzheimer Society of Canada. (2010). Rising tide: The impact of dementia on Canadian Society. Retrieved from http://alzheimersociety.sitesystems.ca/sitecore/shell/Controls/Rich%20Text%20Editor/~/media/Files/national/pdfs/English/Advocacy/ASC_Rising%20Tide_Full%20Report_Eng.ashx

American Association of Colleges of Nursing. (2011). Nursing shortage. Retrieved from http://www.aacn.nche.edu/media-relations/fact-sheets/nursing-shortage

American Psychiatric Association. (2000). *Diagnostic and statistical manual of mental disorders* (4th ed., text revision). Arlington, VA: Author.

Andersen, G., & Horvath, J. (2004). The growing burden of chronic disease in America. *Public Health Reports, 119*, 263–270.

Arling, G., Kane, R. L., Mueller, C., Bershadsky, J., & Degenholtz, H. B. (2007). Nursing effort and quality of care for nursing home residents. *The Gerontologist, 47*(1), 672–682.

Baumbusch, J. L., & Andrusyszyn, M. A. (2002). Gerontological content in Canadian baccalaureate nursing programs: Cause for concern? *Canadian Journal of Nursing Research, 34*(1), 119–129.

Beauchamp, T. L., & Childress, J. F. (2009). *Principles of biomedical ethics* (6th ed.). New York, NY: Oxford University Press.

Beck, A. T., Rush, A. J., Shaw, B. F., & Emery, G. (1979). *Cognitive therapy of depression*. New York, NY: Guilford.

Beck, C., Heacock, P., Mercer, S. O., Walls, R. C., Rapp, C. G., & Vogelpohl, T. S. (1997). Improving dressing behavior in cognitively impaired nursing home residents. *Nursing Research, 46*(3), 126–132.

Boult, C., & Wieland, G. D. (2010). Comprehensive primary care for older patients with multiple chronic conditions. *Journal of the American Medical Association, 304*(17), 1936–1943.

Canada Health Act. (R.S.C., 1985, c. C-6). Retrieved from http://laws-lois.justice.gc.ca/eng/acts/C-6/

Canada Mortgage and Housing Corporation. (2011). Senior's housing report: Canada highlights. Retrieved from http://www.cmhc-schl.gc.ca/odpub/esub/65991/65991_2011_A01.pdf?fr=1322004540875

Canadian Healthcare Association. (2009). *New directions for facility-based long term care*. Ottawa, ON: Author.

Canadian Institute for Health Information. (2009). *Health expenditures by year 2009*. Ottawa, ON: Author.

Canadian Institute for Health Information. (2010). Analysis in brief: Depression among seniors in residential care. Retrieved from http://secure.cihi.ca/cihiweb/products/ccrs_depression_among_seniors_e.pdf

Canadian Network for the Prevention of Elder Abuse. (2011). Mandatory reporting. Retrieved from http://www.cnpea.ca/mandatory_reporting.htm

Canadian Nurses Association. (2009). Tested solutions for eliminating Canada's registered nurse shortage. Retrieved from http://www2.cna-aiic.ca/CNA/documents/pdf/publications/RN_Highlights_e.pdf

CARF Canada. (2012). Accreditation. Retrieved from http://www.carf.org/Programs/CARFCanada/

Casada da Rocha, A. (2009). Towards a comprehensive concept of patient autonomy. *American Journal of Bioethics, 9*(2), 37–38.

Castle, N. G., Engberg, J., & Men, A. (2007). Nursing home staff turnover: Impact on nursing home compare quality measures. *The Gerontologist, 47*(1), 650–661.

Centers for Disease Control and Prevention. (2009). National nursing home survey: 2004 overview. Retrieved from http://www.cdc.gov/nchs/data/series/sr_13/sr13_167.pdf

Cherry, B., Ashcraft, A., & Owen, D. (2007). Perceptions of job satisfaction and the regulatory environment among nurse aides and charge nurses in long-term care. *Geriatric Nursing, 28*(3), 183–192.

Chief Public Health Officer. (2010). Report on the state of public health in Canada, 2010. Growing older—adding life to years. Retrieved from http://publichealth.gc.ca/CPHOreport

Cowley, J., Diebold, C., Gross, J. C., & Hardin-Fanning, F. (2006). Management of common problems. In K. L. Mauk (Ed.), *Gerontological nursing: Competencies for care* (pp. 475–560). Sudbury, MA: Jones and Bartlett.

Crain, M. (2001). Control beliefs of the frail elderly. *Case Management Journals, 3*(1), 42–46.

Cummings, S. (2002). Predictors of psychological well-being among assisted-living residents. *Health & Social Work, 27*(4), 293–302.

Dawson, P., Wells, D., & Kline, K. (1993). *Enhancing the abilities of persons with Alzheimer's and related dementias: A nursing perspective*. New York, NY: Springer.

DeSpelder, L. A., & Strickland, A. L. (2011). *The last dance: Encountering death and dying* (2nd ed.). New York, NY: McGraw-Hill.

Donoghue, C., & Castle, N. G. (2006). Voluntary and involuntary nursing turnover. *Research on Aging, 28*(4), 454–472.

Dunbrack, J. (2006). Advance care planning: The glossary project. Final report. Retrieved from http://www.hc-sc.gc.ca/hcs-sss/pubs/palliat/2006-proj-glos/index-eng.php

Eakes, G. G. (2004). Chronic sorrow. In S. Peterson & T. Bredow (Eds.), *Middle range theories* (pp. 165–172). Philadelphia, PA: Lippincott Williams & Wilkins.

Feaster, M. (2006). Financing LTC with life insurance. *Provider, 32*(11), 39–40.

Fernandes, N., & Spencer, B. G. (2010). The private cost of long-term care in Canada: Where you live matters. *Canadian Journal on Aging, 29*(3), 307–316. doi: 10.1017/S0714980810000346

Ferrell, B., & Coyle, N. (2010). *Textbook of palliative nursing.* New York, NY: Oxford University Press.

Fillenbaum, G. G. (1988). *Multidimensional functional assessment of older adults: The Duke older Americans resources and services procedures.* Hillsdale, NJ: Erlbaum.

Fink, R. M., & Gates, R. A. (2010). Pain assessment. In B. Ferrell & N. Coyle (Eds.), *Oxford textbook of palliative nursing* (3rd ed.). New York, NY: Oxford University Press.

Folstein, M. R., Folstein, S. E., & McHugh, P. R. (1975). Mini-mental state: A practical method for grading the cognitive state of patients for the clinician. *Journal of Psychiatric Research, 12,* 189–198.

Fulmer, T. T. (1999). Elder mistreatment. In J. T. Stone, J. F. Wyman, & S. A. Salisbury (Eds.), *Clinical gerontological nursing: A guide to advanced practice* (2nd ed., pp. 665–674). Philadelphia, PA: Saunders.

Gaugler, J. E., & Teaster, P. (2006). The family caregiving career: Implications for community-based long-term care practice and policy. *Journal of Aging & Social Policy, 18*(3–4), 141–145.

Gift, A. (2004). Unpleasant symptoms. In S. Peterson & T. Bredow (Eds.), *Middle range theories* (pp. 78–89). Philadelphia, PA: Lippincott Williams & Wilkins.

Government of Canada. (2007). Report of the National Seniors Council on elder abuse. Cat. No.: 978-0-662-47366-4. Retrieved from http://www.seniorscouncil .gc.ca/eng/research_publications/elder_abuse/2007 /hs4_38/hs4_38.pdf

Hage, A. M., & Lorensen, M. (2005). A philosophical analysis of the concept of empowerment: The fundament of an education-programme to the frail elderly. *Nursing Philosophy, 6,* 235–246.

Harrington, C., Carrillo, H., Blank, B. W., & O'Brian, T. (2010). Nursing facilities, staffing, residents and facility deficiencies, 2004 through 2009. Retrieved from http://www.pascenter.org/nursing_homes/nursing_ trends_2009.php

Harrington, C., Zimmerman, D., Karon, S. L., Robinson, J., & Beutel, P. (2000). Nursing home staffing and its relationship to deficiencies. *Journals of Gerontology Series B: Psychological Sciences and Social Sciences, 55,* S278–S287.

Healthy Aging and Wellness Working Group of the Federal/Provincial/Territorial (F/P/T) Committee of Officials (Seniors). (2006). Healthy aging in Canada: A new vision, a vital investment from evidence to action. Retrieved from http://www.phac-aspc.gc.ca /seniors-aines/alt-formats/pdf/publications/pro /healthy-sante/haging_newvision/vision-rpt_e.pdf

Hirdes, J. P., Mitchell, L., Maxwell, C. J., & White, N. (2011). Beyond the "iron lungs of gerontology": Using evidence to shape the future of nursing homes in Canada. *Canadian Journal on Aging, 30*(3), 371–390. doi:10.1017/S0714980811000304

Houser, A., Fox-Grage, W., & Gibson, M. J. (2009). Across the states: Profiles of long-term care and independent living (8th ed.). Retrieved from http://assets .aarp.org/rgcenter/health/d18763_2006_ats.pdf

Hudson, C., St. Cyr Tribble, D., Bravo, G., & Poitras, M. (2011). Enablement in health care contexts: A concept analysis. *Journal of Evaluation in Clinical Practice, 17*(1), 143–149.

Jonsen, A. R. (2007). A history of bioethics as discipline and discourse. In N. S. Jecker, A. R. Jonsen, & R. A. Pearlman (Eds.), *Bioethics: An introduction to the history, methods, and practice* (pp. 3–16). Sudbury, MA: Jones and Bartlett.

Kaasalainen, S., Brazil, K., Coker, E., Ploeg, J., Martin-Misener, R., Donald, F., . . . Burns, T. (2010). An action-based approach to improving pain management in long-term care. *Canadian Journal on Aging, 29*(4), 503–517.

Kalisch, P. A., & Kalisch, B. J. (2004). *American nursing: A history* (4th ed.). Philadelphia, PA: Lippincott Williams & Wilkins.

Kane, R., Freeman, I. C., Caplan, A. L., Aroskar, M. A., & Urv-Wong, E. K. (1990). Everyday autonomy in nursing homes. *Generations, 14*(Suppl.), 69–71.

Katz, S., Downs, T. D., Cash, H. R., & Grotz, R. C. (1970). Progress in development of the index of ADL. *The Gerontologist, 10,* 20–30.

Kolcaba, K. (2003). *Comfort theory and practice: A vision for holistic health care and research.* New York, NY: Springer.

Komisar, H. L., Feder, J., & Kasper, J. D. (2005). Unmet long-term care needs: An analysis of Medicare-Medicaid dual eligibles. *Inquiry, 42*(2), 171–182.

Koop, C. E., & Schaeffer, F. (1976). *Whatever happened to the human race?* Old Tappan, NJ: Fleming H. Revell.

Law Commission of Ontario. (2009). Canada's traditional and current capacity legal laws. Retrieved from http://www.lco-cdo.org/en/disabilities-call-for-papers-bach-kerzner-partI-sectionV

Leininger, M. (2002). Culture care theory: A major contribution to advance transcultural nursing and practices. *Journal of Transcultural Nursing, 13*(3), 189–192.

Lekan-Rutledge, D. (1997). Gerontological nursing in long-term care facilities. In M. Matteson, E. McConnell, & A. Linton (Eds.), *Gerontological nursing: Concepts and practice* (2nd ed., pp. 930–960). Philadelphia, PA: Saunders.

Lenz, E. R., Suppe, F., Gift, A. G. Pugh, L. C., & Milligan, R. A. (1995). Collaborative development of middle-range nursing theories: Toward a theory of unpleasant symptoms. *Advances in Nursing Science, 17*(3), 1–13.

Lindbloom, E. J., Brandt, J., Hough, L. D., & Meadows, S. E. (2007). Elder mistreatment in the nursing home: A systematic review. *Journal of the American Medical Director's Association, 8*(9), 610–616.

Lomastro, J. A. (2006). The White House conference on aging: A positive view. *Nursing Homes: Long Term Care Management, 55*(1), 14–16, 18.

Maas, M. L., Reed, D., Park, M., Specht, J. P., Schutte, D., Kelley, L. S., . . . Buckwalte, K. C. (2004). Outcomes of family involvement in care interventions for caregivers of individuals with dementia. *Nursing Research, 53*(2), 76–86.

MacAdam, M. (2009). Moving toward health service integration: Provincial progress in system change for seniors. Retrieved from http://www.cprn.org/documents/51302_EN.pdf

McCleary, L., McGilton, K., Boscart, V., & Oudshoorn, A. (2009). Improving gerontology content in baccalaureate nursing education through knowledge transfer to nurse educators. *Nursing Leadership, 22*(3), 33–46.

McGregor, M. J., & Ronald, L. A. (2011). Residential long-term care for Canadian seniors. Non-profit, for-profit or does it matter? *IRPP Study,* 14. Retrieved from http://www.irpp.org/pubs/IRPPstudy/2011/IRPP_Study_no1.pdf

McGuire, L. C., Rao, J. K., Anderson, L. A., & Ford, E. S. (2007). Completion of a durable power of attorney for health care: What does cognition have to do with it? *The Gerontologist, 47*(4), 457–467.

Meenan, R. F. (1985). New approaches to outcome assessment: The AIMS questionnaire for arthritis. *Advances in Internal Medicine, 31,* 167–185.

Melnyk, B. M., & Fineout-Overholt, E. (2010). *Evidence based practice in nursing & healthcare: A guide to best practice* (2nd ed.). Philadelphia, PA: Lippincott Williams & Wilkins.

Mezey, M., Mitty, I., & Ramsey, G. (1997). Assessment of decision making capacity: Nursing's role. *Journal of Gerontological Nursing, 23*(3), 28–34.

Mitty, E., & Flores, S. (2007a). Assisted living nursing practice: The language of dementia: Theories and interventions. *Geriatric Nursing, 28*(5), 283–288.

Mitty, E., & Flores, S. (2007b). Fall prevention in assisted living: Assessment and strategies. *Geriatric Nursing, 28*(6), 349–357.

Mold, J. W. (1995). An alternative conceptualization of health and health care: Its implications for geriatrics and gerontology. *Educational Gerontology, 21,* 85–101.

National Center for Elder Abuse. (2011). Definitions of elder abuse. Retrieved from http://www.ncea.aoa.gov/NCEAroot/Main_Site/FAQ/Basics/Definition.aspx

National Institute of Mental Health. (2010). Older adults: Depression and suicide facts. Retrieved from http://www.nimh.nih.gov/health/publications/older-adults-depression-and-suicide-facts.shtml#how-common

National PACE Association. (2011). About NPA. Retrieved from http://www.npaonline.org/website/article.asp?id=5

Nelson, A. (Ed.). (2006). *Safe patient handling and movement: A practical guide for health care professionals.* New York, NY: Springer.

Nelson, A., Collins, J., Siddharthan, K., Matz, M., & Waters, T. (2008). Link between safe patient handling and patient outcomes in long-term care. *Rehabilitation Nursing, 33*(1), 33–43.

Ontario Ombudsman. (2012). Who we oversee. The MUSH sector. Retrieved from http://www.ombudsman.on.ca/About-Us/Who-We-Oversee/MUSH-Sector.aspx

Peterson, S. J., & Bredow, T. S. (2004). *Middle range theories: Application to nursing research.* Philadelphia, PA: Lippincott Williams & Wilkins.

Registered Nurses' Association of Ontario. (2009). Briefing note: Investing in nursing education. Retrieved from http://www.rnao.org/Page.asp?PageID=122&ContentID=2837&SiteNodeID=467

Registered Nurses' Association of Ontario. (2012). Promoting safety: Alternative approaches to use of restraints. Retrieved from http://www.rnao.org/Storage/88/8224_FINAL_BPG_FOR_WEBSITE.pdf

Remennick, L. I. (2001). All my life is one big nursing home: Russian immigrant women in Israel speak about double caregiver stress. *Women's Studies International Forum, 24*(6), 685–700.

Remsburg, R., & Carson, B. (2006). Rehabilitation. In I. Lubkin & P. Larsen (Eds.), *Chronic illness: Impact and interventions* (pp. 579–616). Sudbury, MA: Jones and Bartlett.

Sikorska-Simmons, E. (2006). Innovations in long-term care: Organizational culture and work-related attitudes among staff in assisted living. *Journal of Gerontological Nursing, 32*(2), 19–27.

Slaughter, S. E., Eliasziw, M., Morgan, D., & Drummond, N. (2009). Incidence and prevalence of excess disability among nursing home residents with middle-stage dementia: A prospective cohort study of functional transitions. *International Psychogeriatrics, 23*(1), 54–64.

Statistics Canada. (2008). The daily. Retrieved from http://www.statcan.gc.ca/daily-quotidien/081021/dq081021a-eng.htm

Statistics Canada. (2010). Population projections for Canada, provinces and territories 2009 to 2036. Cat. No.: 91-520-X. Retrieved from http://www.statcan.gc.ca/pub/91-520-x/91-520-x2010001-eng.pdf

Statistics Canada. (2011a). Canada year book 2011. Cat. No.: 11 - 40 2 -X. Retrieved from http://www.statcan.gc.ca/pub/11-402-x/2011000/pdf/seniors-aines-eng.pdf

Statistics Canada. (2011b). Residential care facilities. Cat. No.: 83-237-X. Retrieved from http://www.statcan.gc.ca/pub/83-237-x/83-237-x2012001-eng.pdf

Statistics Canada. (2011c). Family violence in Canada, A statistical profile. Cat. No.: 85-224-x. Retrieved from http://www.statcan.gc.ca/pub/85-224-x/85-224-x2010000-eng.pdf

Stewart, M. K., Felix, H., Dockter, N., Perry, D. M., & Morgan, J. R. (2006). Program and policy issues affecting home and community-based long-term care

use: Findings from a qualitative study. *Home Health Care Services Quarterly, 25*(3–4), 107–127.

Tarzian, A. J. (2000). Caring for dying patients who have air hunger. *Journal of Nursing Scholarship, 32*(2), 137–143.

Teaster, P. B. (2002). *A response to the abuse of vulnerable adults: The 2000 survey of state adult protective services*. Washington, DC: National Center on Elder Abuse.

Teresi, J. A., & Evans, D. A. (1997). Cognitive assessment measures for chronic care populations. In J. A. Teresi, M. P. Lawton, D. Holmes, & M. Ory (Eds.), *Measurement in elderly chronic care populations* (pp. 1–23). New York, NY: Springer.

Thornlow, D., Latimer, D., Kingsborough, J., & Arietti, L. (2006). *Caring for an Aging America: A guide for nursing faculty*. Washington, DC: American Association of Colleges of Nursing.

Tobin, P., & Salisbury, S. (1999). Legal planning issues. In J. T. Stone, J. F. Wyman, & S. A. Salisbury (Eds.), *Clinical gerontological nursing: A guide to advanced practice* (2nd ed., pp. 31–44). Philadelphia, PA: Saunders.

Tullman, D. F., Mion, L. C., Fletcher, K., & Foreman, M. D. (2008). Delirium. Retrieved from http://consultgerirn.org/topics/delirium/want_to_know_more

Turcotte, M., & Schellenberg , G.(2007). *A portrait of seniors in Canada (2006)*. Cat. No.: 89-519-XIE. Ottawa, ON: Statistics Canada. Retrieved from http://www.statcan.gc.ca/

Varcarolis, E. M., & Halter, M. J. (2010). *Foundation of psychiatric mental health nursing: A clinical approach*. Philadelphia, PA: Saunders.

Wagner, D. L. (2006). Families, work, and an aging population: Developing a formula that works for the workers. *Journal of Aging & Social Policy, 18*(3–4), 115–125.

Willging, P. (2006). Get ready for community-based long-term care. *Long Term Living, 55*(3), 20, 22–23.

World Health Organization. (2008). WHO definition of palliative care. Retrieved from http://www.who.int/cancer/palliative/definition/en/

CHAPTER 19

Hospice Palliative Care

Original chapter by Barbara M. Raudonis
Canadian content added by Gregg Trueman

> *Unfortunately, in end of life care, we do not have a vocal constituency: the dead*
> *are no longer here to speak; the dying often cannot speak, and the bereaved are*
> *often too overcome by their loss to speak.*
> —Harvey Chochinov (May 2000)

INTRODUCTION

According to Curtin and Lubkin (1995), chronic disease is never completely cured and involves the total human environment for supportive and self-care, maintenance of function, and the prevention of further disability. The likelihood of chronic disease not only increases with age (Morrison & Meier, 2004), four chronic diseases in particular—heart disease, cancer, cerebrovascular disease, and chronic respiratory disease—are the leading causes of death for older adults (Statistics Canada, 2011). It is not uncommon for aging Canadians to experience several chronic conditions simultaneously, all of which demand complex care often overwhelming the elder, their family members, and the systems in which chronic disease management and end-of-life care is provided to Canadians.

Chronic diseases share protracted illness trajectories with numerous phases of stability and remission and exacerbation and recovery. Chronic disease is largely a medical matter leading to progressively advanced disease with its own symptom burden, functional decline with disability, and death (Corbin, 2001). *Chronic illness*, or the personal experience of living with chronic disease, is a family matter which can be equally overwhelming (Martin, 2007). Chronic illness is routinely highlighted by vulnerability, suffering, and a host of questions seeking to better understand the uncertainty that lies ahead. The chronic illness experience is not devoid of celebration or meaning making; quite the contrary (Pakenham & Cox, 2009). Elders living with chronic disease celebrate milestones in their lives and those of family members, bring a lifetime of wisdom to their communities, and like all Canadians look forward to the next good day. People living with chronic disease would therefore benefit from hospice palliative care, which seeks to treat, reduce, or prevent symptoms of diseases; relieve suffering; and improve the patient and family's quality of life, without working toward a cure.

The principles of palliative care mirror the regulatory standards underpinning the discipline of nursing. In other words, palliative care is practiced using holistic comprehensive plans of care involving interdisciplinary care teams from the time of diagnosis and throughout the illness trajectory. As our nation ages it behoves practitioners of every stripe to consider how hospice palliative care positively influences aging and the experience of chronic illness. The purpose of this chapter is to provide readers with an overview of the historical roots of hospice palliative care in Canada, a cursory review of Canadian hospice palliative care programming, family caregiving, culturally competent care, and psychosocial assessment, which coalesce to influence Canadians' end-of-life experience. The chapter goes on to describe the role of symptom management and the clinical issues and program opportunities impacting palliative care. The chapter concludes with a review of the professional disciplines operating within hospice palliative care, an emerging research agenda, and a series of guiding questions for self-assessment of learning.

HISTORICAL PERSPECTIVES

"Palliative care" is a term coined by Canadian physician Balfour Mount that grew out of the U.K. hospice movement. Derived from the Latin root *pallium*, palliative refers to an ecclesiastical vestment that *covers* or *cloaks*, alluding to how symptoms are managed. Hospice is both a philosophy of care and a specialized approach to end-of-life care programming. Derived from the Latin root *hospes,* hospice relates to modern-day notions of hospitality. From the 3rd to 15th centuries A.D., pilgrims to the Holy Lands stopped at way stations for food, water, and respite. These way stations (i.e., hospices) were also centres of refuge for people who were poor, sick, and dying. Five hundred years later, Dame Cicely Saunders founded the modern hospice movement after she established St. Christopher's Hospice in Sydenham, England.

St. Christopher's Hospice was the first research and teaching hospice and is known for several innovations, including pain and symptom management, a holistic approach to care, home care, family support throughout the patient's illness, and bereavement follow-up care for family (Meier, 2010). The services delivered by St. Christopher's have evolved over time to include in-patient care, home care, and palliative daycare centres. St. Christopher's Hospice continues to serve as the touchstone for compassionate hospice care around the world. Even so, Dame Saunders, educated as a social worker, then nurse, and finally physician, cautioned clinicians and communities not to clone St. Christopher's but to refine the principles of hospice care within the context of the community in which hospice care is provided. Two years after St. Christopher's Hospice opened Dr. Elisabeth Kubler-Ross's book, *On Death and Dying* (1969), was published. One of the outcomes of this germinal work is what has erroneously come to be known worldwide as "the stages of dying." More importantly, her work inspired a global dialogue on the existential journey of the dying and the bereaved.

Before Dame Saunders died in 2005 she established Cicely Saunders International. This charity's mission is to promote research and best practice in hospice palliative care, and in 2010 the Cicely Saunders Institute of Palliative Care was launched with the goal of improving palliative care and quality of life for people around the world (Cicely Saunders International, 2010; Higginson, 2011). Based on Saunders's work, hospice services have expanded beyond the borders of the United Kingdom, inspiring clinicians around the world (Hansford, 2010). Dr. Balfour Mount, a principal pioneer in the hospice palliative care movement in North America, was equally inspired by Kubler-Ross's work as he was by his visit to St. Christopher's Hospice in the early 1970s. He returned to the Royal Victoria Hospital in Montreal with a new vision for the treatment of persons approaching the end of their lives.

Hospice palliative care in Canada has been described as a complex set of physical, psychological, social, spiritual, and existential approaches to *improve the quality of one's life* in an individualized, flexible, and nonmedical environment. As hospice palliative care philosophy and medical services evolved across Canada, inpatient palliative beds were added in hospitals; community-based and freestanding hospices soon took root across Canada. Mount's work for the next 30 years led the way in translating the English hospice philosophy and models of care into the Canadian context. He has been recognized internationally and has subsequently been made a Member, and later promoted to Officer, of the Order of Canada. In the 1990s Senator Sharon Carstairs championed the cause of hospice palliative care in the upper chamber and initiated a national discussion on the status of end-of-life care in Canada. Although Senator Carstairs's vision and advocacy has placed hospice palliative care on the national healthcare agenda, in 2011 most Canadians who die each year neither received nor had access to hospice palliative care (Collins, 2010; Manitoba Centre for Health Policy, 2007). The typical chronic illness experience of patients and their families demonstrates the need for comprehensive palliative care earlier in the chronic disease

trajectory (National Consensus Project for Quality Palliative Care, 2009).

HOSPICE PALLIATIVE CARE PROGRAMMING

Hospice palliative care programs across Canada (i.e., home care programs, freestanding hospices, drug benefit plans) have necessarily adopted inclusion criteria for enrolment in their programs. Chief among the inclusion criteria is a medical prognosis of 6 months or less, which has created a *de facto* program-based definition of the palliative care patient. Once a patient meets the program admission criteria and is admitted to a local hospice palliative care program, additional resources are brought to bear supporting the holistic care of dying patients. Palliative care resources typically include access to heavily subsidized provincial drug benefits and significantly increased personal care services. In the United States Medicare benefit eligibility criteria for hospice services required a terminal diagnosis and a 6-month prognosis. In addition, Medicare required that patients discontinue curative or life-prolonging treatments to access comprehensive hospice care (Lynn, 2001a). Other definitions of hospice palliative care are described in the literature (Ferris et al., 2002; Passmore, Ho, & Gallagher, 2012), which has informed how hospice palliative care is programmed in Canada.

Defining Hospice Palliative Care

The World Health Organization argues palliative care as the active total care of patients whose disease is no longer responsive to curative treatment. It includes control of pain and other symptoms where psychological, social, and spiritual issues are paramount. Palliative care affirms life and regards dying as a normal human process. Palliative care neither hastens nor postpones death. Instead, it emphasizes relief from spiritual aspects of care and offers a support system to help the family cope during their loved other's illness and their own bereavement (World Health Organization, 1990). The Canadian Hospice Palliative Care Association (CHPCA) describes hospice palliative care as the gestalt of a human philosophy, and professional practice ontology, involving both active and compassionate therapies that may or may not extend survival and is practiced with altruism (2010). Common to all jurisdictions and regulatory authorities is an underlying belief that hospice palliative care provides humane, holistic, comprehensive care to maintain quality of life for the person and family making the transitions at the end of one's life.

The Center to Advance Palliative Care argues that palliative care is not the same as hospice care. Palliative care or interventions that lessen uncomfortable symptoms associated with chronic disease (e.g., pain, loneliness, exercise intolerance) are provided at any time, which may include being an adjuvant to curative treatments. Hospice care, on the other hand, always provides palliative care but is focused on terminally ill patients who no longer seek curative treatments and whose prognosis is 6 months or less. In the United States hospice is a specific type of palliative care and is generally considered a program of care with three primary outcomes: self-determined life closure, safe and comfortable dying, and effective grieving (National Hospice Organization Standards and Accreditation Committee, 1997). In Canada hospice is a specialized freestanding space caring for people during the final weeks

of their life. Hospice programs in Canada provide state-of-the-art palliative care and supportive services to dying persons and their family. This comprehensive care is available 24 hours a day in community and facility-based care settings. An interprofessional team (i.e., patients, family members, professionals, and volunteers) provides holistic care during the final phase of an illness and the period of bereavement (CHPCA, 2005).

Although it appears that hospice and palliative care have much in common, there are two important distinctions. First, palliative care operates in the context of life-prolonging therapies, and second, palliative care is integrated throughout the course of a chronic, progressive, and incurable disease, from diagnosis through death. Hospice care is typically offered only during the final weeks to months of life. Differences in the shared views of what constitutes hospice palliative care are found largely along the trajectory of illness. Earlier in the trajectory more active, often curative, therapies are seen as part of the medical management plan. Later in the illness trajectory, however, care focuses more on symptom management, supporting self-determination, and quality of life. The CHPCA's view of hospice palliative care—as a combination of active and compassionate therapies—means that negotiated goals of care and advance care planning details, illness trajectory, and local resources coalesce to inform which therapies are brought to bear (CHPCA, 2005). Buttressing this view are seven principle and value statements regarding delivery of hospice palliative care services in Canada (**Table 19-1**). Integration of these principles and values into clinical practice enables clinicians to provide a continuum of care otherwise unavailable to patients with advancing illness.

Table 19-1   Canadian Hospice Palliative Care Association Principles and Values

1. The intrinsic value of each person as an autonomous and unique individual

2. The value of life, the natural process of death, and the fact that both provide opportunities for growth and self-actualization

3. The need to address patients' and families' suffering, expectations, needs, hopes, and fears

4. Providing care only when the patient and/or family is prepared to accept it

5. Providing care guided by quality of life as defined by the individual

6. Caregivers enter into a therapeutic relationship with patients and families based on dignity and integrity

7. The knowledge that a unified response to suffering strengthens communities

Shifting Demographics

Shifting demographics in Canada reveal an aging society and the downstream prevalence of chronic disease. The ranks of Canadian elders are swelling into the millions, and in 2007 one in seven Canadians was over the age of 65; the fastest growing demographic in Canada is ages 55 to 64. Canadian octogenarians on their own now exceed 1 million in number—up 25%—making them the second fastest growing demographic (Canadian Institute for Health Information, 2007). Because of the projected fears regarding how elders might impact Canadian health and illness care systems, of which the hospice palliative care system is but one, these combined demographics have been unceremoniously labelled the silver tsunami (Delafuente, 2009; Perry, 2009) and the burgeoning epidemic of dementia (Lunney, Lynn, & Hogan, 2002). Ironically, although much has been written questioning how care systems will cope with an aging society, little has been published about how the collective wisdom of elders living with chronic illness shape the fabric of Canadian society, teaching us all how to bring meaning into the final years, months, weeks, and days of life.

In 2007, 37% of Canadians were diagnosed by a physician or nurse practitioner as having a chronic disease. In 2009, based on medium growth, Statistics Canada projected that the deaths associated with chronic conditions in Canada will increase 33% by the year 2036 to more than 430,000 deaths per year (www.statscan.gc/daily-quotidien/100526/t100526b1-eng.htm). Today, the leading causes of death in Canada are tumours and cancers (29.6%), combined diseases of the cardiovascular and cerebrovascular systems (27.1%), chronic lower respiratory diseases (4.6%), followed by the effects of diabetes mellitus (3.2%), Alzheimer's disease (2.8%), influenza and pneumonia (i.e., acute conditions often associated with chronic illness) (2.3%), and renal disease (1.6%). Hospice palliative care is beneficial for all these groups, which total more than 70% of all cause death (Statistics Canada, 2011). Equally important, the CHPCA (2010) estimates that each death in Canada impacts the immediate well-being of approximately five other people, or more than 1.5 million Canadians, every year.

The Canadian Institute for Health Information (2007) data concerning the end-of-life experience in Atlantic Canada showed that the leading cause of death in the Maritimes was fairly consistent with national patterns: cancers and circulatory disease accounted for most deaths of older adults. These data, however, demonstrated that Maritime Canadians experienced slightly higher percentages of organ failure, followed closely by terminal illness and frailty (Collins, 2011). Across the country the Manitoba Centre for Health Policy (MCHP) conducted a retrospective descriptive cohort analysis (n = 65,503) examining healthcare services in the last year of life (2007). The study demonstrated a discrepancy in utilization of palliative care services in both hospital and community care systems. The report noted that although hospital costs associated with end-of-life care were increasing, as was the average age of patients, palliative care was only provided in 37.2% of terminal illness cases, 7.2% of organ failure patients, and a dismal 3.5% of frailty cases. Additionally, researchers acknowledged variations in drug use at the end of life related to differences in planning and symptom management knowledge among physicians (Manitoba Centre for Health Policy, 2007).

Approximately 16% to 30% of Canadians, depending on where they reside, have access to palliative care, and even fewer receive grief and bereavement care (Canadian Institute for Health Information, 2007). These data represent a marginal improvement from 2000 when a Senate report, entitled "Quality End of Life Care: The Right of Every Canadian," indicated that although Canadians prefer the idea of a home death, surrounded by their loved others, more than 75% of Canadians still die in hospitals and long-term care facilities (Carstairs & Beaudroin, 2000). Not surprisingly, Canadians living with chronic illness–related disabilities are among those most severely impacted when access to hospice palliative care programming is limited.

Quality Improvement in Hospice Palliative Care

Researchers have argued that too many people suffer needlessly at the end of life both from errors of omission when caregivers fail to provide palliative and supportive care that are known to be effective (Peto, Tenerowicz, Benjamin, Morsi, & Burger, 2009). Suffering can also be brought on by errors of commission when caregivers do what is known to be ineffective and even harmful (Field & Cassel, 1997). Research has identified four broad deficiencies in the care of persons with life-threatening and incurable illnesses (**Table 19-2**). The report concluded with optimism that a "vigorous societal commitment . . . would motivate and sustain individual and collective efforts to create a humane care system that people can trust to serve them well as they die" (Field & Cassel, 1997, p. 13).

Quality improvement is a philosophical commitment to an organizational methodology that works to continuously improve the processes underlying an organization's ability to exceed customer expectations (Schroeder, 1994). From a leadership perspective, quality improvement clarifies the work patterns of an organization's employees and practitioners, establishing mechanisms to identify and measure root causes of problems and foster innovation in service delivery for the purpose of improving customer services. Change in hospice palliative care services occurs in part because of an increased involvement of consumers in issues related to quality of life and the burdens of caregiving (Berry, 2004).

Quality improvement has been well described by American end-of-life care organizations and researchers, including the landmark SUPPORT study arguing for the integration of palliative care for all individuals with

Table 19-2   Deficiencies in End-of-Life Care
1. Legal, organizational, and economic obstacles conspire to obstruct reliably excellent care at the end of life.
2. The education and training of physicians and other healthcare professionals fail to provide them with the knowledge, skills, and attitudes required to care well for the dying patient.
3. Current knowledge and understanding are inadequate to guide and support the consistent practice of evidence-informed medicine at the end of life.
4. Healthcare professionals, patients, families, health plan administrators, agency administrators, and policy-makers must work together to change attitudes, policies, and actions to surmount the deficiencies in palliative care.

chronic, debilitating, and life-limiting illnesses (Gillick, 2009). Approximately 100 articles have been published based on the findings of the SUPPORT study. Implications of the data for future reform suggest that improved individual, patient-level decision making may not be the most effective strategy for improving end-of-life care. The SUPPORT investigators recommended systems-level innovations and quality improvement in routine care as effective strategies for change (Lynn et al., 2000; Lynn, Schuster, Wilkinson, & Simon, 2008).

In the Canadian context, academic and clinical coalitions at both the provincial and national levels, founded by nursing, social work, and a range of allied disciplines, have advanced the quality improvement dialogue. Two organizations are identified here as exemplars that support quality improvement in Canadian hospice palliative care.

The Quality Palliative Care in Long Term Care Alliance is a provincial collaboration composed of 38 organizational partners and 27 researchers who actively contribute their expertise to a 5-year comparative case study research project (i.e., Improving Quality of Life for People Dying in Long Term Care Homes). The primary goal of the research is to create a community–university research alliance to develop sustainable, person-focused palliative care programs using a capacity development process consistent with the CHPCA's framework. Similarly, the Quality End-of-Life Care Coalition of Canada (QELCCC) is a group of 33 national associations and organizations with interests in end-of-life care issues. The QELCCC supports the 2000 Senate report in that all Canadians ought to have the right to quality end-of-life care that allows them to die with dignity, free of pain, surrounded by their loved ones, in a setting of their choice. The Coalition believes that to achieve quality end-of-life care for all Canadians there must be a well-funded, sustainable national strategy for hospice palliative and end-of-life care. Toward this end, the QELCCC has established a quality improvement and an advocacy agenda that supports a robust communications strategy among governmental and private sector funders as well as programs of research related to professional education, family and caregiver support, and knowledge translation.

A CHPCA conceptual framework authored by Ferris et al. (2002) works to address deficiencies in end-of-life care by conceptualizing the complexity of relationships among patient needs, interventions, and organizational processes underpinning excellence in hospice palliative care. The framework is organized around the patient and family and organizational outcomes of care. In essence, this framework summarises the major points about hospice palliative care discussed throughout this chapter. Ferris and colleagues' model, the square of care and organization (**Figure 19-1**), was the result of a consensus visioning process among hospice palliative care stakeholders across Canada. Like Wagner's chronic care model, which identifies elements of a care system responsive to chronic disease management (Bernstein, 2008), the square of care comprises two distinct operations that guide patient and family care (i.e., the square of care) as well as organizational functioning and ongoing development (i.e., the square of organization). The square of care integrates hospice palliative care principles and norms of practice to guide (1) assessment, (2) information sharing, (3) decision making, (4) care planning, and (5) care delivery. The square of organization illustrates how resources are combined with operational functions (i.e., governance, administration, quality improvement, and marketing) to develop and facilitate service delivery. An integrated square of care organization depicts how an organization operationalises its clinical and organizational activities, ensuring the patient and family remain at the centre of all activities.

The Ferris et al. (2003) model capably integrates the lexicon of hospice palliative care principles that patients and practitioners can use to guide their work. This, in turn, helps to ensure Canadians have access to consistent, high-quality hospice palliative care. To its credit, Canada is the first country to have developed this kind of a consensus-based road map for hospice palliative care programming.

HEART AND SOUL OF HOSPICE PALLIATIVE CARE

Our family—of choice or of origin—is central to our identity and to the care we require at the end of life. Although death, particularly that of an elder, may not be unexpected, it nonetheless has the potential to create a familial and existential crisis. Family members living the loss of a loved one may find solace in one another creating an unexpected opportunity for growth. The death of a family member may also exacerbate existing issues within the family, calling on clinicians to employ their advanced communication skills, culturally competent psychosocial, spiritual assessment, and care strategies. These strategies are foundational hospice palliative care skill sets that aid clinicians to more fully understand how their altruistic interventions will bring comfort to a patient besieged with unremitting nausea and a family struggling with a crisis of identity.

Family Caregiving

Distinguished by unique caring practices, the patient and family are the primary focus of assessment and care for hospice palliative care practitioners. Family caregivers routinely provide supportive care throughout the chronic illness trajectory, in all care settings, and for all types of needs (McMillan, 2004). Not surprisingly, caregiver burden and burnout are increasing significantly as more complex health care moves into the home setting (Proot et al., 2003). Evidence exists that extended service as a caregiver can negatively impact the physical, social, and emotional well-being of caregivers (Pinquart & Sorenson, 2003). In fact, some caregivers experience sustained stress related to intense periods of caregiving that may

Square of care and organization

PROCESS OF PROVIDING CARE

Domain (COMMON ISSUES)	Assessment	Information-sharing	Decision-making	Care Planning	Care Delivery	Confirmation
(column descriptions)	History of issues, opportunities associated expectations, needs, hopes, fears examination - assessment scales, physical exam, laboratory, radiology, procedures	Confidentiality limits Desire and readiness for information Process for sharing information Translation reaction to information Understanding, desire for additional information	Capacity Goals of care Requests for withholding/ withdrawing, therapy/with no potential for benefit, hastened death issue prioritization Therapeutic choices, options Treatment choices, consent Surrogate decision-making Advance directives Conflict resolution	Setting of care Process to negotiate/ develop plan of care - address issues/opportunities, delivery chosen therapies, dependents, backup coverage, respite, bereavement care, discharge planning, emergencies	Careteam composition, leadership, education, support Consultation Setting of care Essential services Patient, family support Therapy delivery Errors	Understanding Satisfaction Complexity Stress Concerns, issues questions
Disease Management	Primary diagnosis, prognosis, evidence secondary diagnoses - dementia, substance use, trauma co-morbidities - delirium, seizures adverse events - side effects, toxicity allergies					
Physical	Pain, other symptoms cognition, level of consciousness function, safety, aids fluids, nutrition wounds habits - alcohol, smoking					
Psychological	Personality, behavior depression, anxiety emotion, fears control, dignity, independence conflict, guilt, stress, coping responses self image, self esteem					
Social	Cultural values, beliefs, practices relationships, roles isolation, abandonment, reconciliation safe, comforting environment privacy, intimacy routines, rituals, recreation, vocation financial, legal family caregiver protection guardianship, custody issues					
Spiritual	Meaning, value existential, transcendental values, beliefs, practices, affiliations spiritual advisors, rites, rituals symbols, icons					
Practical	Activities of daily living dependents, pets telephone access, transportation					
End of life/death management	Life closure, gift giving, legacy creation preparation for expected death management of physiological changes in last hours of living rites, rituals death pronouncement, certification peri death care of family, handing of body funerals, memorial services, celebrations					
Loss, grief	Loss grief - acute, chronic, anticipatory bereavement planning mourning					

Patient/Family

FUNCTIONS

Function	Details
Governance and administration	Leadership - board, management. Organizational structure, accountability
Planning	Strategic planning Business planning Business development
Operations	Standards of practice, policies and procedures, data collection documentation guidelines Resource acquisition and management Safety, security, emergency systems
Quality management	Performance improvement routine review: outcomes, resource utilization, risk management, compliance, satisfaction, needs, financial audit, accreditation strategic and business plans standards, data collection/ procedures, data collection/ documentation guidelines
Communications/ marketing	Communication marketing strategies Materials Media liaison

RESOURCES

Financial	Human	Informational	Physical	Community
Assets Liabilities	Formal caregivers Consultants Staff Volunteers	Records - health, financial, human resource material, eg. books, journals, internet, intranet resource directory	Environment equipment Materials/supplies	Host organization Healthcare system Partner healthcare providers Community organizations Stakeholders, public

FIGURE 19-1 Square of care and organization.

Source: A Model to Guide Hospice Palliative Care: Based on National Principles and Norms of Practice Attribution/Citation Statement. Ferris, F. D., Balfour, H. M., Bowen, K., Farley, J., Hardwick, M., Lamontagne, C., . . . West P. (2002). *A model to guide hospice palliative care.* Ottawa, ON: Canadian Hospice Palliative Care Association.

negatively impact their bereavement processes (Schulz et al., 2003; Schulz, Newsom, Fleissner, DeCamp, & Nieboer, 1997). Other research from the University of Victoria has established that caregivers are able to simultaneously experience both feelings of burden and feelings of well-being (Chappell & Dujela, 2008), making clear the multiple layers of meaning that are inherent in the palliative caregiving process.

Although resilience has been recognized as a mediating correlate of caregiver risk, more hours of caregiving for the terminally ill, caregiver gender, and dementia care involving disruptive behaviour tend to increase caregiver strain and perceptions of burden or burnout (Barber, 1988; Chappell & Dujela, 2008; Parrish & Adams, 2003; Redinbaugh, Baum, Tarbell, & Arnold, 2003). Successful intervention studies have been carried out with caregivers of patients living with Alzheimer's disease (Lu, 2001) and evidence is emerging relative to caregivers of patients living with other chronic diseases (Proot et al., 2003). The Quality End-of-Life Care Coalition of Canada consensus statement on improving end-of-life care concluded that more research related to caregiver burden is needed. Studies are needed to determine which caregivers are at greatest risk for distress and specific interventions that are most likely to relieve the distress (Quality End-of-Life Care Coalition of Canada, 2010).

Culturally Competent Care

Culture is a defining component of the human experience. Each individual's culture provides a sense of security, belonging, and guidelines regarding how to live and die (End of Life Nursing Education Consortium, 2009b). Cultural diversity refers to differences between people based on shared teachings, beliefs, customs, language, and so forth that influence an individual's and family's response to illness, treatment, death, and bereavement (Showalter, 1998). Despite the enormous differences among individuals, an understanding of common cultural characteristics is helpful in providing culturally competent and effective care (Kemp, 1999). It is beyond the scope of this chapter to describe the cultural perspectives of individual populations regarding dying, death, and bereavement. However, it is important to be aware that culturally sensitive care is critical to family-centred palliative care.

In the United States, Sullivan (2001) identified Latino views regarding end-of-life care using focus groups as the method of data collection. The focus groups were conducted in Latino communities. The Latino participants believed they could not communicate effectively with healthcare providers because of language barriers and they did not understand the concept of informed consent, even with the use of interpreters. It was important for the family to care for their relatives in the home rather than place them in long-term care settings. Religious beliefs, primarily reliance on God, and fatalism were critical components of their decision making regarding end-of-life care. Racial discrimination and cultural insensitivity were perceived by many participants in focus group discussions.

In Canada, aboriginal Canadians' experience of Western medicine has been grounded in the many interconnected factors presently challenging quality hospice palliative care of First Nations patients. Geographical isolation, respectful communication, cultural awareness, and institutional practices were identified in a literature review of aboriginal Canadians receiving hospice palliative care. Other themes included family and community values and traditional and holistic concepts related to health and dying (Kelly & Minty, 2007). Perhaps most meaningful in this review is a clearer understanding that contrasting styles of communication can complicate care. A qualitative study concentrating on communication with First Nations elder patients in rural Ontario described the importance of nonverbal communication with an emphasis on listening and accepting silence as key practitioner competencies (Kelly & Brown, 2002). Traditional family and community values speak to the cultural relevance of caring for each other until death (Kaufert, 1999). Based on the significant body of knowledge in the area of aboriginal health, the CHPCA (2007) and the National Aboriginal Health Organization (2002) both authored reports with recommendations for improving hospice palliative care services for aboriginal Canadians.

A phenomenological study using in-depth interviews was undertaken with bereaved First Nations family members and their experiences of losing a loved one (Kelly, Linkewich, St. Pierre-Hansen, & Antone, 2009). Again, communication with or between physicians and family members involving words of encouragement, words that acknowledge the patient's "courageous fight" along the illness trajectory, were regarded as culturally respectful. Advance care planning was identified as an area that may place family members and the care team in conflict. Some aboriginal families preferred not to speak of the illness and in so doing protected the dying family member from the prognosis. Use of translators was regarded as a culturally sensitive practice and they were noted as important members of the interprofessional team relative to spiritual caregiving. Ensuring that care facilities were sufficient for the large numbers of family member who traditionally attend the final days and hours, including death, of a family member emerged as a key finding (Kelly et al., 2009). **Table 19-3** outlines 10 principles of culturally sensitive care originally developed by the Council on Social Work Education Faculty Development Institute in 2001, as cited in Sherman (2004).

Psychosocial, Spiritual, and Bereavement Needs

Psychosocial, spiritual, and bereavement care are key components of hospice palliative care. Many members of interdisciplinary palliative care teams routinely assess and intervene to meet the psychosocial and spiritual needs of patients and their families. Bereavement support is an equally important part of the follow-up family assessment and care after a loved one dies. Research demonstrates that family members with unresolved spiritual and psychological distress are more likely to experience an extended or complicated grief and bereavement process (McClain, Rosenfeld, & Breitbart, 2003). So, the simple act of acknowledging another person's spiritual distress can be a powerful hospice palliative care intervention. However, a common language and mutual comfort between patient and practitioner must be present for this "simple" exchange to occur (Chochinov, 2004).

Helping patients die with dignity is a basic tenet of palliative care. Empirical work with dying patients found that the paradigm of dignity, which includes matters of spirituality, meaning, purpose, and other psychosocial issues related to dying, included acceptable language and topics for discussion (Chochinov et al., 2004). This work is adding to the growing empirical evidence that palliative care is more than symptom management and must include the spiritual,

Table 19-3	Principles of Culturally Sensitive Care

1. Be knowledgeable about cultural values and attitudes of the persons they serve

2. Attend to diverse communication styles

3. Ask patients for their preferences for decision making early in the care process

4. Recognize cultural differences and varying comfort levels with regard to personal space, eye contact, touch, time orientation, learning styles, and conversation styles

5. Use a cultural guide from the palliative care patient's ethnic or religious background

6. Get to know the community, its people, and its resources available for social support

7. Create a culturally friendly physical environment (e.g., decorate facilities with artwork or pictures valued by the cultural groups to whom care is most commonly provided)

8. Determine the acceptability of patients being physically examined by a practitioner of a different sex

9. Advocate for availability of services, accessibility in terms of cost and location, and acceptability of services that are compatible with cultural values and practices of the person served

10. Conduct a self-assessment of their own beliefs about illness and death

Source: Adapted from Council on Social Work Education Faculty Development Institute (2001) as cited in Sherman (2004).

psychosocial, and existential concerns. It must be person centred and maintain a person's dignity through his or her last breath of life. Chochinov developed a dignity-conserving model and interventions based on the analysis of 50 qualitative interviews of patients with advanced cancer. The interviews were conducted to understand the patients' perceptions of dignity. The dignity-conserving model of care consists of three areas of influence on a person's perception of dignity: (1) influences stemming directly from the illness, (2) influences from the person's psychological and spiritual resources or self (dignity-conserving repertoire), and (3) environmental influences (social dignity inventory) (Chochinov, 2011). The model serves as the basis for the psychotherapeutic intervention called *dignity therapy*.

In dignity therapy dying patients are interviewed about aspects of their life they would like recorded and remembered. The interviews are transcribed and edited to read like an intimate story of one's life. The narratives are returned to the patient and ultimately given to the patient's loved ones. Chochinov reported that 76% of the 100 patients in a clinical trial of the dignity therapy intervention reported a sense of heightened dignity, and 91% were satisfied with the intervention (Chochinov et al., 2005); 95% of the family members of the dignity therapy participants reported they would recommend dignity therapy for other patients and families faced with a terminal illness and 77% would continue to use the recorded narratives as a source of remembrance and comfort (McClement et al., 2007). Chochinov acknowledges that dignity-conserving care must be validated in diverse populations. However, the author urges that the concept of "conserving dignity in end-of-life care should become part of the palliative care lexicon and the overarching

standard of care for all patients nearing death"
(Chochinov, 2011, p. 359).

HOSPICE PALLIATIVE CARE SYMPTOM MANAGEMENT

A core principle of palliation is the relief of pain
and other symptoms (Steinhauser, Christakis,
Clipp, McNeilly, & Tulsky, 2000), which begins
with a thorough assessment. Findings support the
practice of routine and standardized symptom
assessment with validated instruments (Morrison
& Meier, 2004). Benefits attributed to routine assessments include identification of overlooked or
unreported symptoms (Bookbinder et al., 1996;
Manfredi et al., 2000). Dissemination and increased use of validated instruments facilitate
the comparison of findings across practice settings and research studies. The Canadian Virtual
Hospice provides access to clinically useful and
valid instruments through their website (see
Internet Resources at end of chapter) and associated links to regional hospice palliative care
programs across Canada. A comprehensive assessment serves as the foundation for goal setting, developing a plan of care, implementing
interventions, and evaluating the outcomes and
effectiveness of care (Glass, Cluxton, & Rancour,
2001). The Ferris et al. (2002) framework is useful in terms of organizing patient assessment
and care according to six domains: assessment,
information sharing, decision making, care planning, care delivery, and confirmation. Based
on the changing needs of patients and families
across the trajectory of the chronic illness, quality of life should be repeatedly assessed at routine points along the trajectory: (1) at the time
of diagnosis, (2) before and after treatments,
(3) prognosticating long-term survival or terminal phase, and (4) during active dying.

Goals of Care and Advance Care Planning

Palliative care is needed across the lifespan;
assessments and interventions ought to be tailored to the specific population served. Often,
the literature categorises adults as a homog-
enous group needing palliative care. Experts in
gerontology, however, are calling for recognition of the unique palliative care needs of older
adults (Cassel, 2003). Amella (2003) described
the common goal of helping patients experience
the best quality of life as the touchstone for collaboration between geriatric and palliative care
nurse specialists. Symptoms of illness and dying may appear differently, for longer periods,
and in greater numbers in older adults (Amella,
2003). Pain, confusion, dyspnea, fatigue, satiety
and anorexia, gastrointestinal distress, infection
and fever, and fears and depression are symptoms that can present differently in older adults.
Palliative care interventions logically flow from
goals of care. Therefore, the first step in hospice
palliative care is to establish the patient's goals
of care (Morrison & Meier, 2004). In the context of chronic, debilitating, and life-threatening
illness, realistic and attainable goals of care
that relieve pain and other symptoms, improve
quality of life, limit the burden of care, enhance
personal relationships, and provide a sense of
control are crucial to the dying person and their
families (Steinhauser et al., 2000). Professional
palliative care practitioners work with patients
and their families to establish reasonable goals
of care (Vollrath & von Gunten, 2007).

Establishing goals of care, whether daily,
weekly, or monthly, is a shared approach to
honouring the values and beliefs of the patient in the context of direct care activities as
well as meaning-making opportunities. Using
open-ended and probing questions may be

helpful when interviewing the client (Morrison & Meier, 2004). The clinician may ask questions such as the following to illuminate meaningful goals of care: "What makes life worth living for you?", "Given the severity of your illness, what are the most important things for you to achieve?", "What are your most important hopes?", "What are your biggest fears?", or "What would you consider to be a fate worse than death?" (Quill, 2000). Goals of care are dynamic across the trajectory of a chronic disease (EPEC Project, 2004; Quill, 2000). Meier, Back, and Morrison (2001) describe some of the warning signs of ineffective or contradictory goals as frequent or lengthy hospitalizations, physician feelings of frustration, anger or powerlessness, and feelings of caregiver burden.

After establishing patient and family goals of care, the next logical intervention is the completion of an advance care plan. Goals of care reflect the values, beliefs, and culture of the person with a serious, life-threatening illness. Numerous studies (Miles, Koepp, & Weber, 1996) reported that most people do not have advance care plans and that the documents that do exist are ineffective in improving communication between patients and their physicians (Morrison & Meier, 2004). Other authors reported that advance care plans are ineffective related to the decision making relative to cardiopulmonary resuscitation (Teno et al., 1997). Morrison and Meier (2004) suggested that as the number of advance care plans increases, more consumers and healthcare professionals will become familiar with the documents, thus improving their effectiveness. The literature suggests that the focus of advance care planning needs to shift to helping patients engage their loved ones in an authentic dialogue regarding what they regard as an acceptable quality of life (Fried, Bradley, Towle, & Allore, 2002; Meier &

Morrison, 2002). This discussion is the crucial element, not the completion of the advance care planning forms.

Consumers and healthcare professionals can use a variety of resources for advance care planning as numerous programs have developed thoughtful advance care planning processes. Alberta Health Services developed an integrated program using the "My Voice" workbook and videos (see Internet Resources) as the platform to engage the family conversation, which is at the heart of advance care planning. Workbooks and goals of care designation documents are available online (see Internet Resources) that help families discuss their values and wishes regarding medical treatment if they cannot speak for themselves. It is also important to be aware of the provincial regulations related to advance care planning because documentation and process can vary from province to province.

Clinical Practice Guidelines for Hospice Palliative Care

The prevalence of symptom burden at the end of life is high for patients with chronic disease such as COPD and renal disease (Nazir & Erbland, 2009; Yong et al., 2009). According to the National Institutes of Health (2004), assessment and management of symptoms have been studied most thoroughly in patients with cancer. Patients with other life-limiting illnesses, such as congestive heart failure, have their own challenges. Regardless of the diagnosis, symptoms common to advanced disease include anorexia and cachexia, anxiety, constipation, depression, delirium, dyspnea, nausea, and pain (Morrison & Meier, 2004). It is beyond the scope of this chapter to describe in detail the assessment and management recommendations for these symptoms; however, there are numerous resources in the literature with specific protocols and interventions (American Geriatrics Society Panel on Persistent Pain in Older Persons, 2002; Block, 2000; Casarett & Inouye, 2001; Luce & Luce, 2001; Strasser & Bruera, 2002). These clinicians and researchers have worked diligently to integrate the evidence in the form of clinical practice guidelines that are outcome driven. Clinical practice guidelines are evidence-informed care management tools developed by experts in disciplines such as nursing, pharmacy, and medicine. These tools are intended for use by palliative care consultants as well as other healthcare professionals who are involved in the palliation of symptoms. **Table 19-4** refers the reader to a series of clinical practice guidelines commonly associated with select chronic disease symptoms.

The Center to Advance Palliative Care identified major outcomes of palliative care, including: (1) relief of pain and other distressing symptoms, (2) clear communication and decision making regarding goals of care and development of treatment plans, (3) completion of life-prolonging or curative treatments, and (4) increased patient and family satisfaction. The next steps in palliative care are to develop the science, the care delivery systems, and the instruments to deliver and evaluate the outcomes of quality palliative care.

Table 19-4 Clinical Practice Guidelines for Common Symptom Experiences

Chronic Disease	Common Issue	Advocacy Organization	Clinical Practice Guidelines
Chronic obstructive pulmonary disease	Dyspnea	Canadian Thoracic Society	http://www.respiratoryguidelines.ca/2011-cts-slide-kit-copd-dyspnea-management-en
Diabetes mellitus	Neuropathy	Canadian Diabetes Association	http://www.diabetes.ca/forprofessionals/resources/2008-cpg/
Cerebrovascular accident	Seizure	Edmonton Palliative Care Program	http://www.palliative.org
Congestive heart failure	Transitional care	Canadian Heart Failure Network	http://www.chfn.ca/practice-guidelines
Hypertension	Detection and management	BC Ministry of Health	http://www.bcguidelines.ca/guideline_hypertension.html#algorithm1
Alzheimer's disease	Delirium	National Guideline Clearinghouse	http://www.guidelines.gov/content.aspx?id=11533
Parkinson's disease	Advance care planning	Canadian Virtual Hospice	http://www.virtualhospice.ca
Addiction	Compulsive thoughts	Behavioural Health Recovery Management	http://www.bhrm.org/guidelines/addguidelines.htm

CASE STUDY

www

Mr. James is an 80-year-old widower who resides alone in his first-floor apartment. He has a history of cardiac disease requiring a pacemaker and medication for hypertension. Mr. James was diagnosed with congestive heart failure 4 years ago after increasing episodes of fatigue and dyspnea. He was recently discharged from the hospital after an episode of extreme short-ness of breath and fluid retention. His daughter is visiting from out of town and brought him to his post-discharge appointment with his nurse practitioner. His recent hospitalization occurred because of his most severe exacerbation of his symptoms to date. His cardiologist changed his congestive heart failure classification to the New York Heart Association Functional Class III. His nurse practitioner reviews his medical record, medication profile, and family care confer-ence notes. An advance directive has been completed and is now part of his medical record. His daughter is the designated healthcare power of attorney.

Mr. James's daughter is very concerned about her father's physical and emotional health. He seems depressed and "ready to go home to be with his wife." The daughter suggested that Mr. James consider moving so that the family could take care of him. Mr. James wants to re-main in his own apartment and manage his symptoms at home rather than in the hospital. His nurse practitioner realizes this is an opportunity to discuss Mr. James's future, his options, and goals of care. Available treatment options include medication changes, antidepressants, home oxygen therapy, nutrition, physical therapy, home health care, and support groups for persons with heart failure (some are online). After the discussion with Mr. James and his daughter, the nurse practitioner will write up the plan chosen by Mr. James and document it in his medical chart to maintain continuity of care with all of his healthcare providers.

Discussion Questions

1. Would you describe this situation as responsive to palliative care (provide rationale)?
2. Based upon the information provided, what is your recommended plan of care for Mr. James?
3. What are some examples that may indicate the need for a change in location of care for Mr. James?
4. What is the relevance of having Mr. James's daughter, his designated agent for healthcare decisions, involved in the discussion regarding his goals of care?
5. How would you respond to Mr. James when he states, "I want to go home and be with my wife"?
6. Based on this case study how would you negotiate changes in Mr. James's goals of care?

HOSPICE PALLIATIVE CARE ISSUES AND OPPORTUNITIES ____

Limited understanding of the options available to dying patients and their families results in delayed access to hospice and palliative care services (Field & Cassel, 1997). Surveys consistently indicate patients prefer to die at home. Consumers' and communities' lack of understanding of what comprehensive palliative care programs offer, poor communication about patient and family preferences, and a societal denial of death all impede timely referrals to palliative care services (End-of-Life Nursing Education Consortium, 2009a). Communication is a core competency underpinning excellence in hospice palliative care; however, many clinicians are uncomfortable sharing bad news and poor prognoses. Ineffective communication among patients, families, and their physicians led to undesired resuscitation efforts, extensive use of hospital resources, and additional suffering. Other studies suggested that "patient-centred" interviews are associated with improved levels of satisfaction on the part of patients and their families (Dowsett et al., 2000; Steinhauser et al., 2000).

Issues in palliative care exist for numerous reasons. The major underlying resistance stems from a biomedical philosophy that emphasizes cure and prolongation of life over quality of life and relief of suffering (Morrison & Meier, 2004). Physician reimbursement plans (e.g., fee for service), particularly in primary care, influence medical practice patterns related to palliative care. Regionally, in British Columbia and Alberta, for example, provincial medical associations have negotiated alternative payment plans for physicians that tend to support the development of interprofessional teams. Research evaluating how these payment plans actually influenced the practice patterns of physicians who choose to work in the interprofessional context has, however, not been undertaken.

Prognostication in chronic, debilitating, and life-threatening illness presents a major challenge for professional practitioners and is a barrier to adequate palliative care (Christakis & Lamont, 2000). Our current care systems often force patients and families to choose between curative treatment and comfort care. However, there is growing recognition that hospice palliative care is needed from diagnosis through the process of dying (Foley, 2001). To reiterate, palliative care can be defined as interdisciplinary care focused on the relief of suffering with the goal to improve one's quality of life. This focus, some have argued, reasonably should remove the burden of prognostication and the requirement of a terminal diagnosis (von Gunten & Romer, 1999) in favour of a more laissez-faire practice ontology. Still, prognostication remains an important part of Canadian hospice palliative care service delivery for clinicians and patients alike (Glare et al., 2008).

Education for Healthcare Professionals

Research suggests a critical need for improvement in the education and training of healthcare professionals in palliative and end-of-life care (Field & Cassel, 1997). Healthcare professionals have traditionally received inadequate education and training in the safe and effective management of pain and other symptoms. They also lack the skills and confidence to address the psychological, social, and spiritual aspects of care (Sullivan, Lakoma, & Block, 2003). Nursing curricula and textbooks are deficient in palliative and end-of-life content and clinical learning opportunities. If registered nurses are not taught that their professional role includes providing quality palliative and end-of-life care, then they cannot practice it (Ferrell, Virani, & Grant, 1999). In response to these identified needs, resources for teaching palliative care nursing to students and practicing nurses have been and continue to be developed and disseminated (CASN, 2011).

Ferrell and Coyle (2001, 2006) wrote a comprehensive volume entitled *Textbook of Palliative Nursing*; the third edition was re-named the *Oxford Textbook of Palliative Nursing* to recognize it as a leading resource in the field of palliative nursing. Recognizing the special needs of older adults, Matzo and Sherman authored *Gerontologic Palliative Care Nursing* (2004). Morrison and Meier, two palliative medicine specialist physicians, authored the textbook *Geriatric Palliative Care* (2003). Experienced clinicians and researchers continue to share their knowledge, skills, and passion for palliative care through diverse publications, websites, conferences, and now social media such as Facebook and Twitter.

The Pallium Project received major funding from the Health Canada Primary Care Transition Funds for the development and dissemination of the Learning Essential Approaches to Palliative and End of Life Care (LEAP) curriculum (Pereira et al., 2008). Hospice palliative care education seminars were developed for interprofessional teams across Canada. Geriatric and acute medicine nurses, pharmacists, physicians, social workers, volunteers, and palliative care program coordinators were invited to a 3-day weekend gathering and educated with the LEAP curriculum using a Train-the-Trainer methodology, which was then taken back to the local program. Collegial sharing is in the spirit

of improving and disseminating the science and the art of palliative care. One of the outcomes of the Pallium Project was an award-winning series of clinical palliative care videos, organizational presentations using PowerPoint format, and 10 podcasts entitled "Conversations on Caring." Physicians have a parallel program within Pallium; however, the mission of the Pallium Project is to educate all healthcare professionals on the essential clinical competencies in palliative care. The Education on Palliative and End of Life Care curriculum was developed for physicians in the United States and is available online (www.epec.net). Its purpose is advancing end-of-life care through an online community of educational scholars. Case studies, presentations, and articles are a few of the resources available.

Professional Practice Specialties in Hospice Palliative Care

Hospice palliative care is organized around the concepts of holism and an engaged interprofessional team. Complete care of the whole person begins and ends with the patient and family, who are supported by registered and practical nurses, social workers, chaplains, volunteers, and other rehabilitation professionals. Palliative medicine is the specialty practiced by physicians and is an important part of the interprofessional team relative to medical management of symptom load (Derek, Hanks, Cherny, & Calman, 2004).

HOSPICE PALLIATIVE CARE NURSING

Hospice palliative care closely parallels the discipline of nursing, honouring and assessing the health and illness experience of persons, including the families of origin and of choice, in the environment in which they live. Individuals and families experiencing life-limiting progressive illness are the focus of the hospice palliative care nurse's evidenced-informed physical, emotional, psychosocial, spiritual, and existential assessments and interventions. Coyle (2010) described the distinctive features of hospice palliative care nursing as "a whole person" philosophy of care that is provided across care settings throughout the illness trajectory, including the patient's death and the ensuing family bereavement. A nurse's relationship with the patient and family is a critical component of the healing relationship that, together with empiric knowledge (e.g., effective pain and symptom management) and clinical skill (e.g., addressing the emotional, psychosocial, spiritual needs, and cultural values), is the essence of hospice palliative care nursing specialty (Coyle, 2010).

In 2001, CHPCA supported the development of a national examination administered by the Canadian Nurses Association to certify advanced hospice palliative care competencies among registered nurses. The CHPCA Nurses Group, a national nursing coalition, was formed in 2003 to serve the networking and support needs of nurses caring for terminal patients and their families. The CHPCA Nurses Group provides representative leadership, advocacy, and education to advance quality hospice palliative care for the benefit of all Canadians.

ALLIED HOSPICE PALLIATIVE CARE DISCIPLINES

The CHPCA's valuing of the whole interprofessional team has resulted in norms and standards of practice for several identified members of the interprofessional team, including volunteers, pharmacists, social workers and counsellors, spiritual advisors, and physiotherapists. Interest

groups have been established across Canada and are supported with a biennial learning institute that provides clinicians with advanced clinical education related to hospice palliative care. See Internet Resources later in the chapter for website addresses that will inform allied hospice palliative care clinicians across Canada. The norms and standards of practice documents can be found under the professionals tab on CHPCA's main web page at www.chpca.net /about_igs.

PALLIATIVE MEDICINE

Gelfman and Morrison (2008) defined palliative medicine as "a sub-specialty that focuses on relieving suffering and improving quality of life for patients with serious illness and their families" (p. 36). The Canadian Society of Palliative Care Physicians was formed in 1993 to advance the quality of life of dying patients and their families and ensure the provision of interdisciplinary palliative care of the dying by primary care physicians who are supported by palliative medicine and palliative care experts. Arising from the work of a group of dedicated physicians, a growing number of universities are now providing training programs for medical students in palliative medicine. In Canada two universities have established 1-year palliative medicine fellowships. Most of the physicians finishing these fellowships work in any number of salaried consultant positions in acute care hospitals across Canada. In 2006 the American Board of Medical Specialties announced the addition of a new subspecialty certificate in Hospice and Palliative Medicine joining members of the international community including Great Britain, Canada, Ireland, and Australia in formally recognizing palliative medicine as a subspecialty (von Gunten & Lupu, 2004).

RESEARCH

Goldstein and Morrison (2005) called for a new research agenda for geriatric palliative care. Their premise, based on the National Institutes of Health (2004) and Institute of Medicine (Cleeland, 2001; Field & Cassel, 1997) reports, was that the evidence base for palliative care in older adults is sparse. Adults 75 years or older with comorbidities and noncancer diagnoses have repeatedly been excluded from palliative care research. Their proposed research agenda for palliative care in geriatrics includes the following: (1) establishing the prevalence of symptoms in patients with chronic disease, (2) evaluating the association between symptom treatment and outcomes, (3) increasing the evidence base for symptom treatment, (4) understanding patients' psychological/spiritual well-being and quality of life, (5) elucidating sources of caregiver burden, (6) reevaluating service delivery, (7) adapting research methodologies specifically for palliative care, and (8) increasing the number of geriatricians trained in palliative care research (Goldstein & Morrison, 2005).

The continued evolution of hospice palliative care to meet the needs of an aging population rests in part on knowledge generation and translation. Aging adults' care needs include interventions to manage the symptoms and distress of chronic illness. However, the knowledge base to support symptom management, communication, and decision-making skills and models for the delivery of palliative care are often inadequate. As the science supporting the practice of palliative care is built, it is imperative to determine whether the research, education, and clinical interventions already funded to improve hospice palliative care for individuals with life-limiting or terminal illnesses were effective. Measuring the effectiveness of palliative care is a challenge that requires both prospective and retrospective studies (Steinhauser, 2004). Four challenges exist related to outcome measurement in palliative care: (1) end of life is a complex multidimensional experience in which understanding of the interrelatedness of domains is unclear; (2) the period "end of life" is ill defined; (3) both patient and family are the unit of care, yet little is known about the correlations between the trajectories of their experiences; and (4) patients, the primary focus of care, are often unable to communicate in their last days or weeks, rendering their subjective experience unable to be evaluated (Steinhauser, 2004).

Outcomes research in palliative care continues to develop, generating consensus about the broad domains related to end-of-life care: physical or psychosocial symptoms, social relationships, spiritual or philosophical beliefs, hopes, expectation and meaning, satisfaction, economic considerations, and caregiver and family experiences. Quality of life is also considered an outcome, but quality of life needs a clearer definition and consistent measurement to strengthen the relationship. The Palliative and End-of-Life Care (PELC) Initiative was developed by the Canadian Institutes of Health Research's Institute of Cancer Research to support the development of a prioritized research agenda, develop infrastructure, enhance interdisciplinary research collaboration, and encourage the development of early hospice palliative care career researchers. PELC research presents unique methodological, logistical, and ethical challenges unique to a population of participants who are also living their dying. PELC research involves extremely vulnerable populations and thus needs highly trained personnel, increasing its cost and complexity. The PELC practice community is itself nascent, and few practitioners in PELC have research training. With a total investment of $16.5 million over 6 years, the Canadian Institutes of Health Research's PELC Initiative is the largest research investment of its type in the world.

Finally, a nursing research collaborative, involving the University of Victoria, the Fraser Health Authority, Trinity Western University, the Vancouver Coastal Health Authority, University of British Columbia-Okanagan, the Interior Health Authority, and the Vancouver Island Health Authority, has mobilized nurses to consider their care practices for chronic disease patients who are accessing community and acute care but who fall within the 70% of Canadians who do not routinely have access to palliative care. These Canadian researchers endeavour to learn how nurses can bring a *palliative approach* to their care in settings where palliation would add depth and quality to a person's life, but where the person does not meet admission criteria to the local hospice or palliative care program. The palliative approach involves physical, psychological spiritual and social care, which is not delayed until the end stages of an illness. Instead, the palliative approach is applied earlier in the illness trajectory to provide active, comfort-focused care aimed at relieving suffering, facilitating quality life experiences that are directed by patient and family, and shaping intentional therapeutic space for expressions of loss and bereavement (Kristjanson, Toye, & Dawson, 2003). The ongoing work of the iPANEL collaborative can be viewed at www.iPANEL.ca.

SUMMARY

In summary, chronic disease, like any other disease process, has its own natural history. With few exceptions, the illness trajectory of most chronic diseases can be described by periods of general wellness punctuated with exacerbations of potentially life-threatening disease. A multiplicity of issues exists in the setting of symptom burden and functional decline that influence the personal context underpinning the chronic illness experience. Pain management, symptom control, advance care planning, celebration and connection, meaning making, and comfort all coalesce within a caring practice ontology known as the palliative approach. By routinely utilizing a palliative approach across care settings, hospice palliative care extends a compassionate hand to people who are often struggling through the myriad transitions associated with chronic disease at the end of life

INTERNET RESOURCES   **WWW**

The Canadian Virtual Hospice organization has developed a website providing information and support on palliative and end-of-life care and loss and grief issues for patients, their families, and the professionals who serve them (www.virtualhospice.ca). The website features articles of interest (e.g., Talking with Children), books, links, FAQ sheets, and information on hospice palliative care programs and services.

Palliative Care Resources

Alberta Health Services for Advance Care Planning:
    www.calgaryhealthregion.ca/programs
    /advancecareplanning/acp_tools.htm
Canadian Geriatrics Society:
    www.canadiangeriatrics.ca/default/
Canadian Hospice Palliative Care Association:
    www.chpca.net/about_igs
Canadian Hospice Palliative Care Association
    Aboriginal Issues:
    www.chpca.net/become-a-member
    /aboriginal-issues.aspx

(continues)

INTERNET RESOURCES (Cont.)

www

Canadian Hospice Palliative Care Association Nurses Interest Group:
www.chpca.net/become-a-member/nurses.aspx

Canadian Hospice Palliative Care Association Strategic Plan:
www.chpca.net/canadian_strategy_for_palliative_and_eol_care

Canadian Virtual Hospice:
www.virtualhospice.ca/en_US/Main+Site+Navigation/Home.aspx

Centre for Advancement of Palliative Care:
www.capc.org

Edmonton Regional Palliative Care Program:
www.palliative.org

Education in Palliative and End-of-Life Care:
www.epec.net

National Guideline Clearing House:
www.guideline.gov

National Palliative Care Research Center:
www.npcrc.org

Pain Resource Center:
www.prc.coh.org

Palliative Care:
www.getpalliativecare.org

Pallium Project:
www.pallium.ca

Quality End of Life Care Coalition of Canada:
chpca.net/projects-and-advocacy/the-quality-end-of-life-care-coalition-of-canada.aspx

Toolkit of Instruments to Measure End of Life Care (TIME):
www.chcr.brown.edu/pcoc/-toolkit.htm

Evidence-Informed Practice Box

Ninety-two community-based caregivers on Vancouver Island for persons aged 65 and older and also experiencing heavy caregiving demands were studied with respect to role-specific burden and two quality of life measures. Data were collected at two different times, 1 year apart, using face-to-face interviews and several structured questionnaires to measure role-specific *burden*, *life satisfaction*, and *overall perceived stress*. Multiple regression analyses were conducted with each of the preceding outcomes to assess each as a predictor of role-specific burden. Findings support the claim that despite levels of burden, most caregivers cope with the care of their loved one and high levels of burden do not necessarily mean a low quality of life. Demands of the caregiving role turned out to be the best predictors of caregiver burden. Overall quality of life, however, was best predicted by the caregivers' personal resources and their perception of burden. Interestingly, researchers were not able to identify any differences in burden or overall quality of life relative to either age or gender. Instead, individual management of the varied roles that caregivers find themselves occupying as well as a sense of personal resilience helped to determine how the demands of caregiving impact one's overall well-being.

Source: Chappell & Dujela (2008).

STUDY QUESTIONS

1. Reflect on the following statement: Hospice care is palliative care but not all palliative care is hospice care. What does it mean to you as a provider and to the recipient of your care?

2. List the domains of end-of-life care developed by the CHPCA.

3. Identify barriers to palliative care for an individual with a serious, life-limiting illness.

4. What is your vision of hospice palliative care?

5. Identify three online resources to further your education in hospice palliative care of the older adult.

6. Go online and find support information appropriate for the family caregiver of a palliative care patient.

7. Describe how you could you use Nolan and Mock's (2004) "A Conceptual Framework for End-of-Life Care" as an organizing framework in your clinical practice.

8. Describe how the goals of care might differ for an 85-year-old man diagnosed with prostate cancer versus a 65-year-old man diagnosed with stage 3 lung cancer.

For a full suite of assignments and additional learning activities, use the access code located in the front of your book and visit this exclusive website: **http://go.jblearning.com/kramer-kile**. If you do not have an access code, you can obtain one at the site.

REFERENCES

Amella, E. J. (2003). Geriatrics and palliative care: Collaboration for quality of life until death. *Journal of Hospice and Palliative Nursing, 5*(1), 40–48.

American Geriatrics Society Panel on Persistent Pain in Older Persons. (2002). The management of persistent pain in older persons. *Journal of the American Geriatrics Society, 50*(Suppl.), S205–S224. Retrieved from http://www.eapc.org/building-a-hospital-based-palliative-care-program/case/outcomes

Barber, C. (1988). Correlates of subjective burden among adult sons and daughters caring for aged parents. *Journal of Aging Studies, 2*(2), 133–144.

Bernstein, S. J. (2008). A new model for chronic-care delivery. *Front Health Serv Manage, 25*(2), 31–38; discussion 43, 45–46.

Berry, P. H. (2004). Promoting quality of life during the dying process. In M. L. Matzo & D. W. Sherman (Eds.), *Gerontologic palliative care nursing* (pp. 1–2). St. Louis, MO: Mosby.

Block, S. D. (2000). Assessing and managing depression in the terminally ill patient. *Annals of Internal Medicine, 132*(3), 209–218.

Bookbinder, M., Coyle, N., Kiss, M., Goldstein, M. L., Holritz, K., Thaler, H., Gianella, A., . . . Portenoy, R. K. (1996). Implementing national standards for cancer pain management: Program model and evaluation. *Journal of Pain and Symptom Management, 12*(6), 334–347.

Canadian Hospice Palliative Care Association. (2005). *Applying a model to guide hospice palliative care: An essential companion toolkit for planners, policy makers, caregivers, educators, managers, administrators and researchers.* Ottawa, ON: Author.

Canadian Hospice Palliative Care Association. (2007). *Moving forward by building on strengths: A discussion document on aboriginal hospice palliative care in Canada.* Ottawa, ON: Author.

Canadian Hospice Palliative Care Association. (2010). *CHPCA fact sheet: Hospice palliative care in Canada* (pp. 1–12). Ottawa, ON: Author.

Canadian Institute for Health Information. (2007). Canada's greying anatomy. *CIHI Directions, 14*(3), 1–8.

Carstairs, S., & Beaudroin, G. (2000). Quality end of life care: The right of every Canadian. Final report Retrieved from http://www.parl.gc.ca/Content/SEN /Committee/362/upda/rep/repfinjun00-e.htm

Casarett, D. J., & Inouye. S. K. (2001). Diagnosis and management of delirium near the end of life. *Annals of Internal Medicine, 135*, 32–40.

Cassel, C. K. (2003). Foreword. In R. S. Morrison & D. E. Meier (Eds.), *Geriatric palliative medicine* (pp. vii–ix). Oxford, UK: Oxford University Press.

Center to Advance Palliative Care. (2011). Improving clinical outcomes. Retrieved from http://www.capc.org /building-a-hospital-based-palliative-care-program /case/outcomes/

Chappell, N., & Dujela, C. (2008). Caregiving: Predicting at-risk status. *Canadian Journal on Aging, 27*(2), 169–179.

Chochinov, H. M. (2000, May). Testimony at recent senate subcommittee hearing to update "Of life and death." *Canadian Physicians for Life.* Retrieved from http://www.physiciansforlife.ca/html/life/palliative /articles/pallcarecomments.html

Chochinov, H. M. (2004). *Interventions to enhance the spiritual aspects of dying. National Institutes of Health state-of-the-science conference on improving end-of-life care program & abstracts.* Bethesda, MD: U.S. Department of Health and Human Services, National Institutes of Health.

Chochinov, H. M. (2011). Dignity-conserving care—a new model for palliative care: Helping the patient feel valued. In S. J. McPhee, M. A. Winker, M. W. Rabow, S. Z. Pantilat, & A. J. Markowitz (Eds.), *Care at the close of life: Evidence and experience* (pp. 353–362). New York, NY: McGraw-Hill.

Chochinov, H. M., Hack, T., Hassard, T., Kristjanson, L. J., McClement, S., & Harlos, M. (2004). Dignity and psychotherapeutic considerations in end-of-life care. *Journal of Palliative Care, 20*(3), 134–142.

Chochinov, H. M., Hack, T., Hassard, T., Kristjanson, L. J., McClement, S., & Harlos, M. (2005). Dignity therapy: A novel psychotherapeutic intervention for patients near the end of life. *Journal of Clinical Oncology, 23*(24), 5520–5525.

Christakis, N., & Lamont, E. B. (2000). Extent and determinants of error in doctors' prognoses in terminally ill patients: Prospective cohort study. *British Medical Journal, 320*, 469–473.

Cicely Saunders International. (2010). Cicely Saunders Institute. Retrieved from http://www.cicelysaunders foundation.org

Cleeland, C. S. (2001). Cross-cutting research issues. A research agenda for reducing distress of patients with cancer. In K. Foley & H. Gelband (Eds.), *Improving palliative care for cancer* (pp. 233–274). Washington, DC: National Institute of Medicine.

Collins, J. (2011). *Health care use at the end of life in Atlantic Canada.* Ottawa, ON: Canadian Institute for Health Information.

Corbin, J. (2001). Introduction and overview: Chronic illness and nursing. In R. Hyman & J. Corbin (Eds.), *Chronic illness: Research and theory for nursing practice* (pp. 1–15). New York, NY: Springer.

Coyle, N. (2010). Introduction to palliative nursing care. In B. R. Ferrell & N. Coyle (Eds.), *Textbook of palliative nursing* (3rd ed., pp. 3–11). Oxford, UK: Oxford University Press.

Curtin, M., & Lubkin, I. (1995). What is chronicity? In I. Lubkin (Ed.), *Chronic illness: Impact and interventions* (3rd ed., pp. 3–25). Sudbury, MA: Jones and Bartlett.

Delafuente, J. C. (2009). The silver tsunami is coming: Will pharmacy be swept away with the tide? [Opinion]. *American Journal of Pharmaceutical Education, 73*(1), 1–2.

Derek, D., Hanks, G., Cherny, N., & Calman, K. (2004). Introduction. In D. Doyle, G. Hanks, N. Cherny, & K. Calman (Eds.), *Oxford textbook of palliative medicine* (3rd ed., pp. 1–4). Oxford, UK: Oxford University Press.

Dowsett, S. M., Saul, J. L., Buttow, P. N., Dunn, S. M., Boyer, M. J., Findlow, R., & Dunsmore, J. (2000). Communication styles in the cancer consultation: Preferences for a patient-centered approach. *Psychooncology, 9*, 147–156.

End of Life Nursing Education Consortium. (2009a). *Module 1: Nursing at the end of life.* American Association of Colleges of Nursing and City of Hope National Medical Center. Washington, DC: Author.

End of Life Nursing Education Consortium. (2009b). *Module 5: Cultural considerations in EOL care.* American Association of Colleges of Nursing and City of Hope National Medical Center. Washington, DC: Author.

EPEC Project. (2004). Education on palliative and end-of-life care. Retrieved from http://www.epec.net

Fassbender, K., Smythe, J., Carson, M., Finegan, B., & Boothe, P. (2006). *Costs and utilization of health care services at end-of-life.* Report of the Institute for Public Economics Health Research Group to Alberta Health and Wellness. Edmonton, AB: Institute for Public Economics.

Ferrell, B. R., & Coyle, N. (Eds.). (2001). *Textbook of palliative nursing.* New York, NY: Oxford University Press.

Ferrell, B. R., & Coyle, N. (Eds.). (2006). *Textbook of palliative nursing* (2nd ed.). New York, NY: Oxford University Press.

Ferrell, B., Virani, R., & Grant, M. (1999). Analysis of end-of-life content in nursing textbooks. *Oncology Nursing Forum, 26*(5), 869–876.

Ferris, F. D., Balfour, H. M., Bowen, K., Farley, J., Lamontagne, C., Lundy, M., . . . West, P. J. (2002). *A model to guide hospice palliative care.* Ottawa, ON: CHPCA.

Field, M. J., & Cassel, C. K. (Eds.). (1997). *Approaching death: Improving care at the end of life.* Committee on Care at the End of Life, Division of Health Care Services, Institute of Medicine. Washington, DC: National Academies Press.

Foley, K. (2001). Preface. In K. M. Foley & H. Gelband (Eds.), *Improving palliative care for cancer* (pp. xi–xii). Washington, DC: National Academies Press.

Fried, T. R., Bradley, E. H., Towle, V. R., & Allore, H. (2002). Understanding the treatment preferences of seriously ill patients. *New England Journal of Medicine, 346,* 1061–1066.

Gelfman, L. A., & Morrison, R. S. (2008). Research funding for palliative medicine. *Journal of Palliative Medicine, 11,* 36–43.

Gillick, M. R. (2009). Decision making near life's end: A prescription for change. *Journal of Palliative Medicine, 12*(2), 121–125. doi:10.1089/jpm.2008.0240

Glare, P., Sinclair, C., Downing, M., Stone, P., Maltoni, M., & Vigano, A. (2008). Predicting survival in patients with advanced disease. *European Journal of Cancer, 44*(8), 1146–1156.

Glass, E., Cluxton, D., & Rancour, P. (2001). Principles of patient and family assessment. In B. R. Ferrell & N. Coyle (Eds.), *Textbook of palliative nursing.* New York, NY: Oxford University Press.

Goldstein, N. E., & Morrison, R. S. (2005). The intersection between geriatrics and palliative care: A call for a new research agenda. *Journal of the American Geriatrics Society, 53,* 1593–1598.

Hansford, P. (2010). Palliative care in the United Kingdom. In B. R. Ferrell & N. Coyle (Eds.), *Oxford textbook of palliative nursing* (3rd ed., pp. 1265–1274). Oxford, UK: Oxford University Press.

HCIC-SSSC. (2007). 10th Annual Health Care in Canada Survey: A national survey of health care providers, managers, and the public. Toronto, ON: *MediResource Inc.* Retrieved from http://www.hcic-sssc.ca/english/files/CurrentContent/2007/2007_hcic.pdf

Higginson, I. J. (2011). Foreword. In S. J. McPhee, M. A. Winker, M. W. Rabow, S. Z. Pantilat, & A. J. Markowitz (Eds.), *Care at the close of life: Evidence and experience.* New York, NY: McGraw-Hill.

Hospice and Palliative Nurses Association. (2011). Leading the way. Retrieved from http://www.hpna.org/Displaypage.aspx?Title=LeadingtheWay

Kaufert, J. (1999). Cultural mediation in cancer diagnosis and end of life decision-making: The experience of aboriginal patients in Canada. *Medical Anthropology, 6*(3), 405–421.

Kelly, L., & Brown, J. (2002). Listening to native patients. Changes in physicians' understanding and behaviour. *Canadian Family Physician, 48*(10), 1645–1652.

Kelly, L., Linkewich, B., St. Pierre-Hansen, N., & Antone, I. (2009). Palliative care of First Nations people: A qualitative study of bereaved family members. *Canadian Family Physician, 55*(4), 394–395.

Kelly, L., & Minty, A. (2007). End of life issues for aboriginal patients: A literature review. *Canadian Family Physician, 53*(9), 1459–1465.

Kemp, C. (1999). *Terminal illness: A guide to nursing care* (2nd ed.). Philadelphia, PA: Lippincott.

Kristjanson, L., Toye, C., & Dawson, S. (2003). New dimensions in palliative care: A palliative approach to neurodegenerative diseases and final illness in older people. *The Medical Journal of Australia, 179*(6 Suppl.), S41–S43.

Kubler-Ross, E. (1969). *On death and dying.* New York, NY: Macmillan.

Luce, J. M., & Luce, J. A. (2001). Perspective on care at the close of life: Management of dyspnea in patients with far-advanced lung disease: "Once I lose it, it's kind of hard to catch it . . ." *Journal of the American Medical Association, 285*, 1331–1337.

Lunney, J. R., Lynn, J., & Hogan, C. (2002). Profiles of older Medicare decedents. *Journal of the American Geriatrics Society, 50*(6), 1108–1112. doi:10.1046/j.1532-5415.2002.50268.x

Lynn, J. (2001a). Serving patients who may die soon and their families: The role of hospice and other services. *Journal of the American Medical Association, 285*, 925–932.

Lynn, J. (2001b). Perspectives on care at the close of life. Serving patients who may die soon and their families: The role of hospice and other services. *Journal of the American Medical Association, 285*(7), 925–932.

Lynn, J., Arkes, H. R., Stevens, M., Cohn, F., Koenig, B., Fox, E., . . . Tsevat, J. (2000). Rethinking fundamental assumptions: SUPPORT's implications for future reform. *Journal of the American Geriatrics Society, 48*(5), S214–S221.

Lynn, J., Schuster, J. L., Wilkinson, A., & Simon, L. N. (2008). *Improving care for the end of life: A sourcebook for health care managers and clinicians* (2nd ed.). Oxford, UK: Oxford University Press.

Manfredi, P. L., Morrison, R. S., Morris, J., Goldhirsch, S. L., Carter, J. M., & Meier, D. E. (2000). Palliative care consultations: How do they impact the care of hospitalized patients? *Journal of Pain and Symptom Management, 20*, 166–173.

Manitoba Centre for Health Policy. (2007). *Health care use at the end of life in Western Canada.* Ottawa, ON: CIHI.

Martin, C. (2007). Chronic disease and illness care. *Canadian Family Physician, 53*(12), 2086–2091.

Matzo, M. L., & Sherman, D. W. (Eds.). (2004). *Gerontologic palliative care nursing.* St. Louis, MO: Mosby.

McClain, C. S., Rosenfield, B., & Breitbart, W. (2003). Effect of spiritual well-being on end-of-life despair in terminally ill cancer patients. *Lancet, 361*, 1603–1607.

McClement, S., Chochinov, H. M., Hack, T., Hassard, T., Kristjanson, L. J., & Harlos, M. (2007). Dignity therapy: Family member perspectives. *Journal of Palliative Medicine, 10*(5), 1076–1082.

McMillan, S. C. (2004). *Interventions to facilitate family caregiving. National Institutes of Health state-of-the-science conference on improving end-of-life care program & abstracts.* Bethesda, MD: U.S. Department of Health and Human Services, National Institutes of Health.

Meier, D. E. (2010). The development, status, and future of palliative care. In D. E. Meier, S. L. Isaacs, & R. G. Hughes (Eds.), *Palliative care: Transforming the care of serious illness* (pp. 4–76). San Francisco, CA: Jossey-Bass.

Meier, D. E., Back, A. L., & Morrison, R. S. (2001). The inner life of physicians and care of the seriously ill. *Journal of the American Medical Association, 286*, 3007–3014.

Meier, D. E., & Morrison, R. S. (2002). Autonomy reconsidered. *New England Journal of Medicine, 346*, 1087–1089.

Miles, S. H., Koepp, R., & Weber, E. P. (1996). Advance end-of-life treatment planning: A research review. *Archives of Internal Medicine, 156*, 1062–1068.

Morrison, R. S., & Meier, D. E. (Eds.). (2003). *Geriatric palliative care.* New York, NY: Oxford University Press.

Morrison, R. S., & Meier, D. E. (2004). Palliative care. *New England Journal of Medicine, 350*, 2582–2590.

National Aboriginal Health Organization. (2002). *Discussion paper on end of life care for aboriginal peoples.* Ottawa, ON: NAHO.

National Consensus Project for Quality Palliative Care. (2009). *Clinical practice guidelines for quality palliative care* (2nd ed.). Retrieved from http://www.nationalconsensusproject.org/guideline.pdf

National Hospice Organization Standards and Accreditation Committee. (1997). *A pathway for patients and families facing terminal illness.* Arlington, VA: Author.

National Institutes of Health. (2004). *National Institutes of Health State-of-the Conference Statement: Improving end-of-life care.* Washington, DC: Author.

Nazir, S., & Erbland, M. (2009). Chronic obstructive pulmonary disease: An update on diagnosis and management issues in older adults. *Drugs & Aging, 26*(10), 813–831. doi:10.2165/11316760-000000000-00000

Nolan, M. T., & Mock, V. (2004). A conceptual framework for end-of-life care: A reconsideration of factors influencing the integrity of the human person. *Journal of Professional Nursing, 20*(6), 351–360.

Pakenham, K., & Cox, S. (2009). The dimensional structure of benefit finding in multiple sclerosis and relations with positive and negative adjustment: A longitudinal study. *Psychology & Health, 24*(4), 373–393.

Parrish, M., & Adams, S. (2003). Caregiver comorbidity and the ability to manage stress. *Journal of Gerontological Social Work, 42*(1), 41–58.

Passmore, M. J., Ho, A., & Gallagher, R. (2012). Behavioral and psychological symptoms in moderate to severe Alzheimer's disease: A palliative care approach emphasizing recognition of personhood and preservation of dignity. *Journal of Alzheimer's Disease, 29*(1), 1–13.

Perry, D. P. (2009). In the balance: Silver tsunami or longevity dividend? *Quality in Aging in Older Adults, 10*(2), 15–22.

Peto, R., Tenerowicz, L., Benjamin, E., Morsi, D., & Burger, P. (2009). One system's journey in creating a disclosure and apology program. *Joint Commission Journal on Quality and Patient Safety, 35*(10), 487–496.

Pinquart, M., & Sorenson, D. (2003). Differences between caregivers and noncaregivers in psychological health and physical health: A meta-analysis. *Psychology and Aging, 18*(2), 250–257.

Proot, I., Abu-Saad, H., Crebolder, H., Goldsteen, M., Luker, K., & Widdershoven, G. (2003). Vulnerability of family caregivers in terminal palliative care at home: Balancing between burden and capacity. *Scandinavian Journal of Caring Sciences, 17*(2), 113–121.

Quality End-of-Life Care Coalition of Canada. (2010). Blueprint for Action: 2010 to 2020 *Annual Report.* Ottawa, ON: Author.

Quill, T. E. (2000). Perspectives on care at the end of life: Initiating end-of-life discussions with seriously ill patients: Addressing the "elephant in the room." *Journal of the American Medical Association, 284,* 2502–2507.

Redinbaugh, E., Baum, A., Tarbell, S., & Arnold, R. (2003). End-of-life caregiving: What helps family caregivers cope? *Journal of Palliative Medicine, 6*(6), 901–909.

Schroeder, P. (1994). *Improving quality and performance: Concepts, programs, and techniques.* St Louis, MO: Mosby.

Schulz, R., Mendelsohn, A. B., Haley, W. E., Mahoney, D., Allen, R., Zhang, S., . . . Belle, S. H. (2003). End-of-life care and the effects of bereavement among family caregivers of persons with dementia. *New England Journal of Medicine, 349,* 1936–1942.

Schulz, R., Newsom, J. T., Fleissner, K., DeCamp, A. R., & Nieboer, A. P. (1997). The effects of bereavement after family caregiving. *Aging and Mental Health, 1,* 269–282.

Sherman, D. W. (2004). Cultural and spiritual backgrounds of older adults. In M. L. Matzo & D. W. Sherman (Eds.), *Gerontologic palliative care nursing* (p. 11). St. Louis, MO: Mosby.

Showalter, S. (1998). Looking through different eyes: Beyond cultural diversity. *Journal of the American Geriatrics Society, 45,* 500–507.

Statistics Canada (2011). Health trends. *Statistics Canada.* Cat. Nos.: 82-213-XWE. (Released October 25, 2011. ed.).

Steinhauser, K. E. (2004). *Measuring outcomes prospectively. National Institutes of Health state-of-the-science conference on improving end-of-life care program & abstracts.* Bethesda, MD: U.S. Department of Health and Human Services, National Institutes of Health.

Steinhauser, K. E., Christakis, N. A., Clipp, E. C., McNeilly, L., & Tulsky, J. A. (2000). Factors considered important at the end of life by patients, family, physicians, and other care providers. *Journal of the American Medical Association, 284,* 2476–2482.

Strasser, F., & Bruera, E. D. (2002). Update on anorexia and cachexia. *Hematology and Oncology Clinics of North America, 16,* 589–617.

Sullivan, A. M., Lakoma, M. D., & Block, S. D. (2003). The status of medical education in end-of-life care: A national report. *Journal of General Internal Medicine, 18,* 685–695.

Sullivan, M. C. (2001). Lost in translation: How Latinos view end-of-life care. *Plastic Surgery Nursing, 21*(2), 90–91.

Teno, J., Lynn, J., Wenger, N., Phillips, R. S., Murphy, D. P., Connors, A. F., . . . Knaus, W. A. (1997). Advance directives for seriously ill hospitalized patients: Effectiveness with the patient self-determination act and the SUPPORT intervention. SUPPORT investigators. Study to understand prognoses and preferences for outcomes and risks of treatment. *Journal of American Geriatric Society, 45*(4), 500–507.

Vollrath, A. M., & von Gunten, C. F. (2007). Negotiating goals of care: Changing goals along the trajectory of illness. In L. L. Emanuel & S. L. Librach (Eds.), *Palliative care: Core skills and clinical competencies* (pp. 70–82). Philadelphia, PA: Saunders/Elsevier.

von Gunten, C. F., & Lupu, D. (2004). Recognizing palliative medicine as a subspecialty: What does it mean for oncology? *Journal of Supportive Oncology, 2*(2), 166–174.

von Gunten, C., & Romer, A. L. (1999). Designing and sustaining a palliative care and home hospice program: An interview with Charles von Gunten. *Innovations in end-of-life care: An International Journal of Leaders in End-of-Life Care, 1*(5). Retrieved from http://www2.edc .org/lastacts/archives/archivessept99/featureinn1.asp

World Health Organization. (1990). *Cancer pain relief and palliative care.* Technical Report Series 804. Geneva, Switzerland: Author.

Xu, J., Kochanek, K. D., Murphy, S. L., & Tejada-Vera, B. (2010). Deaths: Final data for 2007. *National Vital Statistics Report, 58*(19).

Yong, D., Kwok, A., Wong, D., Suen, M., Chen, W., & Tse, D. (2009). Symptom burden and quality of life in end-stage renal disease: A study of 179 patients on dialysis and palliative care. *Palliative Medicine, 23*(2), 111–119. doi:10.1177/0269216308101099

CHAPTER 20

Rehabilitation

Original chapter by Kristen L. Mauk
Canadian content added by Marnie L. Kramer-Kile

INTRODUCTION

"Rehabilitation refers to services and programs designed to assist individuals who have experienced a trauma or illness that results in impairment that creates a loss of function (physical, psychological, social, or vocational)" (Remsburg & Carson, 2006, p. 579). Rehabilitation is also an approach to care in which persons with chronic illness and disability are "made able" again (Pryor, 2002).

Rehabilitation assists individuals with long-term health alterations to regain independence and adapt to changes that have occurred as a result of deviations in their health status. A popular rehabilitation saying is that "rehabilitation begins day one" and thus should be considered as part of the overall plan of care for most acute illness episodes and throughout the duration of most chronic illnesses.

The primary goal of rehabilitation is to achieve the highest level of independence possible for the client. This goal is highly individualized. For example, a person with a mild stroke may have the goal to walk again and resume gainful employment at the same job she held previously. Another person with a high-level spinal injury may realistically have a different goal of being mobile independently with the use of a mechanically adapted wheelchair, such as a Sip-N-Puff chair. Both persons have achievable goals that are based on their capacity and functional limitations that have resulted from illness or injury.

The goals of rehabilitation may be summarized with a few concepts: restoring or maximizing the level of function, facilitating independence, preventing complications, and promoting quality of life. Rehabilitation typically involves an interdisciplinary team of professionals working toward a common goal. The client and family are considered the most important team members. Professional team members may include physicians, nurses, therapists, social workers, vocational counsellors, nutritionists, orthotists, prosthetists, and chaplains. Additional professionals may be consulted to help meet the unique needs of the individual.

Rehabilitation is commonly associated with certain disorders or illnesses in which therapeutic interventions have been shown to be effective. These include health alterations such as stroke, spinal cord injury, traumatic, or other brain injury; neurological diseases such as Parkinson's disease, coronary artery disease, multiple sclerosis, and Guillain-Barré syndrome; orthopedic problems such as arthritis, fractures, or joint replacements; and, less commonly, burns, cancer, or respiratory disorders. In each condition persons can be assisted to regain maximal functioning that may have been altered because of a disease process, injury, or congenital defect.

One of the foci of the rehabilitation process is community reintegration or reentry, sometimes referred to as resocialisation. This is a process by which individuals are reintegrated into society after a life-altering health condition or situation changes their previous roles and abilities. Within a rehabilitation setting reintegration is an ongoing goal. Rehabilitation professionals work with disabled clients or individuals with chronic illness and their families to help them reenter their communities; they may have to accomplish significant adjustments to adapt to changes that have occurred in every area of their lives. Often, this process involves the client relearning how to do self-care with activities of daily living (ADLs) such as bathing, grooming, toileting, eating, and dressing. However, other self-care goals may be at the forefront, such as behaviour change, learning to exercise, changing diets, and optimizing health. Rehabilitation is a hopeful process that encourages individuals to maximize their strengths while making positive adaptations to their limitations.

DEFINITIONS

Rehabilitation

Rehabilitation refers to services and programs designed to assist individuals who have experienced a trauma or illness that results in impairment that creates a loss of function (physical,

psychological, social, or vocational) (Remsburg & Carson, 2006). Common themes among these definitions should be considered. Concepts include the complex, dynamic interactions among the individual, the disease or health condition, and the environment. Most definitions of rehabilitation include assisting an individual with a limitation to attain his or her maximal independence and function. The Institute of Medicine (IOM) defined rehabilitation as "the process by which physical, sensory or mental capacities are restored or developed. . . . Rehabilitation strives to reverse what has been called the disabling process, and may therefore be called the enabling process" (Brandt & Pope, 1997, pp. 12–13).

Rehabilitation Nursing

Rehabilitation is a continuous process, and clients rehabilitate themselves through the influence of the comprehensive approach to care provided by the rehabilitation nurse. Rehabilitation nurses are leaders who specialize in assisting individuals affected by chronic illness and disability to maximize their health through health restoration, maintenance, and promotion (Association of Rehabilitation Nurses [ARN], 2007). The ARN (2008) defines rehabilitation nursing as "the diagnosis and treatment of human responses of individuals and groups to actual or potential health problems related to altered functional ability and lifestyle" (p. 13). In Canada the Canadian Association of Rehabilitation Nurses define their mission as "promoting the advocacy, art, science and practice of professional rehabilitation nursing practice through education, advocacy, collaboration and research to enhance the health and quality of life of Canadians with chronic illness, disability, frailty and aging" (Canadian Association of Rehabilitation Nurses, 2010, para 1).

General information for rehabilitation nurses and advanced rehabilitation nurses is included in the *Standards and Scope of Rehabilitation Nursing Practice* (ARN, 2008) and *Scope and Standards of Advanced Clinical Practice in Rehabilitation Nursing* (ARN, 1996). In Canada nurses may seek advanced certification through the Canadian Nurses Association, Rehabilitation Nursing Certification program. Because of the growth of the specialty of rehabilitation nursing, there are many subspecialties associated with this field.

Restorative Care

"The purpose of restorative care is to actively assist individuals in long-term care settings to maintain their highest level of function and to assist residents in retaining the gains made during formal therapy" (Remsburg & Carson, 2006, p. 580). Restorative care differs from rehabilitation in that it does not include activities directed by therapists but emphasizes nursing interventions that promote adaptation, comfort, and safety within a long-term care setting. Restorative care focuses on maximizing an individual's abilities, helping to rebuild self-esteem and to achieve appropriate goals (Nadash & Feldman, 2003; Resnick & Fleishall, 2002; Resnick & Remsburg, 2004). Restorative care often focuses on assisting individuals with ADLs as well as walking and mobility exercises, transferring, amputation/prosthesis care, and communication. Self-care skills, such as management of one's diabetes, ostomy care, or medication setup and administration, are also emphasized (Remsburg, 2004). Restorative care, although conceptually similar to rehabilitation, is most appropriate for those individuals who either have already reached their maximal functional level and need to maintain that function or are not appropriate candidates for intensive rehabilitation services.

Vocational Rehabilitation

Vocational rehabilitation assists the disabled individual to return to gainful employment and focus on financial independence through programs specifically designed for this purpose (Kielhofner et al., 2004; Lysaght, 2004; O'Neill, Zuger, Fields, Fraser, & Pruce, 2004; Targett, Wehman, & Young, 2004). In Canada vocational rehabilitation is most often led by occupational therapists, but other health professions such as nursing will centre efforts on this type of rehabilitation. Vocational rehabilitation is appropriate for a myriad of chronic conditions. Menear et al. (2011) completed a qualitative study focusing on supportive employment for people living with psychiatric disabilities. Their goal was to shed light on the organizational and contextual factors influencing supportive employment implementation in three Canadian provinces (British Columbia, Ontario, and Quebec). The study found that the employing agency's exposure to different institutional pressures, interactions, and relationships with other outside groups and organizations, paired with the values and beliefs of the organization shaped the evolution of supportive employment programs in each province.

REHABILITATION MODELS AND CLASSIFICATION SYSTEMS

Models are used to help explain, guide, or direct practice or processes. Rehabilitation models can aid in understanding how chronic conditions and disability develop and progress or how they can be managed. Several major classification systems are used to document rehabilitation processes and outcomes (Brandt & Pope, 1997; World Health Organization [WHO], 1980, 2002). These include the functional limitations system, the enabling–disabling model, and the WHO International Classification of Functioning, Disability, and Health (ICF).

The IOM recommends the use of the enabling–disabling process model, whereas the WHO recommends the use of the ICF to help standardize and effectively communicate information about diagnoses, care, and treatment. The model used may depend largely on the facility and its preferences and choices. The use of standard terminology within these models can help facilitate communication, but rehabilitation professionals must be thoroughly familiar with the chosen model and understand the terminology within it.

Enabling–Disabling Process

The enabling–disabling process was developed at the IOM in 1997 as a framework for professional rehabilitation practice. It emphasizes the uniqueness of each individual client by revising the original Disability in America model generated by the IOM (Pope & Tarlov, 1991). A committee of professionals enhanced the 1991 IOM model "to show more clearly how biological, environmental (physical and social), and lifestyle/behavioral factors are involved in reversing the disabling process, i.e., rehabilitation, or the enabling process" (Brandt & Pope, 1997, p. 13). In the new enabling–disabling process, "disability does not appear in this model since it is not inherent in the individual but, rather, a function of the interaction of the individual and the environment" (Brandt & Pope, 1997, p. 11). Disability is seen as a product of the interaction

of an individual with the environment. The model posits that rehabilitation depends largely on the individual and his or her unique characteristics and that the disabling process may even be reversed with appropriate rehabilitation interventions (Lutz & Bowers, 2003). The basic concepts of the model include pathology, impairment, functional limitation, disability, and society limitation (Brandt & Pope, 1997). **Table 20-1** provides a summary of the concepts of the enabling–disabling process.

Brandt and Pope (1997) urged rehabilitation professionals to adopt a framework that better described the rehabilitation process. Since its introduction, however, the enabling–disabling model has not received the recognition or use within healthcare professions that was probably hoped for by the IOM. A search of several notable scholarly databases over the last 10 years revealed few articles written by rehabilitation professionals in healthcare professions that mentioned this process or used it as a framework for research.

International Classification of Functioning, Disability, and Health

In 1980 the WHO developed a classification system that was widely used for years internationally. The WHO originally defined impairment as a loss related to structure and function; a disability was related to a loss of ability to perform an activity, and a handicap was a disadvantage for a person related to the environment.

The ICF is the WHO's framework for measuring health and disability at both individual and population levels: "ICF is a classification of health and health related domains that describe body functions and structures, activities and participation. The domains are classified from body, individual and societal perspectives"

(WHO, 2007, p. 1). The ICF provides a shift in viewing disability as gradually becoming a part of the majority of persons' lives over time. It provides a holistic look at the process of disability related to health, considering all aspects, not just the medical or physical (WHO, 2007). The four major sections of the classification document are body functions (by system and including mental health), body structures (by system), activities and participation (such as learning,

Table 20-1   Concepts of the Enabling–Disabling Process

Pathophysiology	Impairment	Functional Limitation	Disability	Societal Limitation
Interruption of or interference with normal physiological and developmental processes or structures	Loss and/or abnormality of cognition, and emotional, physiological, or anatomical structure or function, including all losses or abnormalities, not just those attributable to the initial pathophysiology	Restriction or lack of ability to perform an action in the manner or within a range consistent with the purpose of an organ or organ system	Inability or limitation in performing tasks, activities, and roles to levels expected within physical and social contexts	Restriction, attributable to social policy or barriers (structural or attitudinal), that limits fulfilment of roles or denies access to services and opportunities that are associated with full participation in society
		Level of Impact		
Cells and Tissues	Organs and Organ Systems	Function of the Organ and Organ System	Individual	Society
Structural or functional	Structural or functional	Action or activity performance or organ or organ system	Task performance by person in physical, social contexts	Societal attributes relevant to individuals with disabilities
		Patient Examples		
Lacunar infarct of the cerebellum (right hemisphere) related to microvascular changes associated with chronic hypertension	Neuromotor function of the brain	Left hemiparesis or difficulty with spatial–perceptual tasks, difficulty sequencing, memory deficits	Deficits in ambulation, self-care, shopping, work	Lack of adaptations in the work environment that would enable the person to continue employment

Source: Whyte (1998). Reprinted with permission from Elsevier.

communication, self-care, community involvement), and environmental factors (such as products, technology, attitudes, service, and policy) (WHO, 2007). **Table 20-2** provides an overview of ICF.

Other models that can guide rehabilitation practice have emerged from rehabilitation nurse scientists. These middle-range theories are not classification systems for general rehabilitation but provide insight and direction about specific processes or phenomena. An example of an area in which several new frameworks or models have arisen is in stroke rehabilitation and recovery. Secrest and colleagues (Secrest & Thomas, 1999; Secrest & Zeller, 2007) explored the relationship of continuity and discontinuity after stroke. They continue to publish about the relationship of this phenomenon with functional ability, depression, and quality of life. Their work resulted in the development of a tool to measure themes common to the post-stroke experience such as control, connection with others, and independence (Secrest & Zeller, 2003).

Mauk (Easton, 2001; Mauk, 2006) developed a model from grounded theory that identified six phases of post-stroke recovery that may help guide practice and interventions. She found that stroke survivors journey through a predictable pattern, with certain variables influencing the ease of adaptation after stroke. Other rehabilitation nurse scientists have explored the experience of caregivers of stroke survivors (Hartke & King, 2002; Pierce et al., 2004; Pierce, Steiner, Hicks, & Holzaepfel, 2006). Each of these examples suggests that although large, general models and classification systems are necessary and helpful, more manageable models, frameworks, and instruments are also needed to better reflect the unique experiences in rehabilitation and to guide practice.

Table 20-2   Concepts of the International Classification of Functioning, Disability, and Health

Health Condition	Impairment	Activity Limitation	Participation Restriction
Major Concepts			
Diseases, disorders, and injuries, e.g., leprosy, diabetes, spinal cord injury	Problems in body function or structure such as a significant deviation or loss, e.g., anxiety, paralysis, loss of sensation of extremities	Difficulty an individual might have in executing activities	Problems an individual may experience in involvement in life situations, e.g., unable to attend social events, unable to use public transportation to get to church, unable to perform job functions
Example			
Spinal cord injury	Paralysis	Incapable of using public transportation	Unable to attend religious activities

Source: World Health Organization (2002).

REHABILITATION ISSUES AND CHALLENGES

Rehabilitation services provided by an interdisciplinary team within a variety of settings suggest several possible challenges for providers. These include the rising costs of care, caregiver burden, inequities among those with disabilities, the negative image of disability, the changing composition of the disabled population, ethical issues, providing culturally competent care, and professional and informal caregiver issues.

Rising Care Costs

According to Mirolla (2004) direct medical care costs for people living with chronic illness in Canada accounts for 42% of total direct medical care expenditures within the country (averaging $39 billion a year). Indirect productivity losses resulting from chronic illness should also be taken into account. For example, premature death due to cancer results in a loss of $11.6 billion per year, circulatory diseases cost up to $12.8 billion per year, and musculoskeletal disorders (arthritis and osteoporosis) have some of the highest productivity losses, at $14.9 billion per year. Combining both the direct and indirect costs related to chronic illness in Canada nets a staggering $93 billion each year. Given these statistics, major challenges for rehabilitation professionals are to assist persons to attain and regain their health and become productive, working members of society, and to explore other means of providing improved access to health care.

Caregiver Burden

Because an event requiring rehabilitation happens to the entire family and community, not just the client, it is important to address the needs of caregivers throughout the rehabilitation process and/or chronic illness trajectory. Family members comprise the vast majority (72%) of paid and unpaid caregivers of older persons with functional limitations from chronic disease, with adult children caregivers (42%) and spouses (25%) bearing the largest burden of care (Shirey & Summer, 2000). The caregiver's ability to cope with the care demands is influenced by a variety of factors, including the type and severity of illness, the length of quality of recovery, social support, inherent caregiver factors, and coping ability. This may hold true for both formal and informal caregivers (Bushnik, Wright, & Burdsall, 2007). For example, the caregiver spouse of a person with uncomplicated coronary bypass surgery may be able to meet care demands over a limited period of rehabilitation, whereas the older spouse caregiver of a stroke survivor with severe aphasia and functional deficits may be facing years of caregiving—a burden that is often overwhelming.

Caregiver burden, the effects of caregiving-related stress on family members or other care providers, has been associated with a number of health problems in the caregiver. Emotional distress, anxiety, depression, decreased quality of life, hypertension, lowered immune function, and increased mortality are among the concerns noted by researchers of caregivers (Anderson, Linto, & Stewart-Wynne, 1995; Brouwer et al., 2004; Canam & Acorn, 1999; das Chagas Medeiros, Ferraz, & Quaresma, 2000; Grunfeld et al., 2004; Hughes et al., 1999; King, Hartke, & Denby, 2007; Kolanowski, Fick, Waller, & Shea, 2004; Lieberman & Fisher, 1995; Mills, Yu, Ziegler, Patterson, & Grant, 1999; Schulz & Beach, 1999; Shaw et al., 1999; Ski & O'Connell, 2007; Weitzenkamp, Gerhart, Charlifue, Whiteneck, & Savic, 1997; Wu et al., 1999). There is sufficient research since 1995 to demonstrate that the burden of caregiving over time can have a deleterious effect on the health of the family caregiver.

The caregiver burden is thought to be greater when more care is required. Research suggests that although education and training programs have some effect on caregiver stress levels, the benefit is short term and caregivers are likely to need ongoing involvement from care professionals to help maintain their own health (Draper et al., 2007; Halm, Treat-Jacobson, Lindquist, & Savik, 2007; King et al., 2007). Assessment of caregiver burden should be included in the rehabilitation plan of care. Early identification and interventions related to managing caregiver stress may result in better outcomes for the entire family, and appropriate discharge planning and follow-up are an important part of the process.

Inequities Among Disabled Canadians and Stigma of Disability

Although much progress has been made on a national policy level toward dispelling the negative image and stigma associated with disability through modifying rehabilitation models (Brandt & Pope, 1997; WHO, 2002), many persons with disabilities still report feelings of negative reactions from others regarding their differences. The disability could be something as relatively invisible as a hearing aid worn by an adolescent (Kent & Smith, 2006) to obvious employment discrimination for a person with mental illness (Lloyd & Waghorn, 2007; Stuart, 2006). One study found that a positive factor such as exercise performed by a person with a physical disability may undermine the negative impressions that some persons have and fight the stigma of disability (Arbour, Latimer, Ginis, & Jung, 2007).

Changes made in today's rehabilitation models portray disability on a continuum, with a prominent factor being the environment. In a classic work by Zola (1982), the author toured a 65-acre utopia in The Netherlands as a professional visitor. The village was designed for those with disabilities who did not fit well into other existing societies, with complete and full accessibility, environmental adaptation, and removal of barriers. Each of the 400 members of the village had to contribute to their self-crafted society. However, in such an environment persons functioned well and without stigma, because their situation was the new norm. Zola found himself feeling out of place, although able-bodied, suggesting that the environment is a key factor in perception of disability.

Persons with disabilities who have helped to change the perception of the public include role models in the arts, science, politics, and sports. Marla Runyon (Olympic runner), the late actor/director Christopher Reeve, actor Michael J. Fox, scientist Stephen Hawking, and Senator Max Cleland are just a few examples of such role models. Runyon is legally blind yet participated as an Olympic runner in the 2000 games in Sydney, Australia. Christopher Reeve, the actor best known for his role as Superman, had a high-level spinal cord injury resulting in ventilator-dependent tetraplegia. Reeve continued to act and direct movies throughout his life and, along with his late wife, Dana, helped establish services for those with spinal cord injuries.

The actor Michael J. Fox experienced early-onset Parkinson's disease and has been a crusader for research in that area. Stephen Hawking, noted physicist and prolific author, was diagnosed with motor neuron disease (amyotrophic lateral sclerosis) at a relatively young age and yet has continued to work. Even after he was completely paralyzed by his disease, he continued to write with the use of technology and his blink reflex. Cleland, a triple amputee, was a United States senator and director of the Veterans Administration. These individuals may seem remarkable because of their accomplishments; however, thousands of other "everyday" citizens with disabilities are productive members and make significant contributions to society. Theirs are the untold stories.

Ethical and Legal Issues

Rehabilitation professionals are often in positions that require difficult decision making. Masters-Farrell (2006) stated that the "conflict occurs when a choice must be made between two equal possibilities" (p. 590) and that an ethical dilemma is present when a situation forces one to evaluate and choose between two equally unattractive choices. For example, take the situation of a nonterminal rehabilitation client who had just told the nurse he did not wish to be resuscitated if he should "code." However, the paperwork for advance directives had not yet been completed, signed, or placed on the chart and the nurse found him minutes later without a pulse or respirations. Although she must call the code team in this situation, the nurse is in conflict because she has intimate knowledge that this action was contrary to the client's wishes.

Beauchamp and Childress (2001), in their classic text on principles of biomedical ethics, emphasized four cornerstone principles: respect for person, nonmaleficence, beneficence, and justice. These principles play into many aspects of rehabilitation practice and programming. Common ethical (and often legal) issues that pertain particularly to rehabilitation clients may include the following (Ellis & Hartley, 2004;

Kirschner, Stocking, Wagner, Foye, & Siegler, 2001; Masters-Farrell, 2007):

- Withholding or withdrawing treatment
- Determining competence in decision making
- Do not resuscitate orders
- Use of physical or chemical restraints
- Genetic screening
- Organ donation

Ethics committees are becoming more popular in acute care hospitals and even retirement communities to assist in difficult decision making (Hogstel, Curry, Walker, & Burns, 2004; Hughes, 2004; Johnson, 2004; Nelson, 2004). Ellis and Hartley (2004) viewed the ethics committee as an interdisciplinary group of healthcare professionals that is established specifically to address ethical dilemmas that occur in a particular setting. Persons serving on an ethics committee may include physicians, nurses, advanced practice nurses, social workers, therapists, pastoral care personnel, members of the community, and an ethicist. The benefits of an ethics committee include allowing many perspectives to be discussed, providing a forum for communication, fostering development of related policies, promoting awareness of existing and potential issues, and focusing on the patient (Masters-Farrell, 2007). Some disadvantages include the potential for inefficiency and political influence and lack of time for participation.

Cultural Competency

Cultural sensitivity involves an awareness and consideration of a group's beliefs, values, communication styles, language, and behaviour. How clients and families perceive disability and participate in rehabilitation is heavily influenced by cultural norms and expectations

(Campinha-Bacote, 2001). The first step in becoming culturally sensitive is to know one's own self. This involves healthcare professionals taking the time to reflect on their own understandings of culture and how this may influence the care they provide. Because of the vast differences among and within the many cultural groups that rehabilitation professionals serve, it is wise to ask clients about their particular beliefs and practices.

Formal and Informal Caregiver Issues

As the population increases and the oldest of the elderly become the fastest growing age group, there will be a lack of physicians and nurses prepared to meet the care demand for the number of persons with chronic illness and disability. The Canadian Nurses Association has been an advocate for nurses gaining specialty certification in rehabilitation nursing. However, few nursing programs provide rehabilitation education as a separate course or have dedicated content to this specialty area. Getting healthcare professionals such as physicians and nurses interested in the specialty has been difficult because of its limited visibility in traditional educational programs (Neal, 2001; Thompson, Emrich, & Moore, 2003). The European Union has addressed concerns regarding a shortage of physicians trained in physical medicine and rehabilitation through the Union of European Medical Specialists by beginning to standardize training and education throughout its 28 member countries. Within these countries there are 13,000 specialists and more than 2,800 trainees in physical and rehabilitation medicine (Ward & Gutenbrunner, 2006), and the specialty is believed to be robust. Still, there is a concerted effort to recruit and educate physicians in physical and rehabilitation medicine in Europe.

Despite concerted efforts to change it, a negative stigma persists regarding care of older adults among nursing students. Without education in gerontology, healthcare professionals may not realize the rehabilitation potential of many of these older adults. The common rehabilitative disorders often are seen in the older age group, and even small improvements in function and independence can allow older adults to age in place and remain at home. Even those making long-term care or retirement communities their home can improve their strength and function with small lifestyle changes and exercise.

There is also a growing number of persons whose caregiving needs go unmet (Kennedy, 2001; LaPlante, Kaye, Kang, & Harrington, 2004). More than 34 million persons are limited in some way from usual activities because of chronic illness. An estimated 3.8 million adults with disabilities require assistance with ADLs and 7.8 million need help with instrumental ADLs (Adams, Dey, & Vickerie, 2007). Persons who need assistance were more likely to be poor, older, and less educated. Persons whose needs are not met are more likely to experience discomfort, weight loss, dehydration, falls, and burns (LaPlante et al., 2004). Further research is needed to help identify consequences from unmet caregiving needs as well as strategies to address this growing problem.

INTERVENTIONS

Rehabilitation Process

Rehabilitation is both a philosophy and a discipline (Secrest, 2007). Rehabilitation is based on the premise that all individuals have self-worth and are deserving of dignity, respect, and quality health care regardless of their limitations. Many concepts are imbedded in the field of rehabilitation and are reflected through the following common sayings:

- Rehabilitation begins day one
- What you do not use, you lose
- Progress is measured in small gains
- Independence is better than dependence
- Motivation is a key to success
- All care should include rehabilitation principles
- Activity strengthens and inactivity wastes
- If it can be corrected, it probably could have been prevented

Rehabilitation should begin from the first day the person is in the hospital. When healthcare professionals forget the basic principles of rehabilitation, complications such as contractures, pressure sores, and incontinence ensue. Rehabilitation includes nursing, medical therapies, and social services. It is an interdisciplinary team process focused on maintaining or restoring function, preventing complications, promoting independence and self-care, and enhancing quality of life.

Team Approach

The team approach is most effective when working with clients with complex needs such as those requiring rehabilitative services. Although several models are used in this approach, the common threads are that the team members work toward goals that are mutually established with the client.

Prevailing models are either multidisciplinary, interdisciplinary, or transdisciplinary. Multidisciplinary teams involve professionals from different disciplines, each treating the client within their various areas; however, they may not coordinate their efforts in the care of a client (Secrest, 2007). The advantage of this type of model is that all professionals bring their education and expertise to promote the best outcomes for the client. However, the major weakness is that communication between and across the disciplines may be lacking.

In the transdisciplinary model each client has a primary therapist from the team, who may be a nurse, physical therapist, or occupational therapist. One therapist is cross-trained to provide comprehensive care to the client (Secrest, 2007). Although this model may provide for continuity of care, issues surrounding licensure, scope of practice, and accountability abound. In addition, team members are often out of their comfort zone in providing services for which they were not specifically trained. Turf issues often complicate this type of care. Finally, some organizations that have tried this model have given it up for a different approach because the team was not motivated to embrace it.

The most preferred rehabilitation team model is the interdisciplinary team. The interdisciplinary team approach involves each team member communicating on a regular basis with each other and establishing common goals for clients (Secrest, 2007). This is often accomplished through weekly team meetings in which the entire team reviews the progress of each client and mutual goals are discussed and updated. The client and family are an important part of the team as well. Nontraditional team members may be added to the team based on the client's needs.

Evaluation of the Client

An important element in considering rehabilitation as an option for any client is proper evaluation of rehabilitation potential. There are many factors that comprise such an evaluation, but several forces seem to play a major role. These include the severity of the illness, injury, or defect; functional level and cognitive status; willingness to participate; internal or external motivation (Kemp, 1986); social support (Fairfax, 2002); and available resources.

POTENTIAL STRENGTHS OF THE CLIENT, FAMILY, AND ENVIRONMENT

Another important factor in the evaluation process is the identification of the client's and family's strengths. Several questions are important to ask during this assessment: What can the client do for him- or herself? What does the client see as his or her own strengths and weaknesses? What are the family's strengths and weaknesses? What coping mechanisms does the client typically use, and will they be sufficient for the current crisis? What community resources are available to the family and client? What are the client's personal goals? A highly motivated client and supportive family are important to the success of the rehabilitation process.

Functional Assessment

Although functional assessment is important, the evaluator should not forget that a true evaluation of rehabilitation potential must consider all factors, not just physical or function related. Functional assessment includes an evaluation that identifies one's ability to perform self-care and physical activities. The two approaches generally used are asking questions and observation (Guse, 2006).

A number of tools are available to assess function, although these are mainly aimed at screening for disability. Functional assessment tools are as follows: (1) the development of a client problem list, (2) goal setting based on identified strengths and weaknesses of the client, (3) evaluation of the client's progress and outcomes, (4) measurement of treatment interventions, (5) cost–benefit effectiveness of care, (6) assistance in the rehabilitation program's evaluation and audit, and (7) research (Remsburg & Carson, 2006).

CASE STUDY

Dr. Janes, a community dentist, was diagnosed with multiple sclerosis at age 54. His clinical patterns proved to be the relapsing-remitting type with slowly progressive disability and loss of function over time. By age 60 Dr. Janes retired because complications of his multiple sclerosis, such as fatigue, visual problems, and poor balance, made it difficult to continue his busy pediatric dentistry practice. His wife was frustrated with his decline in health and early retirement. Dr. Janes consulted a clinical nurse specialist during the last hospitalization for a severe exacerbation to help better manage his condition after retirement, now that he was "able to focus on his own health more." A new medication in the group of immunomodifiers proved effective in reducing the number and severity of exacerbations per year, and working with the rehabilitation team on an outpatient basis helped to improve Dr. Janes's quality of life.

CASE STUDY   (Continued)

www

Discussion Questions

1. What team members would have been involved in Dr. Janes's rehabilitation in the inpatient rehabilitation unit after an acute exacerbation of his multiple sclerosis?
2. What goals would be appropriate for Dr. Janes in the long term? Short term?
3. Name two tools or classification systems that would be appropriate in evaluating Dr. Janes's functional ability.
4. If you developed a long-term plan of care for Dr. Janes, what outcomes would be appropriate over a 10-year period?

Evaluators may use a variety of methods to complete a functional assessment. Generally, a combination of self-report, whether in the form of a questionnaire completed by the person or the interviewer, and observation are used. An example of an easy tool to assess general geriatric health is the Timed Up and Go (TUG) test. The person is asked to rise up from a chair, walk 10 feet, turn around, and sit back down. Increased TUG times have been associated with falls in the elderly (Podsiadlo & Richardson, 1991).

The FIM (Uniform Data System for Medical Rehabilitation, 1997) is the most widely accepted and most used performance-based measure of ADLs (**Figure 20-1**). A revised version of the FIM (called the Wee-FIM) is available for pediatric patients. The FIM is an instrument that is completed by a trained evaluator to assess 18 performance items on a seven-level scale. The tool is completed upon admission, at discharge, and often several times in between to monitor progress. The total score of all categories can help to show improvement over time. The evaluator may be one person, or different team members may complete various parts of the FIM tool based on their expertise. For example, the nurse may complete the sphincter control item and the speech therapist may complete the communication section. Team members base their evaluation on direct observation of the subject. The items assessed include self-care, sphincter control, transfers, locomotion, communication, and social cognition. The evaluator quantifies each category by determining how much assistance is required in each category. A score of 1 means total assistance was needed and the subject provided less than 25% of the effort. A score of 7 signifies complete independence in a timely and safe manner (i.e., the subject was completely independent in that activity).

The usefulness or accuracy of some of these tools has been called into question by some. It is wise to investigate the development of the instrument and which patient groups were used during its development. In addition, the outcomes of a tool generally somewhat depend on the person using it, so it is essential that evaluators are properly educated in the use of the instrument. Many tools have questionable generalisability to older adults and may not take into consideration the normal effects of aging.

L E V E L S	7 Complete Independence (Timely, Safely) 6 Modified Independence (Device)	**NO HELPER**
	Modified Dependence 5 Supervision (Subject = 100%+) 4 Minimal Assist (Subject = 75%+) 3 Moderate Assist (Subject = 50%+) **Complete Dependence** 2 Maximal Assist (Subject = 25%+) 1 Total Assist (Subject = less than 25%)	**HELPER**

	ADMISSION	DISCHARGE	FOLLOW-UP
Self-Care A. Eating B. Grooming C. Bathing D. Dressing - Upper Body E. Dressing - Lower Body F. Toileting			
Sphincter Control G. Bladder Management H. Bowel Management			
Transfers I. Bed, Chair, Wheelchair J. Toilet K. Tub, shower			
Locomotion L. Walk/Wheelchair M. Stairs	W Walk C Wheelchair B Both	W Walk C Wheelchair B Both	W Walk C Wheelchair B Both
Motor Subtotal Score			
Communication N. Comprehension O. Expression	A Auditory V Visual B Both V Vocal N Nonvocal B Both	A Auditory V Visual B Both V Vocal N Nonvocal B Both	A Auditory V Visual B Both V Vocal N Nonvocal B Both
Social Cognition P. Social Interaction Q. Problem Solving R. Memory			
Cognitive Subtotal Score			
TOTAL FIM Score			

NOTE: Leave no blanks. Enter 1 if patient not testable due to risk.

FIGURE 20-1   FIM instrument.

Source: Copyright © 1997 Uniform Data System for Medical Rehabilitation (UDSmr), a division of UB Foundation Activities, Inc. (UBFA). Reprinted with the permission of UDSmr, University at Buffalo, 232 Parker Hall, 3435 Main Street, Buffalo, NY 14214. All marks associated with IFM and UDSmr are owned by UBFA.

Pain Management

Both acute and chronic pain may be present in rehabilitation clients. Acute pain is thought to be of shorter duration and associated with the insult. Chronic pain, more often seen in those clients with chronic illness and disability, is of longer duration and can result in diminished health, disability, and reduction in quality of life (American Pain Society, 2006; Hertzberg, 2007). Chronic pain has been associated with depression, disability, decreased function, and increased time off of work (Harris, 2000; Lipton, Hamelsky, Kolodner, Steiner, & Stewart, 2000; Walsh, Dumitru, Schoenfeld, & Ramaurthy, 2005). The popularity of pain clinics, whose major purpose is to address chronic, intractable pain, is growing, and referrals are often made to these programs when other interventions fail.

Pain, whether acute and/or chronic, can interfere with rehabilitation goals. Therefore, pain management is a part of most rehabilitation programs. The ARN, in fact, provides specific goals for pain management in clients, stating that rehabilitation nurses should seek to assist clients with acute or chronic pain to improve their physical functioning and thus improve their quality of life (ARN, 1996). Pain is a complex problem that requires a comprehensive approach from an interdisciplinary team using a variety of pharmacological and nonpharmacological interventions.

REHABILITATION SETTINGS

Rehabilitation services are offered in a wide variety of settings. These may include freestanding rehabilitation facilities, acute rehabilitation within hospitals, long-term care facilities, or the home. Regardless of the setting for care, services should be provided by an interdisciplinary team of trained professionals. In the past rehabilitation units, especially those within hospitals, served patients with diverse diagnoses. However, as the specialty has grown and the body of research and evidence-informed practice expands, it is becoming more common for larger rehabilitation facilities to target services for specific diagnostic groups of clients, such as multiple trauma, traumatic brain injury, stroke syndromes, spinal cord injuries, cancer, burns, or HIV, or at least to provide dedicated units for persons with similar diagnoses.

Subacute Care Units

Subacute care units are for patients who require more intensive nursing care than the traditional long-term care facility or nursing home can provide but less than that provided by the acute care hospital or skilled care unit (Mauk, 2006). These units are sometimes referred to as transitional care units. Clients seen in subacute care are typically those who need the following (Easton, 1999, p. 15):

> [A]ssistance as a result of non-healing wounds, chronic ventilator dependence, renal problems, intravenous therapy, and coma management and those with complex medical and/or rehabilitation needs, including pediatrics, orthopedics, and neurologic. These units are designed to promote optimum outcomes in the least expensive cost setting.

Clients may stay from days to several weeks. Persons who need rehabilitation services but would be unable to tolerate the intensive therapy of acute rehabilitation may be candidates for this level of care.

Skilled Nursing Facilities

Skilled nursing facilities may also provide rehabilitation and can be housed in acute care hospitals and on independent specialty units or within long-term care facilities. Remsburg and colleagues caution that not all skilled nursing facilities provide the same level of rehabilitation services, with services ranging from those who are Commission on Accreditation of Rehabilitation Facilities–accredited programs and others that offer some restorative care, so consumers should carefully evaluate options when choosing a facility (Remsburg, Armacost, Radu, & Bennett, 1999; Remsburg, Armacost, Radu, & Bennett, 2001; Resnick & Fleishell, 2002).

Several benefits are seen with skilled nursing facilities. The pace is generally slower. Often patients will have more continuity of care with nursing staff than in an acute care hospital. Length of stay is generally longer, perhaps weeks or months instead of days. The focus of treatment is on individual outcomes with less regard to speed of progress (Osterweil, 1990).

Hospitals and Freestanding Facilities

Acute rehabilitation is often provided in acute care hospitals or freestanding rehabilitation facilities. A person requiring inpatient rehabilitation is not just in need of therapy; if that was the only service required, it could be done on an outpatient basis, as often occurs with such conditions as joint replacement surgery. The person needing intensive inpatient rehabilitation is one who also requires 24-hour nursing care to address such problems as medication management, complex comorbidities, nutrition, swallowing disorders, behaviour issues, skin care, and bowel and bladder retraining. Clients in acute rehabilitation may be admitted for a specific diagnosis such as stroke but also have pre- or coexisting conditions that complicate recovery, such as hypertension, cancer, diabetes, and renal disease. In addition, most clients treated in acute rehabilitation are older adults. Older adults as a population have unique needs with or without undergoing acute rehabilitation. Generally, to qualify for acute intensive rehabilitation services offered in these facilities, clients must be able to tolerate at least 3 hours of therapy per day, have a goal of discharge to home, and be able to demonstrate progress toward mutually established goals (Mauk & Hanson, 2010). They should also have private insurance or Medicare coverage to cover the high cost of the interdisciplinary services provided by multiple therapies and nursing.

Long-Term Care Facilities or Retirement Communities

Although long-term care facilities often carry a negative stigma with the general public, rehabilitative services offered in these facilities may be quite appropriate for assisting adults in regaining independence and function. Long-term care facilities, especially those offering multiple levels of care, may have accredited rehabilitation units housed within them. Persons making a retirement community their home may also avail themselves of therapeutic services offered within the facility. An increasing number of continuous care retirement communities have physical or other therapists available to assist with rehabilitation after an accident, surgery, or illness to help older adults "age in place." In addition, many continuous care retirement communities have begun to offer health promotion activities that include state-of-the-art fitness centres with personal trainers to foster primary prevention as well as rehabilitation.

Community-Based Rehabilitation

Community-based rehabilitation may involve a rehabilitation team or involve only nursing. Community-based nurses may work in outpatient rehabilitation clinics, senior centres, assisted living, home health care, public schools, churches, or function as case managers. According to Parker and Neal-Boylan (2007), community-based rehabilitation is used in a variety of settings including home health care, subacute care, long-term care, and independent living.

Home health care provides services to clients of all ages and emphasizes primary care and case management. It allows individuals and families to remain in the home and still receive services that focus on health restoration and maximizing function. Home care is considered a cost-effective service for those recuperating from an injury or illness who are not able to completely care for themselves (National Association for Home Care and Hospice, 2007). Unique models may even allow continuous care retirement communities to provide home care services covered by Medicare (L. Mullet, personal communication, November 26, 2007).

Subacute care in the community-based model generally provides services to adults through a team-nursing delivery system, with most of the daily care provided by nursing assistants supervised by licensed practical nurses and case management by registered nurses. In the long-term care setting services are offered mainly to geriatric residents using a team approach, with the registered nurse in the role of case manager. In independent living settings older adults may receive care from personal care attendants. Here again the registered nurse serves as a care manager and client advocate (Parker & Neal-Boylan, 2007).

REHABILITATION SPECIALTIES

There are many subspecialties within the discipline of rehabilitation. Although most traditional rehabilitation programs provide care to a mixed case of clients, both population- and diagnosis-specific units cater to the needs of smaller, select groups of patients. These types of specialty programs may be inpatient or outpatient and may include geriatrics, pediatrics, cardiac, pulmonary, cancer, HIV, and Alzheimer's disease programs.

Geriatric Rehabilitation

By 2017 it is estimated that there will be more seniors than children in Canada (Statistics Canada, 2011b). An increase in chronic conditions will also accompany this shift. The top chronic illnesses considered the greatest health burden to society include arthritis, heart disease and stroke, diabetes, cancer, and, more recently, obesity and tobacco-related disease (National Center for Chronic Disease Prevention and Health Promotion, 2007).

Geriatric rehabilitation focuses on restoring and maintaining optimal function while considering holistically the unique effects of aging on the person (Clark & Siebens, 2005). Programs specifically designed for older adults may have adjusted expectations such as requiring less intensive rehabilitation and preventing potential complications such as falls, dehydration, pressure sores, immobility, delirium, and poly pharmacy that occur more frequently in older adults (Beers & Berkow, 2004; Lin & Armour, 2004; Routasalo, Arve, & Lauri, 2004; Worsowicz, Stewart, Phillips, & Cifu, 2004). Geriatric rehabilitation also focuses on enhancing quality of life through the strengthening of social support systems, family involvement, client education, and connection with community resources.

Mauk and Lehman (2007) suggested two ways in which disability affects older adults: acquiring disability at an advanced age and aging with an earlier onset disability. Factors that may affect an older adult's rehabilitation potential include age, frailty, the normal aging process, effects of chronic disease, functional and cognitive status, the use of multiple medications, and the presence of social support (Bagg, Pombo, & Hopman, 2002; Bandeen-Roche et al., 2006; Beaupre et al., 2005; Charles & Lehman, 2006; Yu, 2005). The more common acquired disabilities in older adults include stroke, head injury, and fractures from falls. In addition, the various syndromes (such as delirium, dizziness, incontinence, dehydration, and functional loss) that are seen more often in older adults can negatively impact the rehabilitation process (Mauk & Lehman, 2007).

Persons aging with a disability tend to experience a greater degree of complications over time. For example, a man with a lower extremity amputation that occurred in his 20s is much more likely to have arthritis and range-of-motion problems in his shoulders from overuse of a non–weight-bearing joint than the person who has lost this limb later in life. However, the person with lower extremity amputation later in life as a result of peripheral vascular disease secondary to diabetes is at an increased risk for complications because of advanced age and disease process. Therefore, both the disability and the aging process contribute to one's overall rehabilitation potential. Rehabilitation can positively impact older adults by providing services to strengthen both physical and psychosocial functioning.

Pediatric Rehabilitation

Children with functional limitations have different needs and development concerns than adults do. Pediatric rehabilitation involves the collaboration of an interdisciplinary team of professionals to provide a continuum of care for children from the onset of injury or illness until adulthood. The focus of treatment is on adaptation and maximum function to promote independence within the family and society. The ARN (2007) defines pediatric rehabilitation nursing as "the specialty practice committed to improving the quality of life for children and adolescents with disabilities and their families" (p. 1). Professionals working with children practice family-centred care, must be knowledgeable about normal growth and development, and must be able to work with an interdisciplinary team to address interventions that include physical, emotional, cultural, educational, socioeconomic, and spiritual dimensions (Edwards, Hertzberg, & Sapp, 2007).

Some of the common disorders associated with the need for pediatric rehabilitation include traumatic brain injury, spinal cord injury, burns, cancer, congenital diseases and birth defects, and chronic illness. For example, whether a child sustains a brain injury from an accident or is born with cerebral palsy, the interventions from the interdisciplinary rehabilitation team will be designed to maximize function and help the child attain adulthood as a well-adjusted member of society.

Cardiac Rehabilitation

According to Statistics Canada (2011a), in 2008 heart disease accounted for 29% of the deaths in Canada. Cardiac rehabilitation "enhances recovery, and secondary prevention measures prevent further complications from disease" (Carbone, 2007). The Canadian Association of Cardiac Rehabilitation created guidelines for cardiac rehabilitation and cardiac disease prevention that promote a chronic care approach to cardiovascular disease (CACR, 2009). Cardiac rehabilitation is appropriate for persons with congenital or acquired heart disease such myocardial infarction, chronic angina, heart failure, cardiomyopathy, or postsurgical patients. The aims are to improve functional capacity and to reduce related morbidity and mortality (Singh, Schocken, Williams, & Stamey, 2004).

Cardiac rehabilitation after a myocardial infarction has four phases (Shah, 2005; Singh et al., 2004):

- Phase I: acute phase—during the inpatient stay
- Phase II: convalescent phase—early post-discharge
- Phase III: training phase—structured and supervised exercise program
- Phase IV: maintenance phase—posttraining and lifestyle changes

Measures used in cardiac rehabilitation include risk factor modification along with medication management and medical interventions. Risk factor management focuses on smoking cessation, controlling hypertension, weight loss, decreasing cholesterol, management of diabetes,

increasing physical activity, and decreasing stress (American Heart Association, 2011). Client participation in cardiac rehabilitation is an ongoing problem, with research suggesting that the strength of physician recommendation, gender (men participated more than women), and disease severity may be the best predictors of whether clients initiate cardiac rehabilitation (Ades, Waldmann, McCann, & Weaver, 1992; Shanks, Moore, & Zeller, 2007). Other researchers argue that participation is contingent upon other more complicated social factors and contexts associated with health behaviour change (Angus et al., 2009). What is clear is that the process of cardiac rehabilitation is a complicated one that attempts to balance biomedical frameworks of care within the social lives of its participants.

Pulmonary Rehabilitation

Chronic obstructive pulmonary disease, which includes chronic bronchitis and emphysema, is the fourth leading cause of death in Canada (Public Health Agency of Canada, 2011). When asthma and other pulmonary problems are factored in, chronic respiratory problems are a leading cause of functional disability in Canada. The primary risk factor for chronic obstructive pulmonary disease is smoking, and 80% to 90% of deaths from chronic obstructive pulmonary disease are attributed to this cause (American Lung Association, 2011). Because of the large numbers of North Americans experiencing pulmonary problems, specific programs have been developed to address these needs. The American Association for Respiratory Care (2002) stated that essential components of a pulmonary rehabilitation program include assessment, patient education, exercise, psychosocial interventions, and follow-up. Smoking cessation programs are a major focus in both the prevention and rehabilitative treatment of respiratory problems.

Cancer Rehabilitation

According to the Canadian Cancer Society (2011), the top cancer deaths for males across all races are prostate, lung, and colorectal. For women, the leading causes of cancer deaths are lung, breast, and colorectal (Canadian Cancer Society, 2011). Given these statistics many cancers detected early are highly treatable and do not need to be viewed as a terminal diagnosis. These data suggest that persons with cancer will not only survive but may require rehabilitation to enhance quality of life and return to optimal functioning after their diagnosis and as part of their treatment. "Cancer rehabilitation is the process that assists the person with cancer in obtaining maximum physical, social, psychological, and work-related functioning during and after cancer treatment" (People Living with Cancer, 2006, p. 1).

The goals of cancer rehabilitation include maximizing independence in mobility and ADLs, preserving dignity, and promoting quality of life (Beck, 2003; Gillis, Cheville, & Worsowicz, 2001; Vargo & Gerber, 2005). These goals are individualized to each person, given the stage of their disease. The cancer rehabilitation team includes all the usual team members of rehabilitation as well as the oncologist. Quality of life is enhanced through cancer rehabilitation by assistance with ADLs, pain management, improving nutrition, smoking cessation, stress reduction, and improved coping strategies. In one study of women with breast cancer, exercise therapy was found to significantly enhance quality of life (Dale et al., 2007). Rehabilitation can also assist individuals with terminal cancer to live a better quality of life until end of life.

Dementia or Alzheimer's Programs

Alzheimer's disease is a progressive and fatal brain disease that currently affects more than 5 million Americans (National Institute on Aging, 2010). Research from the National Institutes of Health suggests that one in seven Americans older than age 71 has some type of dementia (Plassman et al., 2007). Generally occurring in older adults, there are still believed to be between 220,000 and more than half a million cases of early-onset Alzheimer's that affect persons in their 30s, 40s, and 50s (Alzheimer's Association, 2007). It is the most common type of dementia and has no cure. Although Alzheimer's disease is not generally considered a rehabilitation diagnosis, it certainly fits the profile of chronic illness. Those with early-onset Alzheimer's disease would certainly avail themselves of all treatment possible to postpone the inevitable effects of this progressive illness. This would include interventions from the rehabilitation team.

Rehabilitation nurses are often found working in long-term care facilities that serve residents with dementia, and the need is likely to grow. Although the focus of care for older persons with Alzheimer's disease includes rehabilitation goals, realistic outcome planning as the disease progresses will not likely include discharge to home. Persons with Alzheimer's disease may receive services from assisted living, nursing homes, and/or special care units (Alzheimer's Association, 2007). The Alzheimer's unit within the nursing home often becomes the last home that a person with dementia will know. The number of Alzheimer's units within long-term care facilities is increasing due to the demand for services as the disease progresses and because family caregivers are no longer able to manage persons at home. As their condition deteriorates with advancing dementia, the fundamental principles of rehabilitation still apply to these residents: to assist individuals to remain as independent as possible for as long as possible, to maintain function, and to prevent complications.

HIV and AIDS

It was estimated that 65,000 people in Canada were living with HIV or AIDS in 2009 (ACT, 2010). It is estimated that between 34.6 million and 42.3 million people in the world have HIV or AIDS (Monahan, Sands, Neighbors, Marek, & Green, 2007), and about 25 million people worldwide have died from AIDS, including about a half million Americans (Centers for Disease Control and Prevention, 2006). Although current treatments have dramatically increased the life expectancy for many persons with HIV, those developing AIDS experience many associated neurological, pulmonary, cardiac, and rheumatological problems.

Rehabilitation programs designed to address all levels of prevention along with the associated health problems inherent with HIV/AIDS are becoming more common. Rehabilitation nurses may work with infected patients from before diagnosis through end of life (Manning & Haldi, 2007). Rehabilitation goals depend on the stage of illness, whether symptomatic, asymptomatic, or terminal, but include interventions such as monitoring client status, careful assessment, addressing psychological needs and responses, balancing energy with rest, medication management, education regarding prevention of transmission, emotional support, and counselling for the person and family.

OUTCOME MEASUREMENT AND PERFORMANCE IMPROVEMENT

According to Black (2007), outcomes of care are being emphasized as never before. She lists the following benefits of monitoring outcomes (p. 395):

- Track efficiency and effectiveness
- Identify trends
- Facilitate communication among the patient, family, treatment team, payers, referral source, and other stakeholders
- Assess follow-up measures to determine whether progress is continuing after discharge
- Identify areas for improvement
- Measure access to programs

In rehabilitation, outcomes are key to ensuring that goals are being met. Goal setting in rehabilitation should be mutual between the client and the healthcare team. Individual goals for clients are reviewed systematically at team conferences. Outcome measurement can be used to look at trends within an organization, can be benchmarked against industry standards, and can be compared with best practices.

Outcomes can be measured in many ways. Accreditation provides one way to ensure that facilities are meeting the industry standards. A variety of tools can also be used to monitor individual and collective rehabilitation outcomes. One of the most commonly used is the FIM instrument (Uniform Data System for Medical Rehabilitation, 1997), which provides a quantitative measure of function on admission, discharge, and follow-up so that data may be compared across time and with other cohorts. This information often proves useful in justifying insurance coverage by demonstrating continued improvement by the client.

There are also many tools and models for performance improvement in health care. Most of these focus on devices to assist team members to improve the quality of care for clients. Diagrams, flow sheets, checklists, charts, and other visuals can enhance performance. Standard setting by national organizations provides an additional means of quality improvement as organizations strive to meet industry aims. Outcomes measurement and documentation of performance improvement are critical because reimbursement under present payment systems requires rehabilitation providers to provide evidence of the effectiveness of their programs and services (Johnson, Eastwood, Wilkerson, Anderson, & Alves, 2005).

Evidence-Informed Practice Box

This qualitative study explored and compared the hopes of caregivers and nurses dealing with adolescent patients with acquired brain injury. Four themes of hope were revealed by 21 caregivers (mean age, 45 years). Fourteen nurses' perceptions of hope for recovery of the adolescent patients were also examined. Nurses were found to have different perceptions of recovery than the caregivers, who believed they knew the patient better than the staff.

The four themes of hope suggested by the caregivers were (1) family as important, (2) taking one day at a time, (3) knowing the patient better, and (4) spiritual strength as a major social support. Rehabilitation nurses can learn from this limited study that caregivers believe they can provide good insight into the patient with brain injury and that social supports in the form of family and spirituality were seen as important to this group.

Source: Gebhardt, M. C., Mcgehee, L. A., Grindl, C. G., & Dufour, L. T. (2011). Caregiver and nurse hopes for recovery of persons with acquired brain injury. *Rehabilitation Nursing, 36*(1), 3–12.

SUMMARY

This chapter has highlighted the various definitions of rehabilitation and identified key issues arising for individuals living with chronic illness who are engaging in rehabilitative practices. It is imperative that all rehabilitative settings take a client-centred interdisciplinary approach to ensure that individuals living with chronic illness conditions receive individualized care and support. Though rehabilitation settings may vary all healthcare professionals must keep the overall goal of having the client achieve the highest level of independence possible as a primary outcome. Outcome measures are central for tracking the success of rehabilitative practices, but it is also important to keep the client's experience of the effectiveness of these interventions and their own self-care goals as a guiding factor for care planning within rehabilitative settings.

STUDY QUESTIONS

1. Rehabilitation is both a philosophy and an approach to treatment. Describe the philosophy of rehabilitation and how it relates to treatment from an interdisciplinary team of professionals.
2. Define the following rehabilitation terms in relationship to chronic illness: *impairment, functional limitation, disability,* and *community reintegration.*
3. Identify three problems in the provision of rehabilitation services to the chronically ill.
4. Describe the different settings where rehabilitation services can be provided.
5. What specific issues in rehabilitation make doing research difficult?
6. Discuss the advantages and disadvantages of the major functional assessment tools mentioned in this chapter.

INTERNET RESOURCES

Alzheimer's Association: www.alz.org
American Heart Association: www.aha.org
American Stroke Association:
    www.strokeassociation.org
Association of Rehabilitation Nurses:
    www.rehabnurse.org
Centers for Disease Control and Prevention:
    www.cdc.gov/aging/saha.htm
Centers for Medicare & Medicaid Services:
    www.cms.hhs.gov/medicare/
National Institute of Neurological Disorders
    and Stroke: www.ninds.nih.gov
National Rehabilitation Association:
    www.nationalrehab.org
National Rehabilitation Information Center:
    www.naric.com
National Stroke Association: www.nsa.org

For a full suite of assignments and additional learning activities, use the access code located in the front of your book and visit this exclusive website: **http://go.jblearning.com/kramer-kile**. If you do not have an access code, you can obtain one at the site.

REFERENCES

ACT. (2010). *HIV and AIDS statistics—Canada.* Toronto, ON: Author. Retrieved from http://www.actoronto.org/home.nsf/pages/hivaidsstatscan

Adams, P. F., Dey, A. N., & Vickerie, J. L. (2007). *Summary health statistics for the U.S. population: National Health Interview Survey, 2005.* National Center for Health Statistics. Vital Health Statistics, 10(233). Hyattsville, MD: U.S. Department of Health and Human Services.

Ades, P. A., Waldmann, M. L., McCann, W., & Weaver, S. O. (1992). Predictors of cardiac rehabilitation participation in older coronary patients. *Archives of Internal Medicine, 152,* 1033–1035.

Alzheimer's Association. (2007). Alzheimer's disease. Retrieved from http://www.alz.org/alzheimers_disease_alzheimers_disease.asp

American Association for Respiratory Care. (2002). AARC clinical practice guideline: Pulmonary rehabilitation. *Respiratory Care, 47*(5), 617–625.

American Heart Association. (2011). Heart disease and stroke statistics: 2011 update. Retrieved from http://cire.ahajournals.org/content/123/4/el8.full.pdf

American Lung Association. (2011). COPD. Retrieved from http://www.lungusa.org/lung-disease/copd/

American Pain Society. (2006). Pain: Current understanding of assessment, management, and treatments. Retrieved from http://www.ampainsoc.org/education/enduring/

Anderson, C., Linto, J., & Stewart-Wynne, E. (1995). A population-based assessment of the impact and burden of caregiving for long-term stroke survivors. *Stroke, 26,* 843–849.

Angus, J. E., Rukholm, E., Michel, I., Larocque, S., Seto, L., Lapum, J., . . . Nolan, R. P. (2009). Context and cardiovascular risk modification in two regions of Ontario, Canada: A photo elicitation study.

International Journal of Environmental Research and. Public Health, 6(9), 2481–2499.

Arbour, K. P., Latimer, A. E., Ginis, K. A., & Jung, M. E. (2007). Moving beyond the stigma: The impression formation benefits of exercise for individuals with a physical disability. *Adapted Physical Activity Quarterly, 24*(2), 144–159.

Association of Rehabilitation Nurses. (1996). *Scope and standards of advanced clinical practice in rehabilitation nursing.* Glenview, IL: Author.

Association of Rehabilitation Nurses. (2007). ARN positional statement on the role of the nurse in the rehabilitation team. Retrieved from http://www.rehabnurse.org/pdf/PS-Role.pdf

Association of Rehabilitation Nurses. (2008). *Standards and scope of rehabilitation nursing practice.* Glenview, IL: Author.

Bagg, S., Pombo, A. P., & Hopman, W. (2002). Effect of age on functional outcomes after stroke rehabilitation. *Stroke, 33,* 179–185.

Bandeen-Roche, K., Xue, Q-L., Ferrucci, L., Walston, J., Guralnik, J. M., Chaves, P., . . . Fried, L. P. (2006). Phenotype of frailty: Characterization in the women's health and aging studies. *Journals of Gerontology series A: Biological Sciences and Medical Sciences, 61,* 262–266.

Beauchamp, T. L., & Childress, J. F. (2001). *Principles of biomedical ethics.* New York, NY: Oxford University Press.

Beaupre, L. A., Cinats, J. G., Senthilselvan, A., Scharfenberger, A., Johnston, D. W., & Saunders, L. D. (2005). Does standardized rehabilitation and discharge planning improve functional recovery in elderly patients with hip fracture? *Archives of Physical Medicine and Rehabilitation, 86,* 2231–2239.

Beck, L. A. (2003). Cancer rehabilitation: Does it make a difference? *Rehabilitation Nursing, 28*(2), 32–37.

Beers, M. H., & Berkow, R. (2004). *Rehabilitation. The Merck manual of geriatrics.* Merck & Co., Medical Services, USMEDA, USHH. Retrieved from http://www.merck.com/mrkshared/mm_geriatrics/home.jsp

Black, T. (2007). Outcomes measurement and performance improvement. In K. L. Mauk (Ed.), *The specialty practice of rehabilitation nursing: A core curriculum* (pp. 395–411). Glenview, IL: Association of Rehabilitation Nurses.

Brandt, E., & Pope, A. (1997). *Enabling America: Assessing the role of rehabilitation science and engineering.* Committee on Assessing Rehabilitation Science and Engineering. Division of Health Policy. Institute of Medicine. Washington, DC: National Academies Press.

Brouwer, W. B. F., van Exel, N. J. A., van de Berg, B., Dinant, H. J., Koopmanschap, M. A., & van den Bos, G. A. (2004). Burden of caregiving: Evidence of objective burden, subjective burden, and quality of life impacts on informal caregivers of patients with rheumatoid arthritis. *Arthritis and Rheumatism, 51*(4), 570–577.

Bushnik, T., Wright, J., & Burdsall, D. (2007). Personal attendant turnover: Association with level of injury, burden of care, and psychosocial outcome. *Topics in Spinal Cord Injury Rehabilitation, 12*(3), 66–76.

Campinha-Bacote, J. (2001). A model of practice to address cultural competence. *Rehabilitation Nursing, 26*(1), 8–11.

Canadian Association of Cardiac Rehabilitation. (2009, May). *Canadian guidelines for cardiac rehabilitation and cardiovascular disease prevention: Translating knowledge into action* (3rd ed.). Winnipeg, MB: CACR.

Canadian Association of Rehabilitation Nurses. (2010). Mission. Retrieved from http://www.carn.ca/about/mission/

Canadian Cancer Society Steering Committee on Cancer Statistics. (2011). *Canadian cancer statistics 2011.* Toronto, ON: Canadian Cancer Society.

Canam, C., & Acorn, S. (1999). Quality of life for family caregivers of people with chronic health problems. *Rehabilitation Nursing, 24*(5), 192–196.

Carbone, L. (2007). Cardiovascular and pulmonary rehabilitation: Acute and long-term management. In K. L. Mauk (Ed.), *The specialty practice of rehabilitation nursing: A core curriculum* (pp. 238–259). Glenview, IL: Association of Rehabilitation Nurses.

Centers for Disease Control and Prevention. (2006). Overview. Retrieved from http://www.cdc.gov/hiv/topics/testing/index.htm

Charles, C. V., & Lehman, C. (2006). Medications and laboratory values. In K. L. Mauk (Ed.), *Gerontological nursing: Competencies for care* (pp. 293–320). Sudbury, MA: Jones and Bartlett.

Clark, G. S., & Siebens, H. (2005). Geriatric rehabilitation. In J. DeLisa & B. Gans (Eds.), *Physical medicine and rehabilitation: Principles and practice* (4th ed., pp. 1531–1560). Philadelphia, PA: Lippincott Williams & Wilkins.

Currie, D. M., Atchison, J. W., & Fiedler, I. G. (2002). The challenge of teaching rehabilitative care in medical school. *Academic Medicine, 77*(7), 701–708.

Dale, A. J., Crank, H., Saxton, J. M., Mutrie, N., Coleman, R., & Roalfe, A. (2007). Randomized trial of exercise therapy in women treated for breast cancer. *Journal of Clinical Oncology, 25*(13), 1713–1721.

das Chagas Medeiros, M., Ferraz, M., & Quaresma, M. (2000). The effect of rheumatoid arthritis on the quality of life of primary caregivers. *Journal of Rheumatology, 27*(1), 76–83.

Doherty, R. B. (2004). Assessing the new Medicare prescription drug law. *Annals of Internal Medicine, 141*(5), 391–395.

Draper, B., Bowring, G., Thompson, C., Van Heyst, J., Conroy, P., & Thompson, J. (2007). Stress in caregivers of aphasic stroke patients: A randomized controlled trial. *Clinical Rehabilitation, 21*(2), 122–130.

Easton, K. L. (1999). *Gerontological rehabilitation nursing*. Philadelphia, PA: Saunders.

Easton, K. L. (2001). *The post-stroke journey: From agonizing to owning*. Doctoral dissertation. Wayne State University, Detroit, MI.

Edwards, P., Hertzberg, D., & Sapp, L. (2007). Pediatric rehabilitation nursing. In K. L. Mauk (Ed.), *The specialty practice of rehabilitation nursing: A core curriculum* (pp. 336–358). Glenview, IL: Association of Rehabilitation Nurses.

Ellis, J. R., & Hartley, C. L. (2004). *Nursing in today's world: Trends, issues, and management* (8th ed.). Philadelphia, PA: Lippincott Williams & Wilkins.

Fairfax, J. (2002). *Theory of quality of life of stroke survivors*. Doctoral dissertation. Wayne State University, Detroit, MI.

Gillis, T. A., Cheville, A. L., & Worsowicz, G. M. (2001). Cardiopulmonary rehabilitation and cancer rehabilitation: Oncologic rehabilitation. *Archives of Physical Medicine and Rehabilitation, 83*(Suppl. 1), S47–S51.

Grunfeld, E., Coyle, D., Whelan, T., Clinch, J., Reyno, L., Earle, C. C., . . . Glossop, R. (2004). Family caregiver burden: Results of a longitudinal study of breast cancer patients and their principal caregivers. *Canadian Medical Association Journal, 170*(12), 1795–1801.

Guse, L. W. (2006). Assessment of the older adult. In K. L. Mauk (Ed.), *Gerontological nursing: Competencies for care* (pp. 265–292). Sudbury, MA: Jones and Bartlett.

Halm, M. A., Treat-Jacobson, D., Lindquist, R., & Savik, K. (2007). Caregiver burden and outcomes of caregiving of spouses of patient who undergo coronary artery bypass graft surgery. *Heart & Lung, 36*(3), 170–187.

Harris, J. A. (2000). Understanding acute and chronic pain. In P. Edwards (Ed.), *The specialty practice of rehabilitation nursing* (4th ed.). Glenview, IL: Association of Rehabilitation Nurses.

Hartke, R. J., & King, R. B. (2002). Analysis of problem types and difficulty among older stroke caregivers. *Topics in Stroke Rehabilitation, 9*(1), 16–33.

Hertzberg, D. (2007). Understanding acute and chronic pain. In K. L. Mauk (Ed.), *The specialty practice of rehabilitation nursing: A core curriculum* (pp. 260–274). Glenview, IL: Association of Rehabilitation Nurses.

Hogstel, M. O., Curry, L. C., Walker, C. A., & Burns, P. G. (2004). Ethics committees in long-term care facilities. *Geriatric Nursing, 25*(6), 364–369.

Hughes, S., Giobbie-Harder, A., Weaver, F., Kubal, J., Henderson, W. (1999). Relationship between caregiver burden and health-related quality of life. *The Gerontologist, 39*(5), 534–545.

Johnson, J. A. (2004). Withdrawal of medically administered nutrition and hydration: The role benefits and burdens, and of parents and ethics committees. *Journal of Clinical Ethics, 15*(3), 307–311.

Johnston, M. V., Eastwood, E., Wilkerson, D. L., Anderson, L., & Alves, A. (2005). Systematically assessing and improving the quality and outcomes of medical rehabilitation programs. In J. DeLisa & B. M. Gans (Eds.), *Rehabilitation medicine: Principles and practice* (3rd ed., pp. 1163–1192). Philadelphia, PA: Lippincott-Raven.

Kemp, B. (1986). Psychosocial and mental health issues in rehabilitation of older persons. In S. Brody & G. Ruff (Eds.), *Aging and rehabilitation* (pp. 122–158). New York, NY: Springer.

Kennedy, J. (2001). Unmet and undermet need for activities of daily living and instrumental activities of daily living assistance among adults with disabilities: Estimates from the 1994 and 1995 disability follow-back surveys. *Medical Care, 39*(12), 1305–1312.

Kent, B., & Smith, S. (2006). They only see it when the sun shines in my ears: Exploring perceptions of adolescent hearing aid users. *Journal of Deaf Studies & Deaf Education, 11*(4), 461–476.

Kielhofner, G., Braveman, B., Finlayson, M., Paul-Ward, A., Goldbaum, L., & Goldstein, K. (2004). Outcomes of a vocational program for persons with AIDS. *American Journal of Occupational Therapy, 58*(1), 64–72.

King, R. B., Hartke, R. J., & Denby, F. (2007). Problem-solving early intervention: A pilot study of stroke caregivers. *Rehabilitation Nursing, 32*(2), 68–76.

Kirschner, K. L., Stocking, C., Wagner, L. B., Foye, S. J., & Siegler, M. (2001). Ethical issues identified by rehabilitation clinicians. *Archives of Physical Medicine and Rehabilitation, 82*(12 Suppl. 2), S2–S8.

Kolanowski, A. M., Fick, D., Waller, J. L., & Shea, D. (2004). Spouses of persons with dementia: Their healthcare problems, utilization, and costs. *Research in Nursing & Health, 27*, 296–306.

LaPlante, M., Kaye, H. S., Kang, T., & Harrington, C. (2004). Unmet need for personal assistance services: Estimating the shortfall in hours of help and adverse consequences. *Journal of Gerontology, Series B, Psychological Science and Social Science, 59*(2), S98–S108.

Lieberman, M., & Fisher, L. (1995). The impact of chronic illness on the health and well-being of family members. *The Gerontologist, 35*(1), 94–102.

Lin, J. L., & Armour, D. (2004). Selected medical management of the older adult rehabilitative patient. *Archives of Physical Medicine and Rehabilitation, 85*(Suppl. 3), S76–S82.

Lipton, R., Hamelsky, S., Kolodner, K., Steiner, T., & Stewart, W. F. (2000). Migraine, quality of life, and depression: A population-based case-control study. *Neurology, 55*(5), 629–635.

Lloyd, C., & Waghorn, G. (2007). The importance of vocation in recovery for young people with psychiatric disabilities. *British Journal of Occupational Therapy, 70*(2), 50–59.

Lutz, B. J., & Bowers, B. J. (2003). Understanding how disability is defined and conceptualized in the literature. *Rehabilitation Nursing, 28*(3), 74–78.

Lysaght, R. M. (2004). Approaches to worker rehabilitation by occupational and physical therapists in the United States: Factors impacting practice. *Work, 23*(2), 139–146.

Manning, K., & Haldi, P. (2007). Specific disease processes requiring rehabilitation interventions. In K. L. Mauk (Ed.), *The specialty practice of rehabilitation nursing: A core curriculum* (pp. 275–322). Glenview, IL: Association of Rehabilitation Nurses.

Masters-Farrell, P. A. (2006). Ethical/legal principles and issues. In K. L. Mauk (Ed.), *Gerontological nursing: Competencies for care* (pp. 589–616). Sudbury, MA: Jones and Bartlett.

Masters-Farrell, P. A. (2007). Ethical, moral, and legal considerations. In K. L. Mauk (Ed.), *The specialty practice of rehabilitation nursing: A core curriculum* (pp. 27–34). Glenview, IL: Association of Rehabilitation Nurses.

Mauk, K. L. (2006). Nursing interventions within the Mauk model of poststroke recovery. *Rehabilitation Nursing, 31*(6), 257–263.

Mauk, K. L., & Hanson, P. (2010). Management of common illnesses, diseases, and health conditions. In K. L. Mauk (Ed.), *Gerontological nursing: Competencies for care* (pp. 382–453). Sudbury, MA: Jones & Bartlett.

Mauk, K. L., & Lehman, C. (2007). Geriatric rehabilitation. In K. L. Mauk (Ed.), *The specialty practice of rehabilitation nursing: A core curriculum* (pp. 359–383). Glenview, IL: Association of Rehabilitation Nurses.

Menear, M., Reinharz, D., Corbiere, M., Houle, N., Lanctot, N., Goering, P., . . . Lecomte, T. (2011). Organizational analysis of Canadian supported employment programs for people with psychiatric disabilities. *Social Science and Medicine, 72*, 1028–1035.

Mills, P., Yu, H., Ziegler, M., Patterson, T., & Grant, I. (1999). Vulnerable caregivers of patients with Alzheimer's disease have a deficit in circulating CD62L-T lymphocytes. *Psychosomatic Medicine, 61*(2), 168–174.

Mirolla, M. (2004). *The cost of chronic disease in Canada*. Chronic Disease Prevention Alliance of Canada. Retrieved from http://www.gpiatlantic.org/pdf/health/chroniccanada.pdf

Monahan, F. D., Sands, J. K., Neighbors, M., Marek, J. F., & Green, C. J. (2007). *Phipps' medical-surgical nursing: Health and illness perspectives* (8th ed.). St. Louis, MO: Mosby Elsevier.

Mpofu, E., & Harley, D. A. (2006). Racial and disability identity: Implications for the career counseling of African Americans with disabilities. *Rehabilitation Counseling Bulletin, 50*(1), 14–23.

Nadash, P., & Feldman, P. H. (2003). The effectiveness of a "restorative" model of care for home care patients. *Home Healthcare Nurse, 21*(6), 421–423.

National Association for Home Care and Hospice. (2007). Basic statistics about home care. Retrieved from http://www.nahc.org/facts/07HC_stats.pdf

National Center for Chronic Disease Prevention and Health Promotion, Centers for Disease Control and Prevention. (2007). Quick facts: Economic and health burden of chronic disease. Retrieved from http://www.cdc.gov/nccdphp/press/#4

National Institute on Aging. (2010). Alzheimer's disease fact sheet. Retrieved from http://www.nia.nih.gov/Alzheimers/Publications/adfact.htm

Neal, L. J. (2001). Using rehabilitation theory to teach medical-surgical nursing to undergraduate students. *Rehabilitation Nursing, 26*(2), 72–75, 77.

Nelson, W. (2004). Addressing rural ethics issues. The characteristics of rural healthcare settings pose unique ethical challenges. *Healthcare Executive, 19*(4), 36–37.

O'Neill, J. H., Zuger, R. R., Fields, A., Fraser, R., & Pruce, T. (2004). The program without walls: Innovative approach to state agency vocational rehabilitation of persons with traumatic brain injury. *Archives of Physical Medicine and Rehabilitation, 85*(4), S68–72.

Osterweil, D. (1990). Geriatric rehabilitation in the long-term care institutional setting. In B. Kemp, K. Brummel-Smith, & J. Ramsdell (Eds.), *Geriatric rehabilitation* (pp. 347–456). Boston, MA: Little, Brown.

Parker, B. J., & Neal-Boylan, L. (2007). Community and family-centered rehabilitation nursing. In K. L. Mauk (Ed.), *The specialty practice of rehabilitation nursing: A core curriculum* (pp. 13–26). Glenview, IL: Association of Rehabilitation Nurses.

People Living with Cancer. (2006). Rehabilitation. Retrieved from http://www.cancer.net/patient/Survivorship/Rehabilitation/#mainContent.idmainContent

Pierce, L., Steiner, V., Govoni, A., Hicks, B., Thompson, T., & Friedemann, M. (2004). Caring-Web Internet-based support for rural caregivers of persons with stroke show promise. *Rehabilitation Nursing, 29*(3), 95–99, 103.

Pierce, L. L., Steiner, V., Hicks, B., & Holzaepfel, A. L. (2006). Problems of new caregivers of persons with stroke. *Rehabilitation Nursing, 31*(4), 166–172.

Plassman, B. L., Langa, K. M., Fisher, G. G., Heeringa, S. G., Weir, D. R., Ofstedal, M. B., . . .Wallace, R. B. (2007). Prevalence of dementia in the United States: The aging, demographics, and memory study. *Neuroepidemiology, 29,* 125–132.

Podsiadlo, D., & Richardson S. (1991). The timed "up & go": A test of basic functional mobility for frail elderly persons. *Journal of the American Geriatric Society, 39,* 142–148.

Pope, A. M., & Tarlov, A. R. (1991). *Disability in America: Toward a national agenda for prevention.* Washington, DC: National Academy Press.

Public Health Agency of Canada. (2011). *Centre for chronic disease prevention and control.* Ottawa, ON: Author. Retrieved from http://www.phac-aspc.gc.ca/ccdpc-cpcmc/index-eng.php

Pryor, J. (2002). Rehabilitative nursing: A core nursing function across all settings. *Collegian, 9*(2), 11–15.

Remsburg, R. (2004). Restorative care activities. In B. Resnick (Ed.), *Restorative care nursing for older adults: A guide for all care settings* (pp. 74–95). New York, NY: Springer.

Remsburg, R., Armacost, K., Radu, C., & Bennett, R. (1999). Comparison of two models of restorative care in the nursing home. *Geriatric Nursing, 20*(6), 321–326.

Remsburg, R., Armacost, K., Radu, C., & Bennett, R. (2001). Impact of a restorative care program in the nursing home. *Educational Gerontology: An International Journal, 27,* 261–280.

Remsburg, R., & Carson, B. (2006). Rehabilitation. In I. Lubkin & P. Larsen (Eds.), *Chronic illness: Impact and interventions* (pp. 579–616). Sudbury, MA: Jones and Bartlett.

Resnick, B., & Fleishell, A. (2002). Developing a restorative care program: A five-step approach that involves the resident. *American Journal of Nursing, 102*(7), 91–95.

Resnick, B., & Remsburg, R. (2004). Overview of restorative care. In B. Resnick (Ed.), *Restorative care nursing for older adults: A guide for all care settings* (pp. 1–12). New York, NY: Springer.

Routasalo, P., Arve, S., & Lauri, S. (2004). Geriatric rehabilitation nursing: Developing a model. *International Journal of Nursing Practice, 10*(5), 207–215.

Santerre, R. E. (2002). The inequity of Medicaid reimbursement in the United States. *Applied Health Economics and Health Policy, 1*(1), 25–32.

Schulz, R., & Beach, S. (1999). Caregiving as a risk factor for mortality: The caregiver health effects study. *Journal of the American Medical Association, 282*(23), 2215–2219.

Secrest, J. A. (2007). Rehabilitation and rehabilitation nursing. In K. Mauk (Ed.), *The specialty practice of rehabilitation nursing: A core curriculum* (5th ed., pp. 2–12). Glenview, IL: Association of Rehabilitation Nurses.

Secrest, J. A., & Thomas, S. P. (1999). Continuity and discontinuity: The quality of life following stroke. *Rehabilitation Nursing, 24*(6), 240–246.

Secrest, J. A., & Zeller, R. (2003). Measuring continuity and discontinuity following stroke. *Journal of Nursing Scholarship, 35*(3), 243–249.

Secrest, J. A., & Zeller, R. (2007). The relationship of continuity and discontinuity, functional ability, depression, and quality of life over time in stroke survivors. *Rehabilitation Nursing, 32*(4), 158–164.

Shah, S. K. (2005). Cardiac rehabilitation. In J. DeLisa & B. M. Gans (Eds.), *Rehabilitation medicine: Principles and practice* (3rd ed., pp. 1811–1842). Philadelphia, PA: Lippincott-Raven.

Shanks, L. C., Moore, S. M., & Zeller, R. A. (2007). Predictors of cardiac rehabilitation initiation. *Rehabilitation Nursing, 32*(4), 152–157.

Shaw, W., Patterson, T., Ziegler, M., Dimsdale, J., Semple, S. J., Grant, I. (1999). Accelerated risk of hypertensive blood pressure recordings among Alzheimer caregivers. *Journal of Psychosomatic Medicine, 43*(3), 215–227.

Shirey, L., & Summer, L. (2000). *Caregiving: Helping the elderly with activity limitations. Challenges for the 21st century: Chronic and disabling conditions.* Washington, DC: National Academy on an Aging Society.

Singh, V. N., Schocken, D. D., Williams, K., & Stamey, R. (2004). Cardiac rehabilitation. Retrieved from http://www.emedicine.com/pmr/topic180.htm

Ski, C., & O'Connell, B. (2007). Stroke: The increasing complexity of carer needs. *Journal of Neuroscience Nursing, 39*(3), 172–179.

Statistics Canada. (2011a). *Mortality, summary list of causes 2008.* Cat. no.: 84F0209X. Retrieved from http ://www.statcan.gc.ca/pub/84f0209x/84f0209x 2008000-eng.pdf

Statistics Canada. (2011b). *An aging population.* Ottawa, ON: Author. Retrieved from http://www.statcan.gc .ca/pub/11-402-x/2010000/chap/pop/pop02-eng.htm

Stuart, H. (2006, September). Mental illness and employment discrimination. *Current Opinion in Psychiatry, 5*, 522–526.

Targett, P., Wehman, P., & Young, C. (2004). Return to work for persons with spinal cord injury: Designing work supports. *Neurorehabilitation. 19*(2), 131–139.

Thompson, T. L., Emrich, K., & Moore, G. (2003). The effect of curriculum on the attitudes of nursing students toward disability. *Rehabilitation Nursing, 28*(1), 27–30.

Uniform Data System for Medical Rehabilitation. (1997). *FIM(tm) instrument.* Buffalo, NY: University at Buffalo.

Vargo, M. M., & Gerber, L. H. (2005). Rehabilitation for patients with cancer diagnoses. In J. DeLisa & B. Gans (Eds.), *Physical medicine and rehabilitation: Principles and practice* (4th ed., pp. 1771–1794). Philadelphia, PA: Lippincott Williams & Wilkins.

Walsh, N. E., Dumitru, D., Schoenfeld, L. S., & Ramaurthy, S. (2005). Treatment of the patient with chronic pain. In J. DeLisa & B. Gans (Eds.), *Physical medicine and rehabilitation: Principles and practice* (4th ed., pp. 493–530). Philadelphia, PA: Lippincott Williams & Wilkins.

Ward, A. B., & Gutenbrunner, C. (2006). Physical and rehabilitation medicine in Europe. *Journal of Rehabilitation Medicine, 38*, 81–86.

Weitzenkamp, D., Gerhart, K., Charlifue, S., Whiteneck, G., & Savic, G. (1997). Spouses of spinal cord injury survivors: The added impact of caregiving. *Archives of Physical Medicine and Rehabilitation, 78*(8), 822–827.

Whyte, J. (1998). Enabling America: A report from the Institute of Medicine on rehabilitation science and engineering. *Archives of Physical Medicine and Rehabilitation, 79*(11), 1477–1480.

World Health Organization. (1980). *International classification of impairments, disabilities and handicaps.* Geneva, Switzerland: Author.

World Health Organization. (2002). Towards a common language for functioning, disability and health ICF. Retrieved from http://www.who.int/classifications /icf/training/icfbeginnersguide.pdf

World Health Organization. (2007). International classification of functioning, disability, and health. Retrieved from http://www.who.int/classifications /icf/en

Worsowicz, G. M., Stewart, D. G., Phillips, E. M., & Cifu, D. X. (2004). Geriatric rehabilitation: Social and economic implications of aging. *Archives of Physical Medicine and Rehabilitation, 85*(Suppl. 3), S3–S6.

Wu, H., Wang, J., Cacioppo, J., Glaser, R., Kiecolt-Glaser, J. K., & Malarkey, W. B. (1999). Chronic stress associated with spousal caregiving of patients with Alzheimer's dementia is associated with down regulation of B-lymphocyte GH mRNA. *Journal of Gerontology: A Biologic Science/Medical Science, 54*(4), M212–215.

Yu, F. (2005). Factors affecting outpatient rehabilitation outcomes in elders. *Journal of Nursing Scholarship, 37*(3), 229–236.

Zola, I. K. (1982). *Disincentives to independent living.* Lawrence, KS: Research and Training Center on Independent Living, University of Kansas.

Index

Page numbers followed by *t* or *f* indicate tables or figures, respectively.

A

abandonment, 475
Aberdeen, Lady, 431
aboriginal peoples
    access to care, 4–5
    health care for, 7–8
    Internet resources for, 513
    views regarding end-of-life care, 502–503
ABSQ. *See* Adult Body Satisfaction Questionnaire
abuse, 474–476
access to care, 4–5, 8, 9–10, 17
access to community resources, 36
access to grief and bereavement care, 498
access to home health care, 430, 439–440
access to hospice care, 440, 498
access to palliative care, 498
Accord on Health Care Renewal, 436
Accreditation Canada, 472
Achieving Health for All: A Framework for Health Promotion (Epp), 12–13
action
    stage of change, 377
    theory of reasoned action, 377–378
action plans
    "My Action Plan," 35
    for self-efficacy, 298
activities of daily living (ADLs)
    adults with disabilities requiring assistance with, 530
    behavioural strategy, 223
    informal caregiver behaviours, 450*t*
    Katz index of, 478
    self-care, 285–286
acupuncture
    for hypertension, 403–404, 405
    regulation of, 398, 401–402

treatment modality, 400–401, 401*t*, 402
use of, 396
acute conditions, 6
adaptation, 99–120
    case study, 110
    contextual variables influencing, 102
    definition of, 100
    evidence-informed practice for, 116–117
    factors associated with, 107
    health-related factors, 108–109
    impact of, 100–102
    individual differences in, 105
    models of, 103–109, 106*f*
    overview of, 111–113
    personal resources for, 107–108, 112
    physical context for, 109
    process of, 105
    psychological, 112
    psychosocial, 112
    of routines, 220
    social context for, 109
    to uncertainty, 218, 219*f*
    women to women conceptual model for, 185–186
adaptive tasks, 109
addiction, 507*t*
adjustment
    to body image, 162–168
    to chronic illness, 100–101
    conceptualization of, 100–102
    in context of individual, 101–102
    definition of, 100, 112
    dynamic process of, 101
    elements of success, 111–112
    indicators of, 112
    individual differences in, 102

in multiple life domains, 100–101
overview of, 111–113
positive and negative outcome dimensions of, 101
ADLs. *See* activities of daily living
admission, in LTC setting, 476–478
adolescents
as caregivers, 353
evidence-informed practice for, 542
adult asthma guidelines for nurses, 193*t*–194*t*
Adult Body Satisfaction Questionnaire (ABSQ), 176
adult literacy, low, 320, 322–324
adults. *See also* older adults
as learners, 311–312, 312*t*, 320, 321*t*
recommended teacher strategies for, 320, 321*t*
advance care planning
with cancer patients, 193*t*–194*t*
for hospice palliative care, 503, 505–506
Internet resources for, 513
advanced practice nursing
CAM treatment issues for, 414–415
definition of, 414–415
advice giving, 221
advocacy
for client empowerment, 277
Ombudsman role, 480
age
and body image, 166
chronological, 319–320
and health promotion, 385
Agency for Healthcare Research and Quality, 22, 325
agenda decisions, 450
aging
with disability, 538
in place, 536–537
stigma of, 75
aging population, 438–439
AIDS. *See* HIV/AIDS
Alberta Children's Hospital, 410
Alberta Health Services
LEAP Project, 410
"Living Well with a Chronic Condition"
programme, 300
"My Voice" workbook and videos, 506
Alberta Health Services for Advance Care
Planning, 513
Alcoholics Anonymous, 142
Ali, Muhammad, 16
alienation, 123–124
alkylating agents, 246
allergies, 395*t*, 397
allied hospice palliative care disciplines, 511
allopathic health care, 414
aloneness, 124
alternative medical systems, 394

alternative medicine. *See also* complementary and
alternative medicine (CAM)
definition of, 394
spending on, 397
use of, 395–396, 395*t*
Alternative Therapies in Health and Medicine, 413
Alzheimer's Association, 543
Alzheimer's disease
case studies, 211–212, 484
clinical practice guidelines for common symptom
experiences in, 507*t*
early-onset, 540
in long-term care, 482–483
rehabilitation programs for, 540–541
Alzheimer's units, 540–541
AMECC, 417
American Association of Colleges of Nursing, 480
American Board of Medical Specialties, 511
American Heart Association, 543
American Medical Association (AMA), 317*t*
American Nurses Association, 232–233
American Stroke Association, 543
American Telemedicine Association, 452
amino acids, 399
amputation desire, 158–159
amputation envy, 158–159
amyotrophic lateral sclerosis (case study), 418–420
andragogy, 311–312, 312*t*
anticipatory guidance
for client empowerment, 278
for managing body image, 177
for managing unpredictability, 223
antioxidant supplements, 406
anxiety
alternative therapy for, 395*t*, 397
with illness uncertainty, 215
appearance, 171–172
ARN. *See* Association of Rehabilitation Nurses
aromatherapy
professional education in, 417
regulation of, 398
arthritis
alternative therapy for, 395*t*, 397
case study, 411–412
Arthritis Impact Measurement Scales, 478
assessment
of behavioural change, 296–297
of body image, 168–170
functional, 532–533
guided care nurse activities, 35
of learners, 313–314
of low literacy, 320, 322–324, 323*t*
in LTC setting, 476–478
PLISSIT model, 251–252, 251*t*

sexual, 249–250
  tools for, 478
assisted living, 467
Association of Rehabilitation Nurses (ARN)
  definition of rehabilitation nursing, 522–523
  goals for pain management, 535
  Internet resources, 543
  Scope and Standards of Advanced Clinical Practice in Rehabilitation Nursing, 523
  Standards and Scope of Rehabilitation Nursing Practice, 523
Asthma Clinic (Alberta Children's Hospital), 410
asthma guidelines, 193*t*–194*t*
Atlantic Canada, 497–498
attitudes
  professional, 84
  sexual attitude reassessments (SARs), 250–251
  toward stigma, 82
audiotapes, 406
autonomy
  versus dependence, 473
  preservation of, 478–479
  promotion of, 478
Ayurvedic medicine, 403, 417

B
back or neck problems, 395*t*, 397
BDD. *See* body dysmorphic disorder
Beck depression rating scale, 478
behaviour
  assessment of, 296–297
  health-related, 46–47
  help-seeking, 51
  illness experience and, 53–55 (*See also* illness behaviour)
  planned, 377–378
  self-determined, 290–292
  sick-role, 46
  stigma-promoting, 90–91
behavioural change
  advising about health risks and benefits of, 297–298
  collaboration for, 298
  5 A's of, 296–299
  for social isolation, 147
  stages of, 297
  strategies for reducing uncertainty, 223
behavioural effect questions, 363*t*
behaviourist framework, 309
beliefs
  assessment of, 296–297
  Illness Beliefs Model (IBM), 336, 340–341, 341–342
belonging, 121
bereavement needs, 503–505
Best Practice Collaborative approach (Kaiser Permanente), 300
bias, 30

bioelectromagnetic-based therapies, 394
biofield therapies
  for cancer, 406
  definition of, 394
  examples, 394
  for hypertension, 404–405
biography, 60
biologically based therapies
  for cancer symptoms, 406
  definition of, 394
  professional education in, 417
biomedical model of adaptation, 103–104
Blood-Based Diagnostic Assay for Breast Cancer, 410
BMC Complementary and Alternative Medicine, 413
body-based methods, 394, 402–403, 403*t*
body dysmorphic disorder (BDD), 159
body image, 157–182
  assessment of, 168–170
  case study, 169
  changes over time in, 164
  conceptualization of, 159–160
  cultural influences on, 165
  definition of, 158–160, 161–162
  evidence-informed practice for, 176
  external changes, 170–171
  factors influencing adjustment to, 162–168
  historical foundations of, 160–161
  indications of improvement, 178–179
  Internet resources for, 179
  interventions for, 174–178
  issues important to chronic illness, 170–174
  meaning of, 162–164
  negative, 176
  significance of, 162–164
  social influences on, 164–165
body schema, 158
bodywork, 417
botanicals, 406, 407
brain injury, 542
breast cancer (case study), 247
breathing techniques
  deep-breathing exercises, 400
  slow breathing, 403–404
Brewster, Mary, 432
Brief Illness Perception Questionnaire, 47
British Columbia Cancer Agency, 405
British North American Act of 1867, 7, 435
bullying, 73
burnout, 355–356

C
CAGE alcoholism scale, 35
calcium supplements, 406
Calgary Health Region, 410

CAM in Undergraduate Medical Education (UME) project, 409
CAMline, 409
Canada Health Act
    access to care provisions, 4, 8, 9–10, 17
    home health care provisions, 430
    limitations, 437
    long-term care provisions, 465
    principles or criteria for medically necessary services, 9, 435–436
    prohibitions against extra billing and user fees, 9
Canada Health Infoway, 450
Canadian Academy of Health Sciences, 23–24
Canadian Association of Rehabilitation Nurses, 522–523
Canadian best practices portal (PHAC), 374
Canadian Best Practices System, 15
Canadian CAM Research Fund, 409
Canadian Cancer Society, 410
Canadian Cancer Society Research Institute, 410
Canadian Community Health Nursing Standards of Practice, 446, 446t
Canadian Council of Examiners, 417
Canadian Geriatrics Society, 513
Canadian Gerontological Nursing Association, 488
Canadian Health Human Resources plan, 11
Canadian Home Care Association, 458
Canadian Hospice Palliative Care Association (CHPCA)
    Aboriginal Issues, 513
    description of hospice palliative care, 496
    Internet resources, 458, 488, 513, 514
    norms and standards of practice, 511
    Nurses Group, 511
    Nurses Interest Group, 514
    principles and values, 497t
    square of care and organization, 499–500, 501f
    Strategic Plan, 514
Canadian Institute of Health Research, 8, 512–513
Canadian Institute of Natural and Integrative Medicine, 410
Canadian Nurses Association
    Advanced Hospice Palliative Care Nursing Certification, 511
    advocacy work, 15, 530
    practice initiatives, 15
    Rehabilitation Nursing Certification, 523
    standards of practice, 232–233
Canadian Patient Safety Institute, 14–15, 488
Canadian Public Health Association, 317t
Canadian Society of Palliative Care Physicians, 511
Canadian Virtual Hospice, 505, 513, 514
cancer
    childhood, 344
    economic and health burden of, 18t
    prevalence of, 3
    and sexuality, 242–246

Cancer and Complementary and Alternative Medicine Research Team, 409–410
cancer care
    advance care planning, 193t–194t
    CAM, 405–408
    for quality of life, 198–199
cancer rehabilitation, 540
cancer surgery, 242–243, 243t–244t
cardiac cripples, 162–163
cardiac rehabilitation, 539
cardiovascular disease
    economic and health burden of, 18t
    management recommendations for, 237, 238t
    prevalence of, 3
care. See also health care
    versus cure, 84
    medical model of, 136
caregiver burden
    definition of, 352–353
    evidence-informed practice for, 514
    family caregiver strain or burden, 352–353
    gender components in, 353
    during rehabilitation, 527–528
caregivers
    adolescents, 353
    behaviours of, 449, 450t
    children, 353
    definition of, 350–351
    double, 465–466
    evidence-informed practice for, 542
    family caregivers, 350–352
    formal, 449–452, 530
    home care benefits for, 358
    informal, 350–351, 449–452, 450t, 530
    for parents, 353
    in rehabilitation, 530
    role satisfaction, 357
    spouses, 353
    support for, 36
    themes of hope suggested by, 542
caregiving
    evidence-informed practice for, 514
    family caregiving, 349–358, 500–502
    financial impact of, 353–355
    live-in, 356
caregiving-related stress, 527–528
CARF Canada, 472
Carstairs, Sharon, 495
CCC system. See clinical care classification system
CCM. See chronic care model
Center for Human Diversity, 317t
Center to Advance Palliative Care, 496
Centers for Disease Control and Prevention, 543
Centers for Medicare & Medicaid Services, 543
Centre for Addiction and Mental Health, 317t

Centre for Advancement of Palliative Care, 514
Centre for Behavioural Research and Program
        Evaluation, 410
Centre for Health Promotion, University of Ottawa, 374
cerebrovascular accident, 507t
change
        advising about benefits of, 297–298
        maintaining, 297
        ongoing, 349–358
        preparation for, 297, 377
        processes of, 377
        readiness for, 319
        stages of, 297, 377
character blemishes, 75
chemotherapy, 246, 247
chest pain, 395t, 397
childhood cancer, 344
children
        as caregivers, 353
        families launching, 346
        with functional limitations, 538
        as learners, 311–312, 312t
        rehabilitation for, 538–539
        young, 343–344
Chinese medicine. See traditional Chinese medicine
chiropractic care
        regulation of, 398
        therapeutic method and rationale for, 402–403, 403t
        use of, 395t, 396
Chochinov, Harvey, 493
CHPCA. See Canadian Hospice Palliative Care Association
CHPCA Nurses Group, 511
chronic care
        case study, 40
        context for, 8–19
        financial impact of, 16–19
        future directions, 23–24
        models of, 29–44
        recommendations for, 24
        social influences, 16
chronic care model (CCM)
        comparison with ECCM, 32, 34t–35t
        expanded chronic care model (ECCM), 32, 33f, 34t–35t
        overview, 30–31, 32f
        theoretical framework, 444–445, 445f
chronic disease. See chronic illness
chronic disease practitioners, 20, 21t. See also
        healthcare providers
Chronic Disease Prevention Alliance of Canada, 307
chronic fatigue syndrome (CFS), 55, 89–90
chronic illness
        adjustment to, 100–101
        body image issues important to, 170–174
        and CAM, 403–408
        chronic phase, 61, 340–341

chronic versus acute conditions, 6
client's view of, 105
crisis phase, 60–61, 339–340
as culture, 15–16
demographics of, 497
disability-related variables, 105
dynamic and unfolding nature of, 339–343
economic burden of, 17, 18t
effects of, 5, 7–8
and families, 335–369, 338f
family management of, 441–442, 441f
health burden of, 17, 18t
health promotion in, 372–374
health-related outcomes of, 106, 106f
home care for, 440–446
identity of, 105
insider perspective of, 61
interventions for, 19–22
key problems of, 59
legitimization of, 55–58
and life cycle, 60–61
management of, 265–266, 440–446
mortality rates, 17, 371, 497
negative aspects of, 101
among older adults, 464–465
perceptions and beliefs about, 6
positive aspects of, 101
powerlessness in, 258–260, 260–261
prevalence of, 3, 379
psychosocial typology of, 338–339
quality of life in, 189–192, 191
role norms for individuals with, 58
self in, 102
self-management of, 36, 441–442, 441f
        (See also self-management)
self-perception in, 125
and sexuality, 236–249
shifting perspectives of, 61–62, 262, 262f
sociodemographic factors, 105
state of, 3
as stigma, 76–77
terminal phase, 61
trajectory phase, 60
uncertainty in, 208–210
variables associated with, 105
ways to decrease the impact of, 19–22
chronic obstructive pulmonary disease (COPD), 18t, 507t
chronic phase, 61, 340–341
chronic sorrow, 54–55
chronicity, 3–28
chronological age, 319–320
Cialis (tadalafil), 241t
Cicely Saunders Institute of Palliative Care, 494–495
Cicely Saunders International, 494–495
cigarette smoking, 375

circular questions, 362–363, 363t
Cleland, Max, 528, 529
client autonomy. *See* autonomy
client-centred interventions, 86–88
client education, 307–334. *See also* education
    case study, 310
    critical questions to ask clients and family, 313
    cultural competence resources for, 316, 317t
    definition of, 311
    for empowerment, 275–276
    evidence-informed practice for, 331
    goal of, 311
    guided care nurse activities, 36
    significance of, 311–320
    teach-back method for, 324
client evaluation, 531–532
clinical care classification (CCC) system, 452–453, 452t
Clinical Evidence, 22
clinical information systems, 34t
clinical practice guidelines, 485, 506–507, 507t
coaching
    guided care nurse activities, 36
    health coaching, 381–382
    for self-management and family management, 442
Cochrane, Archie, 22
Cochrane Library, 22
Cochrane Review, 31
Code of Ethics, 415
coenzyme Q10, 403–404
cognitive adaptation theory, 263–264
cognitive appraisal, 107, 109
cognitive-behavioural strategies, 114
cognitive belief patterns, 86–87
cognitive capacity, 213
cognitive impairment, 482–484
cognitive reframing, 222–223
cognitive schema, 222
cognitive strategies, 218–221
collaboration, 273, 298
commendation practices, 363–364
Commission on Accreditation of Rehabilitation
    Facilities, 536
common sense self-regulation model, 53, 105–106,
    106–107
communication
    for body image, 174–175
    dissemination of information, 412–413
    listening noises, 360
    mass media campaigns, 382
    nonverbal, 503
    about palliative care, 509
    sharing illness narratives, 360–362
    social conversations, 359
    technologies for, 144–147
    therapeutic conversations, 359–360, 363–364

community, 268–270
community-based empowerment, 137
community-based health programs, 386–387
community-based long-term care, 466
community-based rehabilitation, 537
community education programs, 91–92
Community Health Nurses of Canada, 446, 458
community health nursing, 446, 446t
community policies, 35t
community resources
    accessing, 36
    in CCM and ECCM models of care, 35t
    for family networks, 144
"Competencies for Chronic Disease Practice"
    (NACDD), 20, 21t
complementary and alternative medicine (CAM)
    advanced practice nursing issues, 414–415
    benefits of, 394–395
    case studies, 411–412, 418–420
    categories of, 399
    and chronic disease, 403–408
    costs of, 17–19, 397
    cultural considerations, 416
    definition of, 393–394
    evidence-informed practice for, 422
    interventions related to, 420–422
    issues, 408–415
    journals about, 413
    legal implications, 421–422
    legislative matters, 414–415
    other practices, 403, 404t
    paradigm issues, 414
    professional education about, 417
    regulation of practitioners, 397–399
    standards for practice for, 415
    treatment modalities, 399–402
    types of, 394
    users of, 395–397
complementary and alternative therapies, 393–427.
    See also complementary and alternative
    medicine (CAM)
complementary medicine, 394. *See also* complementary
    and alternative medicine (CAM)
Complementary Medicine Education and Outcomes
    Program, 405, 410
Complementary Therapies in Medicine, 413
computer-assisted communication, 144–145
computer-assisted instruction, 326t
confidence, 222
congestive heart failure
    case studies, 289–290, 454–455, 508
    clinical practice guidelines for common symptom
        experiences in, 507t
consciousness raising, 377
Consortium for Spinal Cord Medicine, 252–253

Constitution Act of 1982, 7
constructionist learning theory, 309
contemplation, 297, 377
contingency management, 377
contracts, 382–383
control
    of disease, 105
    locus of, 259
    loss of, 215–216
    perceived, 274–275
    sources of, 263
    vicarious, 274–275
conversations
    social, 359
    therapeutic, 359–360, 363–364
"Conversations on Caring" podcasts, 510
coordination of care
    definition of, 449
    for home health nursing, 449–452
    major issues in, 449
coordination of transitions between sites and
        providers of care, 36
coping
    active, 111
    and body image, 167–168
    cognitive-behavioural strategies for, 114
    description of, 110–111
    emotion-focused, 111
    factors associated with, 107
    indigenist stress coping models, 113–114
    interventions for, 113–114
    overview of, 110–115
    passive, 111
    problem-focused, 111
    process of, 110–111
    with stigma, 83–92
coping effectiveness training, 113–114
coronary artery disease, 237–239
costs. See healthcare costs; healthcare spending
Council on Social Work Education Faculty
        Development Institute, 503, 504t
counselling
    peer counsellors, 142
    PLISSIT model, 251–252, 251t
counterconditioning, 377
covering, 79–80
Criminal Code, 475–476
crisis phase, 60–61, 339–340
cultural diversity, 502
Cultural Human Resources Council, 317t
culturally competent care
    for client empowerment, 278
    definition of, 83
    for hospice palliative care, 502–503
    for rehabilitation, 529–530

resources for, 316, 317t
    tailored, 131
culturally sensitive care, 503, 504t
culture
    and adaptation, 107–108
    and body image, 165
    and CAM, 416
    and chronic care, 15–16
    chronic illness as, 15–16
    concept of, 131
    definition of, 48
    family, 314–316
    and health care, 131
    integration into health care, 140–141
    of poverty, 50
    and powerlessness, 267–268
    role in stigma, 73
    and social isolation, 130–131
    and teaching and learning, 314–316
cure versus care, 84
custodial care, 473–474

D

decision making
    CAM-related, 420–421
    for client empowerment, 277–278
    end-of-life, 474
    ethical, 418
    substitute decision-maker/guardianship, 479
    support for, 34t
deep-breathing exercises, 400
delirium, 482
dementia, 482–483
dementia programs, 483, 540–541
demographics
    aging population, 438–439
    in Canada, 438–439, 497–498
    and illness behaviour, 50–51
    and social isolation, 132–134
demonstration, 326t
dependency
    versus client autonomy, 473
    dealing with, 62
depression, 238–239
devalued self, 54
devaluing, 81
developmental detours, 344
developmental stages, 319–320, 321t
deviance, 70
diabetes mellitus
    case study, 270–271
    clinical practice guidelines for common symptom
        experiences in, 507t
    economic and health burden of, 18t
    incidence of, 239

prevalence of, 3
self-care and self-management outcomes, 302
and sexuality, 239–242
dietary modification
for cancer, 405, 407
for health promotion, 383
dietary supplements, 400
difference questions, 363*t*
digestive problems, 395*t*, 397
dignity-conserving model of care, 503–504
dignity therapy, 504–505
disability
adults with disabilities requiring assistance with ADLs
and IADLs and, 530
aging with, 538
case study, 532–533
enabling–disabling process model for, 524
excess, 473
functional, 127
inequities among Canadians with, 528–529
International Classification of Functioning, Disability,
and Health (ICF), 523–524, 524–526
stigma of, 73, 528–529
Disability in America model, 524
disability-related variables, 105
discharge planning
for client empowerment, 272–273
post-discharge interventions, 324–325
discontent, normative, 162
disease, 5, 52. *See also* illness
disease management
versus illness management, 29–30
interventions for, 30
online, 41
revenues associated with, 30
disease prevention, 481–482
disregard, 80
dissemination of information, 412–413
distress profiles, 102
diversity, cultural, 502
doctor hopping, 55
double caregivers, 465–466
dramatic relief, 377
drug interactions, 400
dying, 494

E
economic abuse, 475
economic burden, 17, 18*t*. *See also* health care costs
ED. *See* erectile dysfunction
Edmonton Regional Palliative Care Program, 514
education. *See also* teaching
for body image, 177*t*
client education, 307–334
for empowerment, 275–276

evaluation of, 327–328
family education, 307–334
guided care nurse activities, 36
for healthcare professionals, 509–510
humanistic framework for, 309
interventions for client and family, 325–329
PLISSIT model, 251–252, 251*t*
post-discharge interventions, 324–325
professional (*See* professional education)
for reducing uncertainty, 219–220
self-management education, 311
starting points for low literacy, 322–324
system factors that influence, 320–322
teaching-learning process, 308–310
tools to assess readability of materials, 323*t*
Education in Palliative and End-of-Life Care, 510, 514
elder abuse, 475
elder exploitation, 475
emotion(s)
feelings that reflect isolation, 123
strategies to control, 222
emotional exhaustion, 355–356
emotional intelligence, 114
emotional/psychological abuse, 475
emotional support, 450*t*
emotive strategies for reducing uncertainty, 221–223
empowerment
community-based, 137
evidence-informed practice for, 279–280
key issues, 271–272
strategies for, 271–272
enablement, 480
enabling–disabling process model, 524, 525*t*
end of life, 512
end-of-life care
deficiencies in, 498, 499*t*
demographics of, 497–498
improving, 502
during the last days and hours (guideline),
193*t*–194*t*
Latino views regarding, 502
pain management in, 481
end-of-life decision making, 474
energetic healing, 417
energy, 394
energy fields manipulation, 403
energy healing, 396
engagement, 222
Engel's biopsychosocial model of adaptation, 105
Enhance-Wellness program, 386–387
environmental factors, 105
environmental reevaluation, 377
environmental strengths, 532–535
environmental support, 298
epilepsy, 170

erectile dysfunction (ED)
in coronary artery disease, 237
in diabetic men, 239–240
in older adults, 236
treatment options for, 240, 241*t*
Erikson, Erik, 166
essential fatty acids, 399, 400
ethical decision making, 418
ethical issues
in long-term care, 472–476
in rehabilitation, 529
ethics committees, 529
ethnicity, 416
European Union (EU), 417, 530
evaluation
of education, 327–328
rehabilitation client, 531–532
evidence, 312–313
evidence-based care guidelines, 193*t*–194*t*
Evidence Based Complementary and Alternative Medicine, 413
evidence-based practice, 22
evidence-based practice movement, 22
evidence-informed guidelines, 192
evidence-informed practice
for adaptation, 116–117
for body image, 176
for CAM, 422
for client education, 331
definition of, 22
for empowerment, 279–280
for guided care, 41
guidelines for, 487
for health promotion, 386–387
for hospice palliative care, 514
for illness experience, 62–63
interventions for quality of life, 192–196
for long-term care, 487
for pain management, 487
for rehabilitation, 542
resources available for, 22
for self-care, 301–302
for sexuality, 252–253
for social isolation, 145–147
for social networks, 145–147
for stigma, 89–90
for uncertainty, 217
excess disability, 473
exclusion, 88
exercise programs
for health promotion, 383
in long-term care, 485
exhaustion, 355–356
expanded chronic care model (ECCM), 32, 33*f*, 34*t*–35*t*
explanatory model of illness perceptions, 47
exploitation, 475

F
Facebook, 88, 144–145
families
case studies, 345, 346–347
chronic illness and, 335–369, 338*f*
community resources for, 144
general factors, 133–134
as heart and soul, 500
illness suffering, 344
influence on teaching and learning, 314
interventions for, 200–201, 358–364
launching children, 346
life cycles, 336–349
low literacy, 322–324
rebuilding, 143–147
self-care and self-management outcomes for,
302–303
strengths of, 363–364, 532–535
structure of, 314
understanding family relationships, 143–144
ways to facilitate common understanding with, 315
with young children, 343–344
family caregivers, 350–352
definition of, 350–351
programs, services, and resources for, 357–358
strain or burden for, 352–353
support for, 350
family caregiving, 349–358
challenges of, 352–358
complexity of, 349–358
excerpt from, 350
experience of, 356–357
growth in, 356–357
hidden costs of, 354–355
hospice palliative care, 500–502
meaning in, 356–357
systems of, 350–352
family culture, 314–315
family education, 307–334
case study, 310
critical questions to ask clients and family, 313
cultural competence resources for, 316, 317*t*
for empowerment, 275–276
interventions for, 325–329
significance of, 311–320
family identity loss, 347–348
family management, 441–442, 441*f*
family members
as caregivers, 350, 351
extended, 351
family nursing, 340–341
family support, 351
family systems-illness model, 336, 337–338, 338*f*
Federal-Provincial Fiscal Arrangements and Established
Programs Financing Act, 9, 436

feelings
    strategies to control, 222
    that reflect isolation, 123
Feldenkrais method, 403
female sexual dysfunction, 240
fibromyalgia, 55
FIM instrument, 533, 534*f*, 541
financial abuse, 475
financial costs. *See also* health care costs
    of caregiving, 353–355
financing. *See* funding
First Ministers' Meeting on the Future of Health Care
    2004, 11
First Nations
    health services for, 435
    home care programs for, 434
    views regarding end-of-life care, 502–503
First Nations Health Program (Whitehorse General
    Hospital), 416
5 A's of behavioural change, 296–299
Flesch formula, 323*t*
Flinders Programme, 38, 299
fluoxetine (Prozac), 247
Fog formula, 323*t*
folk remedies, 396
follow-up: planning for, 298–299
formal caregivers
    in home health care, 449–452
    in rehabilitation, 530
Fox, Michael J., 16, 528–529
France: healthcare expenditures, 16
Frankl, Lee, 432
Fraser Health Authority, 513
fraud, 416
Friends of Alternative & Complementary Therapies
    Society, 414
FSD. *See* female sexual dysfunction
functional ability, 288–289
functional assessment, 532–533
functional disability, 127
functional limitations
    and body image, 173–174
    rehabilitation for, 524
functionality
    and body image, 173
    as determinant of quality of life, 197–198
funding
    for home health care, 435–437, 439
    for long-term care, 470–471
    for public health services, 436
future-orientated questions, 363*t*

G
G-spot (Gräfenberg spot), 235
gaming, 326*t*
GCN. *See* guided care nurse

gender
    and body image, 166–167
    and illness behaviour, 51
    and social isolation, 130–131, 134
gender differences
    in caregiver strain, 353
    in learning, 316–318, 318*t*
generational differences, 348–349
Geriatric Depression Scale, 35
Geriatric Nursing Education Project, 488
geriatric palliative care, 512
Geriatric Palliative Care (Morrison and
    Meier), 510
geriatric rehabilitation, 537–538
Gerontologic Palliative Care Nursing (Matzo
    and Sherman), 510
goal setting, 298
Gräfenberg spot (G-spot), 235
grief and bereavement care, 498
group discussion, 326*t*
group therapy
    for body image disruption, 175
    self-help groups, 115
growth
    in family caregiving, 356–357
    uncertainty as opportunity for, 214–215
guardianship, 479
guided care model, 33–36, 41
guided care nurse (GCN), 33, 35–36
guided imagery, 400
guidelines
    adult asthma guidelines, 193*t*–194*t*
    clinical practice guidelines, 485,
        506–507, 507*t*
    evidence-based care guidelines, 193*t*–194*t*
    evidence-informed, 192, 487
    for health promotion, 386
    for quality of life, 192, 193*t*–194*t*
guilt, 74, 356
gynecological problems, 395*t*, 397

H
Hall, Emmett, 9
Hamilton Health Sciences, 317*t*
hardiness, 112
Hartford Foundation, 480
Hartford Institute for Geriatric Nursing, 488
Hawking, Stephen, 528
HBM. *See* health belief model
HCPs. *See* healthcare professionals
HCSM. *See* Home Care Satisfaction Measure
headache, 395*t*, 397
healing touch
    for cancer, 406
    categorization of, 403
    for hypertension, 404–405

health
definition of, 184–185, 295
as determinant of quality of life, 197–198
as holistic, 295
health (term), 185
health behaviour, 46
health behaviour change
activities for, 377
models and theories relating to, 377–379
processes of, 377
health belief model (HBM), 378
Health Canada
healthcare delivery to aboriginals, 7–8
online resources, 374
Primary Care Transition Funds, 510
10-Year Plan to Strengthen Health Care, 10–11,
11*f*, 13–14, 436
health care
clinical patterns of, 452, 452*t*
components of, 452, 452*t*
integrating culture into, 131, 140–141
key principles in improving, 20
management of, 450*t*
models of care, 29–44
healthcare coordination
definition of, 449
for home health nursing, 449–452
major issues in, 449
transitions between sites and providers
of care, 36
healthcare costs
of alternative medicine, 397
of chronic care, 16–19
of family caregiving, 354–355
global, 307
hidden, 354–355
of medications, 287
for older adults, 463–464
rising, 527
savings with telehomecare, 452
significance of client and family teaching for,
311–320
healthcare expenditures. *See* healthcare spending
Health Care in Canada Survey, 438–439
healthcare providers. *See also* healthcare professionals
(HCPs)
coordination of transitions between sites and, 36
trust and confidence in, 222
healthcare spending
on alternative medicine, 397
in Canada, 16–17, 397
global, 307
on home care, 439
on natural health products, 399
on older adults, 16
on pharmaceuticals, 16–17

health coaching
for client empowerment, 272
to enhance self-management and family
management, 442
health promotion, 381–382
Health Council of Canada, 10–11, 15
health literacy
best practices for improving, 383, 384*t*
definition of, 297–298, 376
for health promotion, 383
interventions for, 383, 384*t*
low levels of, 320
problems with, 375–376
"Health Literacy Map for Canada," 297–298
health promotion, 371–391
active strategies for, 372
barriers to, 375–376
case study, 376
challenges of, 374–375
in chronic illness, 372–374
contracts for, 382–383
definition of, 372–374
evidence-informed practice for, 386–387
frameworks for, 377–379
guidelines for, 386
interventions for, 379–386
in long-term care, 481–482
mass media campaigns, 382
mechanisms relevant to chronicity and health
as collective responsibility, 13
models and theories relating to,
377–379
motivating factors, 381
motivational interviewing for, 380–381
for older adults, 385–386
online resources for, 373
research in, 383–386
web-based programs, 382
health promotion model (HPM), 378
health-related behaviour, 46–47
health-related hardiness, 112
health-related quality of life, 184
health risks, 297–298
health screening, 375, 376–377
healthcare delivery systems
in CCM and ECCM models of care, 34*t*
description of, 7–8
integration with home health care, 440
navigation of, 276–277
and powerlessness, 268–270
healthcare professionals (HCPs)
client interactions for stigma, 83–85
competencies for, 20, 21*t*
definition of, 29
education for, 509–510
home care benefits for, 358

relationships with patients, 57–58
shortage of, 472
healthcare providers. *See also* healthcare professionals
(HCPs)
coordination of transitions between sites
and, 36
trust and confidence in, 222
healthy living, 372
heart disease
alternative therapy for, 395*t*, 397
illness perceptions, 49–50
heart transplant patients, 102
help-seeking behaviour, 51
helping relationships, 377
helplessness, 259
Henry Street Settlement (New York City, NY), 432
herbal therapies
for cancer, 405
professional education in, 417
regulation of, 400
use of, 396, 399
heterogeneity, 102
historical perspectives
on home care, 430–435
on hospice palliative care, 494–495
on long-term care, 465–466
for models of care, 29–30
on public health nursing, 432–433, 433–434
HIV/AIDS
Internet resources for, 93
rehabilitation programs for those with, 541
"holding on," 271–272
Holistic Health Research Foundation, 409
Home Care Healthcare Nurses Association, 458
home care programs, 358, 437–438
Home Care Satisfaction Measure (HCSM), 457
home health care, 429–461
access to, 430, 439–440
approaches to, 437–438
benefits and challenges in, 358
case study, 454–455
challenges for, 438–440
evidence-informed practice for, 456–457
funding for, 435–437, 439
history of, 430–435
integration with healthcare system, 440
Internet resources for, 458
key factors that must be considered in, 358
for older adults, 456–457
organization of, 435–437
outcome measures, 453
outcomes, 453
satisfaction measures, 457
service delivery models, 438
spending on, 439

home health nursing, 446–453
activities of, 446–447
competencies for, 446, 447*t*
coordination of care for, 449–452
goals of, 429
similarities and differences between public health
nursing and, 432–433, 433*t*
as specialty, 430
home healthcare teams, 447–448
homeopathy
for cancer, 405
categorization of, 403
professional education in, 417
regulation of, 398, 400
therapeutic method and rationale for, 404*t*
use of, 396, 399
homes for the aged, 468
hope, 542
Hospice and Palliative Medicine subspecialty, 511
hospice care
access to, 440
definition of, 496
philosophy of, 445–446
hospice palliative care, 493–520
access to, 498
advance care planning, 505–506
case study, 508
clinical practice guideline for, 506–507
culturally competent care, 502–503
definition of, 495–496
description of, 495, 496
evidence-informed practice for, 514
goals of care, 505–506
heart and soul of, 500–505
historical perspectives on, 494–495
Internet resources for, 513–514
issues and opportunities in, 509–510
professional practice specialties in, 510
psychosocial, spiritual, and bereavement needs in,
503–505
quality improvement in, 498–500
research, 512–513
square of care and organization, 499–500, 501*f*
symptom management, 505–507
hospice palliative care nursing, 510–511
hospice palliative care programming, 495–500
Hospital Insurance and Diagnostic Services Act, 8–9
hospitals, 463–464, 536
housing, senior, 130
HPM. *See* health promotion model
humanistic frameworks, 309
hypertension
CAM for, 403–405
clinical practice guidelines for common symptom
experiences in, 507*t*
self-care and self-management outcomes, 302

hypnotherapy, 400, 405
hypothetical/future-orientated questions, 363*t*

I

IADLs. *See* instrumental activities of daily living
IBM. *See* Illness Beliefs Model
ICDC. *See* Interdisciplinary Chronic Disease Collaboration
identity
  of chronic illness, 105
  development of, 139
  family, 347–348
identity belief system, 86–87
identity transformation, 56, 139–140
illness
  causes of, 105
  chronic (*See* chronic illness)
  consequences of, 105
  definition of, 5, 53
  versus disease, 5, 52
  and family life cycles, 343–346
  life beyond, 352–358
  as metaphor, 45
  and social isolation, 134–135
illness behaviour
  case study, 57
  definition of, 46, 47
  impact of, 52–53
  influences on, 50–52
  issues related to, 52–53
  legitimacy of, 56
  professional responses to, 56
Illness Beliefs Model (IBM), 336, 340–341, 341–342
illness experience, 45–68
  evidence-informed practice for, 62–63
  interventions for, 58–64
  patient stories, 5
  research on, 64
  trajectory model of, 60
illness management
  versus disease management, 29–30
  interventions for, 30
illness narratives
  challenges faced by healthcare professionals with, 361–362
  definition of, 360
  sharing of, 360–362
Illness Perception Questionnaire, 47
Illness Perception Questionnaire-revised, 47
illness perceptions, 47–50
illness perspective, 61–62
illness representations, 47
illness uncertainty. *See also* uncertainty
  certainty of, 208–210
  evidence-informed practice for, 217
  forms of, 213

immigrant population, 4
Improving Chronic Illness Care program, 31, 32*f*
IN-CAM. *See* Interdisciplinary Network for Complementary and Alternative Medicine
incentives, 381
inclusion, 88
independence, 288–289
Indian Act, 7–8
Indian and Northern Affairs Canada, 7–8
indigenist stress coping models, 113–114
Indigenous Cultural Competency Programme, 317*t*
individual differences, 105
influencing questions, 362
informal caregivers
  behaviours of, 449, 450*t*
  definition of, 350–351
  in home health care, 449–452
  population of, 354
  in rehabilitation, 530
information
  dissemination of, 412–413
  lack of information, 216–217
  lack of knowledge, 266–267
  PLISSIT model, 251–252, 251*t*
  for reducing uncertainty, 220
information management, 80–81
informed decision making, 220
Innulitsivik Health Centre (Puvirnituq, Nunavik), 416
insider perspective, 61
Institute of Cancer Research, 512–513
Institute of Medicine (IOM)
  Disability in America model, 524
  enabling–disabling process model, 524
  recommendation for rehabilitation model, 524
institutions, 463–464
instruction. *See also* teaching
  computer-assisted, 326*t*
instrumental activities of daily living (IADLs)
  adults with disabilities requiring assistance with, 530
  informal caregiver behaviours, 450*t*
  self-care, 285–286
"Integrative Healing Practices" course (Mount Royal University), 417
integrative medicine, 394
Integrative Medicine Institute, 410
intelligence, emotional, 114
intentionality, 443–444
Interdisciplinary Chronic Disease Collaboration (ICDC), 273
Interdisciplinary Network for Complementary and Alternative Medicine (IN-CAM), 409
interdisciplinary teams
  for home health nursing, 449
  rehabilitation teams, 531
Interior Health Authority, 513

International Classification of Functioning, Disability, and Health (ICF), 523–524, 524–526, 526t
International Conference on Health Promotion, 12–13
Internet resources
    for body image, 179
    for communication, 145
    for health promotion, 373
    for HIV/AIDS issues, 93
    for home health care, 458
    for hospice palliative care, 513–514
    for long-term care, 488
    for mental health issues, 93
    for models of care, 42
    online groups, 145
    for palliative care, 513–514
    for quality of life, 204
    for rehabilitation, 543
    web-based health promotion programs, 382
InterRAI instruments, 477–478
interventions
    client-centred, 86–88
    for coping, 113–114
    for disease management versus illness
        management, 30
    with family, 358–364
    for family quality of life, 200–201
    frameworks for, 59
    health promotion interventions, 379–386
    for illness experience, 58–64
    for long-term care, 476–485
    models for practice, 59
    nursing, 196–197
    for powerlessness, 270–278
    psychosocial, 199–200
    for quality of life, 195–196, 199–200
    rehabilitation, 530–532
    for self-care, 295–296
    for stigma, 83–92, 86–88
    supportive, 199–200
    for uncertainty, 218–223
interventive questions, 362–363, 363t
interviewing
    motivational, 298, 380–381
    patient-centred, 509
intolerance, 73
Inuit peoples
    health services for, 435
    home care programs for, 434
invisibility, 172–173
iPANEL collaborative, 513
isolation
    early isolates, 123
    feelings that reflect, 123
    impact of stigma, 80
    lifelong isolates, 123

nature of, 122–123
as problem, 122
process of, 125
recent isolates, 123
social, 121–155
working definition of, 121–122

J
Joanna Briggs Institute, 22
Johns Hopkins HealthCare, 36
Johns Hopkins University, 33–36
Johnson, Dorothy, 258–259
Johnson, Magic, 16
*Journal of Alternative and Complementary
    Medicine*, 413
Journal of Holistic Nursing, 413

K
Kaiser Permanente, 36, 300
Katz index of activities of daily living, 478
Kirby Report, 10
knowledge
    assessment of, 296–297
    lack of, 266–267
    about self-care, 293, 294f
Kubler-Ross, Elisabeth, 494

L
labelling, 82
labelling theory, 70–72
Lalonde report (*A New Perspective on the Health of
    Canadians*), 12
language, simplifying, 322
Latinos, 502
Lazarus and Folkman model of adaptation, 104
LEAP (Learning Essential Approaches to Palliative and
    End of Life Care) curriculum, 510
LEAP Project—An Online Program for Young People
    Struggling with Depression, 410
learned helplessness, 259
learning
    assessment of, 313–314
    assumptions pertaining to, 312t
    behaviourist framework for, 309
    child versus adult, 311–312
    constructionist theory, 309
    domains of, 325
    influences on, 314–318
    linking with developmental stage, 319–320, 321t
    of older adults, 320, 322t
    online, 326t
    readiness for, 318–319
    resources to facilitate, 320, 322t
    system factors that influence, 320–325
    teaching-learning process, 308–310

learning curves, 327
Learning Essential Approaches to Palliative and End
of Life Care (LEAP) curriculum, 510
learning styles, 316–318
lecture (teaching strategy), 326*t*
legal issues
CAM-related, 421–422
in rehabilitation, 529
legislative matters, 414–415
legitimacy
of chronic illness, 55–58
of illness behaviour, 56
letting go, 271–272, 355–356
Levitra (vardenafil), 241*t*
licensing, 397–398
life cycles
chronic illness and, 60–61
family, 336–349
life expectancy, 17, 371
life structure–maintaining periods, 347–348
life-transition periods, 347–348
lifestyle modification
for cancer, 407
evidence-informed practice for, 176
listening noises, 360
literacy. *See also* health literacy
assessing, 320, 322–324, 323*t*
low, 320, 322–324
"Living Well with a Chronic Condition" programme
(Alberta Health Services), 300
Livneh and Antonak model of adaptation, 105
locus of control, 259
loneliness, 124
long-term care, 463–492
admission to, 476–478
assessment in, 476–478
assessment tools for, 478
case studies, 467–468, 484
community-based, 466
continuum of, 463, 464*f*, 466–469
ethical issues in, 472–476
evidence-informed practice for, 487
funding for, 470–471
historical perspectives on, 465–466
indicators of need for, 465
Internet resources for, 488
interventions for, 476–485
nursing care, 480
problems and issues in, 470–472
provision of care, 470–472
quality of care, 471–472
research in, 486–487
residential settings, 467–469
staffing, 471–472
standards of care, 472

theoretical frameworks for practice, 476
vulnerable recipients of, 469–470
long-term care facilities, 536–537
Lorig, Kate, 36
loss of self, 54
Lotte and John Hecht Memorial Foundation:
2008–2013, 410
Lou Gehrig's disease (case study), 418–420
LSNS. *See* Lubben social network scale
LTC. *See* long-term care
Lubben social network scale (LSNS), 138, 139
lung problems, 395*t*, 397

M
Maclean's, 413
Macleod, Charlotte, 431
magnet therapy, 403
maintenance, 377
management of care, 450*t*
manipulative and body-based methods, 394, 402–403, 403*t*
marginality, 123
marginalization/vulnerability, 267
marital status
and illness behaviour, 50–51
and social isolation, 134
mass media campaigns, 382
massage therapy
for cancer, 406, 407
categorization of, 402
regulation of, 398
therapeutic method and rationale for, 403*t*
use of, 395*t*, 396
mastery, 275
meaning, 356–357
media, mass, 382
Medical Care Act, 9
medical care costs. *See* health care costs
medical model of care, 136
Medical Research Council, 8
medical teams, 447–448
medical treatment, 286–287
Medicare
emergence of, 8–12
hospice palliative care benefits, 495
medications
behaviours to restrict use and costs, 287
and sexuality, 239
meditation
for cancer, 405
categorization of, 400
for hypertension, 403–404
therapeutic method and rationale for, 401*t*
megavitamins, 396, 405
melatonin, 403–404
mental exhaustion, 355–356

mental illness
  and body image, 171
  Internet resources for, 93
  prevalence of, 3
Métis Addictions Council of Saskatchewan Inc., 416
Metropolitan Life Insurance Company, 431–432
middle age
  case study, 346–347
  learner characteristics and recommended teacher
    strategies for, 320, 321*t*
  moving on in, 346
mind-body medicine
  interventions, 394, 401*t*
  professional education in, 417
  treatment modalities, 400–402
mindfulness, 222
mineral supplements
  for cancer, 406, 407–408
  regulation of, 400
  use of, 399
minorities, 4
modelling and role-modeling (MRM) nursing theory
  aims of interventions in, 295
  self-care model, 293, 294*f*
models for practice, 59
models of care, 29–44
  case study, 40
  historical perspectives, 29–30
  Internet resources for, 42
  outcomes, 42
monitoring, 36
Moos and Holohan model of adaptation, 106–109, 106*f*
moral support, 190
moral work, 54
motivational interviewing
  guiding principles, 380–381
  for health promotion, 380–381
  for self-management, 298
motor cortex, 158–159
Mount, Balfour, 495
Mount Royal University, 410, 417
movement therapy, 403
MS. *See* multiple sclerosis
multidisciplinary teams
  for home health nursing, 449
  rehabilitation teams, 531
multigenerational perspectives, 348–349
multiple sclerosis
  adaptation to, 116–117
  case study, 532–533
  and sexuality, 248–249
multivitamins, 407–408
mutual aid, 142
mutual participation model, 84–85
"My Action Plan," 35

"My Voice" workbook and videos (Alberta Health
    Services), 506
myocardial infarction, 539

N

NACDD. *See* National Association of Chronic
    Disease Directors
narrative therapy, 341
National Association for Home Care and Hospice, 458
National Association of Chronic Disease Directors
    (NACDD), 20, 21*t*
National Cancer Institute of Canada, 410
National Center for Cultural Competence, 317*t*
National Guideline Clearinghouse, 22, 514
National Health Council, 10
National Initiative for the Care of the Elderly, 488
National Institute of Neurological Disorders and Stroke,
    543
National Palliative Care Research Center, 514
National Rehabilitation Association, 543
National Rehabilitation Information Center, 543
National Strategy for Investing in Healthy Aging,
    481–482
National Stroke Association, 543
native medicine, 417
Natural Health Products Directorate, 399–400
natural products, 399–400
naturopathy
  categorization of, 403
  professional education in, 417
  regulation of, 398, 399
  use of, 396
neck problems, 395*t*, 397
negative body image, 176
neglect
  definition of, 475
  self-neglect, 475
  of vulnerable adults, 474–476
Netherlands: healthcare expenditures, 16
Network for Multicultural Health Research on Health
    and Healthcare, 317*t*
neutrality, 361–362
A New Perspective on the Health of Canadians (Lalonde
    report), 12
Nightingale, Florence, 311, 431–432
normality, 70
normalization, 221
normative discontent, 162
nursing
  advanced practice nursing, 414–415
  basis of, 443
  community health nursing, 446, 446*t*
  decisions made about, 450
  family nursing, 340–341
  home health nursing, 429, 432–433, 433*t*, 446–453

hospice palliative care nursing, 510–511
long-term care nursing, 480
modelling and role-modeling (MRM) theory,
    293, 294f, 295
overview of, 196–202
public health nursing, 432–433, 433–434, 433t
rehabilitation nursing, 522–523
shortage of registered nurses, 472
standards for practice, 415
nursing homes
    for long-term care, 468
    older adults in, 463–464
    staffing in, 471–472
    standards of, 469
nutritional therapies, 417
Nutritional Therapy & Asthma—New Research
    Project for Asthmatic Children, 410

O

obesity
    and body image, 170–171
    case study, 169
oestrogen deficiency, 240–242
older adults
    abuse and neglect of vulnerable adults, 474–476
    acquired disabilities in, 538
    in Canada, 497
    case study, 128–129, 467–468
    chronic illness among, 7, 464–465
    comorbid health conditions among, 14
    demographics of, 4, 463–464
    diagnostic days, 14
    emergency department visits, 14
    health care costs for, 463–464
    health promotion for, 385–386
    healthcare spending on, 16
    home health care for, 438–439, 456–457
    learner characteristics and recommended teacher
        strategies for, 320, 321t
    in nursing homes and hospitals, 463–464
    physician visits, 14
    resources to facilitate teaching and learning of,
        320, 322t
    and social isolation, 127–130
Older American resources and services, 478
ombudsman, 480
omega 3/essential fatty acids, 399
Oncology Nursing Society, 232–233, 233t
online disease management, 41
online groups, 145
online learning, 326t
online resources. *See* Internet resources
online support groups, 279–280
Ontario Drug Benefit Program, 17
Ontario Volunteer Centre Network, 317t

operational control decisions, 450
orthomolecular therapies, 417
osteoarthritis, 302
osteopathy, 396
Ottawa Charter, 12–13
outcomes
    benefits of monitoring, 541
    models of care, 42
outcomes measurement
    benefits of, 541
    in palliative care, 512
    in rehabilitation, 541–542
overweight/obesity
    economic and health burden of, 18t
    prevalence of, 371–372
Oxford Textbook of Palliative Nursing (Ferrell and
    Coyle), 510

P

PACE (Program of All-Inclusive Care for the Elderly),
    466
pain, 163–164
pain clinics, 535
pain management
    evidence-informed practice for, 487
    goals for, 535
    in long-term care, 481, 487
    in rehabilitation, 535
Pain Resource Center, 514
Palliative and End-of-Life Care (PELC) Initiative,
    512–513
palliative care
    access to, 498
    approach of, 513
    communication about, 509
    core principles of, 505
    definition of, 485, 494, 509
    goals of, 486
    historical perspectives on, 494–495
    hospice palliative care, 493–520
    Internet resources for, 513–514
    issues in, 509
    in long-term care, 485–486
    major outcomes of, 507
    outcomes measurement in, 512
    principles of, 493–494
    proposed research agenda for, 512
Palliative Care, 514
palliative medicine, 511
Pallium Project, 510, 514
Parent-delivered Massage—Randomized-Clinical Trial
    for Children (6–18 years old), 410
parents, 353
Parkinson's disease, 507t
passing, 78

past experience, 51–52
Pathways: Understanding cancer patients'
    pathways of care: An international pilot
    study, 410
patient-centred interviews, 509
patient navigators, 277
patient relationships, 57–58
pedagogy, 311–312, 312*t*
pediatric rehabilitation, 538–539
peer counsellors, 142
peer groups, 164
PELC Initiative. *See* Palliative and End-of-Life
    Care Initiative
penile prostheses, 241*t*
perceived control, 274–275
performance improvement, 541–542
performance incentives, 381
Permission, Limited Information, Specific
    Suggestion, Intensive Therapy (PLISSIT)
    model, 251–252, 251*t*
personal resources, 107–108, 112
personality, 105
PHAC. *See* Public Health Agency of Canada
pharmaceuticals, 16–17
physical abuse, 475
physical activity, 375
physical appearance, 171–172
physical deformity, 74–75
physical environmental factors, 105
physical exhaustion, 355–356
physiology, sexual, 234–236
Pilates, 403
planned behaviour: theory of, 377–378
planned senior housing, 130
planning
    for follow-up, 298–299
    guided care nurse activities, 35
PLISSIT model, 251–252, 251*t*
population, aging, 438–439
positive life skills, 115
poverty, 50
power
    definition of, 260
    individual, 261
    theoretical perspectives of, 261–264
powerlessness, 257–284
    case study, 270–271
    in chronic illness, 258–260, 260–261
    definition of, 258–259
    interventions for, 270–278
    problems and issues associated with, 264–270
    recommendations for further work, 280
    strategies for decreasing feelings of, 62
    theoretical perspectives of, 261–264

prayer
    for cancer, 407
    use of, 395*t*, 396
precontemplation, 297, 377
prejudice, 75
preparation for change, 377
Preparing a Healthcare Workforce for the 21st Century:
    The Challenge of Chronic Conditions (WHO),
    19
preserving self, 54
preventive care
    barriers to, 375, 376–377
    long-term care, 481–482
    strategies for, 19
primary care, 13
primary care services, 436
primary health care (PHC), 12–14
probiotics, 399
problem-solving techniques, 298
professional attitudes, 84
professional education
    CAM curricula, 417
    to decrease the impact of chronic disease, 19–20
    stigma and, 90–91
professional practice
    specialties in hospice palliative care, 510
    stigma and, 89–90
prognostication, 509
program decisions, 450
Program of All-Inclusive Care for the Elderly
    (PACE), 466
Program of Research to Integrate the Services of
    Maintenance of Autonomy (Quebec), 466
prostaglandin, intraurethral, 241*t*
prostheses
    for body image disturbances, 177–178
    penile, 241*t*
providers of care. *See also* healthcare professionals
    (HCPs)
    coordination of transitions between sites and, 36
    trust and confidence in, 222
Prozac (fluoxetine), 247
psychological abuse, 475
psychological adaptation, 112
psychosocial adaptation, 112
psychosocial interventions, 199–200
psychosocial needs, 503–505
psychosocial rehabilitation, 114
psychosocial typology, 338–339
Public Health Agency of Canada (PHAC)
    Canadian best practices portal, 374
    guidelines for health promotion, 386
    online resources, 307, 374
Public Health Network, 11

public health nursing, 432–433, 433–434, 433*t*
public health services, 436
public policy, 470
pulmonary rehabilitation, 539–540

Q

QALY. *See* quality-adjusted life year
QELCCC. *See* Quality End-of-Life Care Coalition
    of Canada
qigong
    categorization of, 400, 403
    for hypertension, 403–404
    therapeutic method and rationale for, 404*t*
Qmentum Program (Accreditation Canada), 472
quackery, 416–417
quality-adjusted life year (QALY), 186
Quality End-of-Life Care Coalition of Canada
    (QELCCC), 499, 502, 514
quality health care, 99
quality improvement, 498–500
quality of care
    in chronic care, 14–15
    in long-term care, 471–472
quality of life, 183–206
    assessment of, 505
    case study, 191
    in chronic illness, 88, 189–192
    conceptualizing, 185–189
    definition of, 184–185
    family interventions for, 200–201
    global, 184
    guidelines for, 192, 193*t*–194*t*
    health-related, 184
    hospice palliative care for, 495
    Internet resources for, 204
    interventions for, 192–196
    measuring, 185–189, 187–189
    psychosocial interventions for, 199–200
    self-care and self-management outcomes, 302
    supportive interventions for, 199–200
    technological interventions for, 201–202
    in terminal illness, 199
    theoretical frameworks for, 185–187
Quality Palliative Care in Long Term Care
    Alliance, 499
questions
    behavioural effect, 363*t*
    circular, 362–363, 363*t*
    difference questions, 363*t*
    hypothetical/future-orientated, 363*t*
    influencing, 362
    interventive, 362–363, 363*t*
    relationally focused, 362–363
    triadic, 363*t*

R

radiation therapy, 243–246, 245*t*
RAI 2.0. *See* Resident Assessment Instrument
randomized controlled trials, 312–313
Rapid Estimate of Adult Literacy in Medicine (REALM),
    323*t*
Rathbone, William, 431
Reach to Recovery, 142
readability, 320, 323*t*
readiness to change, 319
readiness to learn, 318–319
reading comprehension, 320, 323*t*
reality orientation, 483
REALM (Rapid Estimate of Adult Literacy in Medicine),
    323*t*
reasoned action: theory of, 377–378
Red Cross, 431–432
Reeve, Christopher, 16, 528
Reeve, Dana, 16, 528
referral, 251–252, 251*t*
reflexology, 403*t*
registered nurses, 472
Registered Nurses' Association of Ontario, 15, 485, 487
regulation, 397–399
rehabilitation, 521–548
    acute, 536
    cancer, 540
    cardiac, 539
    case study, 532–533
    classification systems, 523–526
    client evaluation, 531–532
    common sayings, 531
    community-based, 537
    definition of, 522
    ethical issues, 529
    evidence-informed practice for, 542
    formal and informal caregiver issues, 530
    geriatric, 537–538
    goals of, 521
    Internet resources for, 543
    interventions, 530–532
    issues and challenges, 527–530
    legal issues, 529
    outcome measurement, 541–542
    pain management in, 535
    pediatric, 538–539
    performance improvement, 541–542
    potential strengths of client, family, and environment
        for, 532–535
    process of, 530–531
    psychosocial, 114
    pulmonary, 539–540
    settings for, 535–537
    specialties in, 537–541

team approach to, 531
vocational, 523
rehabilitation facilities, freestanding, 536
rehabilitation models, 523–526
rehabilitation nursing
definition of, 522–523
Scope and Standards of Advanced Clinical Practice in Rehabilitation Nursing (ARN), 523
Standards and Scope of Rehabilitation Nursing Practice (ARN), 523
Rehabilitation Nursing Certification program, 523
Reiki
for cancer, 406
categorization of, 403
for hypertension, 404–405
therapeutic method and rationale for, 404*t*
rejection, 80
relapse, 297
relationally focused questions, 362–363
relationship-based care, 442–444
relaxation techniques
for cancer, 405
progressive, 400
use of, 395*t*, 396
relief, dramatic, 377
religion, 73
research
on CAM practices, 408–410
health promotion studies, 383–386
in hospice palliative care, 512–513
in illness experience, 64
in long-term care, 486–487
quality of, 312–313
quality of life interventions from, 195–196
Research in Complementary Medicine, 413
Resident Assessment Instrument (RAI 2.0), 477–478
residential LTC settings, 467–469
resilience, 113
resources. *See also* Internet resources
cultural competence, 316, 317*t*
to facilitate teaching and learning of older adults, 320, 322*t*
for family caregivers, 357–358
for natural health products, 400
tools to assess readability and reading comprehension, 323*t*
respiratory diseases, 3
respite, 141–142
respite programs and services, 357–358
response shift, 101
restorative care, 523
restraints, 485
retirement communities, 536–537
retirement homes, 467
return demonstration, 326*t*

rheumatism
alternative therapy for, 395*t*, 397
case study, 411–412
risk reduction, 484–485
Robert Wood Johnson Foundation, 31, 32*f*
role modelling, 295
Rolfing, 403
Romanow, Roy, 10
Romanow Report, 10, 435
routines, 220
"Row Your Own Boat" workshop (Alberta Health Services), 300
Royal Canadian Mounted Police, 434, 435
Royal Commission on Health Services, 9
Royal Victoria Hospital (Montreal), 495
Runyon, Marla, 528

S
safe-handling programs, 485
safety, 484–485
sandwich generation, 351–352
SARs. *See* sexual attitude reassessments
Saunders, Dame Cicely, 494
Scope and Standards of Advanced Clinical Practice in Rehabilitation Nursing (ARN), 523
secondary care services, 436–437
selection bias, 30
selenium, 406
self
in chronic illness, 102
devalued, 54
loss of, 54
preserving, 54
self-awareness, 271–272
self-care, 285–306
as adherence to medical treatments, 286–287
aims of interventions for, 295
anti–self-care, 287
as belief in ability to self-manage, 287–288
for body image, 177
case study, 289–290
with chronic illness, 57–58
definition of, 285–286, 292–293
evidence-informed practice for, 301–302
frameworks for, 286–296, 294*f*
as functional ability and independence, 288–289
Internet resources for, 303–304
key issues, 286–296
knowledge about, 293, 294*f*
as multidimensional concept, 292
nursing interventions for, 480
outcomes of, 302–303
perspectives on, 286–292
resources for, 293–295, 294*f*
as self-determined behaviour that meets unique individual needs, 290–292
versus self-management, 287

self-care actions, 295
self-care activities, 291–292
self-care agency, 293
self-care model, 293, 294f
self-care programmes, 300–301
self-concept
    alterations in, 178
    definition of, 162
    disturbed, 178
self-control, 215–216
self-determination, 271–272, 275
self-determination theory, 262–263
self-determined behaviour, 290–292
self-efficacy, 298, 318–319
self-esteem, 162
self-healing, 394
self-help groups
    for body image, 175–177
    overview of, 115
self-liberation, 377
self-management, 285–306
    anti–self-management, 287
    case study, 289–290
    in CCM and ECCM models of care, 34t
    with chronic illness, 63–64, 441–442
    coaching for, 442
    definition of, 36–37, 441
    for empowerment, 273–274
    evidence-based care guideline for, 193t–194t
    evidence-informed practice for, 301–302
    Flinders program, 38
    framework of, 441, 441f
    guided care nurse activities, 36
    health coaching for, 381–382
    identity development, 139
    Internet resources for, 303–304
    outcomes of, 302–303
    process themes of, 63
    versus self-care, 287
    self-care as belief in ability to self-manage, 287–288
    strategies to support, 296–299
    Tai Chi as technique for, 288
    tasks of, 296
self-management education, 311
self-management interventions (SMIs), 274
self-management programmes
    knowledge of programs, 220
    overview of, 36–39, 115, 299–301
self-neglect, 289, 475
self-perception, 125
self-reevaluation, 377
self-reflection, 420
self-regulation, 105–106
self-worth, 86–87
senior housing, planned, 130
senior population, 4. *See also* older adults

sexual abuse, 475
sexual assessment
    PLISSIT model for, 251–252, 251t
    questions for an initial assessment, 249–250
    after spinal cord injury, 252–253
sexual attitude reassessments (SARs), 250–251
sexual behaviors, 232t
sexual dysfunction
    definition of, 232, 232t
    depression and, 238–239
    female, 240
sexual function
    and body image, 173
    definition of, 232t
sexual physiology, 234–236
sexual response cycle, 234–236
sexuality, 231–256
    case study, 247
    definition of, 231–232, 232t
    effects of alkylating agents on, 246
    effects of cancer surgery on, 242–243, 243t–244t
    effects of chemotherapy on, 246, 247
    effects of medications on, 239, 247
    effects of radiation therapy on, 243–246, 245t
    evidence-informed practice for, 252–253
    interventions for, 249–252
    standards of practice for, 232–233
SF-36-v2, 188, 204
shame, 74
sharing illness narratives, 360–362
shifting perspectives, 61–62, 262, 262f
sick role, 46–47, 58
sick-role behaviour, 46, 56
sildenafil citrate (Viagra), 241t
simulation, 326t
sites of care
    rehabilitation settings, 535–537
    residential LTC settings, 467–469
    transitions between providers of care and, 36
skilled nursing facilities, 536
SMIs. *See* self-management interventions
SMOG formula, 323t
smoking, 375
SNI. *See* social network index
social-cognitive theory, 309
social conversations, 359
social environmental factors, 105
social identity, 70–72
social influences
    on body image, 164–165
    on chronic care, 16
social involvement, 56
social isolation, 121–155
    assessment of, 137–138
    behaviour modification for, 147
    case study, 128–129

characteristics of, 123
description of, 123
distinctions of, 122
early isolates, 123
evidence-informed practice for, 145–147
family factors, 133–134
feelings ascribed to, 123
healthcare perspectives on, 135–137
illness factors, 134–135
interventions for, 137–142
issues of, 124–125
lifelong isolates, 123
and marital status, 134
measurement of, 138–139
patterns of, 123
problems of, 124–125
recent isolates, 123
versus similar states of human apartness, 123–124
social components of, 131–132
socioeconomic factors, 132–133
strategies for, 137
techniques for, 137
social liberation, 377
social network index (SNI), 138, 139
social networks
    evidence-informed practice, 145–147
    family networks, 143–147
    reciprocity in, 132
    and uncertainty, 210–211
social roles, 126–127
social support
    for health promotion, 383
    identifying, 298
    informal caregiver behaviours, 450t
    for reducing uncertainty, 220–221
socialization, 383
Sociobehavioural Cancer Research Network, 410
sociodemographic factors, 105
socioeconomic factors, 132–133
Sontag, Susan, 45
sorrow, chronic, 54–55
special care homes, 468
spending. *See* health care spending
spinal cord injury, 178, 252–253
spinal manipulation, 402
spiritual exhaustion, 355–356
spiritual healing
    for cancer, 405, 406
    professional education in, 417
    use of, 396
spiritual needs, 503–505
spiritual well-being, 142–143
spouses, 353
square of care and organization, 499–500, 501f
St. Christopher's Hospice, 494

staffing, 471–472
Stages of Change Model, 297
Standards and Scope of Rehabilitation Nursing Practice
    (ARN), 523
standards of long-term care, 472
standards of nursing homes, 469
Standards of Nursing Practice, 415
standards of practice
    for allied hospice palliative care clinicians, 511
    for CAM health care, 415
    Canadian Community Health Nursing Standards of
        Practice, 446, 446t
    for nursing practice, 415
    for sexuality, 232–233
    Standards of Nursing Practice, 415
Stanford University, 36
Statement on the Scope and Standards of Oncology
        Nursing Practice (Oncology Nursing Society),
        232–233, 233t
stereotyping, 81–82
stigma, 69–97
    attitudes toward, 82–83
    case studies, 78, 79
    chronic disease as, 76–77
    classifications of, 70
    client-centred interventions for, 86–88
    client outcomes, 92–93
    and community education programs, 91–92
    considerations for, 88
    coping with, 83–92
    definition of, 69, 72
    of disability, 528–529
    effects of, 81–82
    enacted, 76
    evidence-informed practice for, 89–90
    felt, 76
    impact of, 77
    interventions for, 83–92
    living with, 77–83
    perceptions of, 82–83
    and powerlessness, 267
    and professional education, 90–91
    and professional practice, 89–90
    professional responses to, 82–83
    reducing, 83–92
    responses to, 81–82
    role in chronic illness, 70
    and social isolation, 125–126
    theoretical frameworks for, 70–72
    types of, 74–76
    unique aspects of, 72–74
stigma (term), 70
stigma-promoting behaviours, 90–91
stigmatized individuals, 77–83
stimulus control, 377

story telling, 360–362
stress
  caregiving-related, 527–528
  indigenist stress coping models, 113–114
  and uncertainty, 215
structural resources, 218–219
structure providers, 213
subacute care, 537
subacute care units, 535
support groups
  for coping with or reducing stigma, 87–88
  for coping with social isolation, 137, 142
  face-to-face, 279–280
  online groups, 145, 279–280
supportive interventions, 199–200
supportive others, 88
surgery, 242–243, 243t–244t
symptom management
  clinical practice guidelines for, 507t
  hospice palliative care, 505–507
  for reducing uncertainty, 220

T
tadalafil (Cialis), 241t
tai chi, 288, 400
talk therapy, 175
Tanner Family Support Scale, 449
Task Force on Community Preventive Services, 22
teach-back method, 324, 384t
teaching. *See also* education
  assumptions pertaining to, 312t
  influences on, 314–318
  one-to-one, 326t
  recommended strategies for, 319–320, 321t
  resources to facilitate, 320, 322t
  strategies for, 325–327, 326t
  system factors that influence, 320–325
teaching-learning process, 308–310
teaching plans, 325, 328, 329t–330t
team approach
  for adjustment to body image, 165–166
  home healthcare teams, 447–448
  for rehabilitation, 531
technological interventions, 201–202
telehealth
  challenges to, 451–452
  for health promotion, 383
  for home health care, 450–452
  overview, 41
telehomecare, 452
telephone, 144
10-Year Plan to Strengthen Health Care (Health Canada),
  10–11, 11f, 13–14, 436
terminal illness, 198
terminal phase, 61

termination, 377
Test of Functional Health Literacy in Adults (TOFHL),
  323t
Textbook of Palliative Nursing (Ferrell and Coyle), 510
theory of planned behaviour, 377–378
theory of reasoned action, 377–378
therapeutic conversations, 359–360, 363–364
therapeutic massage, 407
therapeutic touch
  for cancer, 406
  for hypertension, 404–405
time, 164
TIME (Toolkit of Instruments to Measure End of Life
  Care), 514
Timed Up and Go (TUG) test, 533
timelines, 105
TOFHL (Test of Functional Health Literacy in Adults),
  323t
Toolkit of Instruments to Measure End of Life Care
  (TIME), 514
touch
  for communication, 147
  healing, 403, 404–405, 406
  therapeutic, 404–405, 406
traditional Chinese medicine
  categorization of, 403
  professional education in, 417
  regulation of, 398
  therapeutic method and rationale for, 404t
  use of, 399
traditional healing
  categorization of, 403
  evidence-informed practice for, 422
  promotion of, 399
Train-the-Trainer methodology, 510
training, coping effectiveness, 113–114
trajectory, 60
trajectory framework, 60
trajectory phase, 60
transdisciplinary teams
  for home health nursing, 449
  rehabilitation teams, 531
"Transforming Care for Canadians with Chronic Health
  Conditions" strategy (Canadian Academy of
  Health Sciences), 23–24
transitional care, 39–40
transitions between sites and providers of care, 36
transtheoretical model (TTM), 377
triadic questions, 363t
Trinity Western University, 513
trust, 222
Try This series (American Association of Colleges of
  Nursing/Hartford Foundation), 478
TTM. *See* transtheoretical model
TUG (Timed Up and Go) test, 533

U

uncertainty
    adaptation to, 218, 219*f*
    behavioural strategies for reducing, 223
    case study, 211–212
    certainty of, 208–210
    cognitive strategies for reducing, 218–221
    emotive strategies for reducing, 221–223
    evidence-informed practice for, 217
    factors that promote, 215–217
    in family caregiving, 349–358
    forms of, 213
    as harm, 215–217
    illness uncertainty, 207–227
    interventions for, 218–223
    introduction, 207
    nature of, 207–208
    neutrality of, 213–214
    as opportunity, 214–215
    with powerlessness, 264–265
    and social networks, 210–211
    sources of, 211
    structural resources for reducing, 218–219
    summary, 223–224
    theoretical underpinnings, 212–214
Union of European Medical Specialists, 530
United States: healthcare expenditures, 16
University of British Columbia-Okanagan, 513
University of British Columbia School of Nursing, 405
University of Calgary, 410
University of Ottawa, 374
University of Victoria, 513
unloading, 249
unpredictability, 223
U.S. Preventive Services Task Force, 22

V

values clarification, 69
Vancouver Coastal Health Authority, 513
Vancouver Island Health Authority, 513
vardenafil (Levitra), 241*t*
Veterans Independence Program, 434
Viagra (sildenafil citrate), 241*t*
vicarious control, 274–275
Victorian Order of Nurses (VON), 431–432, 432–433, 458
visibility, 172–173
visualization, 405
vital signs, fifth, 163–164
vitamin D, 403–404
vitamins
    for cancer, 406
    regulation of, 400
    use of, 399

vocational rehabilitation, 523
VON. *See* Victorian Order of Nurses
vulnerability, 267, 474–476

W

Wagner, Edward, 31
waiting, 216
Wald, Lillian, 432
walking difficulty, 395*t*, 397
watchful waiting, 216
web-based programs, 382. *See also* Internet resources
Wee-FIM tool, 533
well-being
    of caregivers, 357
    self-care and self-management outcomes, 302
    spiritual, 142–143
wellness, 61–62
wellness programs, 383
Whitehorse General Hospital, 416
Wide Range Achievement Test (WRAT), 323*t*
Widow to Widow, 142
"the wise," 88
women to women conceptual model, 185–186
Women-to-Women program, 317–318
Women to Women Project, 63
work participation, 50
work-related enhancements, 137
Working together to end racial and ethnic disparities:
    One physician at a time (AMA), 317*t*
World Economic Forum, 307
World Health Organization (WHO)
    core competencies, 19, 20*t*
    definition of health, 184–185
    definition of health promotion, 372
    definition of palliative care, 485
    goals of palliative care, 486
    International Classification of Functioning,
        Disability, and Health (ICF), 523–524,
        524–526, 526*t*
    objectives, 21–22
    plan for prevention and control of noncommunicable
        disease, 21–22
    Preparing a Healthcare Workforce for the 21st Century:
        The Challenge of Chronic Conditions, 19
    promotion of traditional medicine, 399
    quality of life measure, 188–189
    recommendation for rehabilitation model, 524
WRAT (Wide Range Achievement Test), 323*t*

Y

yoga, 396, 400, 401*t*
young adults, 320, 321*t*
young children, 343–344